World History of Neurointerventional Surgery

nova
Medicine & Health
New York

Neurosurgery Research Progress Series

Essentials of NeuroICU
Ahmet Şen (Editor)
ISBN: 979-8-89113-794-3
eBook ISBN: 979-8-89113-897-1

Understanding and Managing Cerebral Aneurysms
Xianli Lv, MD (Editor)
ISBN: 979-8-89113-608-3
eBook ISBN: 979-8-89113-683-0

Early Onset Scoliosis: A Comprehensive Approach
Ahmed Majid Heydar, MD (Editor)
ISBN: 979-8-89113-600-7
eBook ISBN: 979-8-89113-702-8

Aneurysmal Subarachnoid Hemorrhage: From Diagnosis to Treatment
Irina Alexandrovna Savvina, PhD (Editor)
ISBN: 979-8-88697-251-1
eBook ISBN: 979-8-88697-298-6

Neurosurgery Research: An Update
Amit Agrawal, MD, Pradeep Chouksey, MD, Adesh Shrivastava, MD, Sumit Raj, MD and Rakesh Mishra, MD (Editors)
ISBN: 978-1-68507-837-9
eBook ISBN: 979-8-88697-076-0

Advances in Neurosurgery Research
Amit Agrawal, MD, Pradeep Chouksey, MD, Adesh Shrivastava, MD, Sumit Raj, MD and Rakesh Mishra, MD (Editors)
ISBN: 978-1-68507-859-1
eBook ISBN: 979-8-88697-061-6

The Handbook of Neuromodulation (2 Volume Set)
Albert J. Fenoy, MD, Georgios Matis, MD, PhD, Pritam Majumdar, PhD, Sait Ozturk, MD (Editors)
ISBN: 978-1-68507-617-7
eBook ISBN: 978-1-68507-789-1

Neuroendoscopic Procedures and Challenges
Soner Duru, MD (Editor)
ISBN: 978-1-68507-092-2
eBook ISBN: 978-1-68507-155-4

Craniospinal Vascular Diseases and Endovascular Neurosurgery
Xianli Lv, MD, Guihuai Wang MD and James Wang MD (Editors)
ISBN: 978-1-53619-342-8
eBook ISBN: 978-1-53619-357-2

More information about this series can be found at
https://novapublishers.com/product-category/series/neurosurgery-research-progress/

Xianli Lv
Zhongxue Wu
Editors

World History of Neurointerventional Surgery

nova
Medicine & Health
New York

DOI: https://doi.org/10.52305/MJSF4144

Library of Congress Cataloging-in-Publication Data

Library of Congress Control Number: 2025945991
ISBN: 979-8-89530-792-2 (Hardcover)
ISBN: 979-8-89530-850-9 (eBook)

Published by Nova Science Publishers, Inc. † New York

Contents

Preface

Endovascular neurosurgery has seen a tremendous growth in the management of vascular diseases in the central nervous system. Such lesions include intracranial aneurysms, giant aneurysms, vasospasms, cerebral AVMs, vein of Galen malformations, spinal AVMs, cranio-cervical atherosclerotic disease, stroke, and neoplasms. Currently, neurointerventional applications are mechanical. By publishing this book, Neurosurgery continues in its efforts to develop and enhance this burgeoning surgical subspecialty.

A knowledge of the history of neurointerventional field is important. The stories and discoveries of our predecessors are not only fascinating, but they also provide a deeper understanding of the origins of the neurointerventional field. Furthermore, history highlights the adversities and challenges that were presented to our predecessors; it highlights the grit and ingenuity with which they tackled these challenges. The presence of pioneers in this book is really an honor for me and a big plus for the reader.

This book will be invaluable for the new generation of neurointerventional surgeon, or those who want to understand the creation, history, and evolution of neurointerventional surgery, including neurosurgery, radiology, neuroradiology, neurology, and cardiology. Through a comprehensive historical review of current techniques and concepts in neurointerventional surgery, this unique monograph will lead readers to find another way to solve the challenges in our profession. They have applied new techniques, made new discoveries, and developed new ideas. They have provided a well-documented evolutionary process of neurointerventional surgery, and their narratives of events have had a significant impact on both the present and the future. They not only describe the history of endovascular neurosurgery, but also tell the story of doctors with a strong sense of responsibility and their involvement in a newly developed field, opening new prospects for the future. These are wonderful, heady times for us in interventional neuroradiology or endovascular neurosurgery. Each year seems to bring new advances, new techniques, better tools, and industry is focusing their resources on trying to keep pace.

This collection of 27 chapters provides a timely assessment of where endovascular therapy has been, where it is now and, to some degree, where it is going. The first thirteen chapters provide personal insights into where the field came from and ideas about where technological advancements may take us, as well as the environment for neurointerventional work. The next seven chapters highlight disease-specific topics, concentrating on the management of aneurysms, AVMs and AVFs, ischemic disease, and head and neck tumors. The final seven chapters concentrate on the worldwide development of neurointerventional surgery.

In this book, we have quoted many names of doctors from different countries. We regret not having mentioned the names of other doctors. There are many interventional neuroradiologists who excel in their work, maintain a low profile, and treat people kindly. They do not enjoy traveling, and they rarely attend various conferences abroad. They like to face life in a very relaxed way.

We are fortunate to stand on the shoulders of giants, and their interesting stories are exposed through this book. If we know the past, perhaps we can learn from their success or failure, and see our future more clearly. In addition, the history of neurointerventional surgery is indeed a fascinating story. Stars in the field of neurointerventional surgery shine in the universe. Their contributions have shaped the field of endovascular neurosurgery. Perhaps the most exciting aspect of endovascular neurosurgery is that it is an emerging historical field. What we are doing today may be overwhelmed by even greater achievements in the next decade.

Dr. Lv has specialized in neurosurgery and has practiced endovascular neurosurgery for nearly two decades. As a physician practicing in this field during this time, it has been truly heartening to see how much more we can do for our patients. We would like to thank my professors in Beijing who taught me the fundamentals of endovascular neurosurgery. Thanks to all the experts and scholars who are contributing to this book.

Xianli Lv and Zhongxue Wu
Beijing, China
March 6, 2025

Acknowledgments

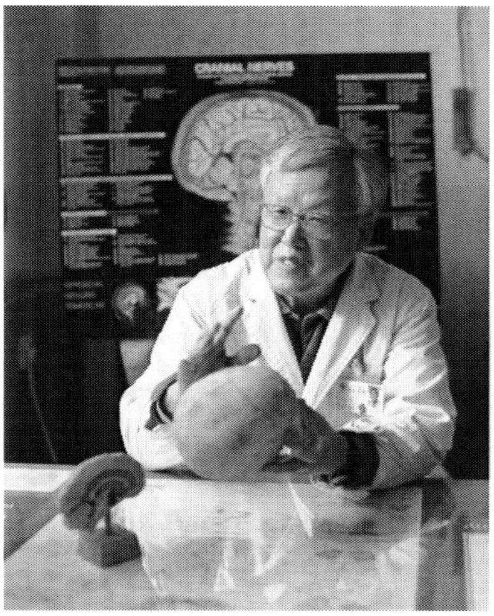

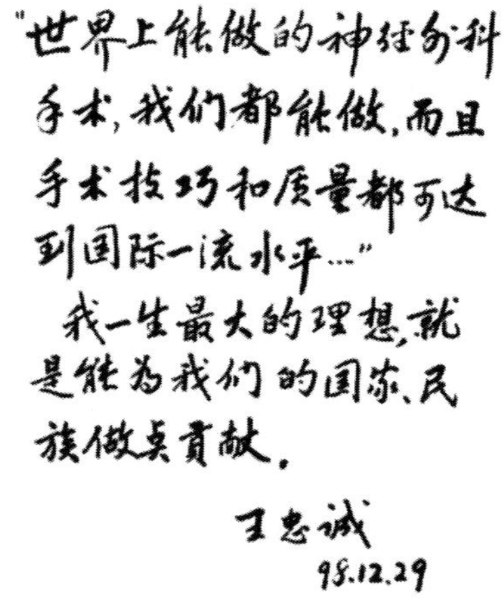

Professor Zhongcheng Wang (December 20, 1925-September 30, 2012), Academician of Chinese Academy of Engineering

Commemorative of Academician Zhongcheng Wang.

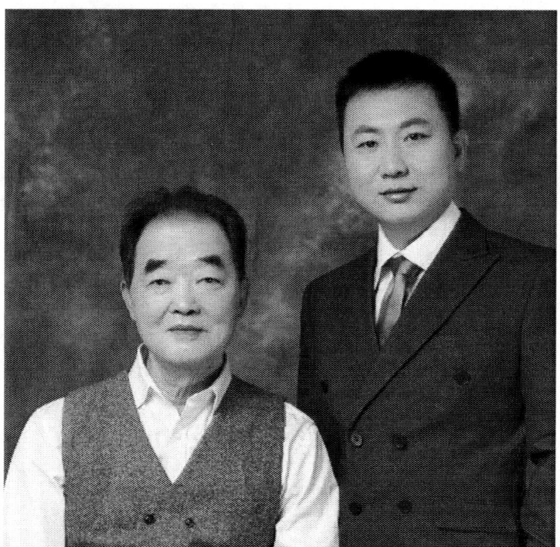

Professor Zhongxue Wu (left) and Xianli Lv (right).

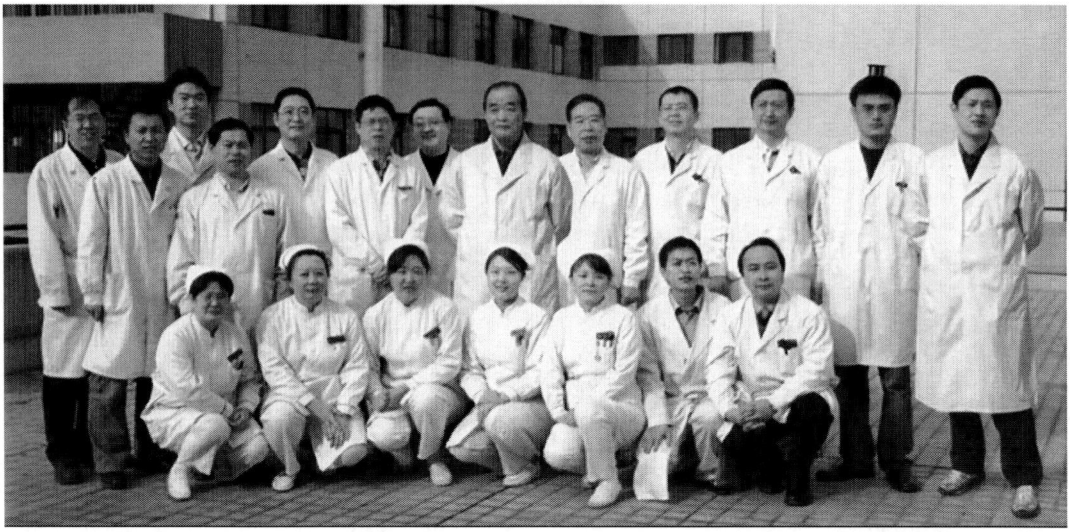

The members of the Beijing Neurosurgical Institute Working-Group in Endovascular Neurosurgery in 2009, Beijing, China.

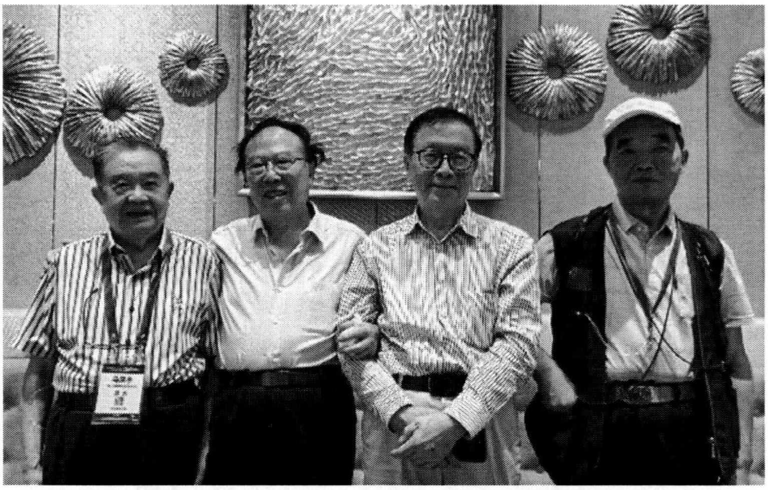

Photo of four pioneers in endovascular neurosurgery in China in 2024. From left to right. Dr. Lianting Ma, Dr. Derang Jiao, Dr. Tielin Li, and Dr. Zhongxue Wu.

Chapter 1

The History of Diagnostic Cerebral Angiography and Early Therapeutic Breakthroughs

Mubashir Ahmad Khan[1]
Weiming Kong[2]
and Xianli Lv[2,*]

[1]The First Affiliated Hospital of Zhengzhou University, Medical College of Zhengzhou University, Zhengzhou, Henan, China

[2]Department of Neurosurgery, Beijing Tsinghua Changgung Hospital, School of Clinical Medicine, Tsinghua University, Beijing, China

Abstract

Cerebral angiography, an essential diagnostic tool in neurosurgery, has undergone significant evolution since its introduction in the 1920s. The pioneering work of Egas Moniz in 1927, along with substantial contributions from Walter Dandy and Sven-Ivar Seldinger, was instrumental in establishing cerebral angiography as a routine technique. Originally developed as a diagnostic method, it provides clear images of blood vessels, enabling the detection of vascular irregularities such as aneurysms and arteriovenous malformations. Technological advancements have led to the development of early therapeutic procedures, including electrocoagulation and embolization. This chapter explores the advancements in cerebral angiography, its transformation from a diagnostic tool to a therapeutic neurointervention, and the groundwork for innovations such as magnetic stereotaxis and endovascular neurosurgery.

Keywords: cerebral angiography, electrothrombosis, detachable balloon, coil, endovascular therapy

Introduction

Before cerebral angiography became a practical procedure, early anatomists like Giovanni Battista Morgagni (1682–1771) emphasized the importance of understanding the brain's

* Corresponding Author's Email: lvxianli000@163.com

In: World History of Neurointerventional Surgery
Editors: Xianli Lv and Zhongxue Wu
ISBN: 979-8-89530-792-2

vascular system for diagnosing neurological conditions [1]. Although Morgagni's dissections and detailed anatomical drawings laid the groundwork for future vascular studies, the technological constraints of his time limited their effectiveness. The idea of visualizing blood flow in living patients was not feasible, as there was no available imaging technology to achieve this.

Advancements in electromagnetism have significantly contributed to the evolution of contemporary neuroimaging. The late 19th century was pivotal, marked by discoveries that shaped the future of electromagnetic technology. Two major breakthroughs—the discovery of X-rays by Wilhelm Conrad Roentgen and the identification of the electron by J. J. Thomson—laid the groundwork for neuroimaging [2, 3].

The scientific investigation of electromagnetism began with Danish physicist and chemist Hans Christian Ørsted in 1820, when he discovered the relationship between electricity and magnetism. Ørsted's experiment, in which an electric current caused movement in a compass needle, demonstrated that an electric current generates a magnetic field. This foundational work laid the groundwork for the study of electromagnetism and its applications in various fields, including medicine.

Following Ørsted's work, Michael Faraday and James Clerk Maxwell significantly advanced our understanding of electromagnetic fields and waves [4-7]. Maxwell's equations provided a comprehensive explanation of electromagnetism in the mid-19th century. These discoveries ultimately influenced the application of electromagnetism in neuroradiology, facilitating the discovery of X-rays and their use in medicine, particularly in cerebral angiography, as well as the initial therapeutic breakthroughs that relied on electricity and magnetism.

Wilhelm Conrad Roentgen's discovery of X-ray technology in 1895 marked the beginning of efforts to image brain structures. Pneumoencephalography, developed in the early 1900s, was a technique that involved replacing cerebrospinal fluid with air to visualize the brain's ventricles in X-ray images [8]. However, this procedure was often painful and produced inadequate resolution, resulting in a limited understanding of the brain's complex vascular systems. Until the 1920s, the limitations of existing techniques impeded detailed visualization of cerebral vasculature [3].

Cerebral Angiography

Cerebral angiography was pioneered by the Portuguese physician Egas Moniz, who performed the first cerebral angiogram in 1927. Moniz introduced contrast media into the carotid and vertebral arteries through direct puncture, enabling X-ray imaging of the brain's vascular structures. This groundbreaking advancement allowed clinicians to detect vascular anomalies in the brain, such as aneurysms and arteriovenous malformations (AVMs). Initially, Moniz used sodium iodide as the contrast agent, which posed significant risks, including toxicity and cerebrovascular accidents [9]. In 1949, Moniz was awarded the Nobel Prize, not for his contributions to cerebral angiography, but for his later discredited frontal lobotomy procedure [10]. His work laid the foundation for future therapeutic interventions, which would not be realized for several decades. The ability to visualize brain vasculature marked the first step toward understanding and ultimately treating disorders that were previously deemed inoperable.

After Egas Moniz's groundbreaking discovery of cerebral angiography, American neurosurgeon Walter Dandy quickly recognized its potential to improve the precision of brain surgery. Dandy, renowned for his advancements in ventriculography, adapted and refined Moniz's technique. He utilized cerebral angiography to map vascular systems before performing complex procedures, particularly for cerebral tumors and aneurysms. Dandy's enhancements to the technique included the development of advanced contrast agents that produced clearer images, which were vital for identifying vascular abnormalities during surgical interventions. His adoption of cerebral angiography as a standard preoperative diagnostic tool marked a significant turning point in neurosurgery, particularly in the United States, and demonstrated the global impact of Moniz's contributions [11].

From Carotid Puncture to Femoral Puncture

In 1953, Swedish radiologist Sven-Ivar Seldinger revolutionized cerebral angiography by introducing a safer and more efficient technique: selective catheterization via femoral artery puncture. Previously, the conventional method involved direct needle puncture of the carotid or vertebral arteries, which posed significant risks of bleeding and arterial injury. Seldinger's approach begins with puncturing the femoral artery with a needle, followed by threading a slender guide wire through the needle, and finally withdrawing the needle while keeping the guide wire in place. An arterial sheath can then be introduced over the guide wire into the femoral artery. This breakthrough enabled more precise and targeted catheter placement, reducing complications and enhancing the safety and accessibility of cerebral angiography for a broader patient demographic. The Seldinger technique has become the gold standard for vascular access, applicable not only in cerebral angiography but also in various other medical imaging and therapeutic procedures [12].

Breakthrough in Neuroimaging

In the 1970s, British engineer Godfrey Hounsfield's discovery of Computed Tomography (CT) revolutionized medical imaging by providing a non-invasive method for examining internal tissues, such as the brain. For the first time, clinicians could visualize cross-sectional images of the brain without the need for invasive procedures like cerebral angiography [13]. This innovation was later followed by the development of Magnetic Resonance Imaging (MRI), which offered improved soft tissue contrast [14]. The introduction of MRI, pioneered by Paul Lauterbur in 1973, represented a significant advancement in medical imaging [15]. MRI enabled real-time, non-invasive imaging of soft tissues, greatly enhancing the accuracy and safety of brain tissue assessment.

These technologies have begun to supplant cerebral angiography as the primary diagnostic tool for neurological diseases, particularly in the identification of tumors, hemorrhages, and strokes. However, cerebral angiography remains essential for obtaining detailed images of the intracranial blood vessels, especially when planning surgical procedures or treatments. The introduction of Digital Subtraction Angiography (DSA) in the 1980s helped bridge this gap. DSA enhanced conventional angiographic images by removing background structures, allowing for clearer visualization of blood vessels with minimal invasiveness (Figure 1) [14]. This advancement reduced patient exposure to contrast agents and radiation while improving diagnostic accuracy [14]. The effectiveness of cerebral angiography in diagnosis and treatment has laid the groundwork for modern neurointerventional surgery.

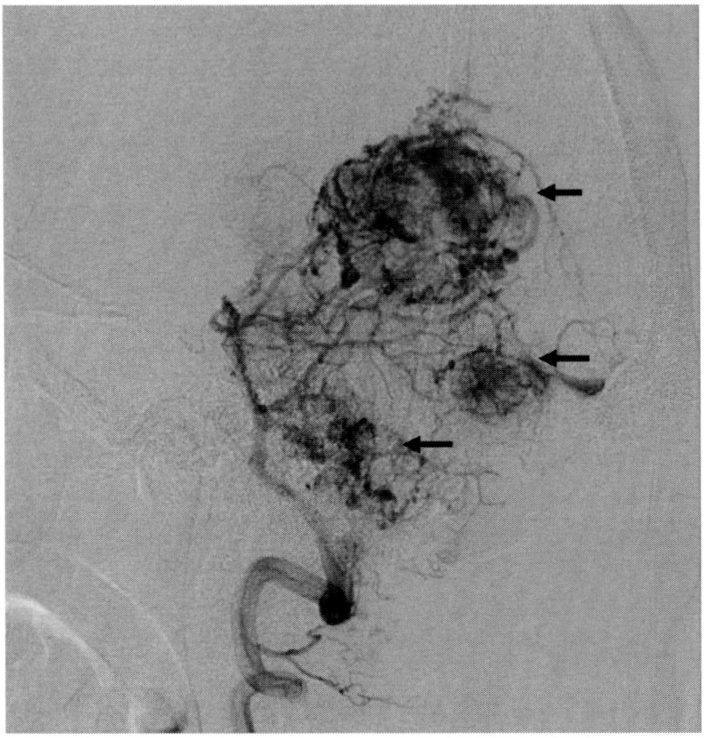

Figure 1. Digital subtraction angiography showing multiple hemangioblastomas in a 54-year-old man (arrows).

The Emergence of Endovascular Therapies

In the pursuit of endovascular treatments as alternatives to open surgical procedures, numerous researchers have explored various technical methodologies. The central concept they developed is a combination of open neurosurgery and endovascular neurosurgery, known as hybrid neurosurgery. This approach involves either exposing the aneurysm or stereotactically identifying it with a probe, followed by puncturing the aneurysm's dome or wall to facilitate intervention. A variety of surgical techniques, including endovascular treatment, stereotactic image guidance, and microsurgical methods, aim to minimize invasiveness in surgical procedures for neurovascular diseases, serving as alternatives or complements to traditional neurosurgery. These early endovascular techniques laid the groundwork for contemporary endovascular treatments, such as coil embolization and the use of liquid embolic agents.

Early experimental efforts in foundational methods of electrothrombosis, conducted by Velpeau and Phillips (1831-1832), were among the first to utilize needles within blood vessels to induce clotting, representing a groundbreaking attempt to control vascular bleeding. Building upon this concept, researchers discovered that they could apply specific metals with a high dissociation constant to treat aneurysms by promoting clot formation within the blood vessel [16, 17].

In 1864, Moore and Murchison improved this technique by permanently inserting a wire into an aortic aneurysm to promote clotting, demonstrating that targeted electric currents can induce controlled thrombus formation. This invention builds upon the original concepts by emphasizing the evolution of methods for longer-lasting and more effective treatments [18].

Notably, in 1847, Ciniselli conducted groundbreaking studies by applying a positive electric current through needles inserted into an aneurysm sac. This technique, known as "wiring and electrothermic coagulation," was further refined by Blakemore, King, Linton, and Hardy in the early 1950s for the treatment of aortic aneurysms. These advancements laid the groundwork for future endovascular treatments designed to minimize invasiveness in neurosurgical procedures [19-21].

In 1941, Sidney C. Werner and his colleagues published their findings in the Journal of the American Medical Association (JAMA) regarding the application of electrocoagulation technology for the treatment of internal carotid artery (ICA) aneurysms. After surgically exposing the aneurysm, a needle was introduced into the aneurysm sac, followed by the insertion of a 9-meter-long silver-coated wire. The wire was electrically heated to 80°C for 40 seconds, resulting in the rapid formation of a clot through electrocoagulation, influenced by the negative charges of white blood cells, red blood cells, platelets, and fibrinogen [22]. The journey continued with the visionary Dr. Irving S. Cooper, who employed electrocoagulation in neurosurgery to address neurological issues using minimally invasive techniques. His method, termed cryothalamotomy, utilized electrical currents to precisely ablate brain tissue, particularly in regions associated with movement disorders such as Parkinson's disease. In the initial phases of his research, Cooper employed a precise electrode on specific areas of the brain, administering a controlled electrical current. This induced thermal coagulation, thereby generating lesions in targeted brain regions to alleviate tremors and involuntary movements in patients [23]. He relied on clinical observation and basic imaging techniques to accurately position the electrodes.

A critical inquiry persisted: what accounted for the consistent formation of thrombi surrounding the positive electrode? The role of positively charged electrodes in thrombus formation was elucidated when Bigelow and De Foyes observed platelet migration toward the positive pole in 1952 [24]. Additionally, Sawyer and Pate demonstrated that blood components, such as red and white blood cells, could aggregate around a positively charged electrode under low currents. The trials revealed that the size of the thrombus correlated with the amount of electric charge administered, with no alteration in blood pH—an essential finding for safe clinical use [25, 26]. The choice of various metals as electrodes influenced the rates of thrombus development. Research indicated that platinum electrodes were highly effective at producing substantial clots and exhibited slower degradation compared to other metals, such as stainless steel or copper. Piton's tests in saline revealed that platinum remained stable under electric current, establishing it as an optimal material for thrombogenic applications. In 1961, Salazar successfully induced total coronary artery thrombosis in dogs with minimal current, demonstrating the potential of electrothrombosis for precise vascular occlusion [27]. In subsequent research, Thompson and Piton obtained similar results in additional arteries, showing that thrombocytopenic blood could still form clots when subjected to electric stimulation [28].

In the 1960s, S. Mullan and his colleagues pioneered the use of electrically induced thrombosis for treating cerebral aneurysms. This method, described in the Journal of Neurosurgery, involved creating a bone window and stereotactically inserting a metal electrode with a tip diameter of 0.1 mm into the aneurysm. A current of 2000 μA was gradually administered, which facilitated imaging and promoted thrombosis within the aneurysm. However, this procedure proved challenging due to the electrode's exceptional thinness, requiring multiple attempts for precise insertion into the aneurysm [29].

In the 1970s, electrocoagulation techniques emerged for the treatment of vascular lesions in the brain. Angiography-guided methods utilized electrical currents to coagulate blood vessels, including those involved in arteriovenous malformations (AVMs). This represented a significant advancement in the therapeutic application of angiographic techniques [30].

In 1974, Mullan et al. first utilized the stereotactic electrocoagulation technique to treat 15 cases of large cerebral aneurysms that were considered unsuitable for conventional clipping surgery. The researchers inserted three slender copper-plated steel needles into the dome of the aneurysm, applied a positive current of 0.5 to 1.0 mA, and performed electrocoagulation for 5 minutes. Although the technique showed initial promise, its limitations—such as significant operational complexity, high equipment costs, and the potential for invasive injury—prevented it from surpassing the effectiveness of clipping surgery, particularly given the lower mortality rates associated with clipping [31].

Despite advancements in electrocoagulation procedures, researchers have focused on utilizing magnetism to promote the formation of blood clots within aneurysms [32]. Stereotactic techniques were employed to position a magnetic probe on the external surface of an exposed aneurysm during the surgical procedure. After puncturing the aneurysm, iron microspheres were introduced into the sac, and the magnetic probe was used to attract these microspheres, with the goal of forming an "iron blood clot." Although this technique is innovative, it has notable drawbacks. Upon removal of the magnetic probe, the clot often dissolved due to its fragility [32].

In the meantime, Fedor Serbinenko emerged as an innovative figure in endovascular neurosurgery, particularly in the management of cerebral aneurysms and arteriovenous malformations (AVMs). Serbinenko's unique approach involved the use of balloon occlusion for treating cerebral aneurysms. His method entailed navigating a catheter through the circulatory system to access the aneurysm. The catheter, typically composed of a flexible material, was carefully maneuvered through the blood vessels with fluoroscopic guidance. Once positioned at the site of the aneurysm, a balloon attached to the catheter could be inflated. This inflation occluded the parent artery, effectively restricting blood flow to the aneurysm and minimizing the risk of rupture. Serbinenko's initial trials indicated that this technique could stabilize aneurysms, providing a crucial option for individuals who were unable to undergo traditional surgical clipping due to associated risks [33]. Following his success with balloon occlusion, Serbinenko introduced the concept of endovascular embolization. This innovative technique involved deploying materials such as coils into the aneurysm through the same catheter system. The coils, often made of soft platinum, would promote thrombosis within the aneurysm, effectively sealing it off from the circulation. This method proved particularly beneficial, as it significantly reduced the need for invasive craniotomies and the associated recovery times [33, 34].

A significant advancement in this strategy occurred in 1980 when John F. Alksne and Randall W. Smith published their research in the Journal of Neurosurgery. They improved upon the previous method by dispersing iron powder in methyl methacrylate, resulting in an organic-metal complex known as "iron acrylic" [31]. This compound polymerizes rapidly, does not fragment, and is nontoxic, thereby reducing the need for prolonged retention of the magnetic probe. It has been tested in a series of experimental animals and in initial clinical cases with promising results. Only two of the 22 patients treated with this approach experienced aneurysm recurrence, and there were no recorded fatalities. The use of this material simplifies and enhances the safety of stereotactic aneurysm treatment. Although this technique was highly effective, it proved to be quite exhausting for the neurosurgeon responsible for its implementation [31]. Despite this achievement, the technique did not gain widespread adoption due to the rise of aneurysm clipping, which had established itself as the conventional treatment during the same period [31].

In the late 20th century, the treatment of intracranial aneurysms primarily relied on surgical clipping, which had become the standard due to its effectiveness in directly addressing the aneurysm. However, this method was associated with severe complications that often stemmed from the invasive nature of the procedure, which required craniotomy. This exposure put patients at risk for infections, neurological deficits, and the physical stress associated with major surgery [35]. During the same period, both surgical clipping and endovascular techniques were developing concurrently. The endovascular method advanced rapidly due to improvements in catheter-based procedures and technology. In fact, the endovascular approach gained prominence and demonstrated substantial potential, leading to a paradigm shift in the treatment of aneurysms [36]. Neurosurgeons began to explore alternative strategies for aneurysm treatment that were less invasive and offered better patient outcomes, recognizing that endovascular treatments could address the limitations of conventional surgical procedures [37].

A significant figure in this transition was Italian-American neurosurgeon Guido Guglielmi, who began to explore endovascular techniques that promised a less invasive alternative to traditional surgical approaches. In the early 1990s, he initially focused on intravascular electrocoagulation, investigating how electric currents could induce coagulation and promote localized clot formation within blood vessels (Figures 2 and 3) [38]. His technique involved developing a catheter system capable of delivering electrical currents directly to aneurysms, along with experiments aimed at optimizing current magnitude and duration to achieve the desired coagulative effect. Based on the current understanding of coagulation and hemostasis, Guglielmi sought to create a device that could assist in the closure of aneurysms by promoting clot formation while minimizing surgical risks. This investigation culminated in the invention of the Guglielmi Detachable Coil (GDC), a soft, flexible coil designed for endovascular deployment, which allows for straightforward catheter navigation to the aneurysm site [39, 40].

The initial clinical application of the Guglielmi Detachable Coil (GDC) took place on March 6, 1990, during the treatment of a patient with a carotid-cavernous fistula. Dr. Guglielmi and Dr. Fernando Viñuela employed the GDC as a last resort after unsuccessful attempts to seal the fistula using arterial and venous balloons. Initially, when two coils—one measuring 40 cm and the other 15 cm—were deployed, there was no immediate visible change, prompting the team to pause and reassess the situation. However, during the follow-up angiogram, they were astonished to discover that the fistula had completely closed [41].

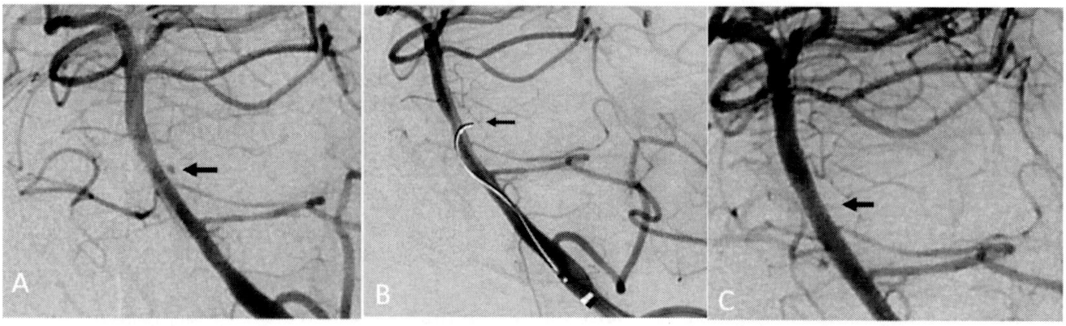

Figure 2. A 54-year-old female patient presented with subarachnoid hemorrhage (SAH). A, the cerebral angiogram revealing a tiny aneurysm (arrow). B, the physician utilizing a micro-guidewire to enter the aneurysm for intravascular electrocoagulation (arrow). C, the postoperative angiogram showing the disappearance of the aneurysm (arrow).

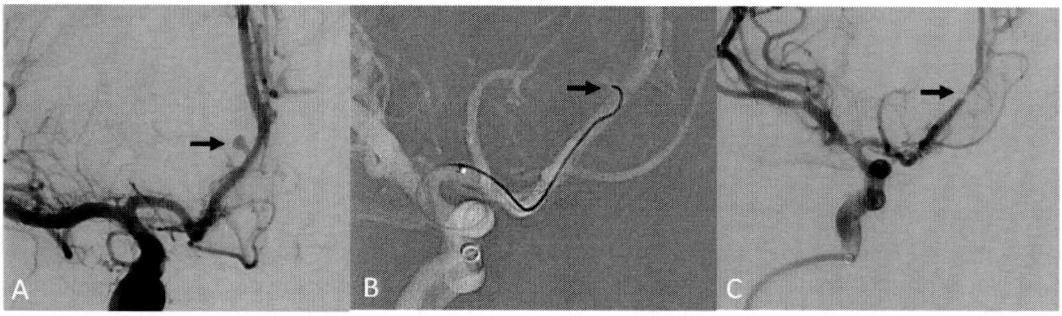

Figure 3. A 46-year-old male patient presented with a subarachnoid hemorrhage (SAH). A, cerebral angiogram showing a small aneurysm. B, the doctor navigating a micro-guidewire to enter the aneurysm and initiates electrocoagulation therapy. C, the postoperative angiogram demonstrates the aneurysm has disappeared.

This unexpected achievement underscored the potential of Guglielmi's coils to bring transformative changes to the field of neurointervention. It ultimately led to the publication of case images on the cover of the journal *Neurosurgery*, marking a significant milestone in this evolving discipline. Following this historic event, major clinical trials were initiated to evaluate the safety and efficacy of the Guglielmi Detachable Coil (GDC) for aneurysm treatment, a crucial step in establishing the device's credibility and addressing concerns within the medical community regarding the practicality of this innovative technique. In late 1990, an Investigational Device Exemption (IDE) was granted, permitting the clinical use of the GDC and paving the way for further exploration of its applications. These studies culminated in the GDC receiving approval from the United States Food and Drug Administration (FDA) on September 8, 1995, representing a significant advancement in neurointervention and the acceptance of endovascular coiling as a primary approach for aneurysm therapy [42].

The Development of Endovascular Therapies

With advancements in diagnostic capabilities, cerebral angiography has evolved into a therapeutic tool. Embolization procedures for the treatment of arteriovenous malformations (AVMs) were developed in the 1940s. These early procedures involved blocking abnormal blood vessels using materials such as silk threads or metallic coils. Although rudimentary, these techniques demonstrated that cerebral angiography could extend beyond mere visualization to include intervention [33].

During the 1960s, innovations in microsurgery and the emergence of stereotactic techniques, informed by angiography, significantly enhanced the accuracy of treatments for aneurysms and vascular anomalies. Microsurgical procedures pioneered by Dr. M. Gazi Yasargil, in conjunction with angiographic guidance, enabled the precise dissection of aneurysms and arteriovenous malformations (AVMs) [43]. In the 1970s, these advancements led to the development of magnetic navigation systems, which utilized external magnetic fields to guide catheters and other instruments within the brain during endovascular procedures.

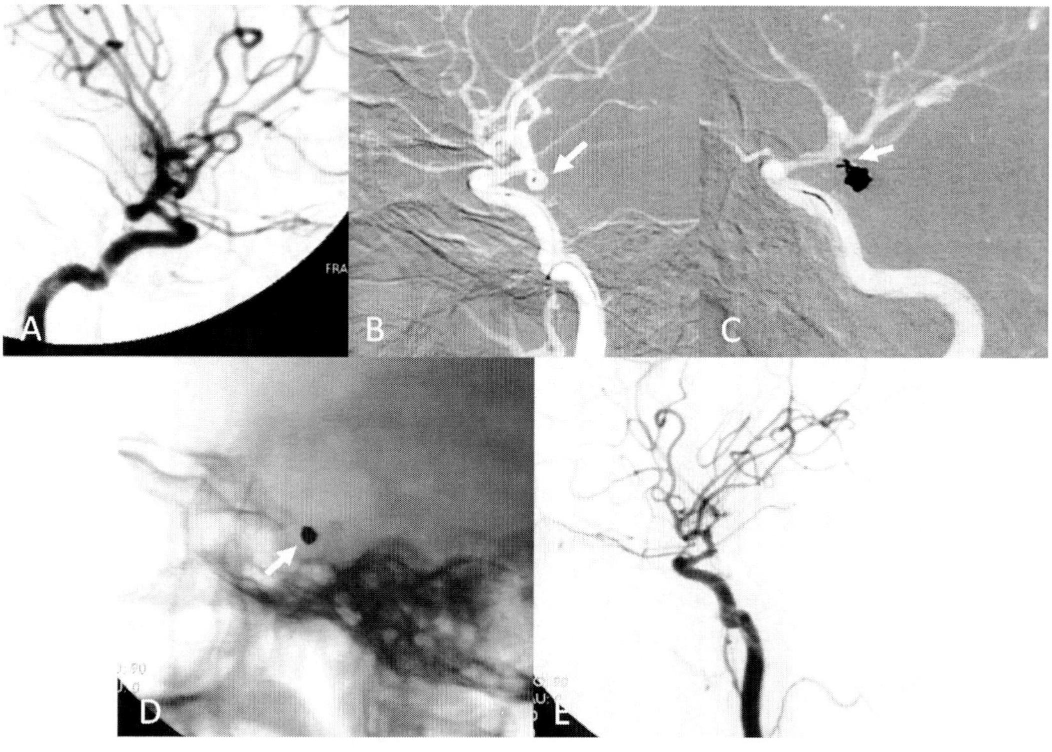

Figure 4. A 40-year-old woman with a posterior communicating artery aneurysm was coiled. A, lateral view of the left internal carotid artery injection showing the aneurysm of the left posterior communicating artery (arrow). B, roadmap image showing a Prowler14 microcatheter (Cordis, USA) was inserted into the aneurysm sac. C, roadmap image showing the aneurysm sac was occluded with coils (Orbit 5mm×10cm, 2mm×2cm, 2mm×1.5cm) and the microcatheter tip was at the aneurysm neck (arrow). D, unsubtracted image showing the coil mass after the last coil (Orbit 2mm×1.5cm) was used to occlude the aneurysm neck (arrow). E, lateral view of the left internal carotid artery injection after aneurysm coiling showing the disappearance of the aneurysm (arrow).

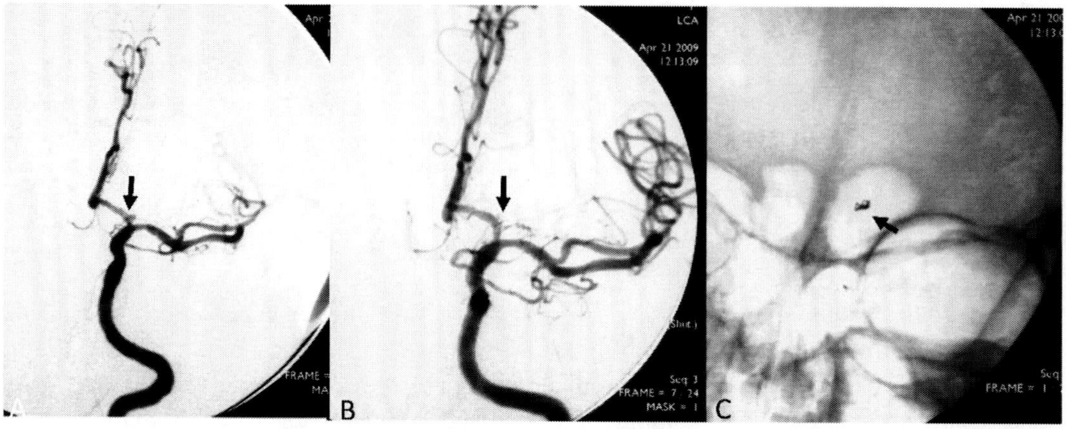

Figure 5. A 45-year-old woman with a ruptured aneurysm of the A1 segment of anterior cerebral artery was coiled. A, frontal view of the left internal carotid artery injection showing the aneurysm of the left A1 segment of the anterior cerebral artery (arrow). B, frontal view of the left internal carotid artery injection after aneurysm coiling showing complete occlusion of the aneurysm (arrow). C, unsubtracted image showing the Orbit 2mm×1.5cm coil (arrow).

Coil embolization played a crucial role in the development of innovative therapies for cerebral aneurysms during the 1990s (Figures 4 and 5) [38]. Starting in 2004, a significant advancement was the introduction of mechanical thrombectomy, a technique that employs a catheter to physically remove a blood clot from a cerebral artery. Angiography was vital in these procedures, enabling real-time visualization of the clot and guiding the catheter's navigation through the blood vessels. In early studies, researchers discovered that mechanical thrombectomy could restore blood flow in stroke patients, leading to significantly better outcomes compared to traditional treatments such as thrombolysis (clot-dissolving drugs). The success of these initial trials led to the widespread adoption of thrombectomy as a standard intervention for large-vessel occlusions in stroke patients, with cerebral angiography serving as the primary guiding tool for this essential technique [44, 45].

In recent years, robotic-assisted methods have begun to transform the field of cerebral angiography. These techniques enable remote-controlled catheter manipulation, enhancing precision and minimizing the risk of human error. The initial successful implementation of robotic assistance in cerebral angiography occurred in neurointervention, where meticulous catheter management is crucial. Angiographic techniques are increasingly incorporating artificial intelligence (AI) alongside robotics. AI algorithms can rapidly analyze angiographic images and provide real-time feedback to physicians, facilitating swift and accurate decision-making during complex procedures such as aneurysm coiling or stroke thrombectomy [46, 47]. These advancements represent the future of cerebral angiography, pushing the boundaries of what is possible in both diagnostic and therapeutic interventions.

Conclusion

The evolution of cerebral angiography and neurointervention has been remarkable, transitioning from initial experimental techniques to a fundamental aspect of contemporary neurovascular therapy. Early efforts, such as electrocoagulation and magnetic stereotaxis, laid the groundwork for minimally invasive approaches, establishing guidelines for safer and more effective interventions. Although these novel techniques were challenging, they catalyzed the development of advanced methods such as aneurysm coiling and hybrid endovascular-surgical procedures. The adaptability of cerebral angiography has underscored its importance, remaining relevant despite the rise of non-invasive imaging techniques like CT and MRI. The integration of robotics and artificial intelligence promises to further enhance the capabilities of cerebral angiography, improving precision and reducing procedural risks. This evolution reflects the power of innovation and the collaborative efforts of scientists and physicians. As imaging and navigation technologies advance, including the emergence of robotic-assisted surgery and improved magnetic systems, cerebral angiography continues to be a vital component in diagnosis and treatment, ensuring its enduring significance in the future of neurointervention.

References

[1] Paleari A, Beretta EP, Riva MA. Giovanni Maria Lancisi (1654–1720) and the modern cardiovascular physiology. *Advances in Physiology Education* (2021) 45 (1):154-159.

[2] Tubiana M. Wilhelm Conrad Röntgen and the discovery of X-rays. *Bull Acad Natl Med* (1996) 180 (1):97-108.

[3] Hoeffner EG, et al. Neuroradiology back to the future: brain imaging. *AJNR Am J Neuroradiol* (2012) 33 (1):5-11.

[4] Stauffer RC. Speculation and Experiment in the Background of Oersted's Discovery of Electromagnetism. *Isis* (1957) 48 (1):33-50.

[5] Wise MN. The Mutual Embrace of Electricity and Magnetism. *Science* (1979) 203 (4387):1310-1318.

[6] Al-Khalili J. The birth of the electric machines: a commentary on Faraday (1832) "Experimental researches in electricity." *Philos Trans A Math Phys Eng Sci* (2015) 373 (2039).

[7] Longair M. "...a paper ...I hold to be great guns": a commentary on Maxwell (1865) "A dynamical theory of the electromagnetic field." *Philos Trans A Math Phys Eng Sci* (2015) 373 (2039).

[8] Towne EB. The Value of Ventriculograms in the Localization of Intracranial Lesions: Three Cases of Obstructive Hydrocephalus and One of Brain Tumor. *Archives of Surgery* (1922) 5:144-158.

[9] Moniz E. L'Encéphalographie artérielle, son importance dans la localisation des tumeurs cérébrales. *Masson* (1927).

[10] Tan SY, Yip A. António Egas Moniz (1874-1955): Lobotomy pioneer and Nobel laureate. *Singapore Med J* (2014) 55 (4):175-176.

[11] Kretzer RM, Coon AL, Tamargo RJ. Walter E. Dandy's contributions to vascular neurosurgery. *J Neurosurg* (2010) 112 (6):1182-1191.

[12] Seldinger SI. Catheter replacement of the needle in percutaneous arteriography; a new technique. *Acta radiol* (1953) 39 (5):368-376.

[13] Bhattacharyya KB. Godfrey Newbold Hounsfield (1919-2004): The man who revolutionized neuroimaging. *Ann Indian Acad Neurol* (2016) 19 (4):448-450.

[14] Derdeyn CP, et al. Intraoperative digital subtraction angiography: a review of 112 consecutive examinations. *AJNR Am J Neuroradiol* (1995) 16 (2):307-318.

[15] Lauterbur PC. Image Formation by Induced Local Interactions: Examples Employing Nuclear Magnetic Resonance. *Nature* (1973) 242 (5394):190-191.

[16] B. A series of experiments performed for the purpose of showing that arteries may be obliterated without ligature, compression, or the knife. *London: Longman & Co. Pamphlet* (1832):66.

[17] A. Mémoire sur la piqûe ou l'acupunture des artères dans le traitement des anévrismes. *Gaz Med Paris* (1881) 2:1-4.

[18] Moore CH, Murchison C. On a new method of procuring the consolidation of Fibrin in certain incurable Aneurisms: With the Report of a case in which an Aneurism of the ascending Aorta was treated by the insertion of Wire. *Med Chir Trans* (1864) 47:129-149.
[19] L. Sulla elettro-puntura nella cura degli aneurysmi. *Gazz Med Ital Lomb Milano* (1847) 6:9-14.
[20] Blakemore AH. Progressive constrictive occlusion of the abdominal aorta with wiring and electrothermic coagulation, a one-stage operation for arteriosclerotic aneurysms of the abdominal aorta. *Ann Surg* (1951) 133 (4):447-462.
[21] Linton RR, H I J. Treatment of thoracic aortic aneurysms by the "pack" method of intrasaccular wiring. *N Engl J Med* (1952) 246:847-855.
[22] Werner SC, Blakemore AH, King BG. Aneurysm of the Internal Carotid Artery within the Skull: Wiring and Electrothermic Coagulation. *JAMA* (1941) 116:578-582.
[23] Das K, et al. Irving S. Cooper (1922-1985): a pioneer in functional neurosurgery. *J Neurosurg* (1998) 89 (5):865-873.
[24] Bigelow F, De Foyes J. Cited by Sawyer P, Pate J. *Am J Physiol* (1953) 175:103-107.
[25] Sawyer PN, Pate JW. Electrical potential differences across the normal aorta and aortic grafts of dogs. *American Journal of Physiology-Legacy Content* (1953) 175 (1):113-117.
[26] Sawyer PN, Pate JW. Bio-electric phenomena as an etiologic factor in intravascular thrombosis. *American Journal of Physiology-Legacy Content* (1953) 175 (1):103-107.
[27] Salazar AE. Experimental myocardial infarction. Induction of coronary thrombosis in the intact closed-chest dog. *Circ Res* (1961) 9:1351-1356.
[28] Piton J, et al. Selective vascular thrombosis induced by a direct electrical current: animal experiments. First clinical trials. *Journal of Neuroradiology= Journal de Neuroradiologie* (1978) 5 (2):139-152.
[29] Alksne JF, Fingerhut AG. Magnetically controlled metallic thrombosis of intracranial aneurysms. A preliminary report. *Bull Los Angeles Neurol Soc* (1965) 30 (3):153-155.
[30] Robles C, Carrasco-Zanini J. Treatment of Cerebral Arteriovenous Malformations by Muscle Embolization. *Journal of Neurosurgery* (1968) 29 (6):603-608.
[31] Alksne JF, Smith RW. Stereotaxic occlusion of 22 consecutive anterior communicating artery aneurysms. *J Neurosurg* (1980) 52 (6):790-793.
[32] Alksne JF, Fingerhut AG, Rand RW. Magnetic probe for the stereotactic thrombosis of intracranial aneurysms. *J Neurol Neurosurg Psychiatry* (1967) 30 (2):159-162.
[33] Serbinenko FA. Balloon catheterization and occlusion of major cerebral vessels. *J Neurosurg* (1974) 41 (2):125-145.
[34] Teitelbaum GP, et al. A tribute to Dr. Fedor A. Serbinenko, founder of endovascular neurosurgery. *Neurosurgery* (2000) 46 (2):462-469; discussion 469-470.
[35] McLaughlin N, Bojanowski MW. Early surgery-related complications after aneurysm clip placement: an analysis of causes and patient outcomes. *J Neurosurg* (2004) 101 (4):600-606.
[36] Molyneux AJ, et al. International subarachnoid aneurysm trial (ISAT) of neurosurgical clipping versus endovascular coiling in 2143 patients with ruptured intracranial aneurysms: a randomised comparison of effects on survival, dependency, seizures, rebleeding, subgroups, and aneurysm occlusion. *Lancet* (2005) 366 (9488):809-817.
[37] Koebbe CJ, et al. Endovascular Management of Intracranial Aneurysms: Current Experience and Future Advances. *Neurosurgery* (2006) 59 (5):S3-93-S3-102.
[38] Dovey Z, et al. Guglielmi detachable coiling for intracranial aneurysms: the story so far. *Arch Neurol* (2001) 58 (4):559-564.
[39] Nesbit GM, Barnwell SL. The use of electrolytically detachable coils in treating high-flow arteriovenous fistulas. *AJNR Am J Neuroradiol* (1998) 19 (8):1565-1569.
[40] Lanterna LA, et al. Treatment of unruptured cerebral aneurysms by embolization with guglielmi detachable coils: case-fatality, morbidity, and effectiveness in preventing bleeding—a systematic review of the literature. *Neurosurgery* (2004) 55 (4):767-775; discussion 775-778.
[41] Strother CM. Electrothrombosis of saccular aneurysms via endovascular approach: part 1 and part 2. *AJNR: American Journal of Neuroradiology* (2001) 22 (5):1011.
[42] Morrison SR. Guglielmi detachable coils: an alternative therapy for surgically high-risk aneurysms. *J Neurosci Nurs* (1997) 29 (4):232-237.

[43] Krayenbühl HA, et al. Microsurgical treatment of intracranial saccular aneurysms. *J Neurosurg* (1972) 37 (6):678-686.

[44] Smith WS, et al. Mechanical Thrombectomy for Acute Ischemic Stroke. *Stroke* (2008) 39 (4):1205-1212.

[45] Munich SA, Vakharia K, Levy EI. Overview of Mechanical Thrombectomy Techniques. *Neurosurgery* (2019) 85 (suppl_1):S60-S67.

[46] Beyar R, et al. Robotics, imaging, and artificial intelligence in the catheterisation laboratory. *Euro Intervention* (2021) 17 (7):537-549.

[47] Bravo J, et al. Robotics and Artificial Intelligence in Endovascular Neurosurgery. *Cureus* (2022) 14 (3):e23662.

Chapter 2

Spinal Angiography: The History of a Diagnostic and Therapeutic Breakthrough

Omar Alwakaa
and Philipp Taussky*, MD
Neurosurgical Service, Beth Israel Deaconess Medical Center, Brain Aneurysm Institute, Harvard Medical School, Boston, MA, USA

Abstract

Spinal angiography remains the definitive imaging modality for evaluating the spinal vasculature, providing high-resolution visualization of the arterial and venous anatomy of the spine. It is essential for the diagnosis of spinal vascular pathology and for preoperative vascular mapping of spinal tumors. The diagnostic and therapeutic capabilities of spinal angiography have evolved from aortography to sophisticated selective catheterization. Spinal angiography emerged in the early twentieth century as a result of breakthroughs in imaging modalities. Between the 1950s and 1970s, significant advances were made with the introduction of selective catheterization techniques that allowed focused visualization of spinal arteries. Another important milestone was the widespread adoption of DSA in the late 1970s, which allowed for improved image resolution by digitally removing background structures. Since the 1980s, technological developments, such as microcatheters, high-resolution fluoroscopy, and three-dimensional imaging, have improved the safety, accuracy, and efficacy of spinal angiography. These advances have made comprehensive evaluation and minimally invasive therapy of complicated vascular pathology more feasible. Despite the development of non-invasive imaging modalities, spinal angiography remains unique in providing dynamic and real-time visualization of the spinal vascular anatomy.

Keywords: spinal angiography, Digital Subtraction Angiography (DSA), Spinal Arteriovenous Malformation (AVM), Spinal Arteriovenous fistula (AVF), spinal tumor embolization

---

* Corresponding Author's Email: philipp.taussky@gmail.com

In: World History of Neurointerventional Surgery
Editors: Xianli Lv and Zhongxue Wu
ISBN: 979-8-89530-792-2

Introduction

Spinal angiography is the gold standard for visualizing the spinal vasculature. This diagnostic procedure visualizes the arterial supply and venous drainage of the spinal cord, vertebrae, and surrounding soft tissues. It includes visualization of the spinal arteries, including the vertebral arteries, radicular arteries, and segmental arteries such as the intercostal and lumbar arteries. In addition, the Adamkiewicz's artery may also be visualized on the spinal angiogram. It usually arises between T8 and L2 and is critical to the supply of the lower two-thirds of the spinal cord. Spinal angiography is often recommended for suspected spinal vascular anomalies such as dural arteriovenous fistulas (AVFs), spinal arteriovenous malformations (AVMs), and spinal cord ischemia. It is also used to map the vascular supply of highly vascularized spinal tumors prior to surgery, which is essential for surgical planning in situations involving spinal cord compression [1].

The role of spinal angiography has evolved from a purely diagnostic tool to an effective therapeutic modality. Specifically, spinal angiography has been used to perform targeted embolization of spinal AVMs, AVFs, and tumor-supplied arteries with liquid embolic agents. In addition, spinal angiographic embolization offers a minimally invasive alternative to surgery. This chapter provides a comprehensive historical overview of spinal angiography. It explains the significant innovations, turning points in history, and technical breakthroughs that have influenced its evolution into the contemporary therapeutic modality that it is today.

Early Developments and Pioneering Work (1920s - 1940s)

The development of vascular imaging in general, and cerebral angiography in particular, is closely related to the development of spinal angiography. The origins of angiography date back to 1927, when the Portuguese neurologist Egas Moniz performed the first cerebral angiography. By developing the basics of using contrast agents to visualize blood vessels through x-ray imaging, Moniz's groundbreaking work created new opportunities for the diagnosis of neurovascular disease [2]. Imaging techniques in the early 20th century were crude due to limited understanding of the spinal vasculature. Early spinal angiographic procedures were indirect, most often involving aortography, the infusion of contrast into the aorta to visualize the spinal vessels. This method faced numerous challenges, including poor image quality, a high prevalence of complications, and limited clinical use. To illustrate, the most common complications were contrast-induced neurotoxicity and spinal cord ischemia [3, 4]. The techniques used during this period laid the foundation for our current understanding of spinal artery imaging and paved the way for subsequent advances.

Development of Selective Spinal Angiography (1950s - 1970s)

Developments in spinal angiography from the 1950s to the 1970s changed the practice forever. This occurred as physicians and researchers sought to develop more specialized and safer techniques for imaging the vascular anatomy of the spinal cord, including the anterior spinal artery, posterior spinal arteries, and Adamkiewicz's artery. Henson and Croft pioneered the angiographic documentation of the first spinal AVM in 1956. Di Chiro reported the first angiographic depiction of a spinal cord tumor. Subsequent advances were also marked by the contributions of Höök and Lindvall in 1958, who used vertebral angiography to illustrate cervical arteriovenous malformations, thus expanding the use of angiography to different spinal segments. Morris further improved this methodology in 1960, illustrating the growing efficacy of angiography in the diagnosis of spinal vascular disease [5]. The most important technological breakthrough of this era was the development of catheter-based techniques, particularly fluoroscopy, which allowed real-time x-ray guidance. During this period, Djindjian, a French neuroradiologist, made fundamental contributions to spinal angiography. His innovative approaches gradually replaced non-selective aortography with selective catheterization techniques [6]. These approaches allowed selective visualization of spinal arteries such as the artery of Adamkiewicz, posterior spinal arteries, and anterior spinal arteries. The use of selective visualization became essential to spinal angiography procedures because of its ability to improve the accuracy and safety of catheter placement. In addition, the ability to selectively catheterize spinal arteries led to a remarkable improvement in diagnostic outcomes, allowing for more accurate detection of vascular pathologies such as AVFs and AVMs.

Djindjian's innovations were complemented by the contributions of other contemporary researchers who improved catheter-based interventions. Innovative techniques were developed to navigate the complex spinal vascular anatomy. Innovative techniques using microcatheters and guidewires specifically designed for spinal endovascular interventions were developed to reduce the risks associated with navigating the complex spinal vascular anatomy, such as vascular injury and spinal cord ischemia [7]. The invention of digital subtraction angiography (DSA) in the late 1970s was a notable milestone in the history of spinal angiography. Drs. Charles Mistretta and Andrew Crummy at the University of Wisconsin were instrumental in the development of DSA. They described computerized fluorography, in which they amplified and digitized images from an image intensifier and displayed them on a monitor. They developed the first digital video image processor (DVIP), which is an essential component of real-time subtraction angiography. In addition, the term "digital subtraction angiography" (DSA) was formally introduced by Meaney et. al. at the Cleveland Clinic in 1980. They paved the way for the first effective clinical use of DSA and contributed to its widespread adoption in clinical practice [8, 9]. DSA revolutionized vascular imaging, allowing digital removal of background structures such as soft tissue and bone from angiographic images. It also enabled a more thorough and accurate evaluation of vascular abnormalities, setting new standards for improved clinical decision making and more specific and successful therapies [10].

Technological Advances and Refinement (1980s - Present)

Rapid technical improvements in the 1980s brought spinal angiography into the modern era, making it safer, more accurate, and more widely used as a diagnostic tool. In particular, advances in high-resolution imaging technology and the development of microcatheters and micro-guidewires made navigation of the complex spinal vasculature easier and more precise. Microcatheters typically have a reduced diameter and improved flexibility. The use of microcatheters in spinal angiography could reduce the hazards associated with catheterization, including vascular damage and spinal cord ischemia. In addition, the use of hydrophilic coatings on catheters has reduced friction, allowing for vessel selectivity and safer navigation through spinal arteries [7].

Advanced imaging techniques have also improved the effectiveness of spinal angiography. These techniques include 3-dimensional rotational angiography and cone beam computed tomography (CBCT). They have made it possible to demonstrate 3-dimensional reconstructions of the spinal vasculature and achieve a comprehensive view of complex lesions and their relationship to adjacent anatomical structures. This detailed imaging modality is essential for planning surgical or endovascular procedures and could help medical providers visualize the exact location and extent of arterial pathology [11].

In general, modern spinal angiography suites are equipped with the most advanced fluoroscopy technology. Current fluoroscopy provides high-resolution imaging with minimal radiation exposure, which can improve patient safety and maintain diagnostic accuracy. In addition, advanced imaging software can help physicians process and interpret images in real time, which may improve their ability to detect small vascular pathologies and allow for immediate intervention. Although non-invasive imaging modalities such as computed tomography angiography (CTA) and magnetic resonance angiography (MRA) have advanced, spinal angiography remains the gold standard for evaluating spinal vascular pathology [1]. Its exceptional ability to provide dynamic and real-time assessment of blood flow makes it an invaluable tool in the diagnosis and management of complicated spinal vascular disease that cannot be adequately assessed by other imaging modalities.

Future Directions and Innovations

Future innovations in minimally invasive treatments, artificial intelligence (AI), and imaging technologies may have a significant impact on the field of spinal angiography. High-resolution CT and MRA are being investigated as potential alternatives or adjuncts to angiography to see if they can provide comparable diagnostic accuracy without invasive catheterization. Interestingly, AI and machine learning are increasingly being integrated into angiographic procedures. They hold great promise for improving the interpretation of DSA images, automating the detection of vascular abnormalities, and optimizing catheter navigation. In addition, future AI algorithms may be able to assess vascular anatomy and flow dynamics in real time, reducing procedure time and improving diagnostic accuracy.

In addition, researchers are working to develop novel contrast agents. Innovations in these contrast agents aim to reduce the risk of neurotoxicity and allergic reactions. The ultimate goal of these innovations is to improve the accuracy, safety and efficacy of spinal angiography. Spinal angiography is expected to remain a fundamental component of spinal vascular diagnosis and treatment as technology evolves and knowledge in the field increases.

Illustrative Case

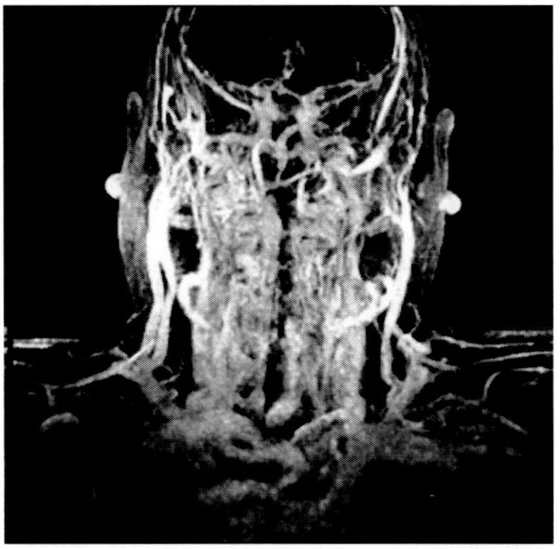

Figure 1. 35-year-old male patient with bilateral progressive upper arm weakness. Neck MRA showing large bilateral venous congestion of the neck vessels.

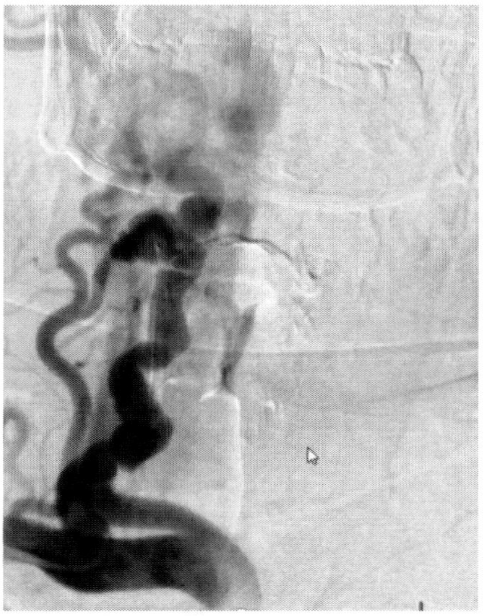

Figure 2. Right vertebral artery injection showing a vertebral-venous fistula at the level of the cervical spine without signs of intracranial vertebral artery filling.

A 35-year-old patient who worked as a handyman in a hotel and was unable to lift his arms presented to our emergency department. A cervical MRA (Figure 1) showed large bilateral venous congestion of the cervical vessels. Injection of the right and left vertebral arteries revealed a complex large vertebral-venous fistula (Figures 2 and 3). The right vertebral artery was then coils occluded (Figure 4). Initially, the patient improved significantly, but six months later he presented with near plegia of his left arm. An MRI of his cervical spine showed almost complete spinal cord compression by a fistulous epidural vein (Figure 5). To locate the fistulous connection in a high-flow situation, a balloon was inflated in the distal left vertebral artery to create a flow occlusion (Figure 6), and a left vertebral artery on balloon inflation revealed a proximal cervical left vertebral artery venous connection that was then coiled (Figure 7). A final vertebral artery injection then showed complete occlusion of the fistula and normal filling of the left vertebral artery extending intracranially (Figure 7). Clinically, the patient improved significantly and was able to return to work without restrictions.

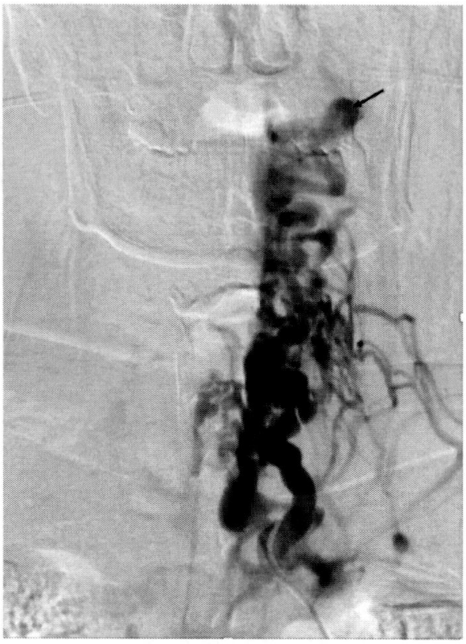

Figure 3. Injection of the left vertebral artery showing also a left vertebral-venous fistula with distal vertebral artery filling (arrow).

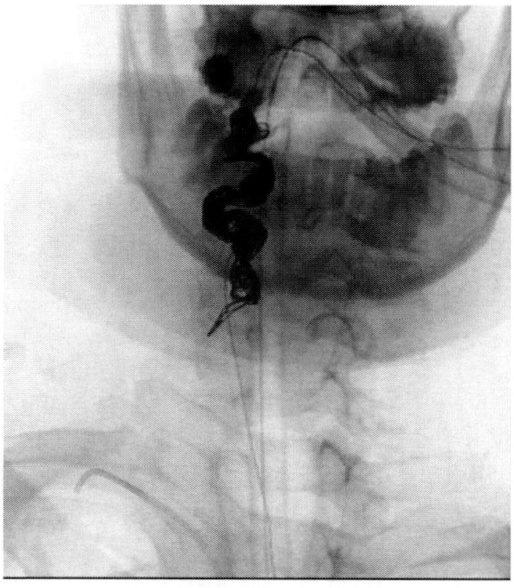

Figure 4. Left vertebral artery was sacrificed with coil occlusion.

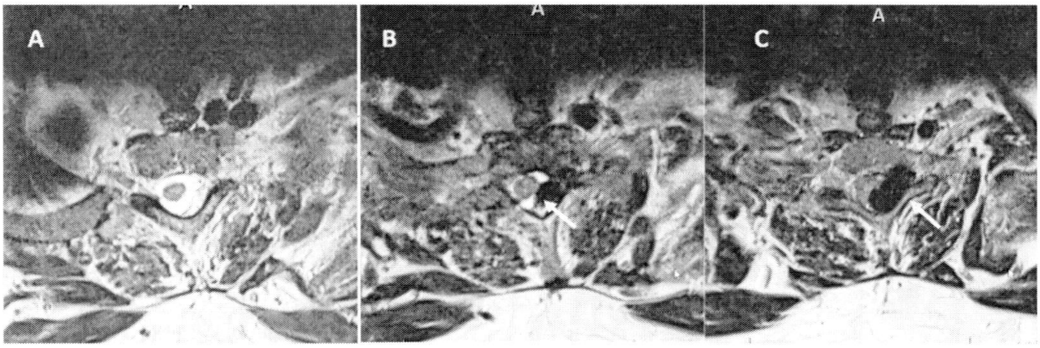

Figure 5. A: 6 months follow-up cervical MRI showing normal spinal cord and CSF flow at lower cervical levels. B: Large dilated epidural fistulous vein (arrow) with compression of the spinal cord. C: Epidural vein with near complete compression of spinal cord due to fistulous vein (arrow).

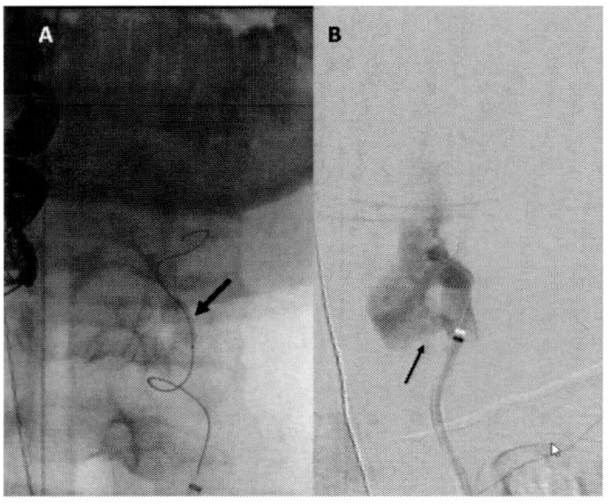

Figure 6. A: Left vertebral artery a balloon (arrow) was used and inflated to arrest flow and assess for the arterial venous fistulous connection. B: Injection of the left vertebral artery with distal balloon occlusion shows the arterial-venous direct fistulous connection (arrow).

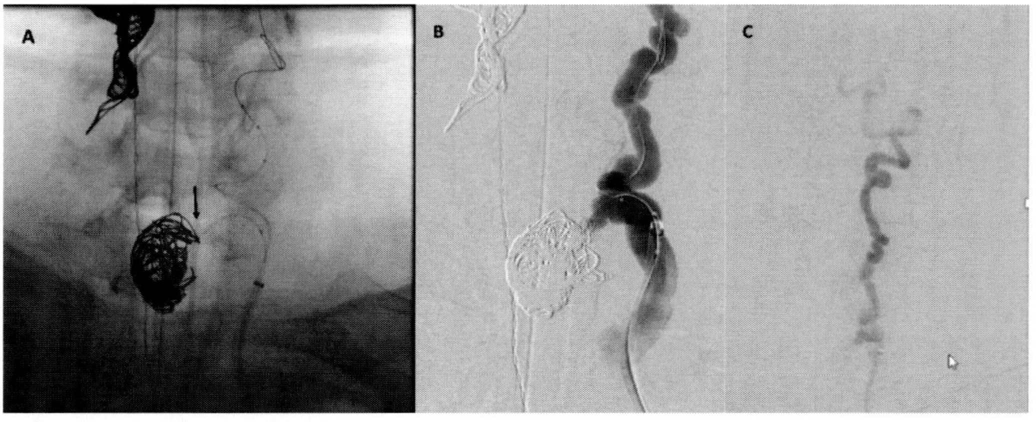

Figure 7. A: Left vertebral artery showing a balloon and wire in the distal vertebral artery guaranteeing distal vertebral access. An additional microcatheter was used to coil off the venous fistulous connection (arrow). B: Final left vertebral artery injection shows normal filling of the vertebral artery without residual fistulous filling. C: Final left vertebral artery injection shows filling intracranially and no fistulous filling.

Conclusion

Spinal angiography emerged in the early twentieth century as a result of breakthroughs in imaging modalities. The developments of microcatheters, high-resolution fluoroscopy, and three-dimensional imaging have improved the safety, accuracy, and efficacy of spinal angiography. The diagnostic and therapeutic capabilities of spinal angiography have evolved from aortography to sophisticated selective catheterization.

Disclaimer

None.

References

[1] Gailloud P. Introduction to Diagnostic and Therapeutic Spinal Angiography. *Neuroimaging Clin N Am* (2019) 29 (4):595-614. doi:10.1016/j.nic.2019.07.008.

[2] Ligon BL. Biography: history of developments in imaging techniques: Egas Moniz and angiography. *Semin Pediatr Infect Dis* (2003) 14 (2):173-181. doi:10.1053/spid.2003.127232.

[3] Margolis G, Tarazi AK, Grimson KS. Contrast medium injury to the spinal cord produced by aortography; pathologic anatomy of the experimental lesion. *J Neurosurg* (1956) 13 (4):261-277. doi:10.3171/jns.1956.13.4.0261.

[4] Killen DA, Foster JH. Spinal cord injury as a complication of aortography. *Ann Surg* (1960) 152 (2):211-230. doi:10.1097/00000658-196008000-00004.

[5] Di Chiro G. Development of spinal cord angiography. *Acta Radiol Diagn (Stockh)* (1972) 13 (0):767-770. doi:10.1177/02841851720130p234.

[6] Djindjian R, Houdart R, Hurth M. [Angiography of the spinal cord]. *Acta Radiol Diagn (Stockh)* (1969) 9:707-726.

[7] Teitelbaum GP. A brief history of angiography and endovascular therapy. *Semin Anesth Perioper Med Pain* (2000) 19 (4):237-240. doi:10.1053/sa.2000.17786.

[8] Meaney TF, Weinstein MA, Buonocore E, et al. Digital subtraction angiography of the human cardiovascular system. *AJR Am J Roentgenol* (1980) 135 (6):1153-1160. doi:10.2214/ajr.135.6.1153.

[9] Jeans WD. The development and use of digital subtraction angiography. *Br J Radiol* (1990) 63 (747):161-168. doi:10.1259/0007-1285-63-747-161.

[10] Crummy AB, Strother CM, Mistretta CA. The History of Digital Subtraction Angiography. *J Vasc Interv Radiol JVIR* (2018) 29 (8):1138-1141. doi:10.1016/j.jvir.2018.03.030.

[11] Chen SH, Sur S, Brunet MC, et al. Advances in 3D angiography for spinal vascular malformations. *J Clin Neurosci Off J Neurosurg Soc Australas* (2020) 72:79-83. doi:10.1016/j.jocn.2020.01.013.

Chapter 3

An Overview of the Vascular Anatomy of the Circle of Willis and Its Variants

Victor Hugo Perez Perez[1,*], MD
Andrew Lee[2,†], DO
and Juan E. Small[2,‡], MD, MSc
[1]Mexican Institute of Social Security, Mexico City, Mexico
[2]Department of Radiology, Lahey Hospital and Medical Center, Burlington, MA, USA

Abstract

The circle of Willis is a vital collateral arterial network at the base of the brain connecting the anterior and posterior circulation. It is a polygon of arterial branches emanating from the internal carotid and vertebrobasilar systems. It possesses significant variability in anatomy and therefore it is important to identify these anatomical variants prior to neurosurgical intervention, to avoid iatrogenic injury. Some variant anatomy types may greatly increase the risk of aneurysm formation as well. A thorough and complete understanding of the anatomical variants of the circle of Willis is essential for the endovascular neurosurgeon as well as the imaging interpreter.

Keywords: circle of Willis, anterior cerebral artery, posterior cerebral artery, recurrent artery of Heubner, anterior communicating artery, posterior communicating artery, Thomas Willis

Introduction

The circle of Willis (COW) is one of the best-known and most famous eponymous structures in human anatomy. Thomas Willis was a physician in the 1600s and recognized as the founder of clinical neurology, neurology being a term that he himself coined. He made pioneering observations of various neural structures, bridging the disciplines of anatomy and clinical

* Corresponding Author's Email: victorhugo2perez@hotmail.com
† Corresponding Author's Email: wingfaiandrew.lee@lahey.org
‡ Corresponding Author's Email: Juan.E.Small@Lahey.org

In: World History of Neurointerventional Surgery
Editors: Xianli Lv and Zhongxue Wu
ISBN: 979-8-89530-792-2

anatomy. He is credited with naming several structures in the brain, including the internal capsule, the vagus nerve, and cerebellar peduncles [1]. However, it may surprise readers that Willis was not the first to describe the eponymous arterial circle, which may have been first described as early as 1561 by the anatomist Gabriel Fallopius or Fallopio [2].

Willis is credited as the first anatomist to illustrate the complete and symmetrical picture of the anastomotic arterial polygon at the base of the brain, that has also been called the arterial circulus or *circulus arteriosus cerebri*. He published *De Cerebri Anatome* in 1664, describing with great accuracy the vascular arrangement at the base of the brain in conjunction with the anatomic drawings of Christopher Wren, Willis' medical assistant and protégé. This work is credited with marking the transition between medieval and modern understanding of the morphology and function of the Circle of Willis [3].

Circle of Willis Anatomical Overview

The arterial circle as described by Willis is comprised of the bilateral A1 segments of the anterior cerebral arteries (ACAs), the bilateral P1 segments of the posterior cerebral arteries (PCAs), the internal carotid arteries (ICAs) at their terminus, and the anastomoses formed by the anterior communicating artery (ACoA) and the posterior communicating arteries (PCoAs) (Figure 1). The arterial circle is formed by the distal branches of the internal carotid artery and the most rostral branches of the basilar artery. The middle cerebral arteries arise from the circle but are not considered to be part of it [4].

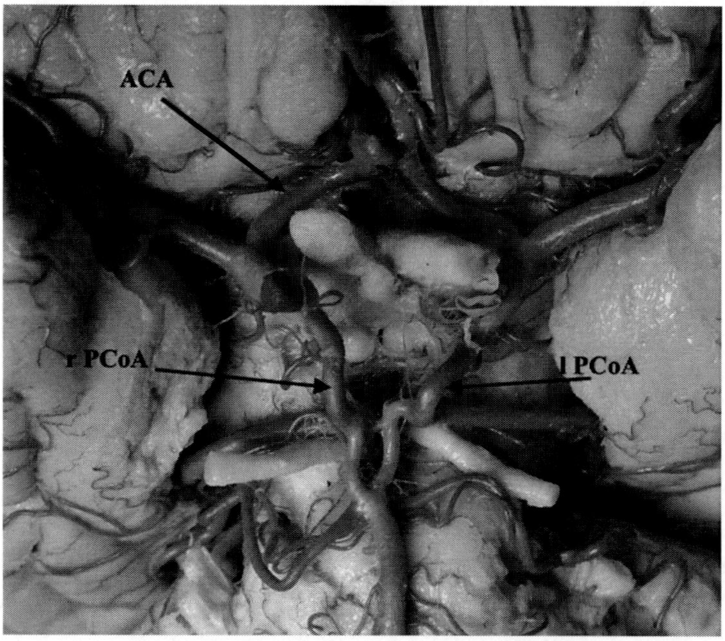

Figure 1. The Circle of Willis. The A1 segments of the anterior cerebral arteries (ACA), the anterior communicating artery, and the posterior communicating arteries (PCoA) connect the anterior and posterior circulations in the polygonal anastamotic network at the base of brain known as the Circle of Willis. Note that both posterior communicating arteries (PCoAs) are fetal variant as their diameter is greater than segment 1 of the posterior cerebral artery.

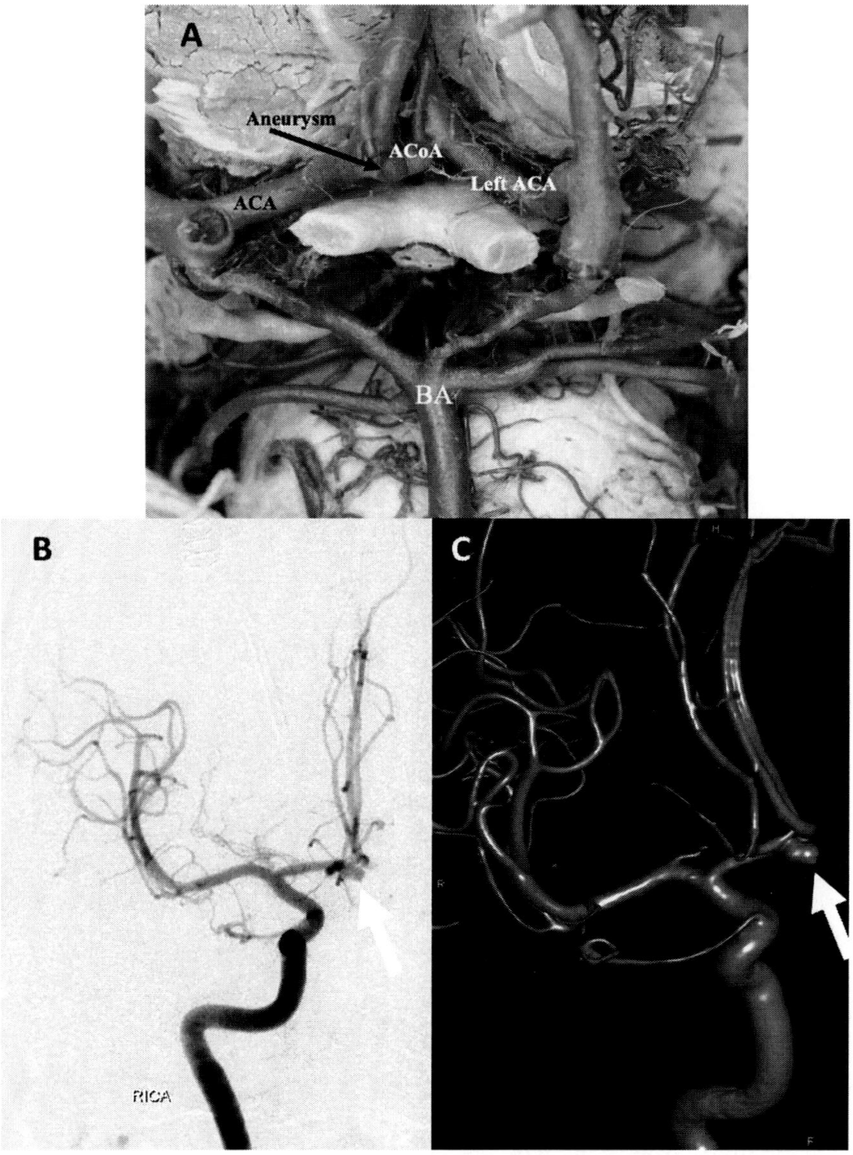

Figure 2. The Circle of Willis. The COW (A) is formed anteriorly by the anterior cerebral arteries (ACA) A1 segments and the anterior communicating artery (ACoA) as well as posteriorly by the posterior communicating arteries (PCoAs), which intersect the posterior cerebral arteries arising from the bifurcation of the basilar artery (BA). A saccular aneurysm is seen at the anterior communicating artery. Right ICA injection DSA image (B) and 3D reconstruction (C) with bilobed anterior communicating aneurysm (arrow).

The COW is an arterial crown that courses adjacent to the optic chiasm, the tuber cinereum and the interpeduncular region. The anterior cerebral arteries follow a rostral and medial direction towards the interhemispheric fissure and are connected by the anterior communicating artery anterior to the optic chiasm (Figures 1 and 2). At the rostral edge of the pons the basilar artery bifurcates, forming the two posterior cerebral arteries. The posterior communicating arteries arise from the internal carotid artery terminus and anastomose with the posterior cerebral arteries (Figure 1) [4].

The internal carotid arteries and the vessels arising from them supply the forebrain through the middle and anterior cerebral arteries and the vertebral arteries, and their branches supply the occipital lobe, the brain stem and the cerebellum. Thus, the circle of Willis serves as the main connection between the anterior and posterior circulation. Willis is credited with first proposing a compensatory mechanism against ischemia guiding the evolutionary development of the COW [4, 5]. It was hypothesized that the COW maintains cerebral blood flow in case one segment becomes occluded or stenosed. Vrselja et al. suggests that this may not be the main function of the COW since cardiovascular disease was unlikely to be a driver of evolution until very recently (global human lifespan was 28.5 years on average at the beginning of the 19th century) [5]. Furthermore, the low percentage of the population that has a complete COW (~20%, the most common anatomy is "variant anatomy" most commonly involving a hypoplastic segment) suggests against the compensatory mechanism as a core function. This is corroborated by another study that found that hypoplastic segments of the COW did in fact lead to decreased upstream flow [6].

Rather, it is thought that this anastomotic structure helps regulate intracerebral blood pressure by minimizing the pressure differences of the blood coming to the brain from anterior and posterior circulations, acting as a pressure absorber that prevents damage to the cranial microvasculature and blood brain barrier [5].

Anterior Cerebral Artery (ACA)

The anterior cerebral artery originates from the bifurcation of the internal carotid artery (Figure 3). It can be divided into 5 segments, first described by Fischer in 1938. The classification presented here slightly modifies the 5 segments described by Fischer and was proposed by Rhoton in 2007, which roughly segments the ACA based on its location relative to the corpus callosum [7]:

- The pre-communicating segment (A1) which originates at the ICA terminus and terminates at the anterior communicating artery.
- The infracallosal segment below the corpus callosum genu segment which originates after the anterior communicating artery and extends anterior to the lamina terminalis and along the rostrum of the corpus callosum (A2).
- The precallosal segment which extends around the genu of the corpus callosum and terminates where the artery turns directly posterior above the body (A3).
- The supracallosal segment which runs above the body anterior to the plane of the coronal suture (A4).
- The postcallosal segment which runs above the body posterior to the plane of the coronal suture (A5).

The ACA may have a rare variant origin, such that the ACA originates from the proximal intradural ICA in close proximity with the ophthalmic artery. In addition, variant anatomy in terms of branching has been described [7].

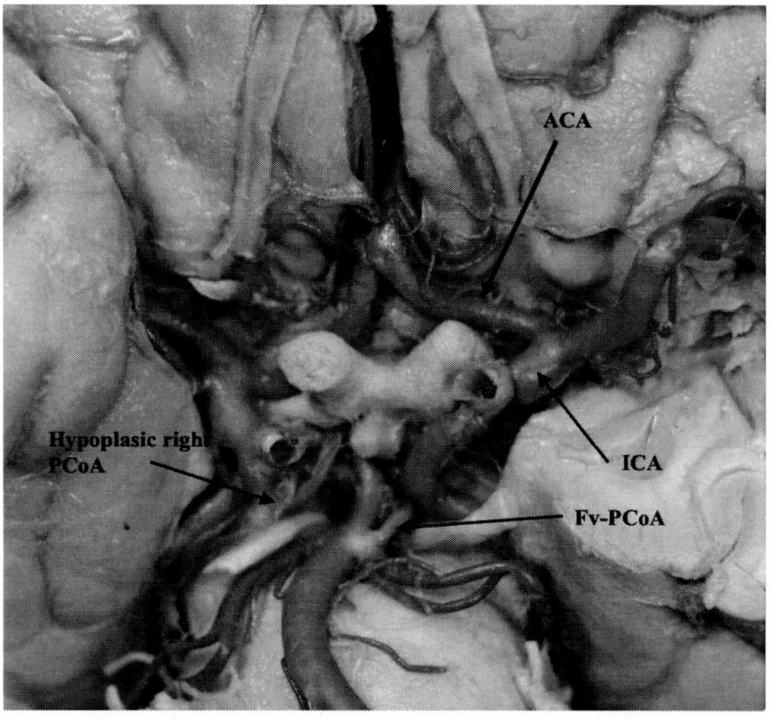

Figure 3. The anterior cerebral arteries (ACA) originate from the bifurcation of the internal carotid artery (ICA). The left temporal pole has been removed to observe this bifurcation in greater detail. This image also shows a left posterior communicating artery, fetal variant (fv-PCoA) and a hypoplastic right posterior communicating artery (PCoA).

A1 and A2 Segment Branches

The ACAs may have a unilateral hypoplastic A1 segment, may be azygous (one branch) or trifurcated with the 2nd/middle ACA A2 segment also known as the Artery of Wilder or "arteria "termatica" (Figure 7). An azygous ACA has been associated with bihemispheric infarcts and has been linked with other midline facial/brain abnormalities such as holoprosencephaly [7]. The unilateral A1 segment hypoplasia is associated with an asymmetric anterior communicating artery diameter, with the larger diameter associated with the non-hypoplastic A1 segment, at which the site of anastomosis predisposes to anterior communicating artery aneurysms [8].

The A1 segment has perforator arteries that can be divided into two groups, posteroinferior and posterior superior. The posteroinferior groups supply the optic nerve, optic chiasm and optic tract. They are generally small and few in number (2-3 perforators), and tend to be oriented more medially than laterally. The posteriorsuperior segments penetrate the anterior perforated substance with a mean of 3 perforators providing supply to the optic chiasm, the anterior commissure, the anterior hypothalamus, genu of the internal capsule, and anterior part of the globus pallidus [9].

The Recurrent Artery of Heubner

First described by Johann Otto Leonhard Heubner in 1872, the recurrent artery of Heubner is the largest medial lenticulostriate branch of the ACA (Figure 4). It supplies the anterior part of the caudate, the anterior third of the putamen, the anterior limb of the internal capsule and globus pallidus [10].

It is important to identify during neurosurgical procedures involving the anterior segment of the COW to avoid iatrogenic occlusion. Isolated damage to the recurrent artery can present as contralateral hemiparesis with facial and brachial predominance. It may also present with significant neuropsychological deficits, such as personality changes. This artery most commonly follows a superior or anterior course relative to A1. The superior course features the recurrent artery running directly above the A1, and the anterior course features it running in front of the A1 [10]. This artery most commonly originates from the A2 segment and ACoA-ACA junction. It least frequently arises from the A1 segment. It is symmetric in origin about half the time. It is rarely seen as a duplicated (17%) or triplicated (2.5%) vessel [10].

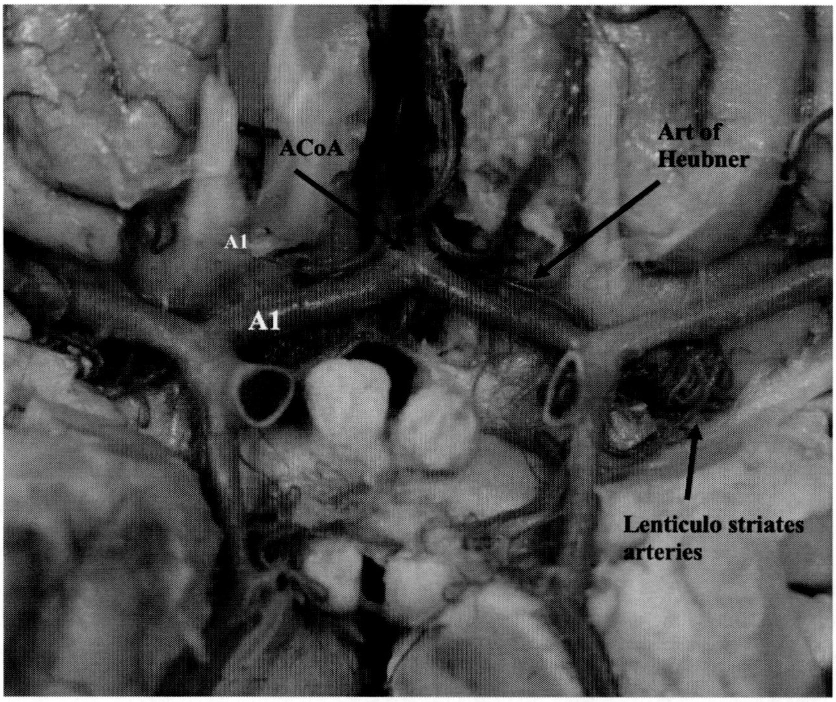

Figure 4. The artery of Heubner can be seen clearly in the left side arising from the A2 segment and coursing posteriorly. A fused anterior communicating artery and an asymmetrically more prominent right ACA A2 segment are also evident.

The Anterior Communicating Artery (ACoA)

The ACoA connects the bilateral anterior cerebral arteries and also marks the boundary between the A1 and A2 segments. The ACoA is located above the optic chiasm and is related to the lamina terminalis of the 3rd ventricle. The microvascular anatomy of the anterior communicating artery presents great variability in its shape, diameter and length (Figures 5 and 6). It is important to understand its variant anatomy, including aplasia, hypoplasia, fenestration, duplication/triplication, and complex types as it is the most common site of intracranial aneurysms (Figure 2). Furthermore, CTA imaging can often misconstrue ACoA variants such as fenestration as aneurysms. Therefore, the possibility of variant anatomy should always be considered along with digital subtraction angiography. Reported average measurements of the ACoA vary widely, however it has been reported to have an average length of 4 mm with an average diameter of 1.7 mm [8]. The ACoA diameter is usually asymmetric and is usually at least 1 mm smaller at the side connected to the larger A1 segment [11]. A single anterior communicating artery is present in 60% of cases. The most common variant is aplasia, seen about 20% of the time (Figure 5) [12].

The ACoA perforating vessels can be organized into three regions: subcallosal, hypothalamic, and chiasmatic. The subcallosal branch is the thickest and most important perforating vessel. It supplies the hypothalamus, lamina terminalis, anterior commissure, and corpus callosum genu among other areas. The hypothalamic branches often coincide in perfusion with the subcallosal branches and are a group of 2-6 perforators that supply the hypothalamus and lamina terminalis. The optic chiasm branch is the rarest perforator, with a probability of existence of approximately10%. It has a diameter of 0.1 to 0.2 mm and is a minor supplier of the optic nerve and the region above the optic chiasm [13].

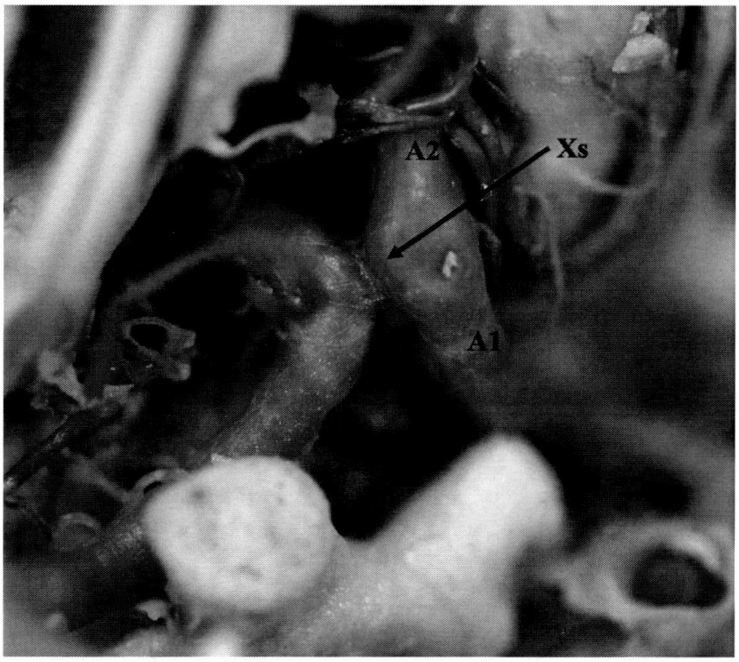

Figure 5. A fused/aplastic variant of the anterior communicating artery (Xs), such that the anterior cerebral arteries appear to be fused together.

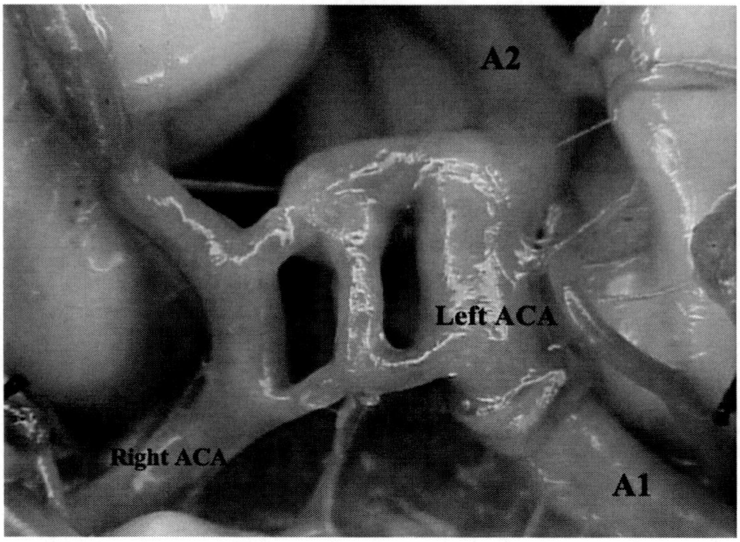

Figure 6. A complex type anterior communicating artery variant, also known as the "H" type is shown. The segmentation of the A1 and A2 segments of the anterior cerebral artery by the complex "H type" anterior communicating artery can also be seen.

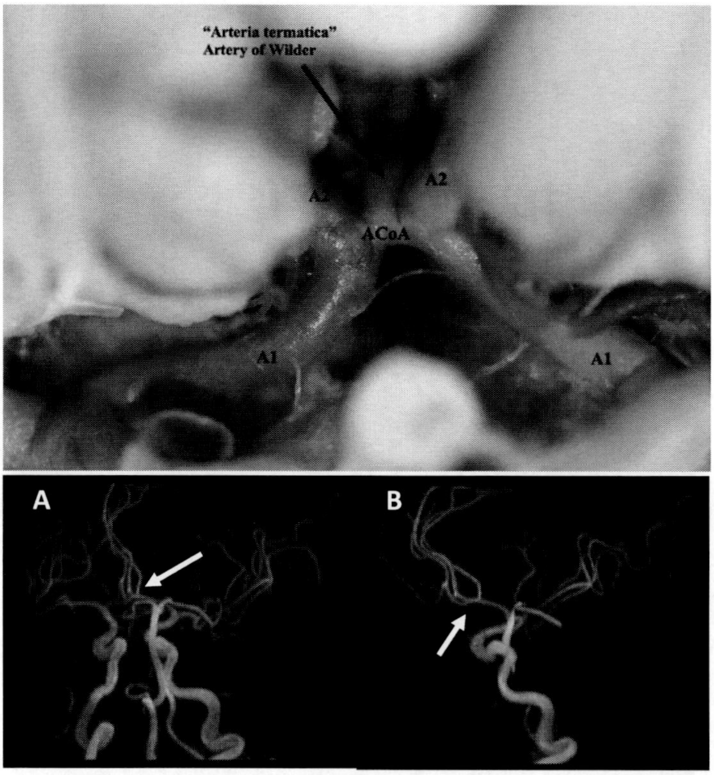

Figure 7. Anterior cerebral artery trifurcation: A. In the specimen above, an "arteria termatica" also known as the artery of Wilder is evident. It is considered as a third A2 artery arising from the anterior communicating artery and is also known as an anterior cerebral artery trifurcation. B. Cranial time-of-flight (TOF) MR angiogram maximum intensity (MIP) images (A and B) demonstrating an anterior cerebral trifurcation (arrow).

Posterior Cerebral Artery (PCA)

The posterior cerebral arteries arise from the basilar artery and course around the cerebral peduncle and over the tentorium cerebelli to supply the occipital lobe, posteromedial temporal lobes, midbrain, thalamus, choroid plexus, and part of the lateral and third ventricles. It may be divided into 5 main segments, with certain cisterns named after the PCA segment [14].

P1: From the basilar artery to the posterior communicating artery.
P2: Post-communicating segment.
  P2A (anterior): sub-segment courses through the crural cistern.
  P2P (posterior or ambient): sub-segment courses through the ambient cistern.
P3: Courses through the quadrigeminal cistern, terminates as it enters the sulci of the occipital lobe.
P4: Within the sulci of the occipital lobe, ends in the calcarine sulcus, giving off the parieto-occipital artery and calcarine artery.
P5: Terminal branches of the calcarine and parieto-occipital artery.

P1 and P2 Segment Branches

The P1 segment gives off small paramedian or mesencephalic arteries that supply the rostral midbrain (Figure 8) and thalamoperforating arteries, which supply part of the thalamus (Figure 8) [14]. The Artery of Percheron is a rare anatomical variant in which a single dominant paramedian artery bifurcates to perfuse the bilateral medial thalami, with varying contributions to the rostral midbrain [15]. Emboli to this anatomic variant can result in bilateral paramedian thalamic infarcts, with or without midbrain involvement that may present with vertical gaze palsy, altered mental status, and memory impairment [16].

The main branch of the P2 segment is the posterior choroidal artery. It also gives rise to peduncular perforating arteries that supply the lateral midbrain and thalamogeniculate arteries that supply the ventrolateral thalamus [14].

Posterior Communicating Artery (PCoA)

The posterior communicating arteries form the lateral border of the COW, arising from the posteromedial wall of the supraclinoid internal carotid artery. It runs posteromedially inferior and lateral to the tuber cinereum, above the sella turcica and oculomotor nerve, and joins the posterior cerebral artery. Rarely, the PCoA origin at the ICA may appear dilated, known as functional dilatation or infundibular widening that may be difficult to distinguish from an aneurysm. It has been described as giving rise to different branches with an average of 8 that can be divided into anterior and posterior. The anterior group of PCoA perforating branches supply the hypothalamus, ventral thalamus, anterior third of the optic tract, and posterior limb of the internal capsule. The posterior group supplies the posterior perforated substance and subthalamic nucleus. The premammillary artery is the largest branch that arises from the PCoA. It enters the floor of the third ventricle in front of or beside the mamillary body and supplies the posterior hypothalamus, anterior thalamus, posterior limb of the internal capsule, and subthalamus [11].

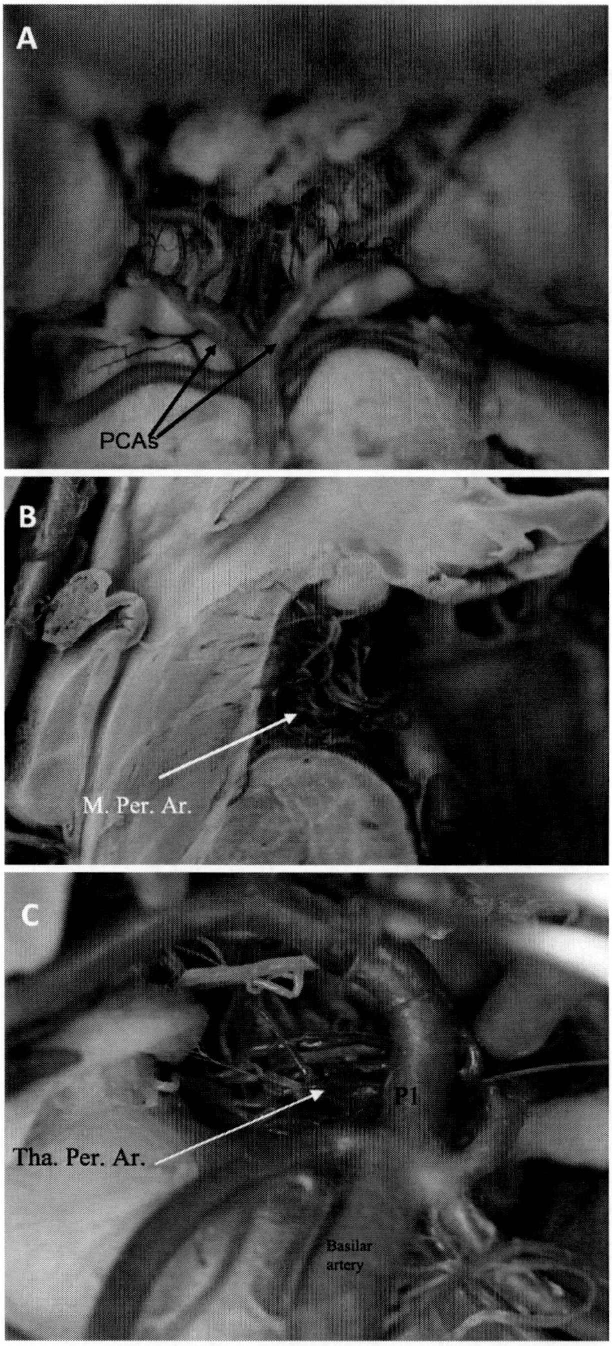

Figure 8. Perforating vessels of the posterior cerebral arteries A. The perforating vessels arising from the P1 segment of the posterior cerebral artery known as paramedian or mesencephalic branches (Mes. Br.). B. Alternate view of the mesencephalic branches showing perforation into the midbrain. C. View of the thalamo perforating arteries arising from the P1 segment of the PCA.

The fetal type variant of the posterior communicating artery is defined as a PCoA which has a larger diameter than the P1 segment of the PCA. This means that the posterior cerebral artery is a continuation of the posterior communicating artery and not the P1 segment [11, 17]. The incidence of the fetal variant is 4-29% and bilateral fetal variants occur in 1-9% of the population [17]. The most common variant overall is hypoplasia (Figure 3) [18].

Conclusion

The circle of Willis has a great deal of anatomical variability. It is important to recognize these anatomical variants prior to endovascular neurosurgery to avoid medical injury. Certain variants are also strongly associated with aneurysm formation. A thorough and comprehensive understanding of the anatomical variants of the Circle of Willis is essential for endovascular neurosurgeons.

References

[1] Molnár, Z. On the 400th anniversary of the birth of Thomas Willis. *Brain* 144, 1033–1037 (2021).
[2] Wolpert, S. M. The circle of Willis. *American Journal of Neuroradiology* 18, 1033–1034 (1997).
[3] Dumitrescu, A. M. et al. The discovery of the circle of Willis as a result of using the scientific method in anatomical dissection. *Rom J Morphol Embryol* 61, 959–965 (2020).
[4] Rosner, J., Reddy, V. & Lui, F. Neuroanatomy, Circle of Willis. In: *StatPearls* (StatPearls Publishing, Treasure Island (FL), 2025).
[5] Vrselja, Z. et al. Function of circle of Willis. *J Cereb Blood Flow Metab* 34, 578–584 (2014).
[6] Hendrikse, J. et al. Distribution of Cerebral Blood Flow in the Circle of Willis. *Radiology* 235, 184–189 (2005).
[7] Tahir, R. A. et al. Anterior Cerebral Artery: Variant Anatomy and Pathology. *J Vasc Interv Neurol* 10, 16–22 (2019).
[8] Chen, J. et al. Anterior Communicating Artery Aneurysms: Anatomical Considerations and Microsurgical Strategies. *Front Neurol* 11, 1020 (2020).
[9] Pai, S. & Kulkarni, R. Microsurgical anatomy of the anterior cerebral artery–anterior communicating artery complex: An Indian study. *Neurol India* 53, 197–202 (2005).
[10] Osiowski, A. et al. The prevalence and anatomy of recurrent artery of Heubner: a meta-analysis with neurosurgical considerations. *Acta Neurochir* 166, 431 (2024).
[11] Rhoton, A. L. J. The Supratentorial Arteries. *Neurosurgery* 51, S1 (2002).
[12] Krzyżewski, R. M. et al. Anatomical variations of the anterior communicating artery complex: gender relationship. *Surg Radiol Anat* 37, 81–86 (2015).
[13] Serizawa, T., Saeki, N. & Yamaura, A. Microsurgical Anatomy and Clinical Significance of the Anterior Communicating Artery and Its Perforating Branches. *Neurosurgery* 40, 1211–1218 (1997).
[14] Javed, K., Reddy, V. & Das, J. M. Neuroanatomy, Posterior Cerebral Arteries. In: *StatPearls* (StatPearls Publishing, Treasure Island (FL), 2025).
[15] Lazzaro, N. A. et al. Artery of Percheron Infarction: Imaging Patterns and Clinical Spectrum. *American Journal of Neuroradiology* 31, 1283–1289 (2010).
[16] Khanni, J. L. et al. Artery of Percheron Infarct: An Acute Diagnostic Challenge with a Spectrum of Clinical Presentations. *Cureus* 10, e2355 (2018).
[17] Golshani, K. et al. A review of the management of posterior communicating artery aneurysms in the modern era. *Surg Neurol Int* 1, 88 (2010).
[18] Capone, S., Shah, N. & George-St Bernard, R. R. A Fetal-type Variant Posterior Communicating Artery and its Clinical Significance. *Cureus* 11, e5064 (2019).

Chapter 4

The History of Spinal Cord Vascular Anatomy and Variation and Its Significance

Victor Hugo Perez Perez*, MD
and Juan E. Small†, MD, MSc
[1]Mexican Institute of Social Security, Mexico City, Mexico
Forensic Sciences Institute, Superior Court of Justice, Mexico City, Mexico
[2]Department of Radiology, Lahey Hospital and Medical Center, Burlington, MA, USA

Abstract

An anatomical understanding of spinal cord vascularity and its variants is crucial for the identification, diagnosis and management of spinal cord vascular abnormalities. In particular, basic knowledge of the dominant radiculomedullary supply to the spinal cord including the artery of Adamkiewicz, the artery of cervical enlargement, the artery of Von Haller, and the great posterior radiculomedullary artery is essential.

Keywords: radiculomedullary arteries, anterior spinal artery, posterior spinal arteries, artery of Adamkiewicz, artery of cervical enlargement, artery of Von Haller, great posterior radiculomedullary artery

Introduction

The spinal cord obtains arterial supply from one ventral (anterior spinal artery) and two dorsal (posterior spinal arteries) trunks [1-7]. In turn, these trunks obtain flow via radiculomedullary arteries. A total of 31 paired radicular arteries exist at each segmental level and they are generally small in size, vary significantly in caliber, and most supply nerve roots, dura or pial plexus. Relatively few radicular arteries contribute meaningfully to the spinal cord and are thus named radiculomedullary arteries (RMA). It is these RMAs that provide the dominant supply to the spinal cord as they are the sole segmental supply both ventrally to the anterior spinal

* Corresponding Author's Email: victorhugo2perez@hotmail.com
† Corresponding Author's Email: Juan.E.Small@Lahey.org

In: World History of Neurointerventional Surgery
Editors: Xianli Lv and Zhongxue Wu
ISBN: 979-8-89530-792-2

artery (ASA) and dorsally to the posterior spinal arteries (PSAs) [1-7]. RMAs specifically contributing to the ASA are referred to as anterior radiculomedullary arteries and those providing flow to the PSAs are named posterior radiculomedullary arteries.

There is marked variability in the number, size and entrance level of both anterior and posterior RMAs. For example, the number of anterior RMAs generally ranges between 2 and 14 in most individuals and approximately 11 to 16 posterior RMAs supply the PSAs. An anastomotic network of flow is thus created by combining these RMAs with circumferential spinal cord arteries thus aiding spinal cord perfusion via a certain degree of collateral flow [1-7].

As one can imagine, an inverse correlation between the number and the caliber of RMAs exists. When few in number they tend to be larger in caliber and are referred as paucisegmental and when they number greater than 6 anteriorly, they are referred as plurisegmental and thus tend to be smaller in caliber [1-7]. Despite the variability in their caliber, important dominant RMAs exist, and these are the focus of our discussion.

The Anterior Spinal Cord Arterial Supply

The ASA courses within the spinal sulcus along the ventral aspect of the cord. This vessel generally changes in caliber along its course ranging in size from 0.2-0.8 mm. The ASA in turn gives rise to central/sulcal arteries, the branches of which provide arterial supply to roughly two thirds of the anterior cord including the anterior horns, spinothalamic and corticospinal tracts. The dominant radiculomedullary supply to the ASA includes the artery of Adamkiewicz, the artery of cervical enlargement, the artery of Von Haller (Dominant anterior thoracic artery) [8-11].

The Artery of Adamkiewicz

The most important RMA is the arteria radiculomedullary magna, most commonly known as the artery of Adamkiewicz (AKA). Albert Adamkiewicz published in 1881 and 1882 the first extensive study on the blood vessels of the spinal cord, and his anatomical discoveries continue to have important implications for clinical practice more than a century later. The eponymically named artery of Adamkiewicz (AKA) provides the major blood supply to the anterior thoracolumbar spinal cord and has immense anatomical and clinical significance. The AKA generally arises in the ventral lower thoracic to upper lumbar segments most often between T8 and L2 and varies in diameter between 0.5-1.2mm (Figure 1a). Nevertheless, much variability in the origin of this vessel exists, rarely arising as high as the level of T3 (Figure 1b) and as low as L2 (Figure1 c and d). Aside from providing dominant anterior supply to the ventral cord, there is also a rich anastomotic network associated with this vessel (Figure 1e). In particular, the arterial basket of the conus medullaris [12] is a critical anastomotic network circumferentially connecting the ASA and PSAs at the level of the conus (Figure 1e).

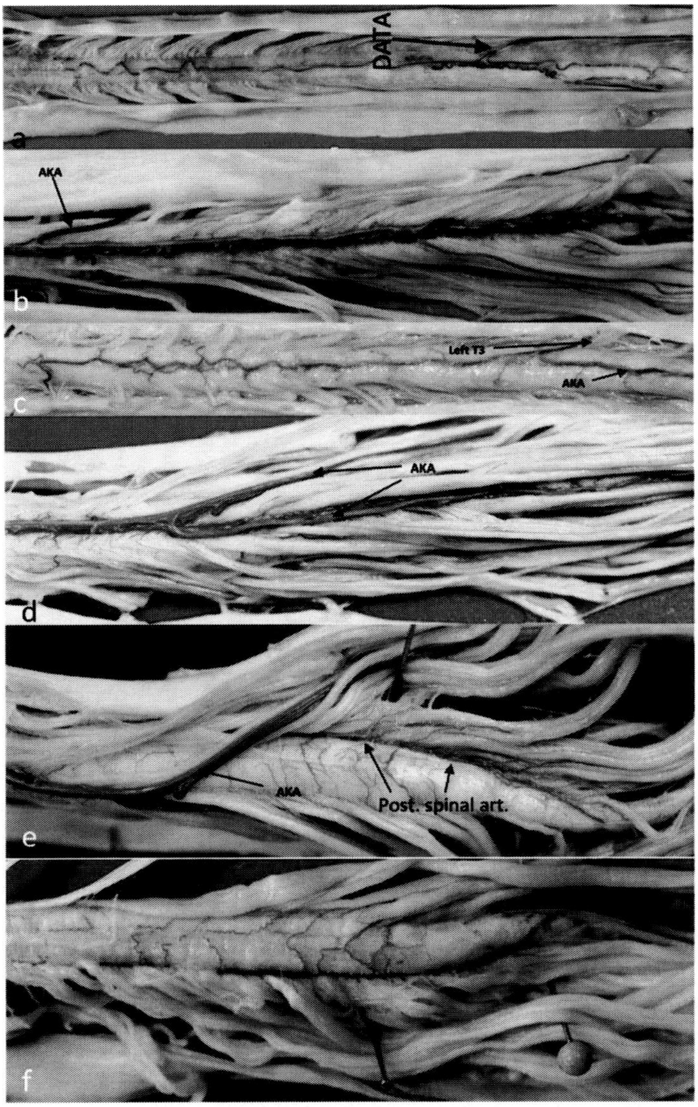

Figure 1. a, artery of Adamkiewicz (AKA) arising from level T9 on the left. b, the artery of Adamkiewicz (AKA) arising at the level of T3. c, the artery of Adamkiewicz (AKA) arising at the level of L2. d, the artery of Adamkiewicz (AKA) arising from left L2. Lumbosacral spinal nerves are displaced to observe the left lateral aspect of this spinal cord and the posterior spinal artery. e, rich anastomotic arch in the lateral aspect of the spinal cord coming from the posterior spinal artery and the great anterior radiculomedullary artery. The arterial basket of the conus medullaris is evident along the inferior conus.

The Artery of Cervical Enlargement

Segmental vessels in the mid to upper cervical spine originate from the vertebral arteries and in the lower cervical region arise from the deep cervical, costocervical, or ascending cervical branches. Typically, one or several dominant unilateral anterior cervical RMAs exist. The dominant anterior cervical RMA is most often in the region of C5-C6 and is referred to as the artery of cervical enlargement (ACE). As previously noted, much variability exists (Figure2, a to c).

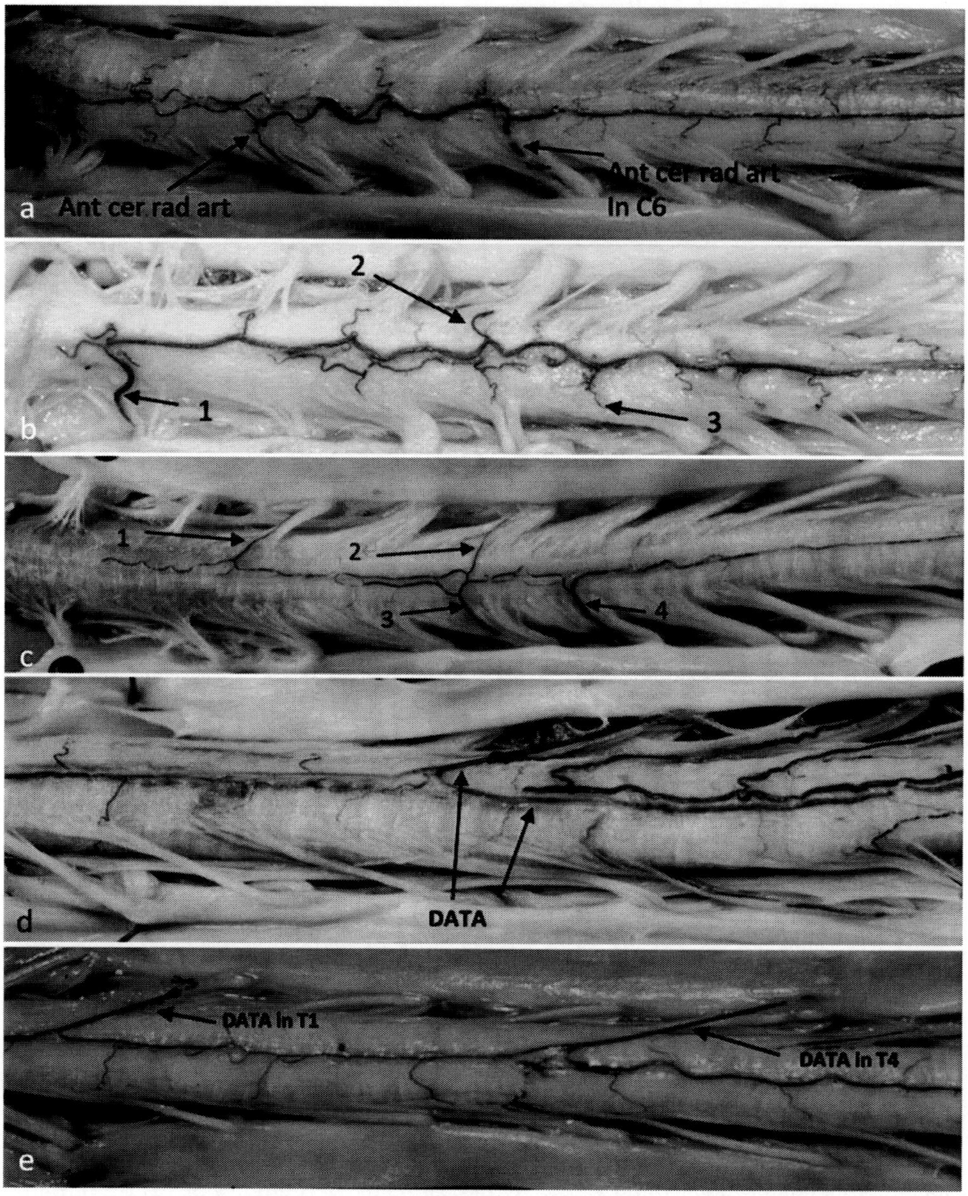

Figure 2. a, two Anterior Cervical Radiculomedullary Arteries (Ant cer rad art), one at C4 and the other at C6 on the right side of cord. b, three anterior cervical arteries, a right C2 (1), left C5 (2) and right C6 (3). c, four Anterior Cervical Radiculomedullary Arteries, with a left C3 (1), a left C5, (2), and right C5 (3) and a right C6 (4) identified. d, a single AVH/DATA at the level of T3 on the left. e, two DATAs in the left side in this spinal cord, at T4 (0.59 mm) and the other at the level of T1 (0.47 mm).

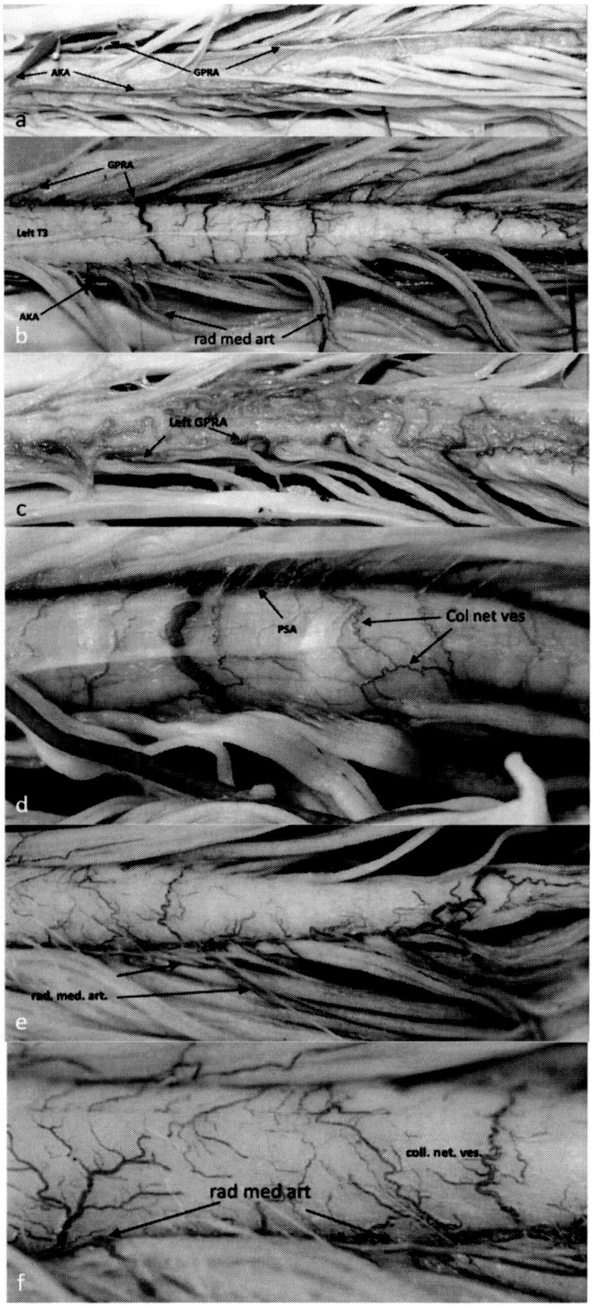

Figure 3. a, in this left anterolateral view of the spinal cord, we see both the artery of Adamkiewicz (AKA) and great posterior radiculomedullary artery (GPRA). b, left lateral aspect of the spinal cord, showing a rich anastomotic arch of veins and arteries. Some fine radiculomedullary arteries (rad med art) are also evident running along the spinal nerves with a dominant artery representing the great posterior radiculomedullary artery (GPRA). c, the Great Posterior radiculomedullary Artery (GPRA) is seen in the left side of this spinal cord. d, collateral network of fine vessels (Col net ves) in the left lateral aspect of the spinal cord and the posterior spinal artery (PSA). Right lateral view of a spinal cord (e) with radiculomedullary arteries (rad. med. art.) that accompany the spinal nerves. The basket of the conus medullaris is visible along the inferior aspect of the conus. A close-up view (f) demonstrates a rich collateral supply of arteries and veins.

The Artery of Von Haller / Dominant Anterior Thoracic Artery

Although the AKA and the ACE have received the most attention clinically and the significant variability in size, number and location of other anterior RMAs still have important implications in the literature. A distinctive upper thoracic anterior radiculomedullary distinguished in caliber and distinct from the AKA and ACE is present in 86% of patients [10-11] and provides important arterial supply to the ventral thoracic cord. This artery is referred to as either the artery of von Haller (AVH) or the dominant anterior thoracic artery (DATA) [10-11]. The eponymical name has been proposed in honor of Albrecht von Haller, who in 1754 documented the arterial supply to the ASA including this vessel as well as the AKA. This vessel is also referred as the dominant anterior thoracic artery (DATA) in order to provide easy recognition and support more reliable terminology. Studies have found that an AVH/DATA is present in 94% of spinal cord specimens and most frequently arises at the level of T4 with average size of 0.446 mm. As previously noted, a large amount of variability exists with a single AVH/DATA present in 66%, two in 26% and three in 2% (Figure2 d and e).

The Posterior Spinal Cord Arterial Supply

Two paired PSAs course along the posterolateral spinal cord to provide dorsal supply. They range in caliber between 0.1-0.4 mm and supply the posterior one third of the cord including the posterior columns, dorsal gray and superficial lateral columns [1-7]. As noted previously, there is also marked variability in the number, size and entrance level of posterior RMAs, in general with approximately 11–16 RMAs supplying the PSAs. Still, most individuals also have a dominant posterior RMA in the region of the lumbar spine, named the great posterior radiculomedullary artery (GPRA) [13] (Figure 3, a to c). Here too, we can find a collateral network of vessels associated with the PSAs (Figure 3, d to f).

Conclusion

Understanding the intricate vascular anatomy of the spinal cord and its variations is critical for addressing spinal cord pathology including vascular malformations. An improved understanding of the spinal cord arterial supply is necessary to reduce the risk of surgical and endovascular aortic and spinal procedures. In addition, thorough knowledge of the dominant radiculomedullary supply to the ASA and PSAs is essential for appropriate imaging interpretation. Attention to the anatomic variations of the dominant RMAs including the AKA, ACE, AVH/DATA and GPRA allows for tailored management of specific patient challenges.

References

[1] Gillian LA. The arterial blood supply of the human spinal cord. *J Comp Neurol* (1958) 110:75–103.

[2] Santillan A, Nacarino V, Greenberg E, et al. Vascular anatomy of the spinal cord. *J Neuronterv Surg* (2012) 4:67–74.

[3] Matthew W. Colman, Francis J. Hornicek and Joseph H Schwab. Spinal Cord Blood Supply and Its Surgical Implications. *J Am Acad Ortop Surg* (2015) 23:581-591.

[4] Vargas MI, Gariani J, Sztajzel R, et al. Spinal cord ischemia: practical imaging tips, pearls, and pitfalls. *AJNR Am J Neuroradiol* (2015) 36:825–30.

[5] Tator CH. Update on the pathophysiology and pathology of acute spinal cord injury. *Brain Pathol* (1995) 5:407–13.

[6] Ahuja CS, Nori S, Tetreault L, et al. Traumatic spinal cord injury-repair and regeneration. *Neurosurgery* (2017) 80:S9–22.

[7] Martirosyan NL, Feuerstein JS, Theodore N, Cavalcanti DD, Spetzler RF, Preul MC. Blood supply and vascular reactivity of the spinal cord under normal and pathological conditions. *J Neurosurg Spine* (2011) 15 (3):238-251.

[8] Gao L, Wang L, Su B, Wang P, Ye J, Shen H. The vascular supply to the spinal cord and its relationship to anterior spine surgical approaches. *Spine J* (2013) 13 (8):966-973.

[9] Manjila S, Haroon N, Parker B, Xavier AR, Guthikonda M, Rengachary SS. Albert Wojciech Adamkiewicz (1850-1921): unsung hero behind the eponymic artery. *Neurosurg Focus* (2009) 26 (1):E2.

[10] Gailloud P. The artery of von Haller: a constant anterior radiculomedullary artery at the upper thoracic level. *Neurosurgery* (2013) 73:1034–43.

[11] J. E. Small and V. H. Perez Perez. The Dominant Anterior Thoracic Artery of the Spinal Cord. *AJNR Am J Neuroradiol* (2023) 44:111-14.

[12] Martirosyan NL, Kalani MY, Lemole GM Jr, Spetzler RF, Preul MC, Theodore N. Microsurgical anatomy of the arterial basket of the conus medullaris. *J Neurosurg Spine* (2015) 22 (6):672-6.

[13] PÉREZ P. V., Juha H., Small J. E. Anatomy of the Great Posterior Radiculomedullary Artery. *AJNR Am J Neuroradiol* (2019).

Chapter 5

A Brief History of Neurointerventional Surgery

Kevin Pierre[1,*], MD
Andre Calixte[2], MD
and Brandon Lucke-Wold[3], MD
[1]University of Florida Department of Radiology, Gainesville, FL, USA
[2]Mount Sinai Health System Department of Neurology, NYC, New York, USA
[3]University of Florida Department of Neurosurgery, Gainesville, FL, USA

Abstract

Neurointerventional surgery has evolved from early cerebral angiography to sophisticated endovascular techniques for managing complex neurovascular conditions. António Egas Moniz laid the foundation for the field after pioneering cerebral angiography in 1927. Subsequent advancements, including safer iodinated contrast agents, the Seldinger technique, and digital subtraction angiography, revolutionized vascular imaging. In the mid-20th century, therapeutic endovascular procedures emerged, with innovations like Serbinenko's flow-directed balloons and Guglielmi's detachable coils. Relatively recent breakthroughs, including mechanical thrombectomy and flow-diverting stents, have also transformed stroke management and aneurysm treatment. Collaborative multidisciplinary training and advancements in robotics, artificial intelligence, and imaging are expected to drive the next phase of progress in neurovascular care. In this chapter, we review the history of neurointerventional surgery.

Keywords: neurointerventional surgery, history, cerebral angiography, endovascular treatment, guglielmi detachable coils, flow diversion, mechanical thrombectomy, robotics, artificial intelligence, imaging technology, multidisciplinary training

Introduction

Neurointerventional surgery, also known as interventional neuroradiology, is an evolving subspecialty that merges neurosurgery, neurology, and radiology to diagnose and treat vascular

---

* Corresponding Author's Email: kpierre150@gmail.com

In: World History of Neurointerventional Surgery
Editors: Xianli Lv and Zhongxue Wu
ISBN: 979-8-89530-792-2

disorders of the central nervous system through minimally invasive, image-guided techniques. The field has undergone a significant transformation from the rudimentary beginnings of cerebral angiography to the sophisticated endovascular procedures of today. In this chapter, we review the historical milestones that have shaped the field.

The Advent of Cerebral Angiography

The foundation of neurointerventional surgery was laid in the early 20th century with the introduction of cerebral angiography. In 1927, Portuguese neurologist António Egas Moniz performed the first cerebral angiogram with direct carotid artery injection using radiopaque contrast material [1]. This work revolutionized the evaluation of vascular anatomy and pathology, such as aneurysms and arteriovenous malformations (AVMs) [2]. Additionally, early cerebral angiography was used to help detect brain tumors by revealing vascular patterns, displacement of vascular structures, and disruptions to the blood-brain barrier. It also facilitated the diagnosis of conditions such as intracranial stenosis, vascular compression syndromes, and traumatic vascular injuries.

Evolution of Intravenous Contrast Agents

Despite its diagnostic value, there were many challenges associated with early neuroangiography. The procedure was invasive and required direct carotid artery puncture or cutdown, which risked vascular injury, hematoma formation, and neurological deficits. Additionally, early contrast agents were often unsafe and poorly tolerated.

António Egas Moniz's first agent was sodium iodide, a radiopaque material that provided sufficient contrast for imaging but was highly irritating to vascular endothelium. It often caused severe pain during injection, vascular spasms, and even thrombosis. Additionally, systemic reactions such as nausea, vomiting, and, in rare cases, anaphylaxis were reported.

By the 1930s, Thorotrast (a colloidal suspension of thorium dioxide) became a popular alternative due to its superior radiopacity and ability to produce detailed images [3]. However, Thorotrast was later found to be radioactive, as it emitted alpha particles with a long biological half-life. It accumulated in the reticuloendothelial system (primarily in the liver, spleen, and lymph nodes) and was strongly linked to delayed carcinogenesis, including angiosarcoma of the liver and hematologic malignancies, which led to its eventual discontinuation in the 1950s [4].

Other early agents, such as iodized oil-based media (e.g., Lipiodol), were introduced but were viscous and poorly water-soluble and thus unsuitable for vascular imaging [5]. The search for safer, water-soluble, iodinated contrast agents led to the development of sodium diatrizoate in the 1950s, which was less toxic and better tolerated, albeit still hyperosmolar and associated with adverse reactions such as transient hypotension, renal impairment, and allergic responses.

In the 1970s, nonionic, low-osmolar iodinated agents were introduced and dramatically improved the safety profile of cerebral angiography and enabled its wider clinical adoption.

The Seldinger Technique and Improved Imaging

Another advancement occurred in 1953 when Swedish radiologist Sven-Ivar Seldinger introduced the percutaneous Seldinger technique for vascular access [2]. This method allowed for safer and more reliable vascular catheterization to minimize complications associated with direct arterial puncture.

Parallel advancements in imaging technology, such as the development of image intensifiers and subtraction angiography in the 1960s, improved the visualization of vascular structures. Digital subtraction angiography (DSA), introduced in the late 1970s, allowed for real-time, high-resolution images with reduced contrast medium volumes.

The Birth of Endovascular Treatment

The concept of using catheters for therapeutic purposes emerged in the mid-20th century. In 1964, American radiologist Charles Dotter performed the first percutaneous transluminal angioplasty to dilate a stenotic femoral artery [6].

In the realm of neurointervention, Russian neurosurgeon Fedor Serbinenko developed flow-directed balloon catheters in the 1970s [7]. He used detachable balloons to occlude intracranial aneurysms and AVMs, which led to the first endovascular treatments for cerebral vascular lesions. Serbinenko's work helped demonstrate that endovascular techniques could effectively manage complex neurovascular conditions. Figure 1 exemplifies the use of a detachable balloon to occlude an ICA aneurysm.

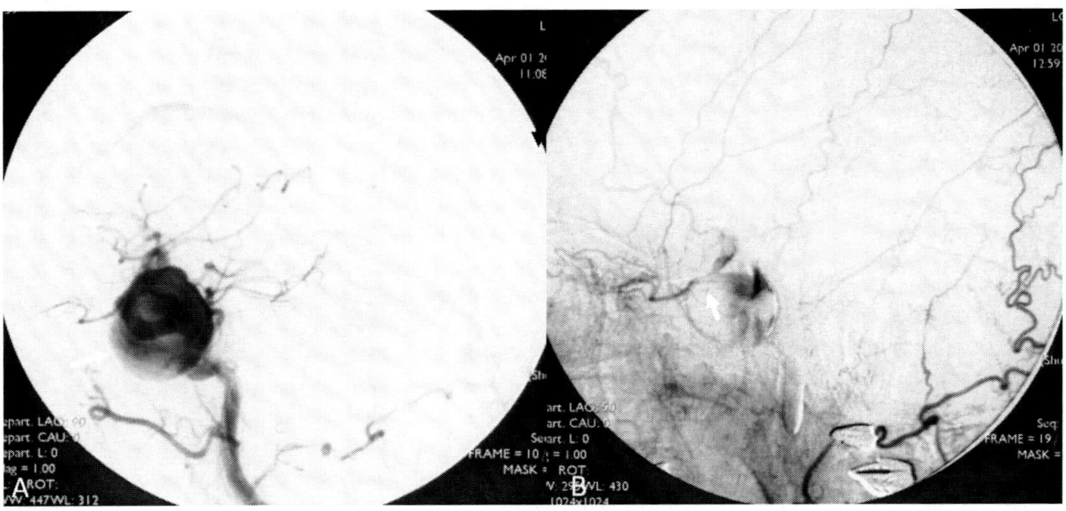

Figure 1. A 59-year-old woman presenting with left oculomotor nerve palsy. A: Lateral view of left carotid artery injection shows a giant aneurysm of the cavernous segment of the internal carotid artery (arrow). B: Lateral view of the late phase left external carotid artery injection demonstrates aneurysm refilling through the ophthalmic artery after occlusion of the internal carotid artery using two detachable balloons.

Microcatheters and Embolic Agents

Microcatheters and advanced embolic materials were introduced in the 1980s and 1990s. Specifically, the development of coaxial microcatheter systems allowed for navigation through tortuous cerebral vessels to reach distal lesions [8-10].

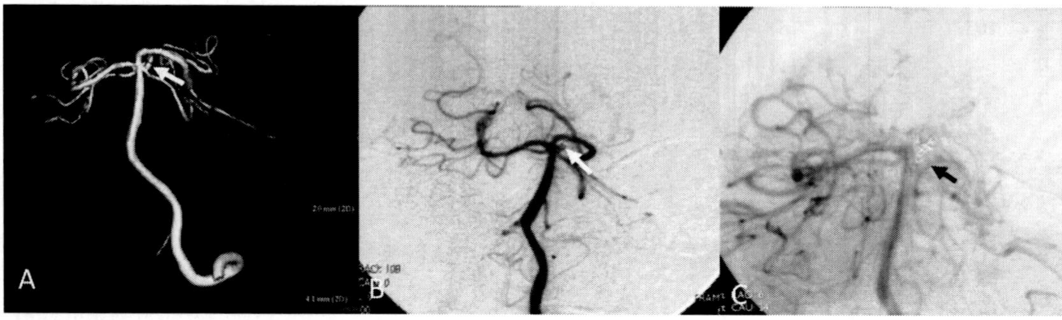

Figure 2. A 53-year-old woman with a ruptured aneurysm at the origin of the left superior cerebellar artery. A: Three-dimensional digital subtraction angiogram showing a 2.0mm×4.0mm aneurysm at the left basilar artery-superior cerebellar artery junction. B-C: The aneurysm was embolized with detachable coils (EDC 3mm×4cm; Microplex 2mm×1cm). C: Postembolization angiogram demonstrates complete obliteration of the aneurysm.

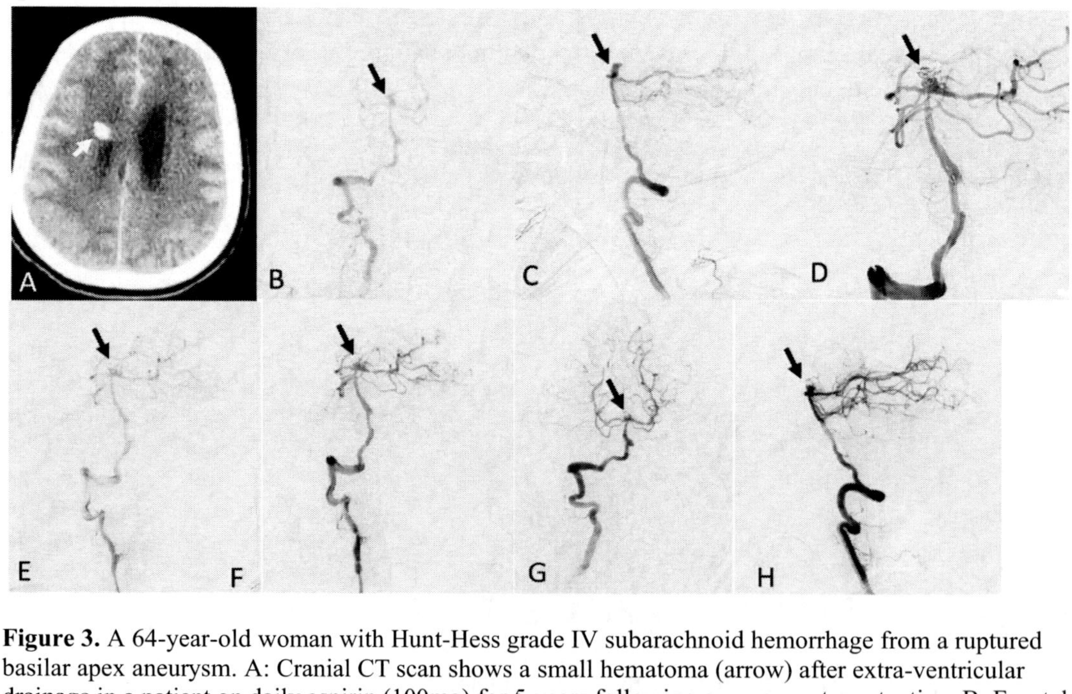

Figure 3. A 64-year-old woman with Hunt-Hess grade IV subarachnoid hemorrhage from a ruptured basilar apex aneurysm. A: Cranial CT scan shows a small hematoma (arrow) after extra-ventricular drainage in a patient on daily aspirin (100mg) for 5 years following coronary artery stenting. B: Frontal view and C: Lateral view of right vertebral artery injection showing an irregular aneurysm of the basilar artery apex (arrows). The aneurysm was coiled without stent placement or cessation of aspirin therapy. D-F: Angiograms at the working angle show stepwise coiling of the aneurysm (arrows). G: Frontal view and H: Lateral view of right vertebral artery injection after embolization showing subtotal occlusion of the aneurysm (arrows).

In 1991, Italian neuroradiologist Dr. Guido Guglielmi introduced the Guglielmi Detachable Coil (GDC) system for the endovascular embolization of intracranial aneurysms [9, 11]. The GDC system utilized electrically detachable platinum coils delivered via microcatheters to induce thrombosis within aneurysms. Similar techniques now serve as a less invasive alternative to surgical clipping (Figures 2 and 3).

Stents and Flow Diversion

The early 21st century marked the integration of stent technology into neurointervention. Wide-neck cerebral aneurysms are defined as those with a dome-to-neck ratio of less than 2 or a neck diameter equal to or greater than 4 mm, and are significantly challenging for endovascular coiling. These challenges include coil herniation into the parent vessel, difficulty delineating the neck-parent vessel interface, and protecting branches originating near the aneurysm neck.

Intracranial stents were initially developed to assist in coil embolization of these wide-neck aneurysms by serving as scaffolds to prevent coil prolapse (Figures 4-6). Stent-assisted coiling allows for increased coil packing density and improves obliteration rates and reduces aneurysm recurrence, particularly for wide-necked and large/giant aneurysms.

Similarly, balloon-assisted coil embolization emerged as another adjunctive technique to reduce the risk of coil prolapse while providing immediate proximal control through balloon inflation in case of intraprocedural rupture.

Flow diversion represented the next evolution, with the Pipeline Embolization Device receiving FDA approval in 2011 [12]. These devices redirect blood flow away from the aneurysm sac to promote thrombosis and vessel reconstruction without requiring coils. This approach has been particularly valuable for complex, fusiform, and giant aneurysms.

Beyond aneurysm treatment, stenting became a viable option for intracranial atherosclerotic disease and extracranial carotid artery stenosis. The development of drug-eluting stents and bioresorbable scaffolds continues to evolve, with general goals of reducing restenosis rates and improving long-term outcomes.

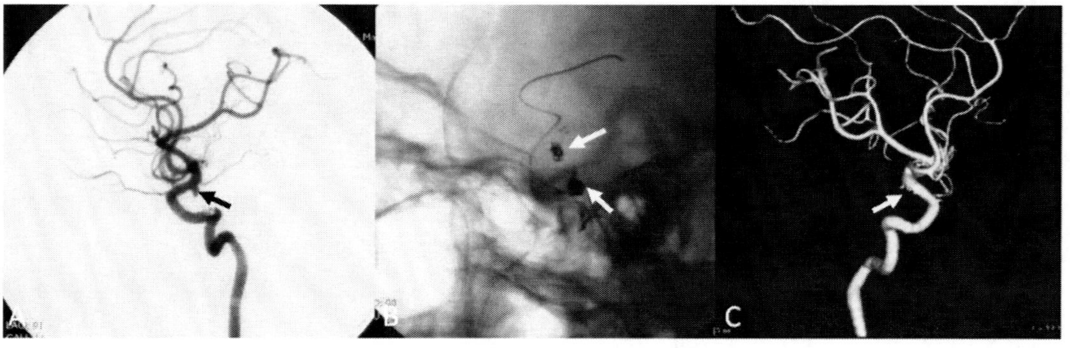

Figure 4. A 38-year-old woman with bilateral posterior communicating artery aneurysms. A: Lateral view of left internal carotid artery injection showing a posterior communicating artery aneurysm (arrow). B: Lateral view of unsubtracted image showing bilateral aneurysms treated with Neuroform stent-assisted coiling (arrows). C: 3D reconstruction of left internal carotid artery injection after treatment showing complete obliteration of the posterior communicating artery aneurysm (arrow).

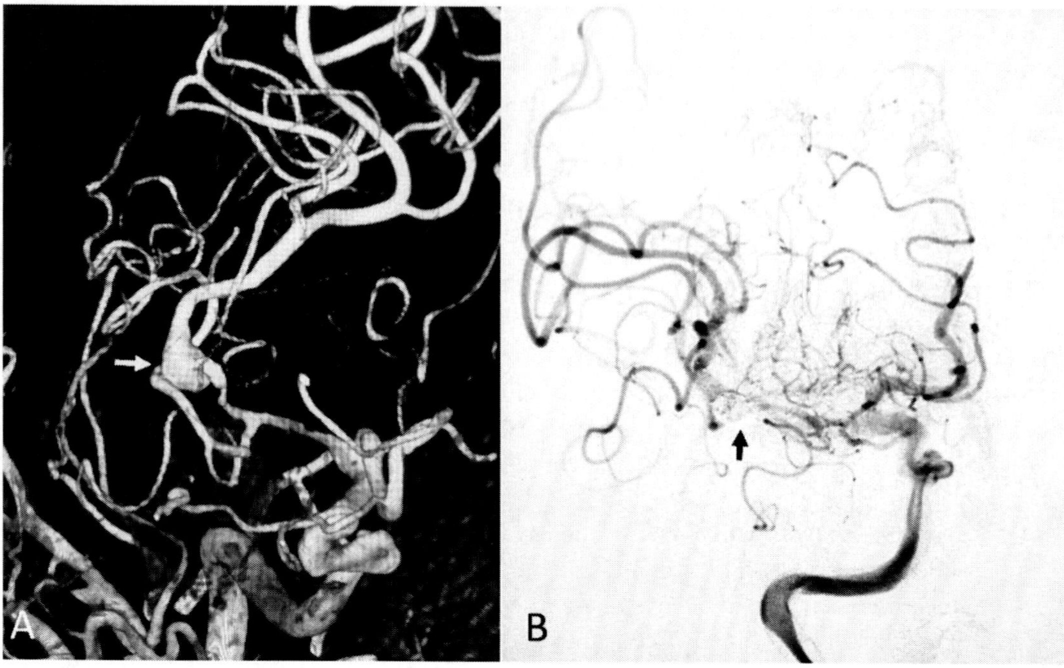

Figure 5. A 70-year-old woman with an incidental middle cerebral artery aneurysm. A: 3D reconstruction of right internal carotid artery injection showing an aneurysm arising from the middle cerebral artery with coexisting proximal atherosclerotic stenosis (arrow), treated with Solitaire AB stent and coils. B: Frontal view of right internal carotid artery injection after coiling showing complete aneurysm occlusion (arrow).

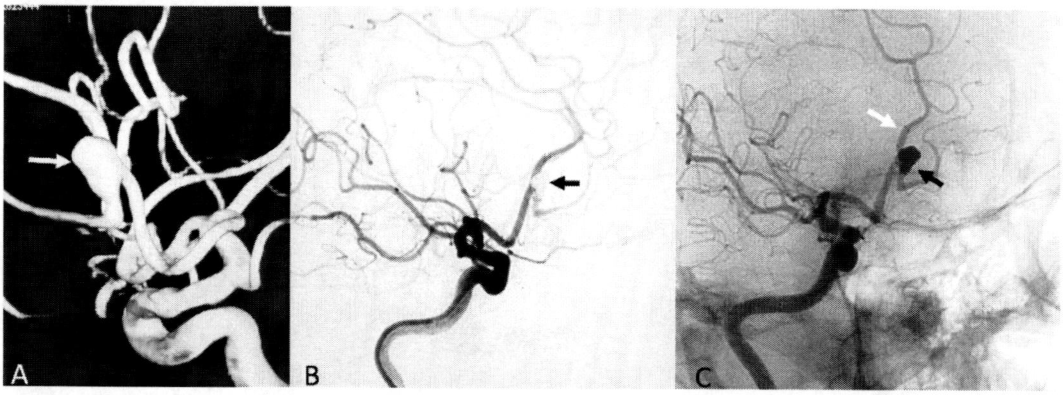

Figure 6. A woman with an incidental A2 aneurysm. A: 3D reconstruction of right internal carotid artery injection showing an A2 aneurysm of the right anterior cerebral artery (arrow). B: Lateral view of internal carotid artery injection after treatment showing complete occlusion of the aneurysm (arrow). C: Oblique view of unsubtracted image showing the aneurysm treated with 4mm×15mm Solitaire AB stent (Medtronic, ev3, USA) (white arrow) and coils (black arrow).

Liquid embolic agents such as N-butyl cyanoacrylate (NBCA) and later Onyx (ethylene-vinyl alcohol copolymer) were also developed primarily for the embolization of arteriovenous malformations (AVMs) and fistulas [10]. These agents can penetrate complex vascular networks to achieve effective obliteration.

Mechanical Thrombectomy

Acute ischemic stroke management underwent a revolution with the advent of mechanical thrombectomy devices [13, 14]. Early attempts using intra-arterial thrombolytics and rudimentary retrieval devices showed limited success. However, the development of stent retrievers and aspiration catheters in the late 2000s significantly improved recanalization rates [15-19].

Landmark clinical trials, including MR CLEAN (2015), ESCAPE, EXTEND-IA, SWIFT PRIME, and REVASCAT, provided robust evidence that mechanical thrombectomy, in conjunction with intravenous thrombolysis, dramatically improves functional outcomes in patients with large vessel occlusions. These findings led to changes in clinical guidelines and subsequently established mechanical thrombectomy as the standard of care within specified time windows for large vessel occlusions.

Advancements in imaging techniques, such as perfusion CT and MRI, have facilitated better patient selection by identifying salvageable brain tissue beyond traditional time constraints. Ongoing research aims to extend treatment windows and refine patient selection criteria further.

Multidisciplinary Collaboration and Training

The complexity of neurovascular disorders necessitated a collaborative approach among neurosurgeons, neuroradiologists, and neurologists [20-23]. To address the need for specialized training, professional societies and accreditation bodies established fellowship programs and certification pathways [24-27]. The Committee on Advanced Subspecialty Training (CAST) and the Society of NeuroInterventional Surgery (SNIS) have contributed to standardizing education and promoting high standards of practice.

The traditional Halstedian model of surgical training, which emphasized extensive hospital time and high surgical volume following the "see one, do one, teach one" philosophy, has transformed to meet modern healthcare demands. This paradigm shift moved training away from a time-based model toward an "intentional practice" approach focused on achieving specific competency milestones, with emphasis on measured outcomes and technical proficiency rather than case volumes alone.

To address the challenges of reduced working hours and increased public scrutiny while maintaining high standards, training programs have incorporated various educational adjuncts such as surgical simulators, focused cadaveric dissections, and structured skills laboratories. Modern fellowship programs typically include both microsurgical and endovascular training to produce practitioners versed in all treatment modalities, though maintaining proficiency in microsurgical techniques requires particular emphasis due to its steeper learning curve.

Technological Integration and Future Directions

The integration of technology continues to propel neurointerventional surgery forward. Innovations such as three-dimensional rotational angiography, flat-panel detector CT, and fusion imaging enhance procedural planning and real-time navigation.

Robotic-assisted endovascular intervention is an emerging field with goals that include increased precision and efficiency, decreased radiation exposure, and improved procedural ergonomics [22]. The use of artificial intelligence and machine learning algorithms in imaging analysis and outcome prediction also holds promise for personalized medicine.

Research into novel embolic materials, bioactive coils, and gene therapy approaches aims to improve treatment efficacy and reduce complications [23]. Nanotechnology and targeted drug delivery systems represent future frontiers that may revolutionize the management of neurovascular diseases.

Conclusion

Neurointerventional surgery has progressed substantially since its inception. The evolution from basic cerebral angiography to current endovascular techniques has significantly broadened treatment options for neurovascular disorders. Ongoing technological advancement and improved understanding of cerebrovascular pathophysiology continue to expand the field's capabilities, particularly for previously untreatable conditions.

References

[1] Moniz E. L'Encéphalographie artérielle, son importance dans la localisation des tumeurs cérébrales. *Masson* (1927).

[2] Seldinger SI. Catheter replacement of the needle in percutaneous arteriography; a new technique. *Acta Radiol (Stockh)* (1953) 39 (5):368-76.

[3] Becker N, et al. Mortality among Thorotrast-exposed patients and an unexposed comparison group in the German Thorotrast study. *Eur J Cancer* (2008) 44 (9):1259-68.

[4] Guimaraes JP, Lamerton LF, Christensen WR. The late effects of thorotrast administration; a review and an experimental study. *Br J Cancer* (1955) 9 (2):253-67.

[5] Bottinor W, Polkampally P, Jovin I. Adverse reactions to iodinated contrast media. *Int J Angiol* (2013) 22 (3):149-54.

[6] Dotter CT, Judkins MP. Transluminal Treatment of Arteriosclerotic Obstruction. Description of a New Technic and a Preliminary Report of Its Application. *Circulation* (1964) 30:654-70.

[7] Serbinenko FA. Balloon catheterization and occlusion of major cerebral vessels. *J Neurosurg* (1974) 41 (2):125-45.

[8] Kerber CW, Bank WO, Manelfe C. Control and placement of intracranial microcatheters. *AJNR Am J Neuroradiol* (1980) 1 (2):157-9.

[9] Guglielmi G, et al. Endovascular treatment of posterior circulation aneurysms by electrothrombosis using electrically detachable coils. *J Neurosurg* (1992) 77 (4):515-24.

[10] Vinters HV, et al. The histotoxicity of cyanoacrylates. A selective review. *Neuroradiology* (1985) 27 (4):279-91.

[11] Molyneux AJ, et al. International subarachnoid aneurysm trial (ISAT) of neurosurgical clipping versus endovascular coiling in 2143 patients with ruptured intracranial aneurysms: a randomised comparison

of effects on survival, dependency, seizures, rebleeding, subgroups, and aneurysm occlusion. *Lancet* (2005) 366 (9488):809-17.

[12] Nelson PK, et al. The pipeline embolization device for the intracranial treatment of aneurysms trial. *AJNR Am J Neuroradiol* (2011) 32 (1):34-40.

[13] Berkhemer OA, et al. A randomized trial of intraarterial treatment for acute ischemic stroke. *N Engl J Med* (2015) 372 (1):11-20.

[14] Campbell BC, et al. Endovascular therapy for ischemic stroke with perfusion-imaging selection. *N Engl J Med* (2015) 372 (11):1009-18.

[15] Goyal M, et al. Randomized assessment of rapid endovascular treatment of ischemic stroke. *N Engl J Med* (2015) 372 (11):1019-30.

[16] Saver JL, et al. Stent-retriever thrombectomy after intravenous t-PA vs. t-PA alone in stroke. *N Engl J Med* (2015) 372 (24):2285-95.

[17] Jovin TG, et al. Thrombectomy within 8 hours after symptom onset in ischemic stroke. *N Engl J Med* (2015) 372 (24):2296-306.

[18] Nogueira RG, et al. Thrombectomy 6 to 24 Hours after Stroke with a Mismatch between Deficit and Infarct. *N Engl J Med* (2018) 378 (1):11-21.

[19] Jauch EC, et al. Guidelines for the early management of patients with acute ischemic stroke: a guideline for healthcare professionals from the American Heart Association/American Stroke Association. *Stroke* (2013) 44 (3):870-947.

[20] Derdeyn CP, et al. The International Subarachnoid Aneurysm Trial (ISAT): a position statement from the Executive Committee of the American Society of Interventional and Therapeutic Neuroradiology and the American Society of Neuroradiology. *AJNR Am J Neuroradiol* (2003) 24 (7):1404-8.

[21] Fiorella D, et al. Usefulness of the Neuroform stent for the treatment of cerebral aneurysms: results at initial (3-6-mo) follow-up. *Neurosurgery* (2005) 56 (6):1191-201; discussion 1201-2.

[22] Mendes Pereira V, et al. Feasibility of robot-assisted neuroendovascular procedures. *J Neurosurg* (2022) 136 (4):992-1004.

[23] McDougall CG, et al. Bioactive versus bare platinum coils in the treatment of intracranial aneurysms: the MAPS (Matrix and Platinum Science) trial. *AJNR Am J Neuroradiol* (2014) 35 (5):935-42.

[24] Chowdhry SA, Spetzler RF. Genealogy of training in vascular neurosurgery. *Neurosurgery* (2014) 74 Suppl 1:S198-203.

[25] Peschillo S, Delfini R. Endovascular Neurosurgery in Europe and in Italy: What Is in the Future? *World Neurosurgery* (2012) 77 (2):248-251.

[26] Riina HA. Neuroendovascular surgery. *J Neurosurg* (2019) 131 (6):1690-1701.

[27] Laurent D, et al. Focused selection of open cerebrovascular cases for residents interested in cerebrovascular neurosurgery. *Neurocirugia (Astur : Engl Ed)* (2023) 34 (2):53-59.

Chapter 6

Testimony of an Interventional Neuroradiology Engineer

Nicolas Plowiecki*
BALT Group, Paris, France

Abstract

This document recounts the transformative journey of neurointerventional surgery, chronicled through the collaborative efforts of engineers and physicians. The narrative begins in 1977 in a Paris suburb, where the beginning of a significant partnership between an engineer, Léopold Plowiecki, and a physician, Professor Jean-Jacques Merland, catalyzed the development of critical medical devices, beginning with the PURSIL. This partnership led to innovations such as the MAGIC catheter, as well as the evolution of tools and techniques that have had a major impact on the management of cerebrovascular disease. Key milestones include the introduction of stent retrievers for clot retrieval and flow diverters for aneurysm treatment, highlighting a history marked by groundbreaking advances in the treatment of AVMs and aneurysms that fundamentally changed the landscape of stroke management and neurointervention.

Keywords: neurointerventional surgery, interventional neuroradiology, medical device innovation, mechanical thrombectomy, flow diverters, aneurysm treatment, stroke management, engineer-physician collaboration, medical R&D, Balt Extrusion

One day in 1977, a man knocked on the door of my father Leopold Plowiecki's extrusion shop. As a doctor, he needed very thin tubes to navigate and deploy small latex balloons to embolize aneurysms in the brain. From that first handshake between my engineer father and Professor Jean-Jacques Merland of the Lariboisière Hospital in Paris, Balt's journey in interventional neuroradiology began. My father developed a complete line of detachable balloons (Figure 1) that enabled the first endovascular aneurysm embolizations and improved physicians' ability to save their patients' lives. Never before had it been possible to penetrate so deeply into the brain. Since then, it has been inconceivable not to.

* Corresponding Author's Email: nicolas.plowiecki@copernic-group.com

In: World History of Neurointerventional Surgery
Editors: Xianli Lv and Zhongxue Wu
ISBN: 979-8-89530-792-2

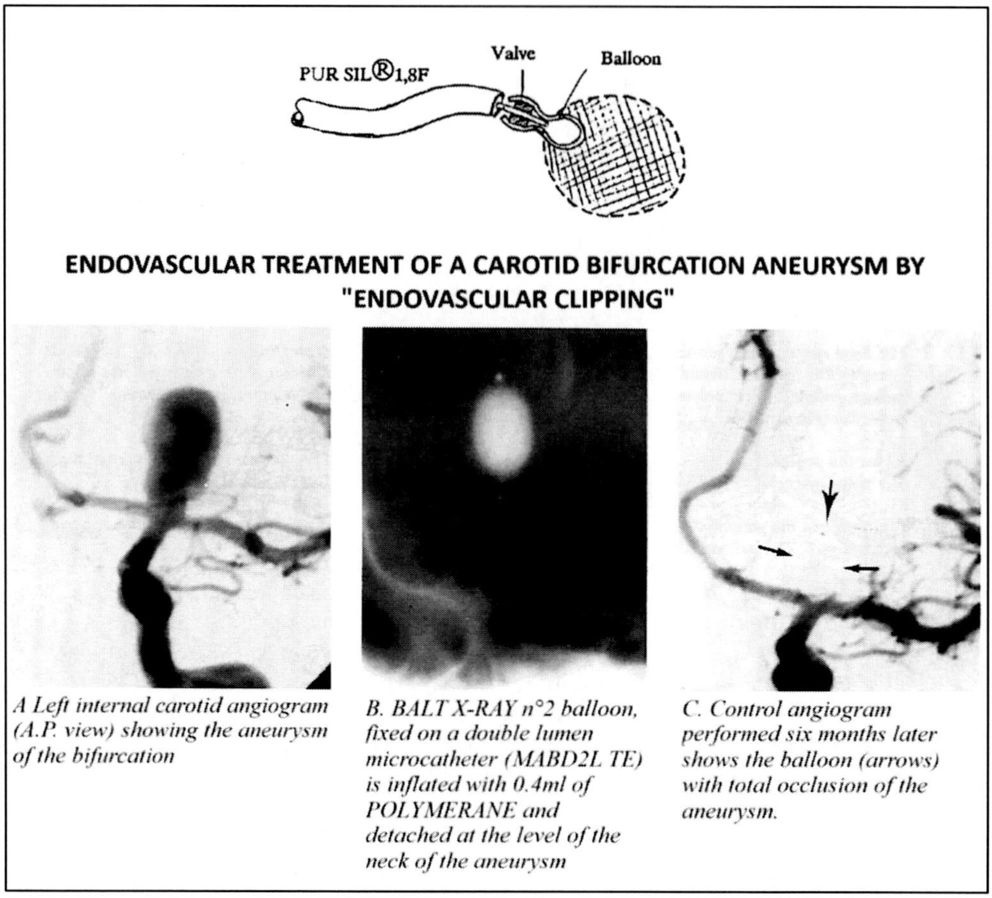

Figure 1. Excerpt from a 1980s brochure presenting BALT's range of detachable balloons.

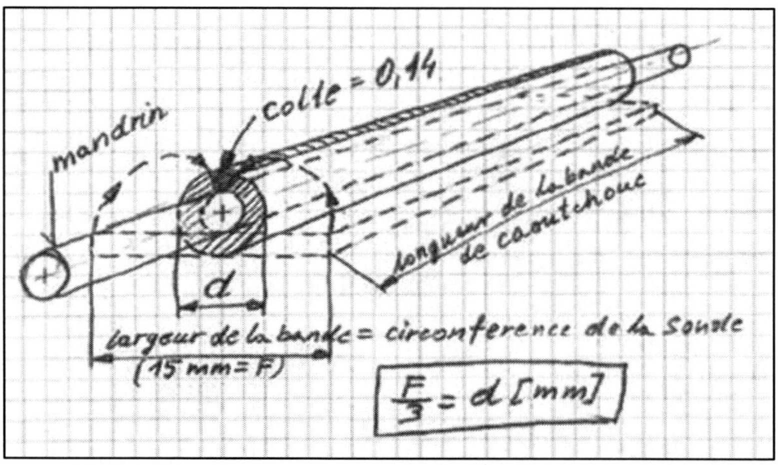

Figure 2. Sketch extracted from Leopold Plowiecki's book "The art and savoir faire of interventional neuroradiology – Memoirs of a manufacturer" explaining the origin of the French Gauge: 3F corresponds to 3mm, the width of the rubber band needed to form a tube measuring a diameter of 1mm.

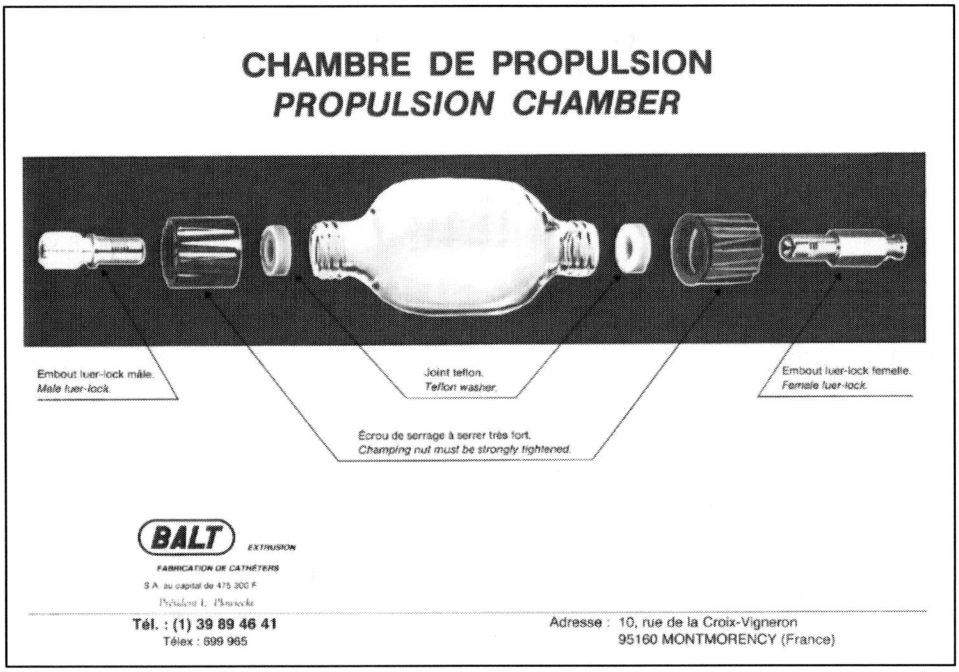

Figure 3. The propulsion chamber used to inject the souple Pursil into the brain arteries.

I'm a witness to how engineers and physicians have pushed the boundaries of interventional neuroradiology. One of the first technological revolutions I remember is the first flow-directed catheter. In 1982, at the request of Dr. Chuck Kerber, a neurosurgeon in San Diego, California, Leopold invented the PURSIL, a 1.2F (0.4 mm diameter - Figure 2) mini-tube that achieved the feat of combining extraordinary flexibility with remarkable strength. This tube was the first flow-directed catheter. It was injected into the internal carotid artery using a propulsion chamber (Figure 3) and then guided by blood flow to reach the most distal parts of the cerebral vasculature [1].

In 1986, Professor Luc Picard of Nancy, France, tired of seeing his hands radiated by the carotid approach routinely used with the Pursil, challenged my father: "You must create a catheter with a rigid proximal end like an angiography catheter and a flow-dependent distal end like the PURSIL." A simple idea, but difficult to realize. A few months later, in the operating room of Professor Jacques Moret at the Rothschild Foundation in Paris, the new catheter navigated through the most tortuous and delicate arteries to reach such distal areas of the brain that Dr. Luca Moschini, who was in the operating room, exclaimed: "It's magic!." More than 35 years later, the MAGIC catheter is still in use around the world and has saved more than 200,000 lives.

I had the privilege of growing up with a passionate man, surrounded by passionate physicians and employees who were dedicated to finding technological solutions to medical needs. Their motivation was never financial. Just as Graham Bell did not do a market study before inventing the telephone, I have always seen Leopold passionately take on the challenges his physician friends gave him without worrying about whether or not there would be a commercial market. My childhood and teenage years were punctuated by technological revolutions: from the first mechanically detachable embolization coils (MDS) to the first remodeling balloon (Figure 4) [2]. I now believe that growing up in such a stimulating environment had a lasting impact on me.

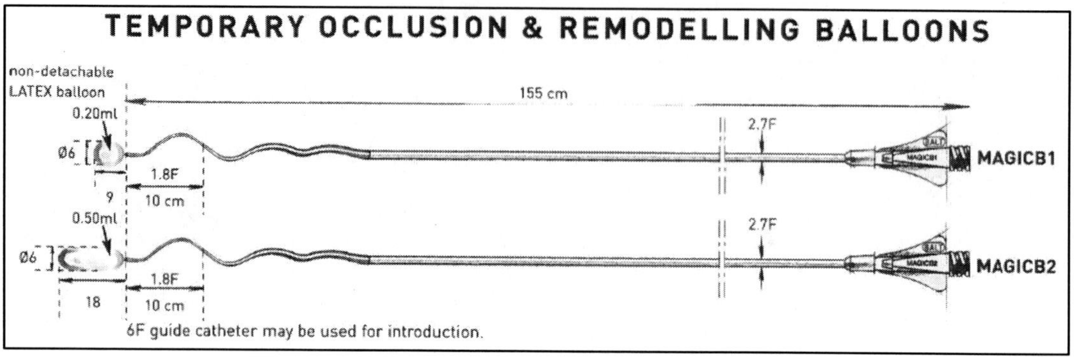

Figure 4. Excerpt of a commercial brochure showing the first remodelling balloons in history MAGIC B1 & B2.

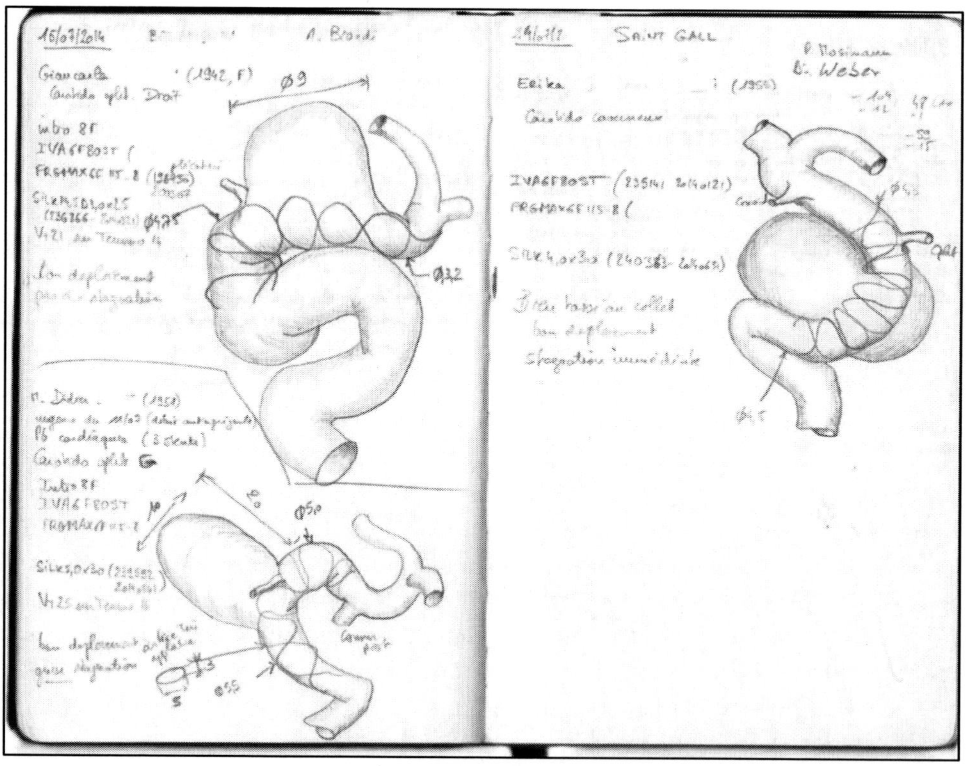

Figure 5. Black notebook.

When I succeeded my father as head of Balt in the early 2000s. It was clear to me that I, in turn, should become a bridge between the world of technology and therapy. So, I split my time between cathlabs around the world, jotting down notes in my black notebook (Figure 5), and Balt labs with my team, designing tools that would meet the needs of doctors and help save their patients' lives.

When I say "team," I am not just referring to R&D. Balt's extraordinary performance was only possible thanks to the passionate involvement of a whole chain of people: the sales team and our highly competent distributors, who maintained a relationship of trust with the doctors; the administrative teams, who always fought to get things done quickly; and, of course, the production teams. The importance of the latter is often underestimated. At Balt, the production operators were fully involved not only in the quality of our products, but also in their technological evolution. It is important to understand that the excellence of a device depends on elements that only the human hand can feel; no testing equipment is sensitive enough for this. And only two people handle the devices to the point of "feeling" them: the doctor and the production operator. Their involvement is therefore fundamental. Balt's products could not have been so innovative and powerful without the passion of its production operators. Elisabeth Pereira, who has passionately led the MAGIC production team for years, is a good example of the people I would like to pay tribute to and without whom nothing could have been achieved.

Together, physicians and technicians, we continued to dream, invent, innovate and create devices to treat three major pathologies: ischemic stroke, AVMs and aneurysms. Together, physicians and technicians, we have gone from revolution to revolution. Here is the story of three innovations that I believe and hope have changed daily life in the neurointerventional cath lab devices:

The Revolution of the First Stent-Retriever

In 2004, during a lively discussion over dinner with Professor René Chapot at the Apicius restaurant in the 17th arrondissement of Paris, René told me about a thromboembolic complication he had encountered in his latest case (Figure6). It was an important issue at the time, when the remodeling technique invented by Pr. Jacques Moret and improved by René, had increased the number of devices present in the arteries during surgery. The idea of using a stent to capture and remove a clot from a cerebral artery suddenly occurred to us.

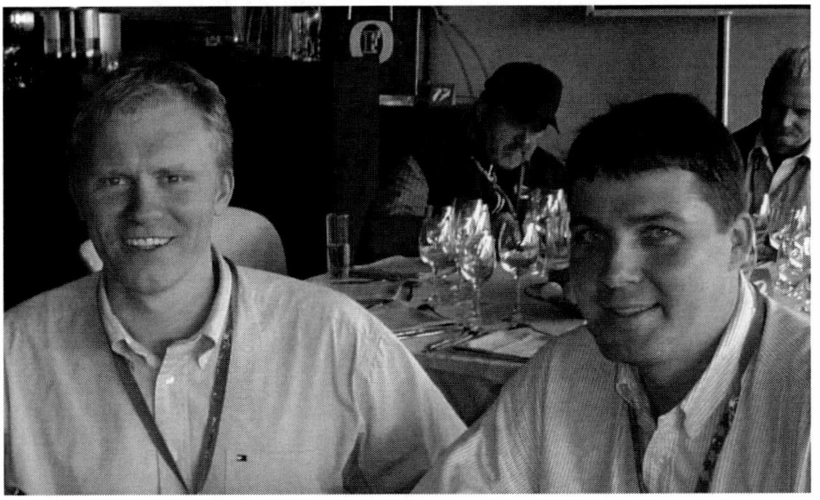

Figure 6. With Professor René Chapot (right) in 2004.

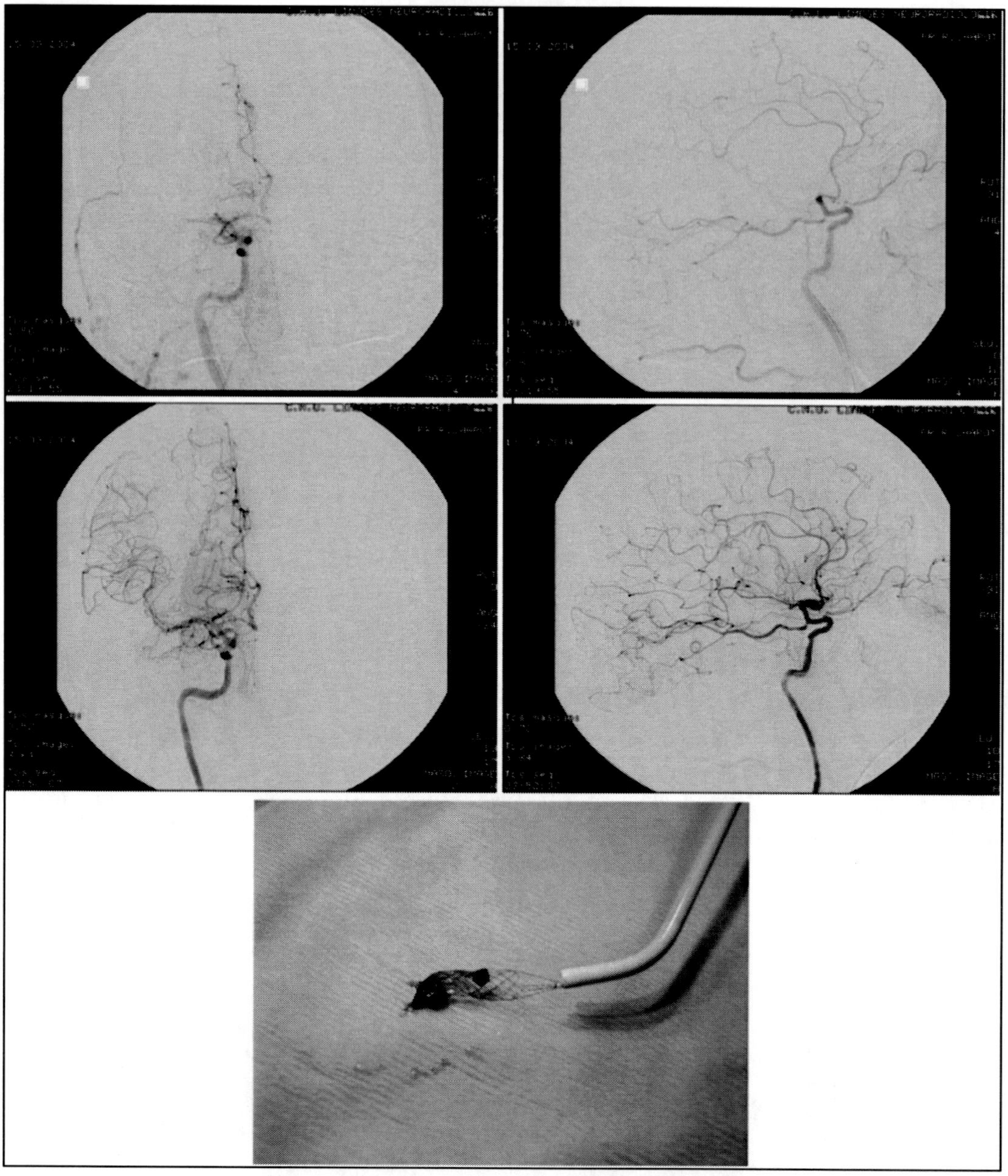

Figure 7. First stentriever case in history by Pr. René Chapot in Limoges, France, on Sept 15th, 2004.

Before dinner was over, we were sketching in my black notebook the first designs of a mechanical thrombectomy system derived from a LEO stent [3]. The first stent-based retriever, the first "stentriever" in history. Its initial goal was to retrieve clots formed during procedures. The next day, at Balt, I gathered Marc Soric and Alain Ramalason from my R&D team to bring these sketches to life, and a few days later, the first prototypes were produced in the workshops, allowing us to begin the series of tests necessary to validate the safety and efficacy of this new device. At that time, obtaining the CE mark was not the ordeal it is today (MDR had not yet wreaked havoc and innovation could still be dynamic in Europe). Within a few months, the first CATCH units were delivered to the Limoges University Hospital. A few days later, René informed me that he had successfully used the device to reopen an occluded M1 artery. His young patient had been transferred by helicopter from another hospital to give him a chance to try a revascularization procedure. For the first time, the CATCH was used for an ischemic stroke rather than a perioperative thrombotic complication (Figure 7). This extraordinary success caught our attention.

At the time, physicians had only chemical thrombolysis and a corkscrew-shaped guide called MERCI, the first design of a mechanical system - but it was not effective enough. A new revolution was underway with the CATCH. The concept of the stent retriever continued to evolve, particularly with the off-label use of EV3's SOLITAIRE stent as a retriever [4]. Originally designed for aneurysm treatment, the performance of this stent was disappointing in this indication. When I saw Pr. Salvatore Mangiafico of Florence, Italy, present very impressive cases using this stent for clot retrieval, I thought: "Yes, a laser-cut stent like the Solitaire is better suited for this use than the braided stent-based CATCH." While the structure of a laser-cut stent in a nitinol tube is less suitable for aneurysm treatment than a braided stent, the opposite is true for clot removal. The laser-cut stent behaves like a spring: the more it is compressed, the greater its radial force. It stretches less when pulled and exerts more force on the clot during removal than the braided stent. With this insight, Balt evolved the CATCH into a laser-cut design, creating the CATCH+ and then the CATCHVIEW (Figure 8).

Later, we developed the first mini stent retriever (CATCHMINI) that could be delivered through a 0.017" microcatheter [5]. This retriever stent was designed for use in small arteries to perform distal thrombectomy several years before the first scientific discussions on the topic. Innovation is always an iterative process, driven by competition.

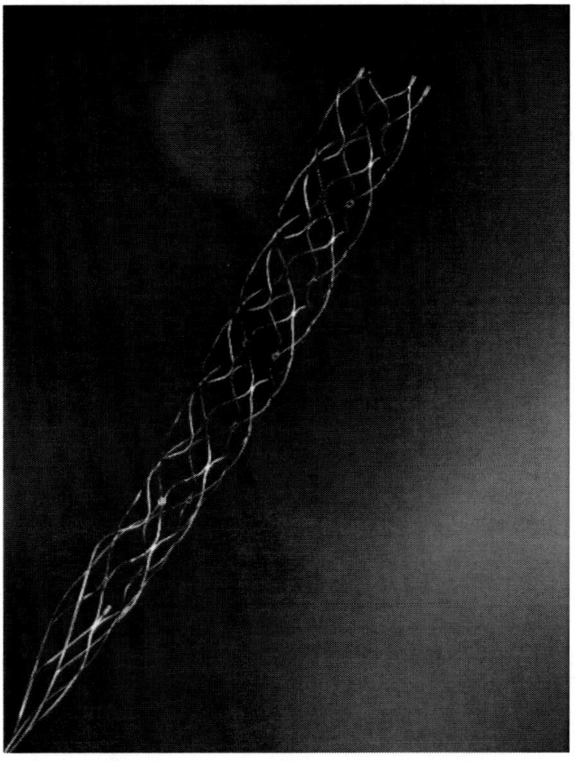

Figure 8. Stentriever CATCHVIEW.

It was only in 2015, 11 years after the first convincing use of the CATCH stent retriever, that the Mr. Clean study scientifically demonstrated the superiority of mechanical thrombectomy. It took 11 years of physician-industry collaboration, evolution, debate, highs and lows for this treatment, born from a discussion at the corner of a restaurant table, to revolutionize the treatment of the most common type of stroke, ischemic stroke.

The Revolution of the First Detachable Tip Catheter

Blockage of the distal extremity of microcatheters used for AVM embolization was a recurring problem. Recurrent and very common: cyanoacrylate glue had been used in most treatments since the 1980s. At that time, Professors Luc Picard, Pierre Lasjaunias, and Alejandro Berenstein urged my father to find a solution that would allow them to extend the injection time of the glue. Alejandro suggested making the tip of the Magic catheter detachable, but no satisfactory technical solution was found. When the distal tip of a catheter was stuck in glue, it had become common practice to cut off the proximal part at the puncture site and leave the remaining length in the patient, extending from the femoral artery to the cerebral arteries.

In the 2000s, the use of ONYX for AVM embolization became popular [6]. This product was actually EVAL, the brainchild of Japanese physician Waro Taki in the 1990s [6]. The idea was revolutionary in two ways: first, the product was non-adhesive, and second, it could be "redissolved" in situ to allow further penetration into the AVM. However, it had two disadvantages. First, the solvent it contained, DMSO, was very aggressive and incompatible with most catheters used at the time, especially the most efficient, the MAGIC. In addition, successful deep embolization required ONYX to reflux onto the distal part of the injection catheter, and even if it was not adhesive, this reflux often caused the catheter to pinch and become blocked in the AVM [7, 8]. In 2005, I discussed the problem again with René Chapot: he insisted that it was becoming essential for physicians treating AVMs to have a microcatheter with the performance of the MAGIC that was compatible with ONYX. It had therefore become essential for Balt, the undisputed specialist in AVM treatment devices, to develop a new generation of microcatheters.

We first developed the BALTACCI, a MAGIC microcatheter made of DMSO-resistant polymers. As its use became more widespread, an unexpected problem arose: ONYX contained tiny aggregates of tantalum powder (the heavy metal used as a radiopaque agent in this product), which eventually clogged the injection microcatheter. The small 1ml syringe used to inject ONYX allowed very high pressures in the catheter, causing the BALTACCI to rupture. It was not strong enough to withstand this type of stress due to the lack of reinforcement. Therefore, we completely redesigned it to improve its resistance without compromising its excellent navigation performance. Balt developed a new exclusive reinforcement process: a flat micro-steel wire wound around the outside of the distal part of the catheter, similar to a "shower hose." The injection pressure resistance was then increased from 7 to 100 bar! The SONIC was born.

However, this innovation had a drawback: the grooved surface of the SONIC's outer braid provided a mechanical grip for the ONYX reflux, increasing the risk of anchoring in the AVM and leaving us no choice but to find a way to dislodge the retained portion. My team and I worked tirelessly to come up with a solution that combined two ideas: the detachable part would be connected to the catheter by a platinum ring, which in turn would be bonded to the catheter with a non-DMSO-resistant adhesive. The ring ensured the cohesion of the two parts of the tube, with excellent pressure resistance at the junction because, like the pipelines seen in deserts, the higher the pressure, the more the inner tube presses against the ring, ensuring tightness and strength (Figures 9a & 9b). Tensile strength was maintained throughout the procedure by the adhesive until the final ONYX reflux reached it, causing it to dissolve and release the tip of the SONIC with a simple pull.

The result was a new revolution: not only did we have a catheter with navigational performance close to that of MAGIC, but it was also resistant to ONYX passage, even under high pressure, and could be released from the embolization site without causing bleeding. Once again, this historic step forward was made possible by the high level of expertise of Balt's technicians. The involvement of our master in extrusion, Akim Maaroufi, with Jarek Marzec and Balt's production operators was fundamental. Gluing the detachable tip of the SONIC under the microscope requires a rare dexterity that only a few people, such as Danièle Maisan or Nelly Maltaverne, possess. Without their passion and professionalism, the SONIC would never have existed.

I remember the enthusiasm of the doctors when I introduced the new SONIC [9]. In particular, Professor Pedro Lylyk from Buenos Aires was a big ONYX user. He immediately wanted to try this new device (Figure 10). I am truly grateful for the trust that our customers and physician friends have shown me so many times. Technically impossible 20 years ago, Professor Alejandro Berenstein's dream became a reality thanks to this continuous collaboration between doctors and technical specialists. The SONIC, along with the FLOWCOILS, MAGIC and SQUID12, is now an essential component of the revolutionary technique developed by Professor Chapot to treat AVMs, the "Pressure Cooker Technique."

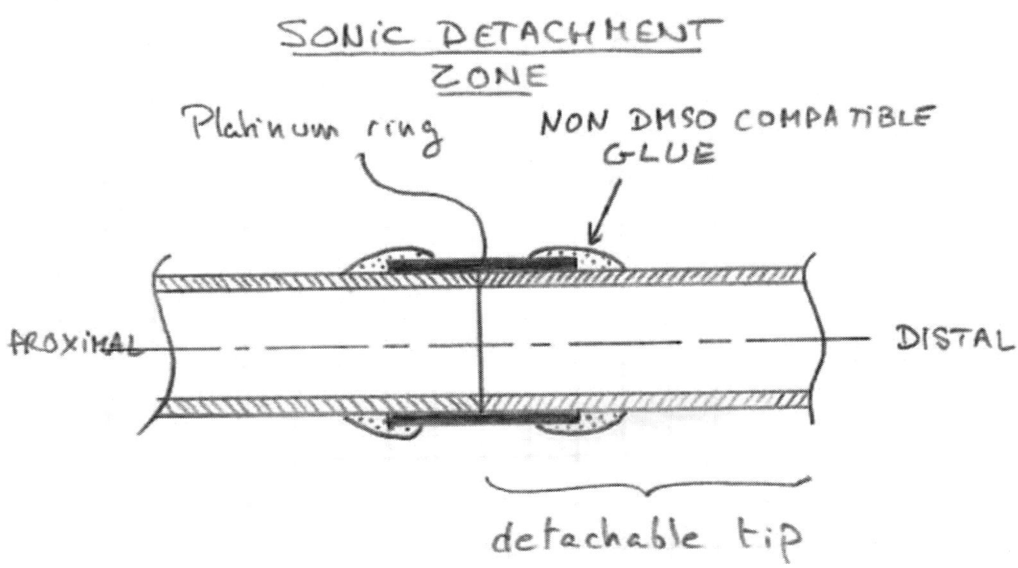

Figure 9a. Illustration of SONIC microcatheter detachment zone.

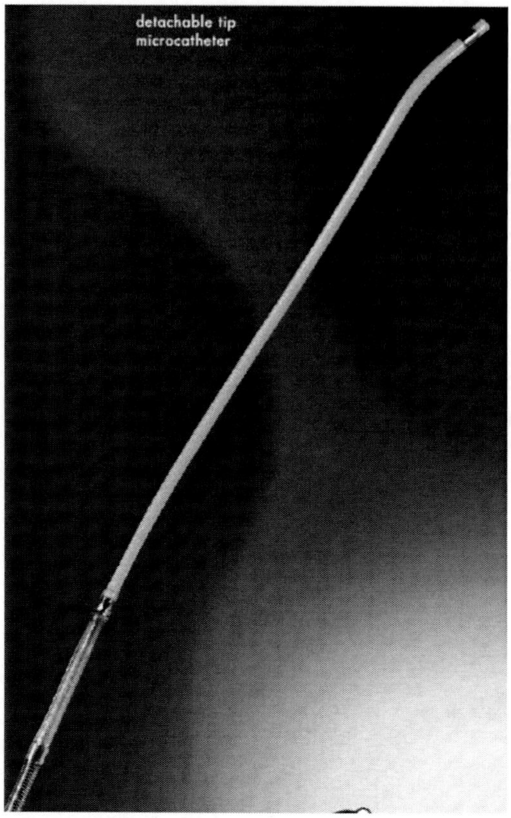

Figure 9b. Distal part of SONIC.

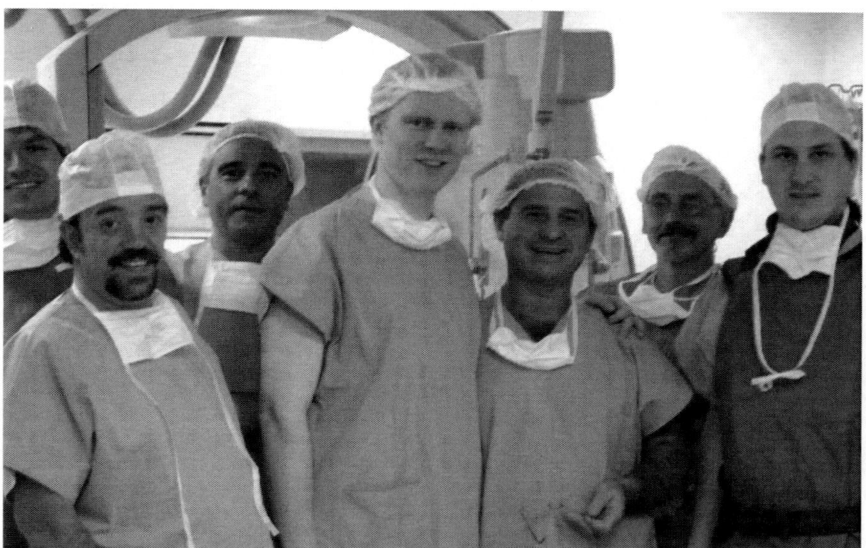

Figure 10. With Pedro Lylyk and his team in Buenos Aires after one of the first uses of the SONIC catheter in 2007.

The Revolution of the First Flow Diverter

Great innovations are always the result of iterative evolution. Such is the case with the concept of flow diversion, the ultimate evolution in intracranial stenting.

- First Evolution:

In the 1990s, Pedro Lylyk was one of the first to perform intracranial stenting trials [10]. He was able to navigate coronary stents through the carotid siphon to deploy them in front of aneurysms up to the middle cerebral artery. The maneuver was delicate and required all of Pedro's expertise; the balloon/stent assembly was too rigid for the tortuosity of the fragile cerebral arteries. This problem needed improvement.

- Second Evolution:

The late 1990s saw the introduction of the first intracranial stents, such as the SMART stent (which later became the NEUROFORM) [11]. The implant itself retained a coronary stent design, but was made of Nitinol, a nickel-titanium shape memory alloy that allowed deployment without a balloon. The innovation was twofold: a change in material and, unlike the coronary stent, which was carried on the distal balloon of a catheter, the SMART stent was delivered inside the delivery catheter after navigation was complete. Therefore, it did not interfere with navigation and its ascent through the vascular tree was atraumatic as it was protected by the catheter. A new step forward was achieved.

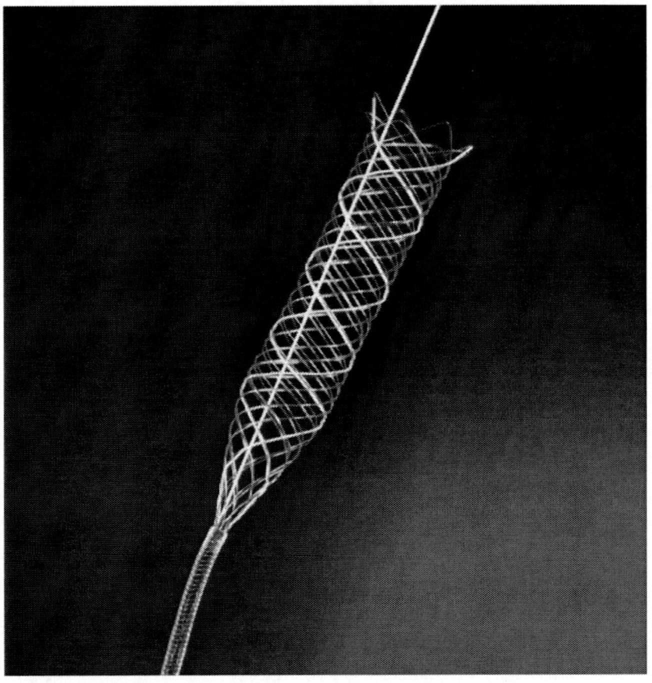

Figure 11. LEO stent, named as a nod to my father Leopold Plowiecki.

- Third Evolution:

The next innovation was to improve the design of the stent itself to make it more suitable for intracranial use: the curves of the arteries are much more pronounced than in the heart, and there is no balloon to help it adhere perfectly to the arterial wall. Balt found the solution in the early 2000s with the development of the LEO stent, the first intracranial stent braided from nitinol wire (Figure 11) [12].

In terms of manufacturing, the drawback was that each stent had to be hand-braided, a task that required meticulous operators, extensive training, and much more time than the automated cutting of "laser-cut" stents, such as the NEUROFORM. Once again, the dedication and motivation of the Balt production team was crucial. But the result was worth it: in addition to much better wall apposition, the system developed by BALT allowed, for the first time, the operator to reposition the LEO as many times as desired to achieve perfect positioning (Figure 12).

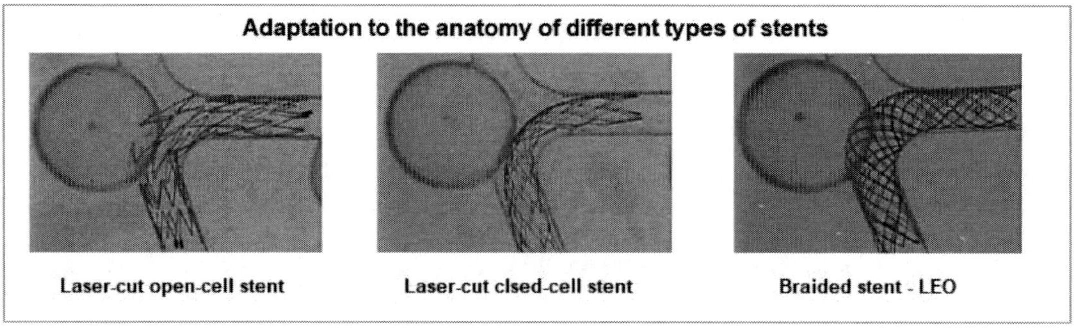

Figure 12. Showing the performance of stents made with different production processes in arterial curves.

Another caveat: the amount of material implanted with a LEO was much greater than with laser-cut stents, resulting in a much better hemodynamic effect but also a more intense thrombotic reaction than with other stents. Pioneers in the use of the LEO, such as Professor Jacques Moret, quickly realized that its implantation had to be accompanied by an anti-aggregation protocol. Surprising as it may seem today, this precaution was not obvious at the time.

The early days of the braided nitinol stent thus presented physicians with a dual training challenge: the deployment technique and the medication protocol, which was a novelty in interventional neuroradiology. The use of the LEO advanced rapidly, and the advances it brought opened up new treatment options for physicians, particularly in the treatment of fusiform aneurysms. I witnessed the first case of this type: the treatment of a giant fusiform aneurysm of the basilar artery by Professors Alfredo Casasco and Carlo Venturi in Siena, Italy, on July 31, 2003, using 3 telescopically placed LEO stents (Figure 13). At the 6-month follow-up, we saw the incredible hemodynamic efficacy of LEO: the artery was completely reconstructed along the stents.

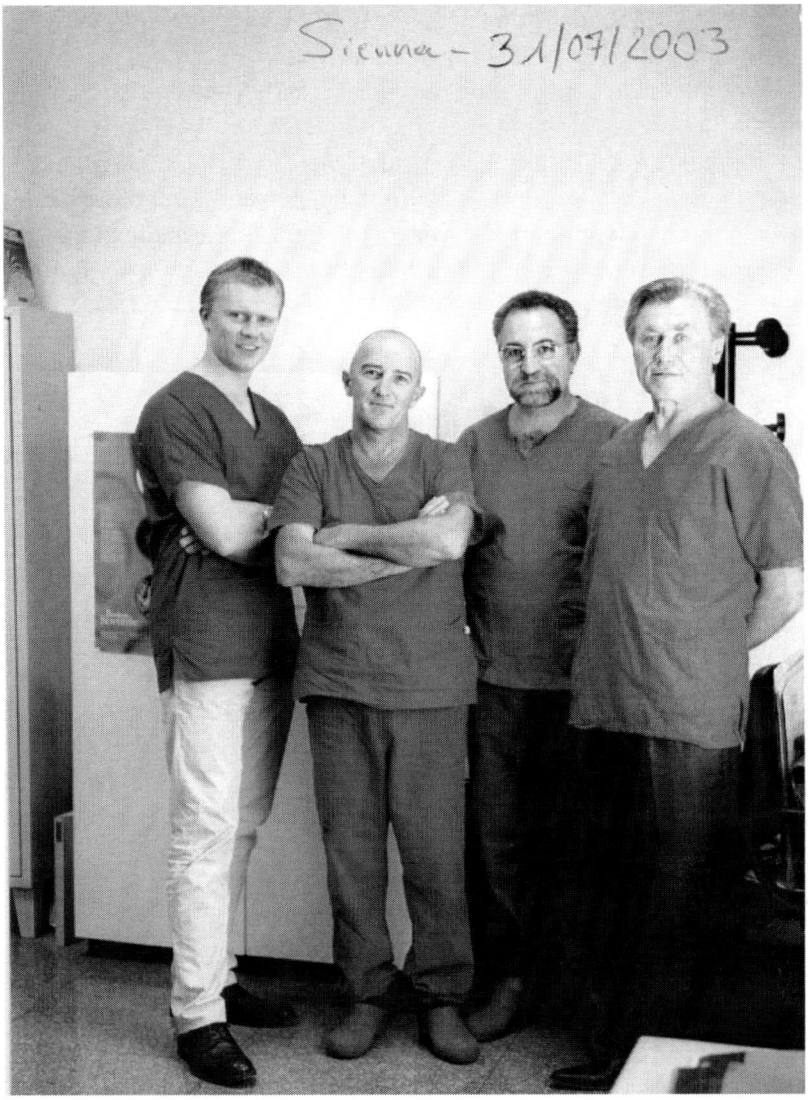

Figure 13. from left to right: Nicolas Plowiecki, Dr. Carlo Venturi, Pr. Alfredo Casasco and Leopold Plowiecki after the first case of treating a fusiform aneurysm with telescopic LEO stenting in Siena, Italy, on July 31, 2003.

- Fourth Evolution:

Amazed by the 6-month follow-up results of the Siena case at the end of 2003, I again challenged my team at Balt to develop a very dense mesh stent that could redirect blood flow and reduce the recanalization rate of embolized aneurysms. Together with Alain Ramalason, fantastic technical experts like Arlindo Esteves or Guillaume Carles would create a new generation of stent, maybe even without coils, who knows? The Siena case was performed with 3 LEO stents, each with 16 wires. 3 times 16 equals 48. 48 wires thin enough to pass through a microcatheter, but even that would have to be specially designed. I knew the Balt teams were up to this titanic challenge.

No operator's hand (no matter how meticulous) can weave these 48 wires together finer than hair. As is often the case, the level of innovation in Balt's products required its experts to invent dedicated and innovative production machines. That's what Guillaume and Arlindo did here by developing a special braiding machine of incredible precision. The catheters and delivery system for this new stent also had to be designed. The Balt teams worked tirelessly to miniaturize everything to the extreme. All of the company's expertise and teams were mobilized to meet this challenge in record time. The result was stunning in its flexibility and delicacy. It was Professor René Chapot who, while handling the stent with his deft hands, said, "It's smooth as silk. This was born the name of this revolutionary new stent: SILK (Figure 14).

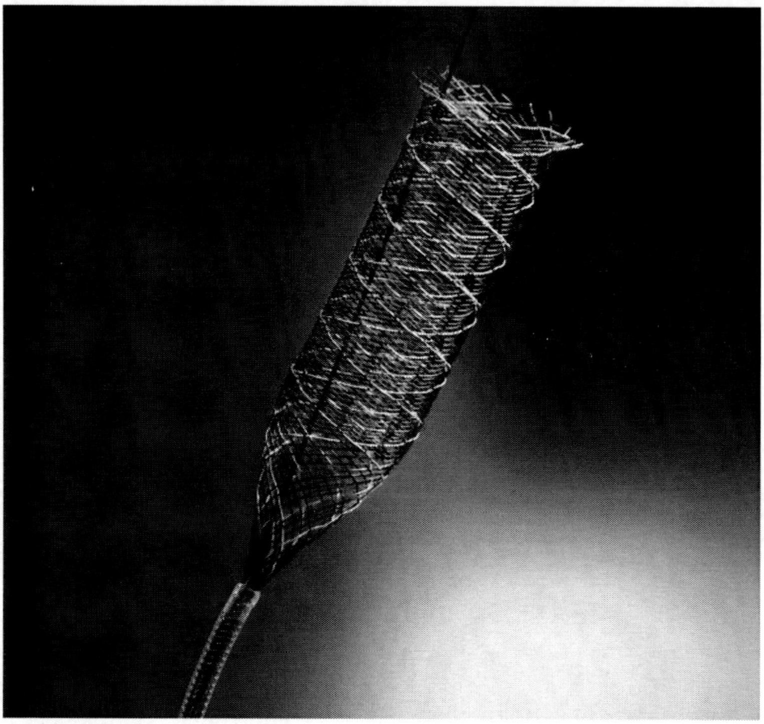

Figure 14. The SILK flow diverter.

While we were working on our flow diverter, an American team led by Dr. Kim Nelson was working on what would become the PIPELINE stent [13]. This competition further motivated us to excel and be first. This was achieved in 2007 when the SILK received CE Mark approval. The first flow diversion aneurysm was treated with a SILK on August 22, 2007 by Professor Patrick Brouwer and his team in Leiden, the Netherlands (Figure 15) [14]. You, the physicians reading this, know the pressure on your shoulders when using a device for the first time. Absolute confidence is essential. The Balt sales team, led by Ludovic Berthelin, has been fantastically supported by distributors such as Georg Landsberg, Zvika Sela or Alexander de Vries (left) to build and maintain the trust that makes this world first possible. Again, a team effort.

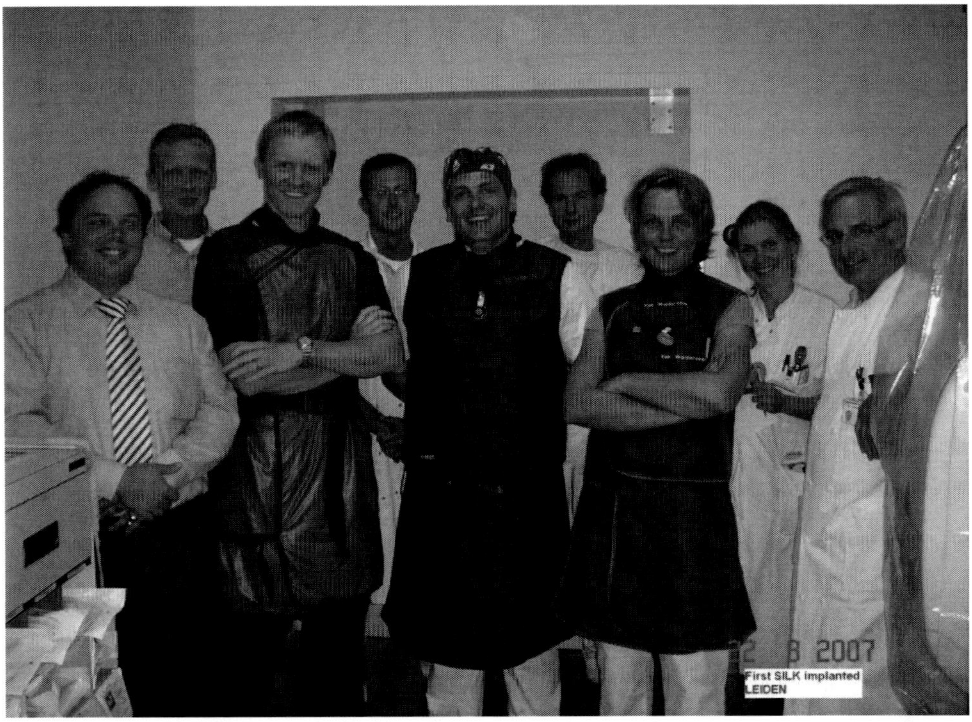

Figure 15. With Patrick Brouwer and his team in Leiden (The Netherlands) after the first flow diversion case in history on August 22, 2007.

SILK, then PIPELINE, opened up a revolutionary new way of treating aneurysms. As with all innovations, there was a learning curve as users became familiar with the characteristics of these new devices, and their widespread use continues to push the envelope. Today, countless braided wire implants are in use: stents, flow diverters, or intrasaccular devices are the heirs of this technique.

Over the past 45 years, from the first detachable balloons to the first low-profile SILK VISTA BABY flow diverter, physicians and technicians have pushed the boundaries of neurointerventional surgery. I don't know if the flap of a butterfly's wing in Brazil can create a tornado in Texas. But I'm sure that the knock of Pr. Merland's knock on my father's extrusion shop door in 1977 changed neurointerventional surgery forever. Never before had it been thought possible to mechanically remove a clot from the blocked artery of an ischemic stroke patient. Never before had it been thought possible to use a catheter with a detachable tip to embolize arteriovenous malformations. And never before had it been thought possible to divert the flow of blood from an aneurysm. Since then, it has become inconceivable not to.

Today, engineers and physicians around the world are working hard to push miniaturization even further, to be able to use molecules like P8RI to coat a stent, or to treat by endovascular approach pathologies that were never imagined to be treatable before (such as spinal CSF leaks, CSDH, pulsatile tinnitus, or chronic migraine...). These are the new frontiers of reality that new technical specialists and physicians will have to push back together. I'm sure that over the next 40 years, from one revolution to the next, technicians and physicians will continue to reinvent the reality of neurointerventional surgery.

Conclusion

This document recounts the transformative journey of neurointerventional surgery, chronicled through the collaborative efforts of engineers and physicians. Key milestones include the introduction of stent retrievers for clot retrieval and flow diverters for aneurysm treatment, highlighting a history marked by groundbreaking advances in the treatment of AVMs and aneurysms that fundamentally changed the landscape of stroke management and neurointervention.

References

[1] Hopkins LN, Ecker RD. Cerebral endovascular neurosurgery. *Neurosurgery* (2008) 62 (6 Suppl 3):1483-501; discussion 1501-2. doi: 10.1227/01.neu.0000333813.95025.a0. PMID: 18695568.

[2] Alaraj A, Wallace A, Dashti R, Patel P, Aletich V. Balloons in endovascular neurosurgery: history and current applications. *Neurosurgery* (2014) 74 Suppl 1:S163-90. doi: 10.1227/NEU.0000000000000220. PMID: 24402485.

[3] Brekenfeld C, Schroth G, El-Koussy M, Nedeltchev K, Reinert M, Slotboom J, Gralla J. Mechanical thromboembolectomy for acute ischemic stroke: comparison of the catch thrombectomy device and the Merci Retriever in vivo. *Stroke* (2008) 39 (4):1213-9. doi: 10.1161/STROKEAHA.107.495614. Epub 2008 Feb 28. PMID: 18309173.

[4] Castaño C, Dorado L, Guerrero C, Millán M, Gomis M, Perez de la Ossa N, Castellanos M, García MR, Domenech S, Dávalos A. Mechanical thrombectomy with the Solitaire AB device in large artery occlusions of the anterior circulation: a pilot study. *Stroke* (2010) 41 (8):1836-40. doi: 10.1161/STROKEAHA.110.584904. Epub 2010 Jun 10. PMID: 20538693.

[5] Barchetti G, Cagnazzo F, Raz E, Barbagallo G, Toccaceli G, Peschillo S. Mechanical Thrombectomy of Distal Occlusions Using a Direct Aspiration First Pass Technique Compared with New Generation of Mini-0.017 Microcatheter Compatible-Stent Retrievers: A Meta-Analysis. *World Neurosurg* (2020) 134:111-119. doi: 10.1016/j.wneu.2019.10.030. Epub 2019 Oct 15. PMID: 31627000.

[6] Richling B. History of endovascular surgery: personal accounts of the evolution. *Neurosurgery* (2006) 59 (5 Suppl 3):S30-8; discussion S3-13. doi: 10.1227/01.NEU.0000226224.79768.83. PMID: 17053616.

[7] Szajner M, Roman T, Markowicz J, Szczerbo-Trojanowska M. Onyx (®) in endovascular treatment of cerebral arteriovenous malformations - a review. *Pol J Radiol* (2013) 78 (3):35-41. doi: 10.12659/PJR.889120. PMID: 24115958; PMCID: PMC3789931.

[8] Zhang H, Liang S, Lv X. Proof-of-Principle for AVM Embolization Complications Caused by the Proximal Occlusion Technique Using Onyx: A Theoretical Basis for Ante-Grade Drifting Technique. *Neurol India* (2022) 70 (4):1443-1447. doi: 10.4103/0028-3886.355140. PMID: 36076641.

[9] Lv XL. Clinical Use of the Sonic Microcatheter with a Detachable Tip. *Journal of Cerebrovascular Disease* (2020) 3 (1):1-9.

[10] Lylyk P, Cohen JE, Ceratto R, Ferrario A, Miranda C. Angioplasty and stent placement in intracranial atherosclerotic stenoses and dissections. *AJNR Am J Neuroradiol* (2002) 23 (3):430-6. PMID: 11901013; PMCID: PMC7975311.

[11] Henkes H, Bose A, Felber S, Miloslavski E, Berg-Dammer E, Kühne D. Endovascular coil occlusion of intracranial aneurysms assisted by a novel self-expandable nitinol microstent (neuroform). *Interv Neuroradiol* (2002) 8 (2):107-19. doi: 10.1177/159101990200800202. Epub 2004 Oct 20. PMID: 20594519; PMCID: PMC3576604.

[12] Zhang J, Lv X, Jiang C, Li Y, Yang X, Wu Z. Endovascular treatment of cerebral aneurysms with the use of stents in small cerebral vessels. *Neurol Res* (2010) 32 (2):119-22. doi: 10.1179/174313209X459110. Epub 2009 Oct 12. PMID: 19825275.

[13] Fiorella D, Woo HH, Albuquerque FC, Nelson PK. Definitive reconstruction of circumferential, fusiform intracranial aneurysms with the pipeline embolization device. *Neurosurgery* (2008) 62 (5):1115-20; discussion 1120-1. doi: 10.1227/01.neu.0000325873.44881.6e. PMID: 18580809.

[14] Byrne JV, Beltechi R, Yarnold JA, Birks J, Kamran M. Early experience in the treatment of intra-cranial aneurysms by endovascular flow diversion: a multicentre prospective study. *PLoS One* (2010) 5 (9):e12492. doi: 10.1371/journal.pone.0012492. PMID: 20824070; PMCID: PMC2932685.

Chapter 7

The History and Development of Coiling

Abdullah M. Al-Qudah[1,*]
Aseel K. Fakhri[2,†]
Ahmed Aljuboori[3,‡]**, MD**
Ahmed Muthana[4,§]**, MD**
and Samer S. Hoz[5,‖]**, MD**

[1]UPMC Stroke Institute, University of Pittsburgh Medical Center, PA, USA
[2]University of Baghdad, College of Medicine, Baghdad, Iraq
[3]Department of Neurosurgery, Geisinger Clinic, PA, USA
[4]Department of Neurosurgery, University of Baghdad, Baghdad, Iraq
[5]Department of Neurosurgery, University of Cincinnati Medical Center, Cincinnati, OH, USA

Abstract

Coiling is a percutaneous endovascular technique used in the management of arterial aneurysms and fistulae with high success rates and minimal associated morbidity. Endovascular coiling continues to evolve and remains a valid modality in managing ruptured and unruptured intracranial aneurysms and high-flow fistulae. The chapter aims to provide a summary of the discoveries and developments that were instrumental in the evolution of the neurointerventional coiling of brain aneurysms. The chapter discusses many key persons who led the development and maturation of this treatment modality. Further, the chapter delves into the indications, potential complications, stent use, mechanisms of action, and future prospects of endovascular coiling, which will provide an indispensable asset for healthcare providers, researchers, and clinicians in the field.

Keywords: coiling, endovascular, aneurysms, high-flow fistula, neurointerventional surgery

* Corresponding Author's Email: qudah.m.a@gmail.com
† Corresponding Author's Email: asilk6195@gmail.com
‡ Corresponding Author's Email: ahmedaljuboori9494@gmail.com
§ Corresponding Author's Email: ahmed.m.najm@gmail.com
‖ Corresponding Author's Email: hozsamer2055@gmail.com

In: World History of Neurointerventional Surgery
Editors: Xianli Lv and Zhongxue Wu
ISBN: 979-8-89530-792-2

Introduction

Overview of Cerebral Aneurysms

Cerebral aneurysms are abnormal dilations of brain arteries, often occurring at vessel bifurcations [1]. With a prevalence of 2-6% in adults, these lesions can rupture, causing life-threatening subarachnoid hemorrhage [2, 3]. Aneurysm formation involves complex interactions between hemodynamic forces, vascular wall degeneration, and genetic factors [4, 5]. High wall shear stress contributes to aneurysm initiation, while both high and low shear stress are associated with progression and rupture [4]. Risk factors include smoking, hypertension, age, and family history [3]. Recent research has identified specific genes, such as THSD1 and SOX17, involved in aneurysm pathogenesis. The interplay between hemodynamics, vascular remodeling, inflammation, and genetics drives aneurysm evolution until stabilization or rupture [6, 7].

Brief Historical Context of Aneurysm Treatment

The treatment of cerebral aneurysms has evolved significantly over the past century, from open surgical techniques to minimally invasive endovascular approaches [8]. Walter Dandy pioneered surgical clipping in 1938, which remained the gold standard for decades [9]. The introduction of the Guglielmi detachable coil in 1991 revolutionized aneurysm treatment, offering a less invasive alternative to open surgery [10]. The International Subarachnoid Aneurysm Trial provided evidence supporting endovascular treatment over surgical clipping [11]. Today, treatment options include microsurgical clipping, endovascular coiling, and advanced techniques such as stent-assisted coiling and flow diversion [12]. The choice of treatment depends on factors like aneurysm characteristics, patient factors, and operator experience [13]. Ongoing technological advancements, including bioactive coils and stents, continue to shape the future of neurointerventional treatment [14].

Early Developments in the Treatment of Cerebral Aneurysms

Surgical Approaches

The surgical treatment of cerebral aneurysms has evolved significantly since Walter E. Dandy pioneered the clipping technique in 1937 [15]. Dandy's contributions included the first surgical clipping of an intracranial aneurysm and descriptions of various vascular malformations [15]. The development of aneurysm clips progressed from malleable metal clips to sophisticated spring clips in the latter half of the 20th century [16, 17]. The introduction of the surgical microscope and advanced clip designs enabled the treatment of complex aneurysms previously considered inoperable [16]. Today, intracranial aneurysms are treated through surgical methods like microsurgical clipping or endovascular techniques such as coiling and flow diversion [12]. Treatment decisions are based on factors including patient characteristics, aneurysm features, and operator experience [12]. The field continues to evolve with ongoing technological advancements and refinement of surgical techniques.

Endovascular Approaches

The development of endovascular techniques, particularly the Guglielmi Detachable Coil (GDC) in 1991, marked a significant shift in the treatment of cerebral aneurysms [18, 19]. This minimally invasive approach offered an alternative to surgical clipping, especially for patients at high surgical risk or with aneurysms in challenging locations [20]. Large clinical trials demonstrated comparable or better outcomes with endovascular coiling for certain aneurysm types [10, 21]. Over time, endovascular treatment has steadily increased, particularly for posterior circulation aneurysms [22]. However, the choice between surgical clipping and endovascular coiling depends on various factors, including aneurysm characteristics, patient health, and physician expertise [23, 24]. Despite advancements in endovascular techniques, surgical clipping remains the preferred option for some aneurysm types, such as those in the middle cerebral artery [25].

Development and Evolution of Endovascular Coiling

Invention of Coiling

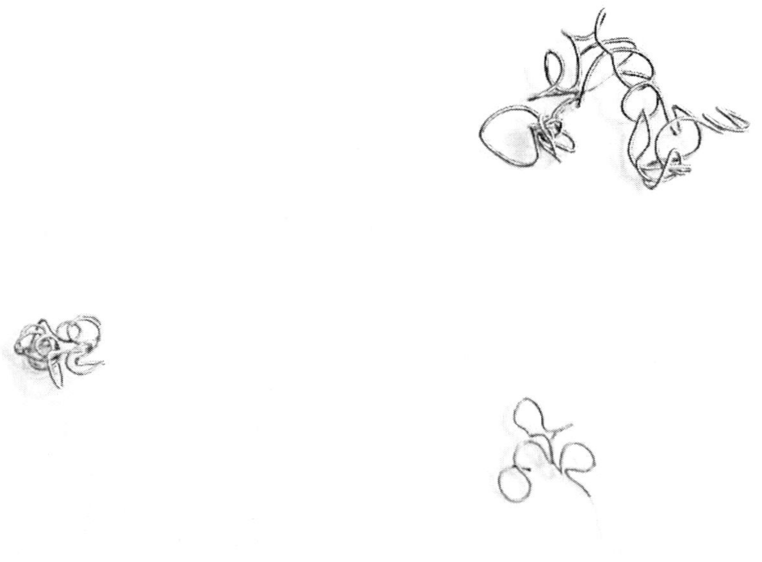

Figure 1. Examples of Guglielmi detachable coils used for intracranial aneurysms.

Endovascular coiling has revolutionized the treatment of intracranial aneurysms since its introduction in 1991 by Dr. Guido Guglielmi [26]. The Guglielmi Detachable Coil (GDC) system allows for minimally invasive aneurysm occlusion through electrolytic detachment of platinum coils [23] (Figure 1). This technique has evolved significantly, with improvements in coil design, including softer coils and multidimensional shapes [27]. The development of GDCs was preceded by earlier attempts using detachable balloons and pushable microcoils [28]. Since its inception, over 7,000 patients had been treated with GDCs by 1996 [29]. The technology continues to advance, with newer coil properties and adjunctive devices improving long-term aneurysm occlusion rates [30]. This evolution has made endovascular coiling a viable alternative to surgical clipping for both ruptured and unruptured aneurysms [31].

Advancements in Coiling Devices

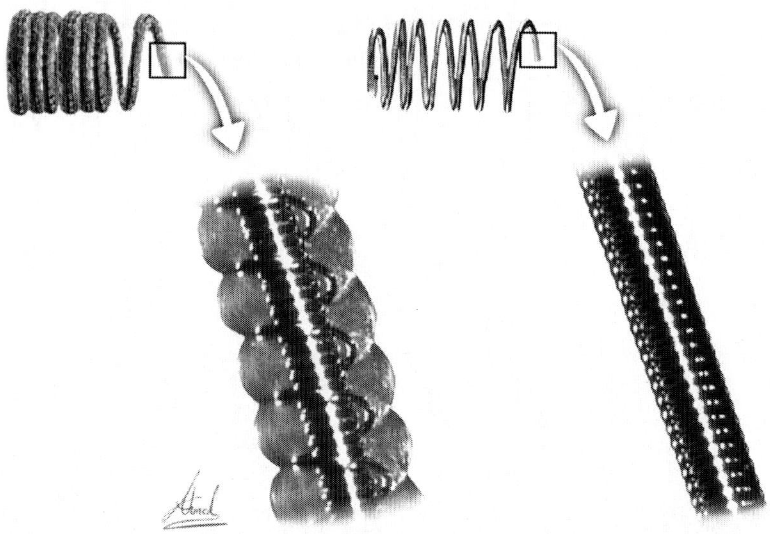

Figure 2. Schematic depiction showing the difference between the platinum coils (Right) and the hydrocoils (Left). Illustration prepared by Ahmed Muthana and courtesy of Samer Hoz.

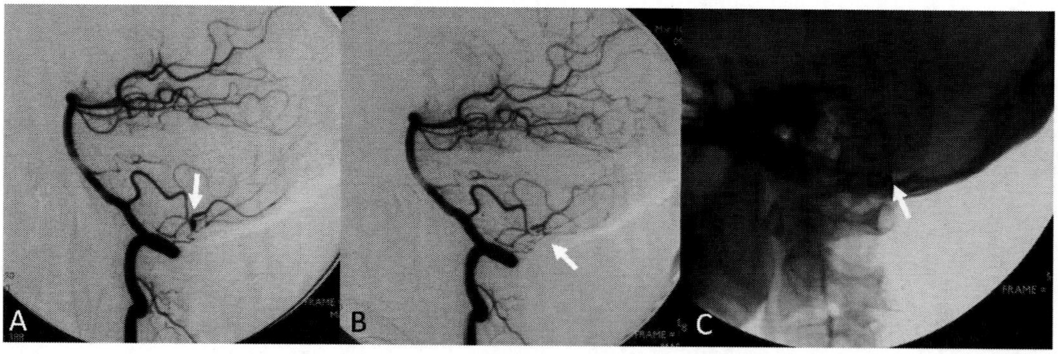

Figure 3. A 33-year-old woman with a ruptured distal posterior inferior cerebellar artery aneurysm was coiled. A, lateral view of the left vertebral artery injection showing a 2mm×3mm aneurysm of the distal posterior inferior cerebellar artery (arrow). B, lateral view of the left vertebral artery injection showing the aneurysm was occluded with coils (arrow). C, unsubtracted image showing the coil mass (arrow).

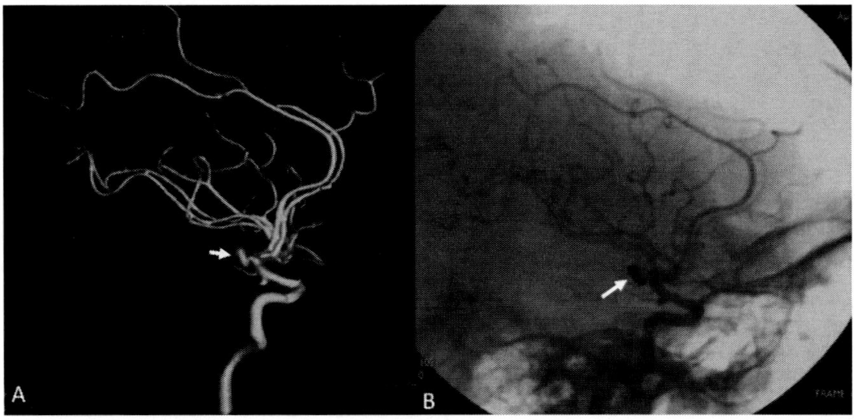

Figure 4. A 38-year-old woman with a ruptured A1 segment aneurysm of the anterior cerebral artery was coiled. A, 3-D reconstruction of the left internal carotid artery injection showing the aneurysm of the origin of A1 segment of the left anterior cerebral artery (arrow). B, lateral view of the unsubtracted angiogram of the left internal carotid artery injection showing the complete occclusion of the aneurysm and coil mass (arrow).

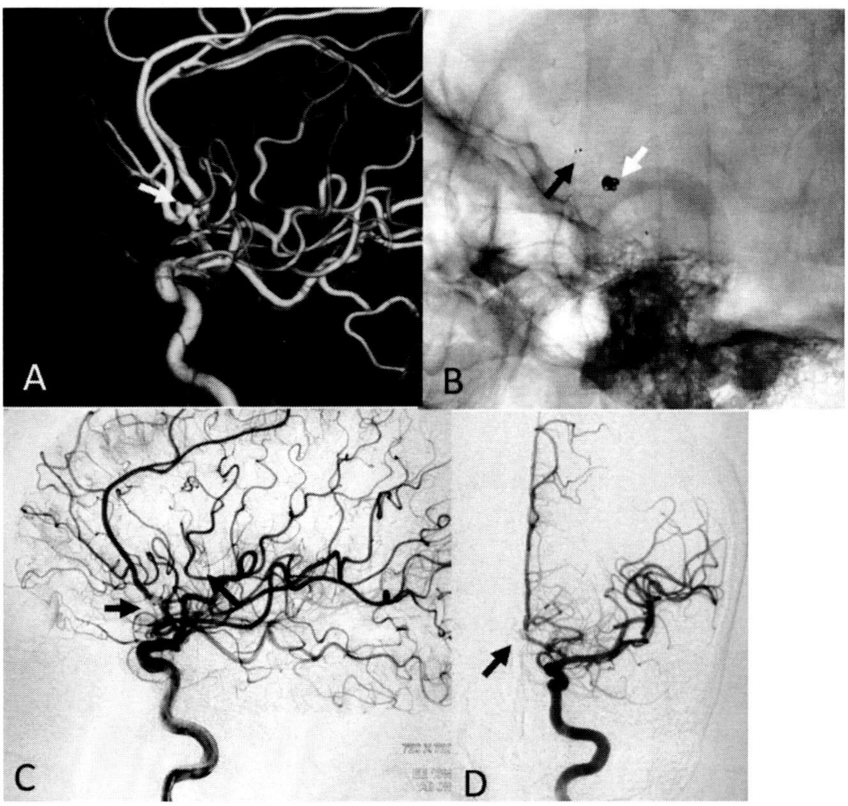

Figure 5. A 56-year-old woman presented with Hunt-Hess grade I subarachnoid hemorrhage. A, 3-D reconstruction of the left internal carotid artery injection showing an aneurysm arising from the anterior communicating artery (arrow), which was treated with 4.0mm×15mm Solitaire AB stent and coils. B, the unsubtracted image showing the head (black arrow) of the Solitaire AB stent and the coil mass (white arrow). Lateral view (C) and frontal view (D) of the left internal carotid artery injection after coiling showing the aneurysm was occluded completely (arrow).

Advancements in coiling technology have improved the treatment of intracranial aneurysms. Hydrocoils, which expand upon contact with blood, provide better aneurysm filling and potentially reduce recurrence rates [32, 33] (Figure 2). Bioactive coils promote endothelial growth and vessel wall reconstruction [34]. A meta-analysis showed that bioactive coils increase complete aneurysm occlusion rates compared to bare platinum coils [35]. Hydrogel coils, in particular, have demonstrated reduced residual aneurysms [35]. Advances in coil delivery systems and imaging technologies have enhanced procedural precision [30]. Additionally, adjunctive devices like balloons and stents have facilitated the treatment of complex aneurysms [36]. While these innovations show promise, long-term follow-up is needed to determine their clinical significance [35]. Overall, these advancements have expanded treatment options and improved outcomes for patients with intracranial aneurysms (Figure 3-5) [37].

Key Contributors to the Field

Pioneers of Neurointerventional Radiology

Neurointerventional radiology has evolved significantly since its inception in the 1960s, with pioneers like Lussenhop introducing intravascular embolization techniques [38]. Key figures such as Alejandro Berenstein and Pierre Lasjaunias made groundbreaking contributions to endovascular treatments for complex neurovascular conditions [39, 40]. The field has seen rapid advancements in technology, including the development of liquid embolics, innovative catheters, and imaging techniques [41, 42]. Multidisciplinary collaboration between radiology, neurosurgery, and neurology has been crucial in driving progress [43]. The scope of neurointerventional procedures has expanded to include treatments for aneurysms, arteriovenous malformations, and ischemic stroke [44]. As the field continues to evolve, emerging technologies like robotic-assisted techniques and artificial intelligence are expected to further enhance patient care and treatment outcomes [43].

Institutions and Centers of Excellence

Neurointerventional radiology is a rapidly evolving multidisciplinary field focusing on minimally invasive therapies for neurological disorders [43]. Research in this area has shown slow growth, high interdisciplinary collaboration, and low funding levels [45]. Academic centers have been at the forefront of neurointerventional procedures, performing the majority of treatments like aneurysm coiling, thrombolysis, and stent placements [46]. The field faces challenges such as low dissemination rates of research results and high rates of study non-completion [47]. To address these issues, initiatives like the International Consortium of Neuro Endovascular Centers have been proposed to support research and collaboration [48]. Despite challenges, the field has seen significant advancements, particularly in stroke treatment, largely driven by industry collaborations. Continued interdisciplinary cooperation and the adoption of innovative technologies are crucial for the future of neurointerventional radiology [43].

Critical Gaps and Challenges in Device Technology

Device Evolution and Limitations

Endovascular coiling technology for treating intracranial aneurysms has evolved significantly, addressing initial limitations like incomplete occlusion and coil compaction [30, 49]. Advancements include improved coil materials, such as hydrocoils and bioactive coils, and adjunctive devices like stents and balloons [30, 50]. Despite progress, challenges persist in achieving complete and durable aneurysm occlusion [51]. Emerging technologies like shape memory polymers and intrasaccular flow disruptors show promise for patient-specific treatments and improved occlusion rates [36, 51]. Flow diverters have revolutionized complex aneurysm treatment, offering an alternative approach to remodeling the aneurysm-vessel interface [36]. While endovascular approaches have shown benefits over open repair in the short term, long-term durability remains a concern [52]. Ongoing research focuses on addressing these limitations and improving long-term outcomes [53].

Treatment Selection and Guidelines

The management of intracranial aneurysms has evolved significantly, with guidelines playing a crucial role in shaping clinical practice. Treatment options include surgical clipping and endovascular techniques, with decision-making based on factors such as aneurysm characteristics, patient health, and clinician experience [12, 13]. The American Heart Association has published comprehensive guidelines for both ruptured and unruptured aneurysms, emphasizing evidence-based approaches to diagnosis, treatment, and management [54, 55]. These guidelines have shifted from consensus-based to evidence-based recommendations over time, with consistent support for nimodipine use and a trend towards earlier treatment and endovascular coiling [56]. However, adherence to guidelines varies across institutions, highlighting the need for personalized approaches in aneurysm management [56].

The Last Decade: Advances in Technique and Safety

Innovations in Imaging and Navigation

Over the past decade, significant advancements in imaging and navigation technologies have revolutionized endovascular and spine procedures. Three-dimensional imaging techniques, such as cone-beam CT and 3D rotational angiography, have improved visualization and procedural outcomes [57, 58]. Image-guided navigation systems, incorporating pre-operative 3D CT images and real-time tracking of surgical tools, have enhanced accuracy and reduced radiation exposure [57]. Robotic assistance has further improved precision and efficiency in spine surgery [59, 60]. Emerging technologies like fluorescence-guided surgery and optical coherence tomography offer higher-resolution imaging of the central nervous system [61]. These innovations have made complex procedures safer and more efficient, reducing the reliance on traditional fluoroscopy [62]. As technology continues to evolve, intraoperative navigation and robotics are expected to play an increasingly significant role in minimally invasive procedures.

Three-dimensional rotational angiography (3DRA) has emerged as a valuable tool in the evaluation and treatment of cerebral aneurysms. Compared to conventional digital subtraction angiography (DSA), 3DRA provides more detailed information on aneurysm morphology, neck size, and relationships with parent and adjacent vessels [63-66]. This improved visualization aids in surgical planning, reducing procedural risks and enhancing decision-making for endovascular or surgical interventions [63, 67, 68]. 3DRA has demonstrated higher sensitivity in detecting aneurysms, with studies reporting additional aneurysms compared to DSA alone [63]. Image fusion techniques, combining preoperative 3D models with intraoperative fluoroscopy, provide real-time guidance and have been shown to decrease radiation exposure, contrast agent use, and procedure times [69, 70]. These technologies have proven beneficial in various applications, including endovascular aneurysm repair, carotid stenting, and neurosurgery [71]. Augmented reality systems, such as HoloLens, offer radiation-free 3D holographic visualization of the vascular system during interventions [72]. As these technologies continue to evolve, they are expected to further improve surgical outcomes, reduce complications, and enhance the learning curve for novice practitioners [73].

Biplane fluoroscopy has emerged as a valuable tool in neurointerventional procedures, offering simultaneous imaging from two angles for improved visualization of complex vascular structures [74, 75]. This technique enhances the precision of catheter navigation and device deployment, potentially reducing procedure time, radiation dose, and complications [76, 77]. Biplane imaging allows for better evaluation of aneurysm morphology and flow dynamics, especially when combined with high-speed angiography [78]. It also facilitates 3D reconstruction and visualization of vascular structures, improving spatial orientation during interventions [79]. The advantages of biplane systems include enhanced operator confidence, particularly in complex procedures [76], and reduced need for additional angiographic views. These advancements have contributed to the widespread adoption of endovascular treatments for cerebral aneurysms.

Refinement of Technique

The refinement of endovascular techniques has led to significant advancements in the treatment of cerebrovascular diseases. New devices and techniques have enhanced the safety and efficacy of interventions for various conditions, including intracranial aneurysms, carotid artery stenosis, and arteriovenous malformations [80]. The development of embolic protection devices (EPDs) has significantly contributed to making carotid angioplasty and stenting (CAS) a viable alternative to endarterectomy for treating carotid artery stenosis [81, 82]. These technological advancements have expanded the scope of endovascularly treatable conditions, offering new hope to patients who may not have been candidates for surgical intervention previously (Figure 6).

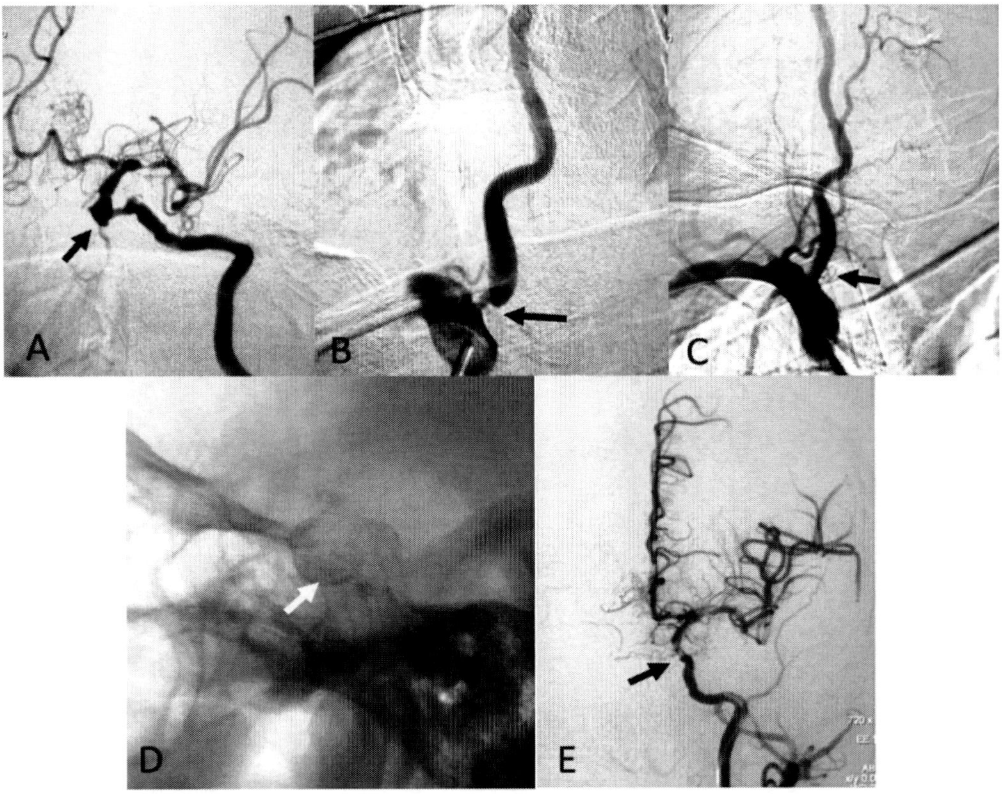

Figure 6. A 70-year-old man presented with dizziness. A, oblique view of the left internal carotid artery injection showing a cavernous aneurysm of the internal carotid artery (arrow). B, frontal view of the right subclavian artery injection showing the stenosis of the vertebral artery orifice (arrow). C, frontal view of the right subclavian artery injection showing the stenosis of the vertebral artery orifice was treated with a 5mm×15mm Express stent (arrow) (Boston Scientific, USA). D, unsubtracted image showing the cavernous aneurysm was treated with a Pipeline flow diversion (arrow). E, frontal view of the left carotid artery angiography showing the disappearance of the aneurysm (arrow).

Procedural Techniques

The evolution of endovascular techniques has revolutionized the treatment of cerebral aneurysms. Advancements in imaging technology have improved diagnosis and treatment planning. The development of microwires, microcatheters, and coils has expanded treatment options for complex aneurysms [12, 83]. Coil technology has progressed with improvements in flexibility and occlusion rates [30]. Flow diversion devices have emerged as a novel endovascular treatment for intracranial aneurysms, particularly for large, giant, and complex cases [84]. Balloon-assisted coiling (BAC) and stent-assisted coiling (SAC) have significantly improved the treatment of wide-necked intracranial aneurysms. Studies comparing these techniques have shown that SAC generally achieves higher rates of complete aneurysm occlusion and lower rates of retreatment than BAC [75, 85, 86]. SAC also demonstrates better long-term stability and progression of occlusion [85]. However, both techniques have similar overall complication rates [86, 87]. A newer approach, stent plus balloon-assisted coiling, has shown promising results for complex wide-necked bifurcation aneurysms, with high rates of complete occlusion and relatively low retreatment rates [88, 89]. Despite these advancements, large and bifurcation aneurysms still present challenges for both BAC and SAC, with higher complication and recurrence rates (Figure 7) [86, 90]. As endovascular therapy continues to evolve, it is becoming a mainstay in aneurysm treatment, complementing traditional surgical approaches.

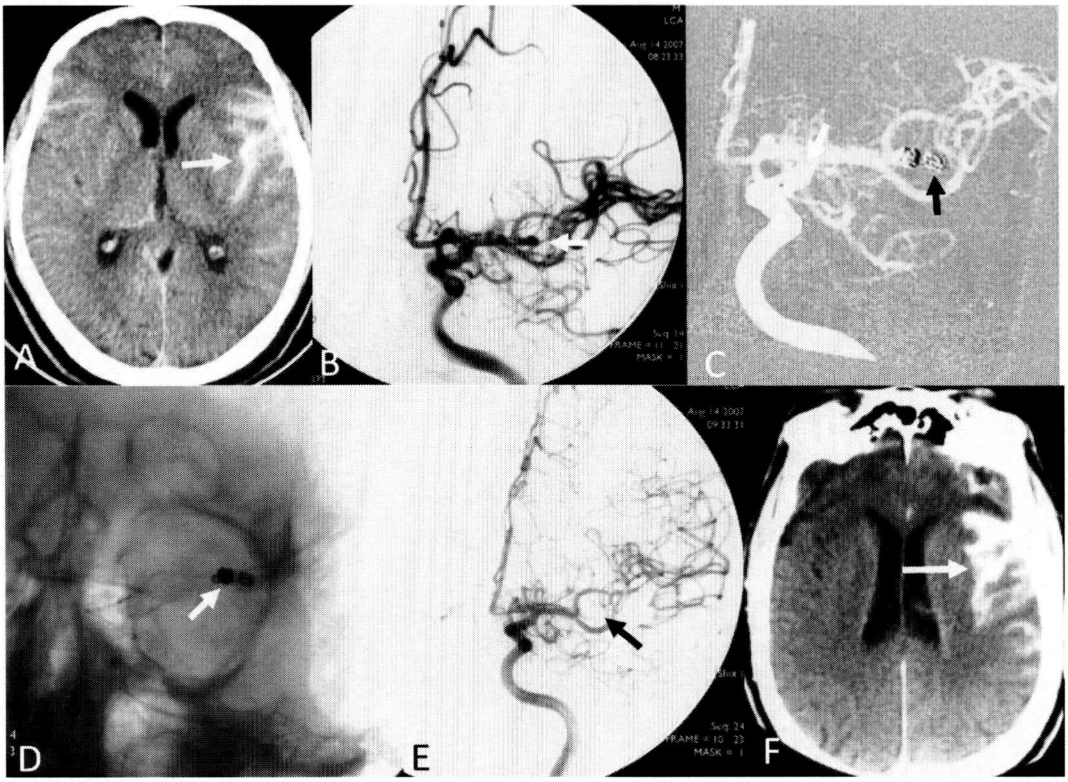

Figure 7. Intraoperative rupture during aneurysm coiling. A 58-year-old man presenting with subarachnoid hemorrhage from a middle cerebral artery bifurcation aneurysm. A, cranial CT image showing subarachnoid hemorrhage in the left Sylvian fissure (arrow). B, a digital subtraction angiogram showing a ruptured middle cerebral artery bifurcation aneurysm (arrow). C, roadmapping image showing the coil protruded out of the aneurysm sac (arrow). D, unsubtracted image showing the aneurysm sac was coiled. E, final angiogram showing complete aneurysm obliteration. D. Postprocedural CT image showing focal contrast medium extravasation.

Current Guidelines and Management Strategies

Modern Guidelines for Endovascular Management

Modern guidelines for endovascular management of cerebral aneurysms have evolved significantly, reflecting the latest evidence-based research and technological advancements. Endovascular coiling has become the mainstay of treatment, often preferred over surgical clipping [91] (Figure 8). Flow diversion has revolutionized the treatment of complex intracranial aneurysms, offering a viable alternative to traditional surgical clipping and endovascular coiling [92-94]. Large clinical trials, such as ISAT, have demonstrated the safety and efficacy of endovascular treatment [10]. Guidelines recommend treatment for symptomatic aneurysms and those larger than 5mm in patients under 60 years [95]. A multidisciplinary approach involving neurosurgeons, interventional radiologists, and neurologists is crucial for optimal patient outcomes [96].

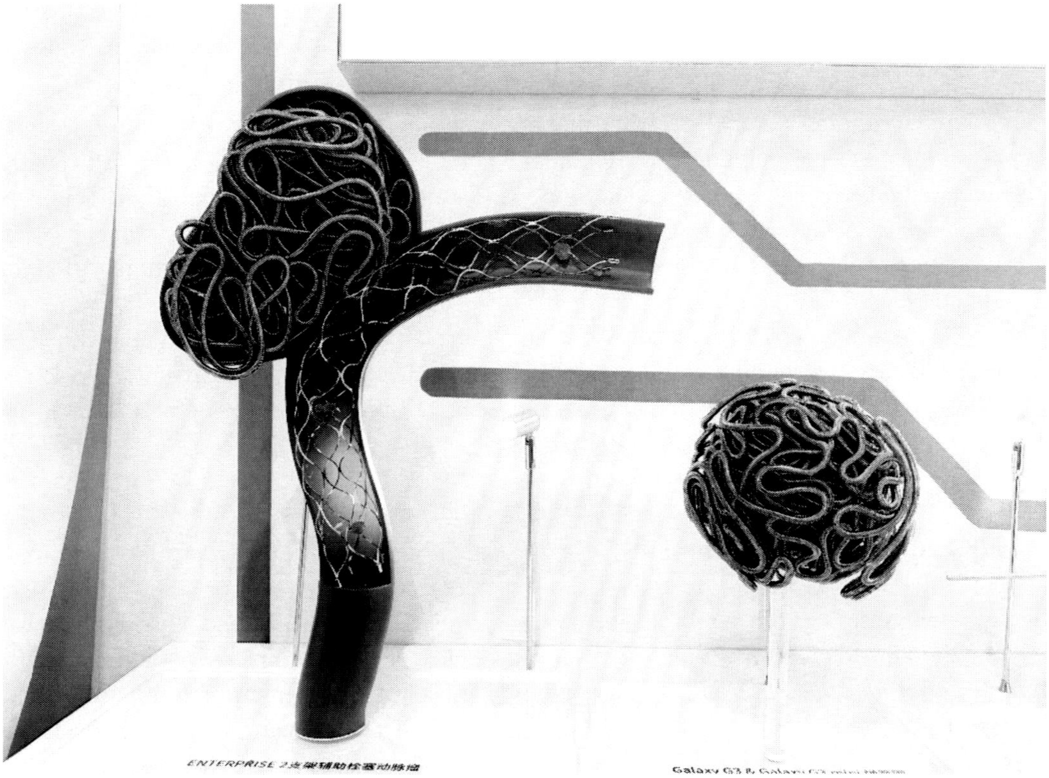

Figure 8. The use of endovascular coiling for treatment of cerebral aneurysms.

The American Heart Association/American Stroke Association has established comprehensive guidelines for managing aneurysmal subarachnoid hemorrhage (aSAH) and unruptured cerebral aneurysms [55]. These guidelines emphasize early intervention, detailed assessment of aneurysm characteristics, and endovascular coiling as a primary treatment option for many patients. The guidelines have evolved from consensus-based to evidence-based approaches, addressing various aspects of aSAH care, including diagnosis, prevention of rebleeding, surgical and endovascular repair, and management of complications [54]. Recent updates have incorporated new evidence and recommendations. However, adherence to these guidelines in clinical practice remains inconsistent, with variations in treatment protocols across institutions [56]. The use of nimodipine has remained a consistent recommendation, while there has been a shift from surgical clipping to endovascular coiling for aneurysm treatment [56].

The European Society of Minimally Invasive Neurological Therapy (ESMINT) has collaborated with other organizations to develop guidelines for mechanical thrombectomy in acute ischemic stroke [97]. These guidelines emphasize patient selection, timely reperfusion, and the importance of best medical management alongside thrombectomy [97]. The society contributes to standards for training in interventional neuroradiology [97]. Reporting standards for endovascular aneurysm repair have been established to ensure consistency in clinical trials and publications [98].

Influence of Evolving Guidelines on Clinical Practice

Current guidelines from leading organizations play a crucial role in managing cerebral aneurysms and guiding clinical decision-making based on recent evidence. These guidelines address various aspects, including presentation, natural history, epidemiology, risk factors, screening, diagnosis, and treatment outcomes [55]. Treatment options include surgical clipping and endovascular techniques, with the choice depending on factors such as patient age, medical history, aneurysm characteristics, and operator experience [12]. Guidelines recommend treating symptomatic aneurysms, conservatively managing small incidental aneurysms (<5mm), and considering treatment for larger aneurysms in younger patients [95]. The management of unruptured aneurysms remains controversial, requiring a balance between rupture risk and intervention risks [99]. A multidisciplinary approach at high-volume centers is advised for optimal treatment outcomes [13].

Role of Multidisciplinary Teams

Effective management of cerebral aneurysms requires a coordinated, multidisciplinary approach. Integrated cerebrovascular programs have been shown to improve patient outcomes, reduce hospital stays, and decrease complications [13, 100]. These programs combine expertise in microsurgery, endovascular techniques, neurology, and critical care. Treatment decisions should consider various factors, including the patient's medical history, aneurysm characteristics, and available interventions. Advanced imaging and biomechanical modeling can aid in patient-specific treatment planning and device evaluation. Risk management and precision care during interventional procedures have been shown to improve surgical safety and outcomes, particularly in elderly patients. The incorporation of artificial intelligence for aneurysm growth monitoring and rupture risk prediction, along with the development of nationwide radiographic and biological registries, may further enhance aneurysm management in the future [101].

Future Directions in the Field

Emerging Technologies and Treatments

Neurointerventional radiology is experiencing rapid advancements in technology and treatments. Emerging technologies include robotic-assisted techniques, artificial intelligence for diagnosis and treatment planning, and innovative devices for endovascular thrombectomy [43]. Novel approaches in interventional neuro-oncology, such as direct arterial infusion of chemotherapy and stem cell-mediated delivery of nanoparticles, are being explored [102]. Improvements in aneurysm treatment involve new coil designs, balloon- and stent-assisted embolization, and advanced imaging technologies [92-94]. The field is also witnessing progress in the treatment of arteriovenous malformations through enhanced microcatheter navigation and improved embolization materials. These advancements are expanding the scope of neuroendovascular interventions and improving patient outcomes [103].

Flow Diverters

Flow diverters represent a significant advancement in treating intracranial aneurysms, particularly large, complex, and previously untreatable cases [93]. These devices, such as the Pipeline Embolization Device, redirect blood flow away from the aneurysm, promoting thrombosis and endothelial growth [94]. Studies have shown high occlusion rates, with 91.2% at 6 months and 94.6% at 1-2 years [104]. Flow diverters demonstrate low complication rates, with severe hemorrhagic complications reported at 2% for PED and 0.8% for SILK [105]. Overall morbidity and mortality rates are 10.4% and 3.9%, respectively [106]. While antiplatelet therapy is necessary, flow diverters have expanded treatment options for aneurysms previously managed by traditional surgical or coil-based methods [107]. Studies comparing flow diverters to traditional coiling techniques have shown higher aneurysm occlusion rates and lower retreatment rates with flow diversion, without significant differences in complication rates or clinical outcomes [108]. This advantage extends to both large unruptured saccular aneurysms and small, noncomplex aneurysms [108, 109]. Flow diverters, such as the Pipeline Embolization Device, have demonstrated high cure rates with low complication rates [94]. However, the risk of severe hemorrhagic complications remains a concern, with reported rates of 2% for the Pipeline device and 0.8% for the SILK flow diverter [105]. Ongoing clinical trials aim to further evaluate their efficacy and safety compared to other treatments.

Intrasaccular Devices

Intrasaccular devices, such as the Woven EndoBridge (WEB), offer a promising treatment option for wide-necked and complex intracranial aneurysms. These devices create a scaffold within the aneurysm sac, promoting thrombosis and vessel remodeling. The WEB device has shown good safety profiles and encouraging occlusion rates in systematic reviews and meta-analyses. Compared to stent-assisted coiling, WEB embolization demonstrates similar midterm complete and adequate occlusion rates for unruptured wide-neck bifurcation aneurysms [110-112]. Other intrasaccular devices, including the Artisse and Contour Neurovascular System, are also being developed and studied [113]. These devices aim to address the limitations of traditional endovascular techniques, offering simpler deployment and potentially reducing thromboembolic risks associated with intraluminal devices [114, 115].

Machine Learning and AI

Artificial intelligence (AI) and machine learning (ML) are rapidly advancing fields with significant potential in interventional radiology and stroke imaging. AI techniques, particularly supervised ML and deep learning, can enhance workflow, image acquisition, reconstruction, and interpretation in acute stroke management [116, 117]. In interventional radiology, AI applications include image analysis, clinical predictive modeling, and trainee education [118]. AI can assist in various tasks such as lesion detection, segmentation, classification, large vessel occlusion detection, and prognostication [116, 119]. Despite challenges in implementation, AI in interventional radiology continues to advance, with potential applications in oncology, neurology, and cardiology [120]. Integration of AI with augmented reality, virtual reality, and radiogenomics may further enhance diagnostic accuracy and treatment planning [121]. As AI technologies evolve, they are expected to significantly improve interventional treatments' processes and efficacy [120, 122].

Looking forward, the field is poised for further advancements. Emerging technologies, such as flow diverters and intrasaccular devices, promise to address current limitations in aneurysm treatment, offering new options for complex cases. Additionally, the integration of machine learning and AI into clinical practice holds the potential to revolutionize treatment planning, device design, and outcome prediction. These innovations are likely to further improve procedural precision and patient care.

Conclusion

This chapter summarizes the discoveries and developments of neurointerventional coiling for cerebral aneurysms. Many of the key persons who led the development and maturation of this treatment modality are discussed. In addition, an in-depth look at the indications, potential complications, stent use, mechanisms of action, and future prospects for endovascular coiling would provide an indispensable asset to healthcare providers, researchers, and clinicians in the field.

References

[1] Sadasivan C, et al. An original flow diversion device for the treatment of intracranial aneurysms: evaluation in the rabbit elastase-induced model. *Stroke* (2009) 40 (3):952–958.

[2] Keedy A. An overview of intracranial aneurysms. *McGill Journal of Medicine: MJM* (2006) 9 (2):141.

[3] Tromp G, et al. Molecular basis and genetic predisposition to intracranial aneurysm. *Annals of Medicine* (2014) 46 (8):597–606.

[4] Munarriz PM, et al. Basic principles of hemodynamics and cerebral aneurysms. *World Neurosurgery* (2016) 88:311–319.

[5] Sforza DM, Putman CM, Cebral JR. Hemodynamics of cerebral aneurysms. *Annual Review of Fluid Mechanics* (2009) 41 (1):91–107.

[6] Cebral JR, Raschi M. Suggested connections between risk factors of intracranial aneurysms: a review. *Annals of Biomedical Engineering* (2013) 41:1366–1383.

[7] Penn DL, et al. The role of vascular remodeling and inflammation in the pathogenesis of intracranial aneurysms. *Journal of Clinical Neuroscience* (2014) 21 (1):28–32.

[8] Kanaan Y, et al. Evolution of endovascular therapy for aneurysm treatment: Historical overview. *Neurosurgical Focus* (2005) 18 (2):1–4.
[9] Prestigiacomo CJ. Historical perspectives: the microsurgical and endovascular treatment of aneurysms. *Neurosurgery* (2006) 59 (5):S3-39.
[10] Koebbe CJ, et al. Endovascular management of intracranial aneurysms: current experience and future advances. *Neurosurgery* (2006) 59 (5):S3-93.
[11] Maurice-Williams R, Lafuente J. Intracranial aneurysm surgery and its future. *Journal of the Royal Society of Medicine* (2003) 96 (11):540–543.
[12] Lee KS, et al. The evolution of intracranial aneurysm treatment techniques and future directions. *Neurosurgical Review* (2022) 45 (1):1–25.
[13] Shivashankar R, et al. Treatment of cerebral aneurysms—Surgical clipping or endovascular coiling: The guiding principles. *Seminars in Neurology* (2013).
[14] Jiang B, et al. Cerebral aneurysm treatment: modern neurovascular techniques. *Stroke and Vascular Neurology* (2016) 1 (3).
[15] Kretzer RM, Coon AL, Tamargo RJ. Walter E. Dandy's contributions to vascular neurosurgery: historical vignette. *Journal of Neurosurgery* (2010) 112 (6):1182–1191.
[16] Acciarri N, et al. Clipping techniques in cerebral aneurysm surgery. *Journal of Neurosurgical Sciences* (2015) 60 (1):83–94.
[17] Louw DF, Asfora WT, Sutherland GR. A brief history of aneurysm clips. *Neurosurgical Focus* (2001) 11 (2):1–4.
[18] Gkogkas C, et al. Endovascular treatment of intracranial aneurysms. *Minimally Invasive Neurosurgery* (2005):151–173.
[19] Guglielmi G. History of endovascular endosaccular occlusion of brain aneurysms: 1965–1990. *Interventional Neuroradiology* (2007) 13 (3):217–224.
[20] Rasmussen PA, Mayberg MR. Defining the natural history of unruptured aneurysms. *Stroke* (2004) 35 (1):232–233.
[21] Delgado AF, Andersson T, Delgado AF. Clinical outcome after surgical clipping or endovascular coiling for cerebral aneurysms: a pragmatic meta-analysis of randomized and non-randomized trials with short- and long-term follow-up. *Journal of NeuroInterventional Surgery* (2017) 9 (3):264–277.
[22] Bender MT, et al. Shifting treatment paradigms for ruptured aneurysms from open surgery to endovascular therapy over 25 years. *World Neurosurgery* (2017) 106:919–924.
[23] Dovey Z, et al. Guglielmi detachable coiling for intracranial aneurysms: the story so far. *Archives of Neurology* (2001) 58 (4):559–564.
[24] Rahal JP, Malek AM. Benefit of cone-beam computed tomography angiography in acute management of angiographically undetectable ruptured arteriovenous malformations. *Journal of Neurosurgery* (2013) 119 (4):1015–1020.
[25] Regli L, et al. Endovascular coiling compared with surgical clipping for the treatment of unruptured middle cerebral artery aneurysms: an update. 2002: Springer.
[26] Guglielmi G. Endovascular treatment of intracranial aneurysms with detachable coils and electrothrombosis, in *Interventional Neuroradiology*. 1993, Springer. p. 111–121.
[27] Hui P-j, et al. Intraoperative microvascular Doppler monitoring in intracranial aneurysm surgery. *Chinese Medical Journal* (2013) 126 (13):2424–2429.
[28] Viñuela F, Duckwiler G, Mawad M. Guglielmi detachable coil embolization of acute intracranial aneurysm: perioperative anatomical and clinical outcome in 403 patients. *Journal of Neurosurgery* (1997) 86 (3):475–482.
[29] Guglielmi G. The GDC system in the treatment of intracranial aneurysms. *Rivista di Neuroradiologia* (1996) 9 (4):463–470.
[30] Campos JK, et al. Advances in endovascular aneurysm management: flow modulation techniques with braided mesh devices. *Stroke and Vascular Neurology* (2020) 5 (1).
[31] Plowiecki L. From the Detachable Balloon to the Endothelial Prosthesis, SILK. *Interventional Neuroradiology: Journal of Peritherapeutic Neuroradiology, Surgical Procedures and Related Neurosciences* (2009) 15 (4):470–474.

[32] Berenstein A, et al. Treatment of cerebral aneurysms with hydrogel-coated platinum coils (HydroCoil): early single-center experience. *American Journal of Neuroradiology* (2006) 27 (9):1834–1840.

[33] Deshaies EM, et al. Determination of filling volumes in HydroCoil-treated aneurysms by using three-dimensional computerized tomography angiography. *Neurosurgical Focus* (2005) 18 (2):1–5.

[34] Reinges M, et al. Bare, bio-active and hydrogel-coated coils for endovascular treatment of experimentally induced aneurysms: long-term histological and scanning electron microscopy results. *Interventional Neuroradiology* (2010) 16 (2):139–150.

[35] Broeders JA, et al. Bioactive versus bare platinum coils for the endovascular treatment of intracranial aneurysms: systematic review and meta-analysis of randomized clinical trials. *Journal of NeuroInterventional Surgery* (2016) 8 (9):898–908.

[36] Fatania K, Patankar DT. Comprehensive review of the recent advances in devices for endovascular treatment of complex brain aneurysms. *The British Journal of Radiology* (2022) 95 (1129):20210538.

[37] Linfante I, Wakhloo AK. Brain aneurysms and arteriovenous malformations: advancements and emerging treatments in endovascular embolization. *Stroke* (2007) 38 (4):1411–1417.

[38] Higashida RT, et al. Treatment of unruptured intracranial aneurysms: a nationwide assessment of effectiveness. *American Journal of Neuroradiology* (2007) 28 (1):146–151.

[39] Bhattacharya J. *Pierre Lasjaunias*. 2008, British Medical Journal Publishing Group.

[40] Sahoo A, et al. History of neurointervention. *Seminars in Neurology* (2023). Thieme Medical Publishers, Inc.

[41] Crowley RW, et al. Endovascular advances for brain arteriovenous malformations. *Neurosurgery* (2014) 74:S74–S82.

[42] Higashida R, Hieshima G, Halbach V. Advances in the treatment of complex cerebrovascular disorders by interventional neurovascular techniques. *Circulation* (1991) 83 (2 Suppl):I196–206.

[43] Calixte A, et al. Neurointerventional radiology: History, present and future. *Journal of Radiology and Oncology* (2023) 7 (2):026–032.

[44] Peschillo S, et al. A systematic review and meta-analysis of treatment and outcome of blister-like aneurysms. *American Journal of Neuroradiology* (2016) 37 (5):856–861.

[45] Lee J, et al. Neurointerventional research between 2003 and 2012: slow growth, high interdisciplinary collaboration, and a low level of funding. *American Journal of Neuroradiology* (2014) 35 (10):1877–1882.

[46] Friedman DP, Maitino AJ. Endovascular interventional neuroradiologic procedures: who is performing them, how often, and where? A survey of academic and nonacademic radiology practices. *American Journal of Neuroradiology* (2003) 24 (9):1772–1777.

[47] Saber H, et al. Predictive analytics and machine learning in stroke and neurovascular medicine. *Neurological Research* (2019) 41 (8):681–690.

[48] Raymond J, et al. The TEAM trial: safety and efficacy of endovascular treatment of unruptured intracranial aneurysms in the prevention of aneurysmal hemorrhages: a randomized comparison with indefinite deferral of treatment in 2002 patients followed for 10 years. *Trials* (2008) 9:1–11.

[49] Yuki I, Murayama Y, Viñuela F. Endovascular management of dissecting vertebrobasilar artery aneurysms in patients presenting with acute subarachnoid hemorrhage. *Journal of Neurosurgery* (2005) 103 (4):649–655.

[50] Oushy S, et al. Recent advances in stent-assisted coiling of cerebral aneurysms. *Expert Review of Medical Devices* (2020) 17 (6):519–532.

[51] Pineda-Castillo SA, et al. Shape memory polymer-based endovascular devices: design criteria and future perspective. *Polymers* (2022) 14 (13):2526.

[52] Hulsbergen AF, et al. Long-term durability of open surgical versus endovascular repair of intracranial aneurysms: a systematic review and meta-analysis. *World Neurosurgery* (2019) 132:e820–e833.

[53] Szatmary Z, et al. Bioactive refinement for endosaccular treatment of intracranial aneurysms. *The Neuroradiology Journal* (2021) 34 (6):534–541.

[54] Hoh BL, et al. 2023 Guideline for the management of patients with aneurysmal subarachnoid hemorrhage: a guideline from the American Heart Association/American Stroke Association. *Stroke* (2023) 54 (7):e314–e370.

[55] Thompson BG, et al. Guidelines for the management of patients with unruptured intracranial aneurysms: a guideline for healthcare professionals from the American Heart Association/American Stroke Association. *Stroke* (2015) 46 (8):2368–2400.

[56] Gritti P, et al. A narrative review of adherence to subarachnoid hemorrhage guidelines. *Journal of Neurosurgical Anesthesiology* (2018) 30 (3):203–216.

[57] Eagleton MJ. Updates in endovascular procedural navigation. *Canadian Journal of Cardiology* (2022) 38 (5):662–671.

[58] Reid AW, Reid DB, Roditi GH. Vascular imaging: an unparalleled decade. *Journal of Endovascular Therapy* (2004) 11 (6_suppl):II-163–II-179.

[59] Hussain I, et al. Evolving navigation, robotics, and augmented reality in minimally invasive spine surgery. *Global Spine Journal* (2020) 10 (2_suppl):22S–33S.

[60] Johnson N. Imaging, navigation, and robotics in spine surgery. *Spine* (2016) 41:S32.

[61] Farooq H, et al. High-resolution imaging of the central nervous system: how novel imaging methods combined with navigation strategies will advance patient care. *Progress in Brain Research* (2015) 218:55–78.

[62] Kagadis GC, et al. Emerging technologies for image guidance and device navigation in interventional radiology. *Medical Physics* (2012) 39 (9):5768–5781.

[63] Hochmuth A, Spetzger U, Schumacher M. Comparison of three-dimensional rotational angiography with digital subtraction angiography in the assessment of ruptured cerebral aneurysms. *American Journal of Neuroradiology* (2002) 23 (7):1199–1205.

[64] Ishihara S, et al. 3D Rotational angiography: recent experience in the evaluation of cerebral aneurysms for treatment. *Interventional Neuroradiology* (2000) 6 (2):85–94.

[65] Tanoue S, et al. Three-dimensional reconstructed images after rotational angiography in the evaluation of intracranial aneurysms: surgical correlation. *Neurosurgery* (2000) 47 (4):866–871.

[66] Wong SC, et al. Benefits of 3D rotational DSA compared with 2D DSA in the evaluation of intracranial aneurysm. *Academic Radiology* (2012) 19 (6):701–707.

[67] Mohammed MAA, et al. A role for virtual reality in planning endovascular procedures. *Journal of Vascular and Interventional Radiology* (2018) 29 (7):971–974.

[68] Gering DT, et al. An integrated visualization system for surgical planning and guidance using image fusion and an open MR. *Journal of Magnetic Resonance Imaging* (2001) 13 (6):967–975.

[69] Jones DW, et al. Image fusion and 3-dimensional roadmapping in endovascular surgery. *Annals of Vascular Surgery* (2018) 52:302–311.

[70] Stangenberg L, et al. A novel tool for three-dimensional roadmapping reduces radiation exposure and contrast agent dose in complex endovascular interventions. *Journal of Vascular Surgery* (2015) 62 (2):448–455.

[71] Mitha AP, et al. Simulation and augmented reality in endovascular neurosurgery: lessons from aviation. *Neurosurgery* (2013) 72:A107–A114.

[72] Kuhlemann I, et al. Towards X-ray free endovascular interventions–using HoloLens for on-line holographic visualisation. *Healthcare Technology Letters* (2017) 4 (5):184–187.

[73] Schoenhagen P, et al. Three-dimensional imaging in the context of minimally invasive and transcatheter cardiovascular interventions using multi-detector computed tomography: from pre-operative planning to intra-operative guidance. *European Heart Journal* (2010) 31 (22):2727–2740.

[74] Vanderbilt E, et al. Evaluation of aneurysm flow diverter (stent) treatment using multi-angled 1000 fps high-speed angiography (HSA) and optical flow (OF). *Proceedings of SPIE* (2024).

[75] Wagner MG, et al. Biplane reconstruction and visualization of virtual endoscopic and fluoroscopic views for interventional device navigation. *Proceedings of SPIE* (2016).

[76] Bellemare C, Poder T. Effectiveness of biplane angiography compared to monoplane angiography for vascular neuro-interventions: a systematic review of the literature. *Clinical Radiology* (2017) 72 (7):612.e1–612.e5.

[77] Jang D-K, et al. Monoplane 3D overlay roadmap versus conventional biplane 2D roadmap technique for neurointerventional procedures. *Neurointervention* (2016) 11 (2):105–113.

[78] Nagesh SS, et al. Simultaneous biplane high speed 1000 fps x-ray angiography (HSAngio). *Proceedings of SPIE* (2022).

[79] Santillan A, et al. E-058 Technical note: BI-plane 3D guidance technique for neuro-interventional procedures: feasibility and potential benefits. *Journal of Neurology, Neurosurgery & Psychiatry* (2018) 89:e1.

[80] Nunna R, et al. Advances in the Endovascular Management of Cerebrovascular Disease. *Missouri Medicine* (2024) 121 (2):127.

[81] Eskandari MK. Cerebral embolic protection. *Seminars in Vascular Surgery* (2005) 18 (2):103–110.

[82] Loftus M, Schumacher H, Meyers P. Interventional therapy for carotid artery disease using angioplasty and stenting with embolic protection. *Minerva Cardioangiologica* (2006) 54 (5):679–685.

[83] Lauzier DC, et al. A review of technological innovations leading to modern endovascular brain aneurysm treatment. *Frontiers in Neurology* (2023) 14:1156887.

[84] Fargen KM, Hoh BL. Flow diversion technologies in evolution: a review of the first two generations of flow diversion devices. *World Neurosurgery* (2015) 84 (2):254–256.

[85] Chalouhi N, et al. Stent-assisted coiling versus balloon remodeling of wide-neck aneurysms: comparison of angiographic outcomes. *American Journal of Neuroradiology* (2013) 34 (10):1987–1992.

[86] Consoli A, et al. Assisted coiling of saccular wide-necked unruptured intracranial aneurysms: stent versus balloon. *Journal of NeuroInterventional Surgery* (2016) 8 (1):52–57.

[87] Cai K, et al. Comparison of stent-assisted coiling and balloon-assisted coiling in the treatment of ruptured wide-necked intracranial aneurysms in the acute period. *World Neurosurgery* (2016) 96:316–321.

[88] Aydin K, et al. Safety, efficacy, and durability of stent plus balloon-assisted coiling for the treatment of wide-necked bifurcation intracranial aneurysms. *Neurosurgery* (2021) 88 (5):1028–1037.

[89] Gunkan A, et al. Stent plus balloon-assisted coiling with low-profile braided stents in the treatment of complex wide-necked intracranial bifurcation aneurysms. *The Neuroradiology Journal* (2024).

[90] Piotin M, Blanc R. Balloons and stents in the endovascular treatment of cerebral aneurysms: vascular anatomy remodeled. *Frontiers in Neurology* (2014) 5:41.

[91] Gupta AK, et al. Real-world evidence of superiority of endovascular repair in treating ruptured abdominal aortic aneurysm. *Journal of Vascular Surgery* (2018) 68 (1):74–81.

[92] Al-Mufti F, et al. Flow diversion for intracranial aneurysm management: a new standard of care. *Neurotherapeutics* (2016) 13 (3):582–589.

[93] Chancellor B, et al. Flow diversion for intracranial aneurysm treatment: trials involving flow diverters and long-term outcomes. *Neurosurgery* (2020) 86 (Supplement_1):S36–S45.

[94] Walcott BP, et al. Flow diversion for the treatment of intracranial aneurysms. *JAMA Neurology* (2016) 73 (8):1002–1008.

[95] Komotar RJ, et al. Controversies in the endovascular management of cerebral vasospasm after intracranial aneurysm rupture and future directions for therapeutic approaches. *Neurosurgery* (2008) 62 (4):897–907.

[96] Patsalides A, et al. Standard of practice: embolization of ruptured and unruptured intracranial aneurysms. *Journal of NeuroInterventional Surgery* (2013) 5 (4):283–288.

[97] Turc G, et al. European Stroke Organisation (ESO)-European Society for Minimally Invasive Neurological Therapy (ESMINT) guidelines on mechanical thrombectomy in acute ischemic stroke. *Journal of NeuroInterventional Surgery* (2023) 15 (8):e8–e8.

[98] Meyers PM, et al. Reporting standards for endovascular repair of saccular intracranial cerebral aneurysms. *Stroke* (2009) 40 (5):e366–e379.

[99] Ajiboye N, et al. Unruptured cerebral aneurysms: evaluation and management. *The Scientific World Journal* (2015) 2015:954954.

[100] Krishna V, et al. Impact of integrated cerebrovascular program on outcomes in patients with intracranial aneurysms. *Journal of NeuroInterventional Surgery* (2013) 5 (3):264–268.

[101] Tjoumakaris SI, et al. ARISE I Consensus Review on the Management of Intracranial Aneurysms. *Stroke* (2024) 55 (5):1428–1437.

[102] Qiao Y, et al. Current and future directions in interventional neuro-oncology—are we there yet? *Journal of NeuroInterventional Surgery* (2024).

[103] Linares G. On the Horizon: Innovative Techniques and Procedures, in *Neurointervention in the Medical Specialties: A Comprehensive Guide*. 2022, Springer. p. 273–277.

[104] Saatci I, et al. Treatment of intracranial aneurysms using the pipeline flow-diverter embolization device: a single-center experience with long-term follow-up results. *American Journal of Neuroradiology* (2012) 33 (8):1436–1446.

[105] Wong GK, et al. Flow diverters for treatment of intracranial aneurysms: current status and ongoing clinical trials. *Journal of Clinical Neuroscience* (2011) 18 (6):737–740.

[106] Giacomini L, et al. Neurovascular reconstruction with flow diverter stents for the treatment of 87 intracranial aneurysms: clinical results. *Interventional Neuroradiology* (2015) 21 (3):292–299.

[107] Crobeddu E, et al. Marked decrease in coil and stent utilization following introduction of flow diversion technology. *Journal of NeuroInterventional Surgery* (2013) 5 (4):351–353.

[108] Chalouhi N, et al. Matched comparison of flow diversion and coiling in small, noncomplex intracranial aneurysms. *Neurosurgery* (2017) 81 (1):92–97.

[109] Chalouhi N, et al. A single pipeline embolization device is sufficient for treatment of intracranial aneurysms. *American Journal of Neuroradiology* (2014) 35 (8):1562–1566.

[110] Hecker C, et al. Comparison of the Contour Neurovascular System and Woven EndoBridge device for treatment of wide-necked cerebral aneurysms at a bifurcation or sidewall. *Journal of Neurosurgery* (2023) 139 (2):563–572.

[111] Islim FI, Saleem N, Patankar T. A review and journey in intrasaccular treatment of intracranial aneurysms. *Interventional Neuroradiology* (2023).

[112] Kashkoush A, et al. Comparative effectiveness of stent-assisted coiling and Woven EndoBridge embolization for the treatment of unruptured wide-neck bifurcation intracranial aneurysms. *Journal of Neurosurgery* (2022) 138 (6):1487–1493.

[113] Heiferman DM, et al. A new era in the treatment of wide necked bifurcation aneurysms: Intrasaccular flow disruption. *Interventional Neuroradiology* (2024) 30 (1):31–36.

[114] Mine B, et al. Stent-assisted coiling of unruptured intracranial aneurysms: long-term follow-up in 164 patients with 183 aneurysms. *Journal of Neuroradiology* (2014) 41 (5):322–328.

[115] White R, et al. Investigating angiographic injection parameters for cerebral aneurysm hemodynamic characterization using patient-specific simulated angiograms. *Proceedings of SPIE* (2023).

[116] Soun J, et al. Artificial intelligence and acute stroke imaging. *American Journal of Neuroradiology* (2021) 42 (1):2–11.

[117] Yedavalli VS, et al. Artificial intelligence in stroke imaging: current and future perspectives. *Clinical Imaging* (2021) 69:246–254.

[118] Meek RD, Lungren MP, Gichoya JW. Machine learning for the interventional radiologist. *American Journal of Roentgenology* (2019) 213 (4):782–784.

[119] Zhu G, et al. Artificial intelligence and stroke imaging: a west coast perspective. *Neuroimaging Clinics of North America* (2020) 30 (4):479–492.

[120] Zhang J, et al. How AI and Robotics Will Advance Interventional Radiology: Narrative Review and Future Perspectives. *Diagnostics* (2024) 14 (13):1393.

[121] von Ende E, et al. Artificial intelligence, augmented reality, and virtual reality advances and applications in interventional radiology. *Diagnostics* (2023) 13 (5):892.

[122] Iezzi R, et al. Artificial intelligence in interventional radiology: a literature review and future perspectives. *Journal of Oncology* (2019) 2019:6153041.

Chapter 8

The History and Development of Flow Diversion

Modhi A. Alhussenan[1,*]
Ahmed Aljuboori[2,†]**, MD**
Ahmed Muthana[3,‡]**, MD**
and Samer S. Hoz[4,§]**, MD**
[1]King Saud Medical City, Riyadh, Saudi Arabia
[2]Department of Neurosurgery, Geisinger Clinic, PA, USA
[3]Department of Neurosurgery, University of Baghdad, Baghdad, Iraq
[4]Department of Neurosurgery, University of Cincinnati Medical Center, Cincinnati, OH, USA

Abstract

Flow diversion is one of the most revolutionary treatment options that has shifted the endovascular techniques for the management of aneurysms, cavernous-carotid fistula, and coexisting aneurysms in case of arteriovenous malformation. It has emerged as a great choice for recurrent aneurysms or aneurysms with complex shapes such as fusiform aneurysms or bifurcated aneurysms where other management options are deemed difficult or impossible. They work mainly by remodelling the parent artery and excluding the affected aneurysm or fistula from the circulation by providing a scaffold for endothelialisation which causes blood stagnation and gradual thrombosis of the artery. This chapter provides an overview of the historical evolution and development of flow diversion in the management of intracranial aneurysms, highlighting the indications, types, mechanisms of actions, possible complications, and future directions.

Keywords: flow diversion, pipeline embolization device, endovascular, aneurysms, fistula

* Corresponding Author's Email: alhussinan.modhi@yahoo.com
† Corresponding Author's Email: ahmedaljuboori9494@gmail.com
‡ Corresponding Author's Email: ahmed.m.najm@gmail.com
§ Corresponding Author's Email: hozsamer2055@gmail.com

In: World History of Neurointerventional Surgery
Editors: Xianli Lv and Zhongxue Wu
ISBN: 979-8-89530-792-2

Introduction

In recent years, the field of neurointerventional surgery has undergone substantial evolution, with new methodologies and strategies aimed at improving patient outcomes and mitigating procedural risks. This advancement is particularly notable in the realm of endovascular treatments for intracranial aneurysms. Historically, endovascular techniques such as coil embolization have proven effective for a range of aneurysm types. However, these methods face significant limitations when dealing with large (15–25 mm) and giant (>25 mm) wide-neck cerebral aneurysms. These aneurysms present considerable challenges due to their size, complex anatomy, and difficult surgical access, often leading to less favorable outcomes even in the hands of expert neurosurgeons [1].

The primary goals in managing intracranial aneurysms include preventing rebleeding, alleviating mass effects, and avoiding thromboembolic complications [2]. Despite the effectiveness of coils in many cases, they are less successful in achieving the aforementioned desired outcomes for wide-neck and complex aneurysms, where recurrence rates of up to 20% have been reported [3]. Recent advancements in neurointerventional techniques have highlighted the potential of endoluminal devices, such as flow diverters, to offer significant improvements over traditional endosaccular therapies. Unlike conventional coil embolization methods, which often face limitations with wide-necked aneurysms and carry risks of aneurysm perforation, flow diverters present a promising alternative. The initial theory behind flow diverters proposed that these intraluminal specialized stents could effectively occlude aneurysms by redirecting blood flow without the need to fill the aneurysm sac with coils [4]. This approach aims to achieve aneurysm occlusion while preserving the integrity of the parent artery and adjacent smaller vessels [5].

Flow diverters feature higher metal coverage and lower porosity compared to traditional stents, allowing them to effectively redirect blood flow away from the aneurysm, whether it is saccular or fusiform in shape [6]. They were specifically designed to overcome the limitations of earlier endovascular techniques. These advanced devices offer a more effective solution by addressing the challenges posed by complex aneurysm anatomy and providing improved outcomes compared to traditional methods [7]. Their introduction has marked a significant advancement in the treatment of cerebrovascular disorders, providing a new approach to managing aneurysms that are challenging to treat with conventional methods [8]. The evolution of flow diverter technology highlights the ongoing progress in this field, reflecting continued innovation aimed at improving treatment outcomes and expanding the range of aneurysms that can be effectively managed [9]. Despite these advances, recurrence rates and other challenges are still faced, but improvements stimulate the neurointerventional community and developers to continue addressing these issues through ongoing research and exploration [1].

Types of Flow Diversion

Each type of flow diverter has unique features tailored to specific clinical needs and vessel characteristics, and the choice of device often depends on factors such as aneurysm size, location, and the patient's vascular anatomy [7]. Among the prominent flow diverters is the Pipeline device from Medtronic, USA (Figure 1). Known for its high metal coverage, the

Pipeline stent is FDA-approved and widely used due to its effectiveness in managing aneurysms by creating a dense mesh that diverts blood flow away from the aneurysm. Similarly, the Surpass device by Stryker, USA, also FDA-approved, offers the highest metal coverage among flow diverters, enhancing its efficacy in reducing aneurysm flow. In contrast, the Silk Vista stent from BALT, Germany, is designed to provide flexibility and adaptability, making it particularly useful for small vessels. The FRED (Flow Re-Direction Endoluminal Device) by Microvention, USA, stands out for its unique design that effectively facilitates flow diversion. The Derivo flow diverter from Acandis, Germany, is a newer device tailored for specific aneurysm types, offering advanced technological features. Lastly, the p64 and p48 stents from Phenox, Germany, are specifically designed for smaller vessels and are recognized for their reduced thrombogenicity, which minimizes the risk of clot formation [8].

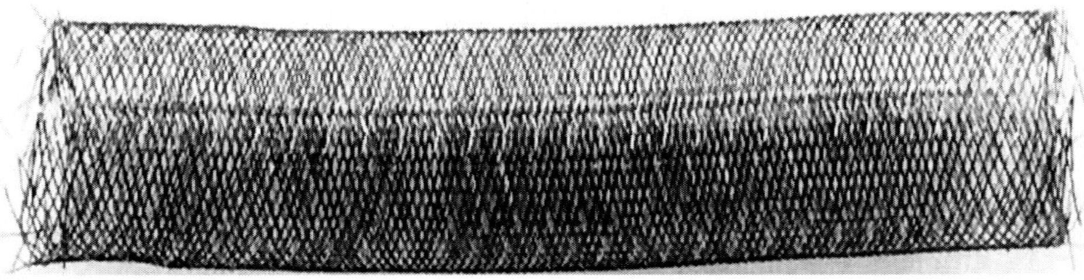

Figure 1. Pipeline embolic device (Medtronic, USA).

The technological advancements in these devices include improved fluoroscopic visibility, which allows for precise deployment and positioning of the stent, thereby ensuring accurate placement and optimal treatment outcomes [9]. Reduced thrombogenicity is another critical feature, as it helps prevent complications such as vessel occlusion or embolism by minimizing the risk of clot formation on the stent [10]. Furthermore, the flexibility and conformability of these stents are essential for navigating complex anatomical configurations and adapting to varying vessel diameters, which contributes to their success in treating challenging aneurysms [11]. These technological innovations collectively enhance the efficacy and safety of flow diverter stents, offering improved outcomes for patients with intracranial aneurysms.

Mechanism of Action of Flow Diversion

Generally, the mechanisms of action for flow diverters (FDs) involve three key phases: the hemodynamic phase, the thrombus formation phase, and the endothelialization phase. Initially, the hemodynamic phase involves the FD's mesh creating resistance to blood flow into the aneurysm, which reduces pressure within the aneurysm sac [12]. This reduction in blood flow leads to the thrombus formation phase, where the altered hemodynamics activate clotting mechanisms, resulting in the formation of a thrombus inside the aneurysm. This thrombus acts as a barrier, preventing further blood entry and stabilizing the aneurysm (Figure 2). Finally, in the endothelialization phase, endothelial cells migrate from the parent artery over the thrombus and FD surface, forming a new layer of endothelial tissue. This process integrates the FD into the arterial wall, ensuring long-term occlusion of the aneurysm and minimizing the risk of rupture [12].

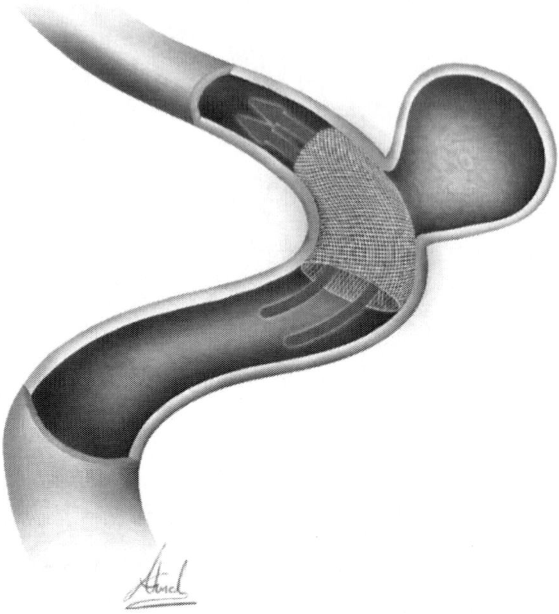

Figure 2. Schematic illustration depicts the concept of flow diversion in the treatment of intracranial aneurysms—illustration prepared by Ahmed Muthana and courtesy of Samer Hoz.

By using the Pipeline Embolization Device (PED) as a primary example to elucidate the general concept of how to flow diverters function due to its pioneering use and extensive study, the PED represents a sophisticated approach to aneurysm treatment that is conceptually closer to surgical aneurysm clipping than to endosaccular coil occlusion. Both the PED and surgical clipping share the fundamental goal of excluding the aneurysmal segment by bridging healthy segments of the parent artery [13].

The PED operates as an endovascular scaffold that effectively reconstructs the artery across the diseased segment. By placing the PED, the aneurysm is excluded, and the device creates a new, structurally secure segment of the artery linking the normal proximal and distal segments [14]. The process involves a gradual transition from initial flow disruption to complete angiographic occlusion, ultimately restoring the parent artery to a normal anatomical configuration. Over time, the PED becomes covered with neointima and endothelium, forming a healthy new endoluminal surface and isolating the abnormal segment [15].

In contrast, endosaccular coil occlusion addresses the aneurysm differently. This method involves filling the aneurysm sac with coils to induce thrombosis and seal off the aneurysm but does not directly address or reconstruct the underlying diseased segment of the parent artery. After coil placement, the aneurysm is sealed biologically, but the segment of the artery containing the disease remains untreated.

Thus, while the PED and surgical clipping both focus on creating a new, healthy artery segment to exclude the aneurysm, endosaccular coils primarily target the aneurysm sac without addressing the underlying arterial pathology.

Complications of Flow Diversion

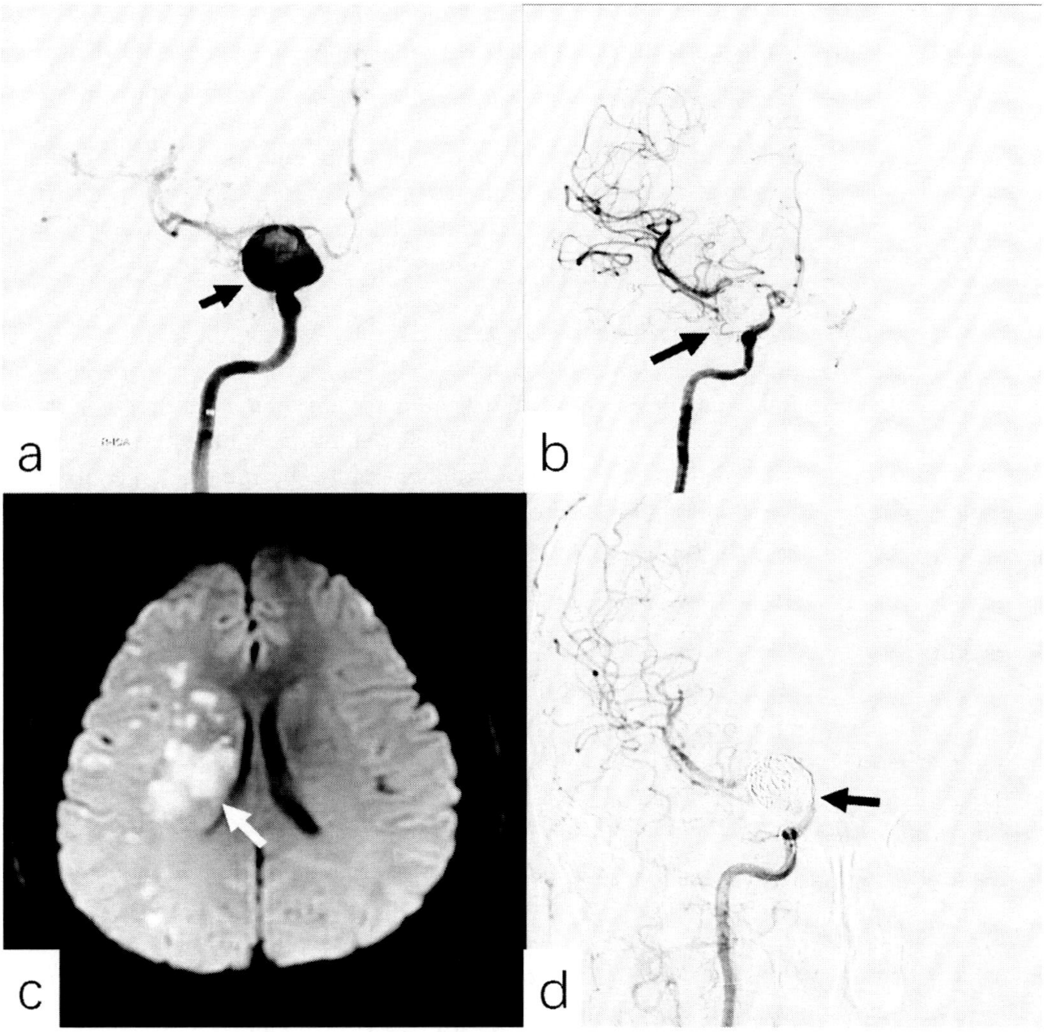

Figure 3. A 52-year-old female patient presented with transient ischemic attack. a, the right internal carotid artery angiogram, frontal view, showed a giant aneurysm in the ophthalmic segment of the internal carotid artery (arrow). b, the post Pipeline flow diverter treatment, the carotid artery angiogram showed that the aneurysm was almost completely occluded on the frontal view of the angiogram. c, MR imaging, DWI, axial view, showed multiple cerebral infarction in the right hemisphere, which was related to thrombus shedding after a Pipeline flow diverter placement (arrow). The patient developed left limb paralysis after treatment. The patient recovered completely after 12 months. d, the right internal carotid artery angiogram at 12 months showed complete occlusion of the aneurysm and vascular stenosis due to endothelial hyperplasia (arrow).

Flow diverters have significantly advanced the treatment of complex intracranial aneurysms, offering promising outcomes for various challenging aneurysm types with complication rates comparable to traditional methods [12]. Despite these advancements, their use entails several inherent risks. Complications can arise at any phase of the treatment timeline, including during the periprocedural period, immediately after the procedure, or as delayed sequelae. Notable thromboembolic and ischemic complications include acute and hyperacute stent thrombosis, large-vessel occlusion, and perforator or side-branch occlusion, with symptomatic thromboembolic events occurring in 2-8% of cases and asymptomatic ischemic events detected by diffusion-weighted imaging reaching up to 63% (Figure3) [16]. Hemorrhagic complications such as intraoperative hemorrhage, delayed aneurysm rupture, and remote hematomas are also significant concerns [7]. Additionally, other complications include in-stent thrombosis or stenosis, perforator infarction—particularly with posterior circulation aneurysms—and vessel perforation during device deployment, with delayed occlusion of covered collateral branches also reported [7]. Although flow diverters are associated with a higher incidence of thromboembolic events due to their high-surface-coverage ratio, which can trigger platelet activation and thrombus formation, dual antiplatelet therapy is employed both prior to and for at least three months following the procedure to mitigate these risks [17].

Despite the inherent risks, the clinical advantages of flow diverters in treating complex aneurysms frequently outweigh the potential complications, particularly when patients are carefully selected. Ongoing advancements are focused on enhancing these devices and mitigating associated risks. For example, innovations like the Shield technology for the Pipeline Embolization Device aim to decrease stent thrombogenicity before endothelialization, potentially offering alternative strategies to dual antiplatelet therapy. However, these innovations also carry a risk of hemorrhagic complications [8].

Conclusion

Flow diverters have represented a revolutionary advance in the treatment of intracranial aneurysms, offering a sophisticated approach to managing complex aneurysm types that were previously challenging to treat. Their ability to redirect blood flow and facilitate aneurysm occlusion while preserving the parent artery has been a significant breakthrough. However, their use is not without risks. Complications such as thromboembolic events, hemorrhagic issues, and device-specific challenges must be carefully managed. The evolution of flow diverter technology continues to enhance their efficacy and safety profile, contributing to improved patient outcomes and expanded treatment possibilities. Ongoing research and technological innovations are essential for further optimizing these devices and minimizing associated risks, ensuring that flow diverters remain a valuable tool in the neurointerventional arsenal.

References

[1] Briganti F, et al. Endovascular treatment of cerebral aneurysms using flow-diverter devices: a systematic review. *The Neuroradiology Journal* (2015) 28 (4):365–375.

[2] Ruan C, et al. Endovascular coiling vs. surgical clipping for unruptured intracranial aneurysm: a meta-analysis. *British Journal of Neurosurgery* (2015) 29 (4):485–492.

[3] Zhao B, et al. Endovascular coiling of wide-neck and wide-neck bifurcation aneurysms: a systematic review and meta-analysis. *American Journal of Neuroradiology* (2016) 37 (9):1700–1705.

[4] Darsaut TE, et al. Flow diverters failing to occlude experimental bifurcation or curved sidewall aneurysms: an in vivo study in canines. *Journal of Neurosurgery* (2012) 117 (1):37–44.

[5] Gentric J, et al. The success of flow diversion in large and giant sidewall aneurysms may depend on the size of the defect in the parent artery. *American Journal of Neuroradiology* (2014) 35 (11):2119–2124.

[6] Suzuki T, et al. Selection of helical braided flow diverter stents based on hemodynamic performance and mechanical properties. *Journal of NeuroInterventional Surgery* (2017) 9 (10):999–1005.
[7] Lv X, et al. Flow-diverter devices in the treatment of intracranial aneurysms: a meta-analysis and systematic review. *The Neuroradiology Journal* (2016) 29 (1):66–71.
[8] Kühn AL, Gounis MJ, Puri AS. Introduction: history and development of flow diverter technology and evolution. *Neurosurgery* (2020) 86 (Supplement_1):S3–S10.
[9] Enriquez-Marulanda A, Young MM, Taussky P. Flow diversion: a disruptive technology coming of age. Lessons learned and challenges for the future. *Journal of Neurosurgery* (2023) 139 (5):1317–1327.
[10] Brinjikji W, et al. Endovascular treatment of intracranial aneurysms with flow diverters: a meta-analysis. *Stroke* (2013) 44 (2):442–447.
[11] Shin D-S, et al. The evolution of flow-diverting stents for cerebral aneurysms; historical review, modern application, complications, and future direction. *Journal of Korean Neurosurgical Society* (2020) 63 (2):137–152.
[12] Alderazi YJ, et al. Flow diverters for intracranial aneurysms. *Stroke Research and Treatment* (2014) 2014:415653.
[13] Twitchell S, et al. Analysis of cerebrovascular aneurysm treatment cost: retrospective cohort comparison of clipping, coiling, and flow diversion. *Neurosurgical Focus* (2018) 44 (5):E3.
[14] Leung G, Tsang A, Lui W. Pipeline embolization device for intracranial aneurysm: a systematic review. *Clinical Neuroradiology* (2012) 22:295–303.
[15] Deutschmann H, et al. Long-term follow-up after treatment of intracranial aneurysms with the Pipeline embolization device: results from a single center. *American Journal of Neuroradiology* (2012) 33 (3):481–486.
[16] Guédon A, et al. Very late ischemic complications in flow-diverter stents: a retrospective analysis of a single-center series. *Journal of Neurosurgery* (2016) 125 (4):929–935.
[17] Hohenstatt S, et al. Prasugrel Single Antiplatelet Therapy versus Aspirin and Clopidogrel Dual Antiplatelet Therapy for Flow Diverter Treatment for Cerebral Aneurysms: A Retrospective Multicenter Study. *American Journal of Neuroradiology* (2024) 45 (5):592–598.

Chapter 9

The History and Development of Neck-Bridging Devices

Alexander Sirakov[1,*]
Kristina Sirakova[2]
and Stanimir Sirakov[1]
[1]Department of Radiology, University Hospital St. Ivan Rilski, Sofia, Bulgaria
[2]Medical University, Sofia, Bulgaria

Abstract

This chapter reviews the historical and technical aspects of the Comaneci and Cascade devices in the context of temporary stent-assisted coiling for cerebral aneurysms. It includes insights from our clinical experiences, highlighting our tips and tricks that can enhance procedural success and mitigate complications. By examining both devices, the chapter aims to provide readers with a comprehensive understanding of their applications, as well as practical recommendations that can be beneficial in real-world settings.

Keywords: comaneci device, cascade device, stent-assisted coiling, cerebral aneurysms, tips and tricks

Introduction

This chapter aims to explore the current state of temporary stent-assisted techniques, along with newly developed temporary neck-bridging stent-like devices for the treatment of intracranial aneurysms. The content presented here is drawn from a comprehensive review of the latest literature and the authors' own clinical experiences. Additionally, case examples and illustrative figures related to these devices will be featured. Key deployment techniques, troubleshooting strategies, and practical tips will also be outlined.

* Corresponding Author's Email: sirakovalex@yahoo.com

In: World History of Neurointerventional Surgery
Editors: Xianli Lv and Zhongxue Wu
ISBN: 979-8-89530-792-2

Historical Overview

Just over two decades ago, the endovascular treatment of intracranial aneurysms primarily relied on straightforward endosaccular coil obliteration. This approach is particularly suitable for aneurysms with a well-defined neck that serves as a clear boundary to the parent artery, eliminating the need for additional devices. However, in some cases, achieving durable and complete aneurysm occlusion remains challenging. Additionally, certain aneurysmal morphologies can lead to complications, including coil herniation, migration, and even occlusion of the parent artery. A meta-analysis performed in 2011 concluded that despite the enthusiasm of the endovascular therapy the conventional coiling yields debatable results with over 20% risk of aneurysm recurrence and nearly 10% of the aneurysm mandate following retreatment. The authors pointed out that larger aneurysms, those with unfavourable morfologpy and wider neck seemed untreatable [1]. Neurointerventionalistst were pondering about a minimally invasive strategy that could safely and permanently exclude such technically obstructing aneurysmsm and offer a durable solution to the surgical clipping [2].

Initially the limitations of the conventional coiling techniques have lead to conseptual and technical improvements of the coil technology [3, 4]. For example, coils with specific geometrical desings that were meant to fill the aneurysm tightly and ehance the durability of the coil mass inside aneurysms with irregular shape. Secondly, coils with three-dimensional preshaped frame were designed to ensure stable initial coil structure that could facilitate the subsequent embolizational coiling process with other coils that were specifically designed to fill tight and small gaps insde the anerurysms.

To better address the challenges associated with endovascular treatment of wide-neck aneurysms, balloon remodeling and stent-assisted techniques (SAC) were developed to improve occlusion rates during coil embolization [5-7]. These advancements have expanded treatment options, making it possible to successfully manage aneurysms with complex geometries. Balloon remodeling, also known as the balloon-assisted coiling (BAC) technique, involves the temporary inflation and positioning of a balloon catheter across the aneurysm neck. This approach facilitates safe coil placement and the formation of a stable, three-dimensional coil structure in aneurysms with unfavorable neck-to-dome ratios.

The permanent placement of an intraluminal implant within an intracranial vessel necessitates the initiation of platelet inhibition, which increases procedural risks. This is particularly concerning for patients requiring intensive care, such as those with acute subarachnoid hemorrhage (SAH), where minimizing bleeding risk is crucial. Furthermore, the use of antiplatelet therapy, often in the form of dual antiplatelet therapy (DAPT) recommended for cases involving permanent stent placement, raises the likelihood of cerebral hemorrhage in areas of ischemic brain tissue affected by post hemorrhagic vasospasm [8, 9]. Therefore, avoiding permanent stent placement is advantageous for patients with acute SAH and those who may require external ventricular drainage as a complication of the ruptured aneurysm. That's probably why many interventionalists favor BAC over SAC for treating ruptured wide-neck aneurysms, as it eliminates the need for antiplatelet therapy. While balloons are a viable option for managing ruptured intracranial aneurysms, meta-analyses indicate that their occlusive effectiveness tends to be lower compared to stent therapy at six months or more following the procedure [7]. In cases of bifurcation IAs, there has been interest in the combined use of multiple stents or balloons, which not only enhances aneurysm occlusion rates but also theoretically increases the possible risk of ischemic and technical complications [10].

Temporary stent-assisted coiling for aneurysm treatment combines the benefits of stent-assisted coiling and balloon-assisted coiling techniques, enhancing support and stability during the coiling procedure [11]. The idea of temporary stent scaffolding has gained significant attention globally, with techniques such as "semi-jailing" being utilized. This technique involves the partial deployment of a stent across the aneurysm neck to provide temporary support during coiling [12].

For this procedure, two microcatheters are utilized. The first microcatheter is positioned to cover the aneurysm neck while deploying the stent. The second microcatheter is then advanced into the aneurysm for coil embolization. This advancement can occur either before or after the stent is deployed. The stent is positioned to cover the aneurysm neck but is not completely released at this stage. Once coil embolization is complete, the stent can be retracted (Figure 1). In the rare event of coil protrusion during stent retrieval, the retraction is halted, the stent is redeployed, and then it can be permanently implanted if necessary [13].

The reversible nature of this technique offers a significant advantage by eliminating the need for DAPT. This is particularly advantageous for patients with subarachnoid hemorrhage, as avoiding DAPT can simplify their management and facilitate treatment for complications such as hydrocephalus [14].

Temporary stent-assisted coiling has become a recognized standard technique for treating wide-neck aneurysms. Initial experiences primarily involved the Enterprise stent, followed by various Solitaire device iterations [11]. It didn't take long for the market to establish a dedicated subset of devices designed specifically for scaffolding, which are temporary, fully resettable, and recapturable. Currently, there are two specific devices available on the market that are designed to provide temporary assistance during endovascular coil embolization: the Comaneci and Cascade devices.

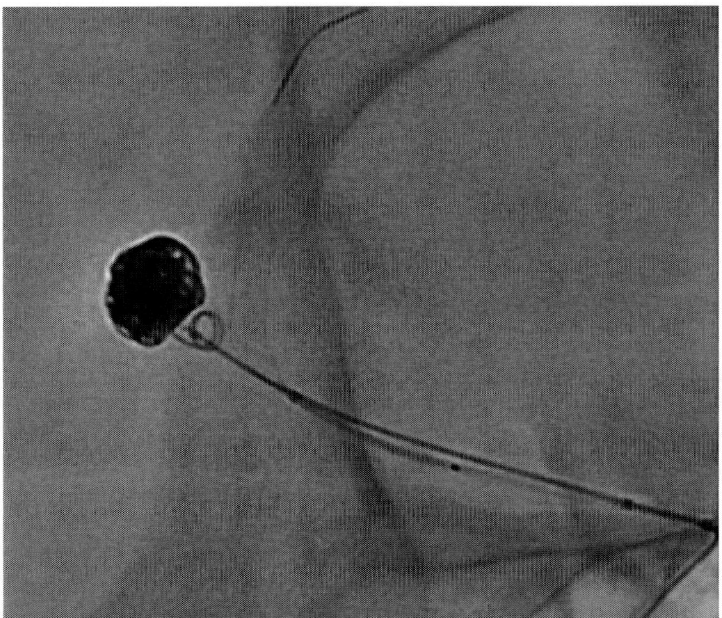

Figure 1. Conseptual application of the temporary stent-assisted coiling technique where a partially depylied retrievable stent has been deployed to facilitate the coiling of a residual cerebral aneurysms.

Dedicated Devices for Temporary Stent-Assisted Coil Embolization of Cerebral Aneurysms

In recent years, temporary neck bridging devices, particularly the Comaneci device (Rapid Medical, Yokneam, Israel) and the Cascade device (Perflow Medical, St. Netanya, Israel), have garnered significant attention. Both devices can be viewed as advancements of the traditional temporary stent technique, which previously utilized the Enterprise and Solitaire stents in off-label applications.

While both devices share a similar appearance, featuring a non-occlusive and highly compliant temporary mesh designed to provide mechanical support during the coil embolization of the target aneurysm, they possess distinct differences in their design and functionality. Specific device characteristics and designs will be described below and in detail.

The Comaneci Device

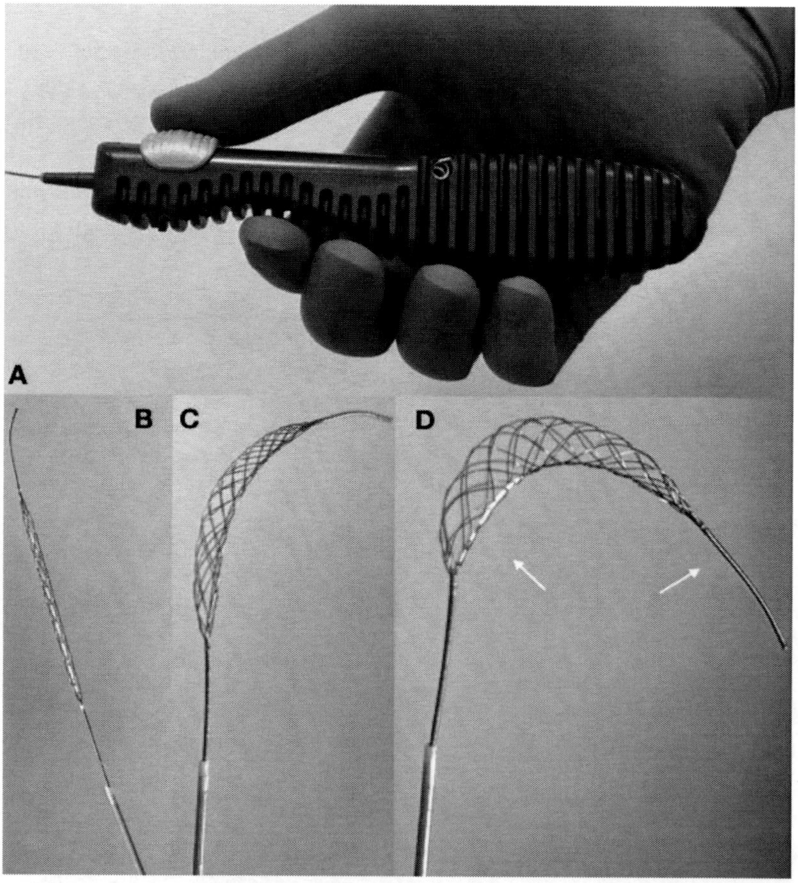

Figure 2. The Comaneci 17 device seen straightened and deployed out of the 0.017-inch microcatheter. The sliding of the manually controlled button starts to (a) inflate and expand the device as it curves outward to its crescent-like form (b, c, d). Contraction is achieved by manipulation of the core wire within the braided mesh. Note how the device's tip follows the convex shape of the remodelling reticulation (c, d, (white arrow)).

The Comaneci device is engineered to serve as a temporary mechanical scaffold for saccular aneurysms and has received both CE and FDA approval. There are three commercially available versions of the device: Comaneci, Comaneci Petit, and Comaneci 17, all of which are compatible with modern 0.021-inch and 0.017-inch microcatheter technologies.

This device features a compliant and braided metallic neck-bridging mesh constructed from fully radiopaque nitinol wire. It is mounted on a 182-cm core wire, equipped with a flexible distal tip that measures 7 mm in length. The device is operated using a manually controllable grip handle that allows for precise inflation and deflation maneuvers. Once fully inflated, the device adopts a semi-compliant crescent-like shape, providing effective support during the coil embolization process (Figure 2).

The procedure for employing the Comaneci device begins with rotational angiography to accurately visualize the target aneurysm and understand the anatomy of the parent vessel. A coiling microcatheter is advanced over a microwire into the aneurysmal sac, where a partial deployment of the initial coil secures the microcatheter in place.

Following this, the chosen Comaneci device is prepared within a second microcatheter, which has an internal diameter of either 0.0165 inches (for the Comaneci 17) or 0.021 inches (for the other two versions). This microcatheter is then navigated to the optimal position across the neck of the aneurysm. The deployment of the neck-bridging mesh requires the careful retraction of the microcatheter while keeping the Comaneci wire fixed. The operator utilizes a control grip handle to manually inflate the device until the desired expansion is achieved.

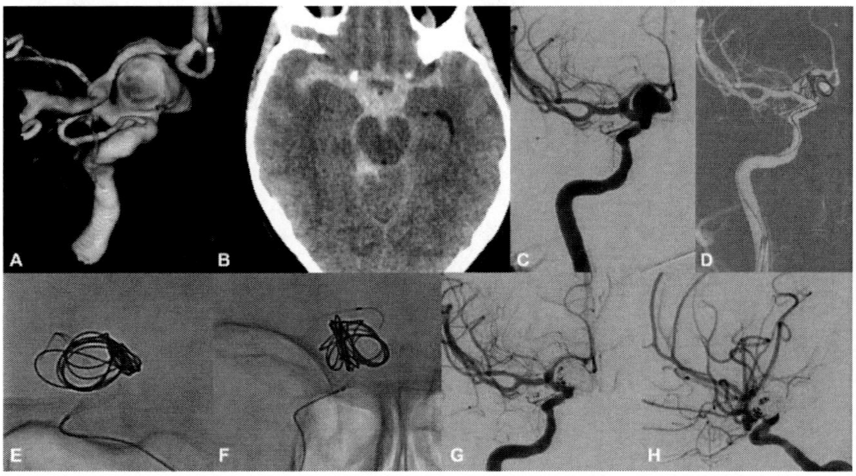

Figure 3. The Comaneci device was utilized for the coil obliteration of an acutely ruptured cerebral aneurysm with a notably wide neck, as illustrated in the rotational angiography images (a, b, c). The crescent shape of the device's mesh provides durability for the regional anatomy, allowing for safe navigation of the catheter into the anterior cerebral artery, from which the implant was carefully deployed (d). Once expanded, the device facilitated stable formation of the initial coil (e, f). Adequate obliteration was observed in the final angiograms, with a small aneurysmal remnant but a secured dome (g, h).

The high radiopacity of the device facilitates clear visualization under fluoroscopy, allowing the operator to observe any potential interactions between the deployed coils and the mesh. Just before detaching the final finishing coil, the Comaneci device is gradually deflated to confirm the stability of the coil basket within the aneurysmal dome. Once sufficient coil stability is established, the neck-bridging device is carefully retracted back into the microcatheter and safely removed from the target artery. This meticulous approach demonstrates the effectiveness of the Comaneci device in providing temporary support during the coiling of saccular aneurysms.

Case example: A 44-year-old woman presented with a World Federation of Neurosurgical Societies (WFNS) grade 2 and Fisher grade 4 acute subarachnoid hemorrhage. This was caused by a 6.5mm wide-necked aneurysm located in the right internal carotid artery (Figure3).

The Cascade Device

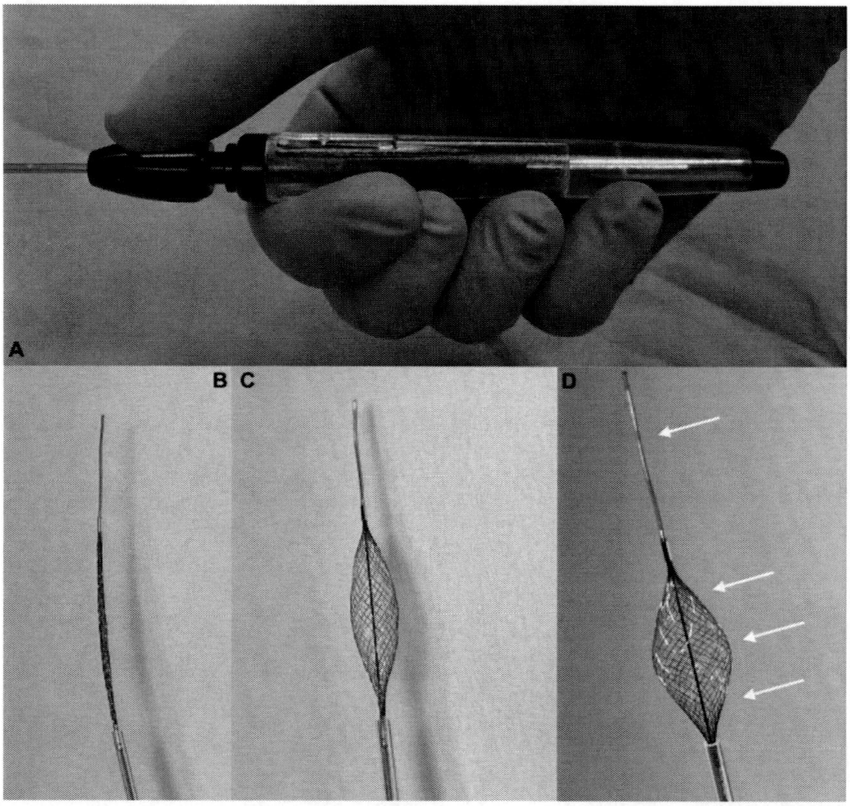

Figure 4. The Cascade M device, shown straightened and deployed out of the 0.021-inch microcatheter, is delivered in a collapsed form through a microcatheter and subsequently expanded using the control grip handle (a, b). The device expands by contracting at both the back and front while the tip remains straight and immobile (c, d). Note how the density of the mesh changes but remains consistently denser than the Comaneci braided mesh during expansions (white arrows).

The Cascade device is a non-occlusive, fully retrievable neck-bridging support system designed to provide temporary assistance during the coil embolization of intracranial aneurysms. It received its CE mark in late 2018, highlighting its regulatory approval for clinical use. Constructed from 42 braided nitinol and platinum wires, the Cascade features a compliant net-like structure that enhances its functionality (Figure 4). The incorporation of platinum wires ensures excellent visualization of the device under fluoroscopy. Additionally, the design includes a short, flexible distal wire and radio-opaque markers located at both the proximal and distal ends of the braided structure. The Cascade is delivered through a 0.021-inch microcatheter and comes in two primary sizes: Cascade M, intended for vessel diameters ranging from 2 to 4 mm, and Cascade L, suitable for vessels measuring 4 to 6 mm in diameter. Agile models are available as shorter versions of both M and L devices. A smaller version, the Cascade-17, compatible with 0.017-inch microcatheters, was introduced, expanding the lineup to a total of five models. The device is initially delivered in a compressed form via the microcatheter and can then be inflated or deflated using the control handle. The handle features two operational modes: auto-lock mode, which allows for stepwise radial expansion, and continuous mode, which enables smoother and more gradual expansion while providing tactile feedback to the operator. In auto-lock mode, each 'click' of the handle corresponds to a controlled expansion of the device. The Cascade can be fully deployed or partially deployed, depending on the specific requirements of the procedure.

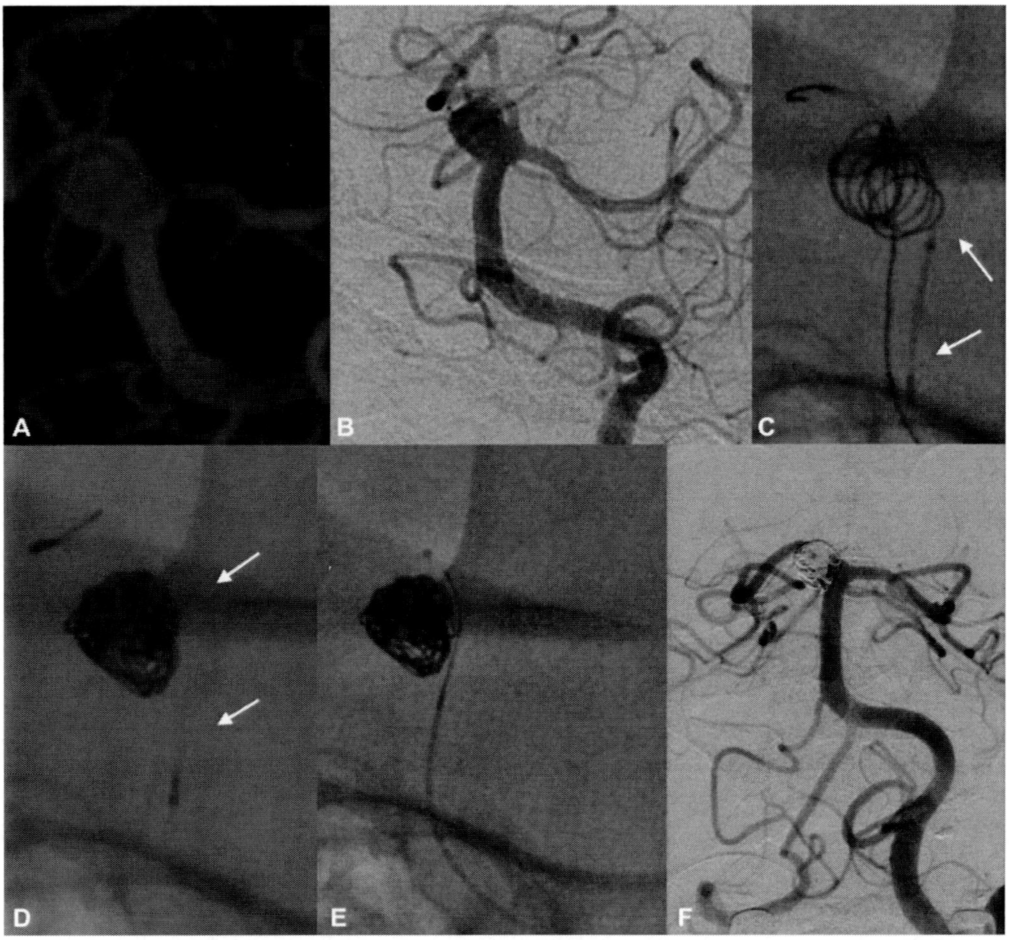

Figure 5. The Cascade M was deployed to secure the embolization of an acutely ruptured, wide-necked cerebral aneurysm (a, b). The images illustrate the device being partially deployed and over-expanded to enhance neck coverage and support during the embolization process (c, d; white arrows). Once coil insertion is complete, careful retraction of the device under fluoroscopy should be performed to avoid any potential interactions (e, f).

The Cascade device, similar in application technique to previously described methods, is introduced through a 0.021-inch microcatheter and positioned across a jailed 0.010-inch microcatheter to provide robust coverage over the aneurysm neck. Initially deployed in a collapsed form by fully retracting the microcatheter, the device is expanded using the proximal control handle, which allows the operator to inflate it to the desired size. The Cascade's variable porosity adjusts with the stent's elongation and foreshortening, offering precise control via the handle. This feature facilitates targeted over-expansion and increased neck coverage, which is especially useful in certain cases to enhance aneurysm obliteration.

Compared to the Comaneci device, the Cascade has a densely braided mesh that virtually eliminates any interaction with the inserted coils. Additionally, the expansion and deflation mechanics of the Cascade differ significantly from the crescent-like structure of the Comaneci device. The Cascade's design allows for straightforward back-and-forth inflation and deflation, ensuring the distal tip remains stable during these adjustments, unlike the pivoting motion observed with the Comaneci's distal tip. This immobility of the distal tip enhances control during the procedure and provides a more stable platform for aneurysm treatment.

Case example: A 54-year-old woman presented with a World Federation of Neurosurgical Societies (WFNS) grade 1 and Fisher grade 4 acute subarachnoid hemorrhage. This was caused by a 5mm wide-necked aneurysm located on the basilar artery (Figure 5).

Discussion

Key Results and Interpretations

The earliest documented use of dedicated devices for temporary stent-assisted coiling appears in an animal study by Gupta et al. which investigated aneurysm coiling facilitated by the Comaneci device in comparison with a conventional microcatheter balloon [15]. Both methods achieved similar aneurysm obliteration rates, with comparable levels of endothelial damage to the parent artery during manipulation. This research likely laid the foundation for the subsequent clinical applications of this technique, beginning with the first successful use of the Comaneci device in the treatment of cerebral aneurysms. Lawson et al. were the first to report the clinical use of a dedicated temporary stent-assisted implant [16]. Since then, multiple reports have documented promising results for this technique in both ruptured and unruptured aneurysm cases (Table 1) [17-25].

Our experience with the device is among the earliest and largest in treating ruptured cerebral aneurysms [21, 26]. In our view, the device offers a manageable learning curve, allowing operators to build confidence and improve technical and clinical outcomes with relative ease. The Comaneci device is available in three versions; notably, the Comaneci 17 is the most commonly used due to its smaller profile, which enables its application beyond the circle of Willis and in more distal cerebral vessels. Recent meta-analyses have shown that using the Comaneci device yields clinical and angiographic results comparable to conventional assisted techniques, such as balloon-assisted coiling (BAC) and stent-assisted coiling (SAC) [18, 27].

Table 1. Summary of published articles reporting on the utilization of both devices in the treatment of cerebral aneurysms

Series, Year	Implant	Time period	Patients number (No)	No. of Total Aneurysms, Acute	Location	Aneurysm Diameter, Mean ± SD (mm)	Aneurysm Neck Width, Mean ± SD (mm)	Dome-to-Neck, Mean ± SD (mm)
Fischer et al. (2017)	Comaneci	2014.12–2015.11	18	18, 0	ICA, 18	6.0 ± 2.76 (2.0–12.0)	3.9 ± 1.6 (2.0–8.0)	-
Sirakov et al. (2018)	Comaneci	2017.5–2017.7	29	29, 29	AComA, 9; ACA, 1; MCA, 7; ICA, 6; BA, 6	5.38 ± 2.41 (2.7–11)	4.28 ± 1.53 (1.9–7.4)	-
Sirakov S. et al. (2020)	Cascade	2019.5–2019.6	12	12, 12	AComA, 3; ICA, 2; MCA, 3; PComA, 2; SCA, 2	6.18 ± 2.08 (3–9.1)	4.49 ± 1.93 (2.3–7.9)	1.46 ± 0.5 (1.06–2.8)
Molina-Nuevo et al. (2020)	Comaneci	2017.3–2019.3	16	18, 14	AComA, 2; PComA, 8; ICA, 8	6.02 ± 2.74 (2.5–13)	NA	1.73 ± 0.8 (0.83–4.30)
Tomasello et al. (2020)	Cascade	2018.7–2019.5	15	15, 5	ICA, 13; VA-V4, 1; SCA, 1	6.27 ± 2.33 (2.8–11)	3.64 ± 1.19 (1.9–6)	1.77 ± 0.5 (0.8–2.4)
Sirakov A. et al. (2020)	Comaneci	2017.8–2019.1	118	118, 118	AComA, 45; ACA, 15; MCA, 21; ICA, 24; BA, 5; PCA, 1; SCA, 4; PICA, 3	6.2 ± 4.1 (2.6–17.3)	4.31 ± 3.1 (2.1–8.6)	-
Lim et al. (2021)	Comaneci	2019.5–2020.4	5	5, 2	MCA, 3; PICA, 1; OA, 1	6.98 ± 1.71 (5.1–9.0)	4.4 ± 0.8 (3.6–5.4)	1.2 ± 0.3 (0.97–1.6)
Taqi et al. (2021)	Comaneci	2019.7–2020.5	26	26, 15	AComA, 10; MCA, 5; PComA, 4; BA, 3; ICA, 1; VA, 1; AchA, 1; SHA, 1	6.59 ± 2.14 (3–11.8)	3.91 ± 1.34 (1.9–6.5)	1.57 ± 0.45 (0.59–3.39)
Vinacci Et al. (2022)	Comaneci	2015.10–2021.5	14	14, 11	AComA, 7; ICA, 5; MCA, 1; PICA, 1	6.77 ± 3.54 (2.2–15.6)	3.14 ± 1.87 (2–8.2)	-

No. = Number; ICA = Internal Carotid Artery; ACA = Anterior Cerebral Artery; AchA = Anterior Choroidal Artery; AcomA = Anterior Communicating Artery; BA = Basilar Artery; MCA = Middle Cerebral Artery; OA = Ophthalmic Artery; PCA = Posterior Cerebral Artery; PcomA = Posterior Communicating Artery; PICA = Posterior Inferior Cerebellar Artery; SCA = Supracerebellar Artery; SHA = Superior Hypophyseal Artery; VA = Vertebral Artery; SD = Standard Deviation; mm = Millimeters; "-" = Not Available.

With over 200 cases in our experience, we believe the key advantages of the device include its ability to preserve normal cerebral blood flow due to its non-occlusive mesh design. The low-metal, compliant braided mesh, combined with the short deployment duration (typically a few minutes), eliminates the need for antiplatelet therapy. This is particularly crucial in cases of acutely ruptured cerebral aneurysms, where antiplatelet avoidance is essential for patient safety.

The Cascade device serves as a key contender in the field of temporary stent-assisted coiling, designed specifically as a neck-bridging support device. While conceptually similar to the Comaneci device in providing temporary stabilization during aneurysm coiling, the Cascade stands apart as an entirely different implant with distinct characteristics. Recent clinical reports on its use have emerged from both our group and Tomasello et al. In our early and steadily growing experience, the Cascade has shown comparable clinical, technical, and angiographic outcomes to the Comaneci device.

A primary distinction in the initial experience with the Cascade is that it was predominantly utilized in its 0.021-inch versions. Due to its denser braided structure and stable, non-movable distal tip, the Cascade has slightly higher rigidity, making it less optimal for distal vessel delivery. However, these same properties enhance its compliance and neck coverage, particularly in aneurysms with unfavorable aspect ratios and wide necks. The Cascade's denser mesh occasionally induces stagnation within the aneurysm sac, which, rather than posing an issue, actually reduces the risk of coil entanglement—especially important when using delicate finishing coils.

In terms of clinical safety, the Cascade device has shown similar outcomes to the Comaneci, maintaining patency of the parent artery and allowing unimpeded blood flow during use. This non-occlusive nature makes it well-suited for applications in cases of subarachnoid hemorrhage (SAH) and ruptured cerebral aneurysms. Enthusiasm for the Cascade's potential has also extended to its use in managing post-hemorrhagic vasospasm, where its unique characteristics are advantageous. Despite being a metallic device, the Cascade exerts a lower radial force on the parent artery than microcatheter balloons, which adds to its safety profile. Bhogal et al. further demonstrated that the Cascade can be effectively and safely employed as a tool for managing post-hemorrhagic vasospasm, broadening its clinical utility [28, 29].

Technical Details, Tips and Troubleshooting

In our experience, we can offer several technical considerations for the on-label use of both the Comaneci and Cascade devices in assisting coil embolization of cerebral aneurysms.

- Comaneci Device Considerations: First, it's important to note that the distal tip of the Comaneci device can sometimes display a degree of "flickering" during manipulation. Although the tip is designed to be movable, careful observation is advised—particularly when the device is positioned near perforating artery openings, such as those in the lenticulostriate complex or the posterior circulation's delicate vessels. This consideration becomes even more critical in cases of subarachnoid hemorrhage (SAH) or when arterial narrowing, like vasospasm, is present.

- Device-Specific Technical Benefits: Both the Comaneci and Cascade devices are highly compliant and generally atraumatic; however, in certain cases—such as larger-diameter internal carotid arteries or aneurysms with complex parent-vessel interfaces—the mesh of these devices may not provide optimal neck coverage. Enhanced neck-bridging can be achieved by applying gentle tension on the microcatheter at the proximal end of the device upon full expansion. This maneuver increases the crescent form of the Comaneci device and enhances the spherical shape of the Cascade device, potentially improving neck coverage. However, these adjustments should only be made after gaining experience with the devices, as they can alter the density of the mesh braid, create bulging into the aneurysm, and increase the risk of coil entanglement. For this reason, we do not recommend using very small finishing coils (under 2 mm in diameter) with the Comaneci device, as they could potentially interact with and become entangled in the device's openings. Although we have not observed such incidents in our clinical practice, vigilance during manipulation is advised, with continuous fluoroscopic monitoring. However, case reports of coil interactions and entaglements have already been published.

Each device also offers distinct benefits depending on the aneurysm's location and anatomical configuration. The Comaneci's crescent shape may be advantageous for specific cases, such as posterior communicating artery (PCom) aneurysms, where the device's semi-lunar form can be used strategically—e.g., by deploying it from the M1 segment to the proximal C7 segment of the internal carotid artery to create a mechanical barrier for safer coiling. However, this configuration may pose challenges in distal vasculature or in vessels with sharp angulation, where the device's convex shape could lead to distal or proximal migration or incomplete neck coverage if the surrounding vasculature does not accommodate it.

In contrast, the Cascade device's spherical, non-crescent shape provides consistent coverage that is less dependent on the vessel's shape, reducing the risk of migration or incomplete neck coverage in complex anatomies. This uniform expansion can be particularly useful in aneurysms where the geometry does not support the Comaneci's crescentic configuration.

Off-Label Applications

Initially, the Comaneci device was introduced to the neurovascular community with a specific purpose: to simplify and enhance coil embolization of wide-necked cerebral aneurysms. However, the device's versatility became apparent with its first reported off-label application in 2020, as documented by Wessels L et al. where it was used to facilitate microcatheterization of the distal cerebral vasculature [30]. Although this initial report covered only two cases, its off-label potential gained further attention through live transvenous demonstrations by Professor René Chapot at the 2019 ALICE (Advanced Live Interventional Course of Essen) meeting. The device's off-label journey continued with the U.S. FDA's recognition over a year ago, granting it breakthrough designation for treating cerebral vasospasm after hemorrhagic stroke—a capability later explored in the COMMAND study and its findings [31]. Interestingly, one might speculate that the device's name, Comaneci, is a nod to retired

Romanian gymnast Nadia Comăneci, whose versatility and perfection in performance resonate with the device's multitool-like abilities.

Our Clinical Experience and Discoveries

Since we integrated the Comaneci device into our practice in July 2017, we have accumulated experience with hundreds of cases across a range of applications. Our usage has gone beyond aneurysm treatment, as we discovered the device's utility in enhancing wall apposition in cases of suboptimal flow diverter stent (FD) deployment, as well as addressing structural irregularities like twisting, critical segmental stenosis, and narrow openings at the distal or proximal ends of flow diverters. However, we have not observed the same vasospasm-modulating effects reported by other users.

An unexpected benefit emerged when we used the non-occlusive mesh of the Comaneci device as a stent retriever. In cases of thrombotic occlusions or inadvertent release of embolic agent fragments (such as PHIL, MicroVention), the Comaneci's mesh was able to capture these obstructions effectively, functioning similarly to a stent retriever (Figure 6).

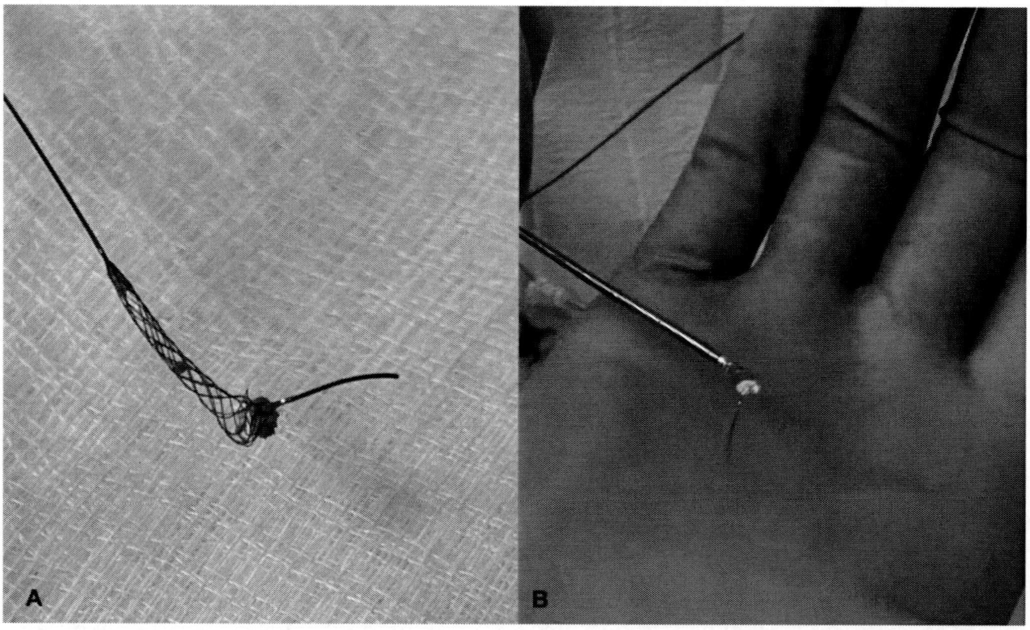

Figure 6. Off-label applications of the Comaneci device in real-world scenarios. The device mesh captured a thrombus within the distal portion of the braided mesh (a) and successfully retrieved fragments of PHIL that had unintentionally entered critical cerebral circulation (b).

When using the Comaneci to address structural irregularities in endoluminal implants or to augment wall apposition in partially deployed stents, it's crucial to apply sufficient radial force. The device, when fully expanded, exerts a radial force of 0.05 to 0.06 N/mm in a 1 mm vessel, slightly decreasing in a 3 mm vessel. According to the manufacturer, this device can generate forces up to 23 kPa (around 172.5 mmHg), which we have found sufficient to address even critical stenoses in defective flow diverters while minimizing the risk of damage to the vessel segment. By comparison, modern compliant and non-compliant balloons can exert significantly higher pressures—up to 579.5 mmHg or 77.2 kPa—especially in curved vessel segments, which may increase the risk of vessel injury [32].

The smallest variant, the Comaneci 17, has proven particularly useful in challenging cases where navigating through a stenotic site of a defective stent is difficult. Its compatibility with 0.017" microcatheters provides enhanced maneuverability within distal vasculature, especially beneficial in complex flow diversion settings.

One consideration with the Comaneci device, particularly during deflation and retraction, is the potential interaction between its braided metallic mesh and certain flow diverters [33,34]. This can result in unintended entanglement with the proximal or distal ends of some flow diverters, including the proximal markers of the p64 FD (phenox), the braided structures of the Silk FD (Balt Extrusion), or the outer layer ends of the Flow-Redirecting Endoluminal Device (MicroVention). Being mindful of these possible interactions is essential, as they are more likely to occur during deflation or retraction maneuvers.

Conclusion

In conclusion, both the Comaneci and Cascade devices represent significant advancements in the field of temporary stent-assisted coiling for wide-necked cerebral aneurysms. Each device offers unique advantages—the Comaneci with its flexible, crescent-shaped design allowing for adaptable neck coverage and navigability, and the Cascade with its denser mesh and immobile distal tip providing enhanced neck coverage and reduced risk of coil entanglement. Our experience highlights the safety and efficacy of these devices in preserving blood flow during aneurysm coiling, especially in challenging cases involving acutely ruptured aneurysms. As such, both devices broaden the toolkit available to neurointerventionalists, enabling more tailored and effective treatment options for complex aneurysms

Disclaimer

None.

References

[1] Ferns SP, et al. Late reopening of adequately coiled intracranial aneurysms: Frequency and risk factors in 400 patients with 440 aneurysms. *Stroke* (2011) 42 (5):1331–1337. https://doi.org/10.1161/STROKEAHA.110.605790.

[2] Henkes H, Weber W. The Past, Present and Future of Endovascular Aneurysm Treatment. *Clinical Neuroradiology* (2015) 25 (S2):317–324. https://doi.org/10.1007/s00062-015-0403-1.

[3] Campos JK, Lien BV, Wang AS, Lin L-M. Advances in endovascular aneurysm management: Coiling and adjunctive devices. *Stroke and Vascular Neurology* (2020) 5 (1):14–21. https://doi.org/10.1136/svn-2019-000303.

[4] Pai AM, Kameda-Smith M, van Adel B. A Review of Recent Advances in Endovascular Therapy for Intracranial Aneurysms. *Critical Reviews in Biomedical Engineering* (2018) 46 (4):369–397. https://doi.org/10.1615/CritRevBiomedEng.2018027003.

[5] Amenta PS, et al. Stent-Assisted Coiling of Wide-Necked Aneurysms in the Setting of Acute Subarachnoid Hemorrhage. *Neurosurgery* (2012) 70 (6):1415–1429. https://doi.org/10.1227/NEU.0b013e318246a4b1.

[6] Chalouhi N, et al. Stent-Assisted Coiling Versus Balloon Remodeling of Wide-Neck Aneurysms: Comparison of Angiographic Outcomes. *American Journal of Neuroradiology* (2013) 34 (10):1987–1992. https://doi.org/10.3174/ajnr.A3538.

[7] Wang F, et al. Stent-assisted coiling and balloon-assisted coiling in the management of intracranial aneurysms: A systematic review & meta-analysis. *Journal of the Neurological Sciences* (2016) 364:160–166. https://doi.org/10.1016/j.jns.2016.03.041.

[8] Lee DH, et al. Dual Antiplatelet Therapy Monitoring for Neurointerventional Procedures Using a Point-of-Care Platelet Function Test: A Single-Center Experience. *American Journal of Neuroradiology* (2008) 29 (7):1389–1394. https://doi.org/10.3174/ajnr.A1070.

[9] Mahaney KB, et al. Risk of hemorrhagic complication associated with ventriculoperitoneal shunt placement in aneurysmal subarachnoid hemorrhage patients on dual antiplatelet therapy. *Journal of Neurosurgery* (2013) 119 (4):937–942. https://doi.org/10.3171/2013.5.JNS122494.

[10] Kuwajima T, et al. Usefulness and problems of Y-Stent and T-Stent assisted coiling for unruptured cerebral aneurysms. *Journal of Stroke and Cerebrovascular Diseases* (2022) 31 (10):106668. https://doi.org/10.1016/j.jstrokecerebrovasdis.2022.106668.

[11] Almekhlafi MA, Hockley A, Wong JH, Goyal M. Temporary Solitaire stent neck remodeling in the coiling of ruptured aneurysms. *Journal of NeuroInterventional Surgery* (2013) 5 (Suppl 3):iii76–iii78. https://doi.org/10.1136/neurintsurg-2013-010737.

[12] Signorelli F, Gory B, Turjman F. Temporary Solitaire Stent-Assisted Coiling: A Technique for the Treatment of Acutely Ruptured Wide-Neck Intracranial Aneurysms. *American Journal of Neuroradiology* (2014) 35 (5):984–988. https://doi.org/10.3174/ajnr.A3798.

[13] Müller M, et al. Temporary Stent-Assisted Coil Embolization as a Treatment Option for Wide-Neck Aneurysms. *American Journal of Neuroradiology* (2017) 38 (7):1372–1376. https://doi.org/10.3174/ajnr.A5204.

[14] Almekhlafi MA, Goyal M. Antiplatelet Therapy prior to Temporary Stent-Assisted Coiling. *American Journal of Neuroradiology* (2014) 35 (10):E6. https://doi.org/10.3174/ajnr.A4090.

[15] Gupta R, et al. Comaneci neck bridging device for the treatment of cerebral aneurysms. *Journal of NeuroInterventional Surgery* (2016) 8 (2):181–185. https://doi.org/10.1136/neurintsurg-2014-011518.

[16] Lawson ALD, et al. Initial experience of coiling cerebral aneurysms using the new Comaneci device. *BMJ Case Reports* (2015) bcr2015011726. https://doi.org/10.1136/bcr-2015-011726.

[17] Fischer S, et al. Coiling of wide-necked carotid artery aneurysms assisted by a temporary bridging device (Comaneci): Preliminary experience. *Journal of NeuroInterventional Surgery* (2017) 9 (11):1039–1047. https://doi.org/10.1136/neurintsurg-2016-012664.

[18] Lim J, et al. Coiling Variations for Treatment of Ruptured Intracranial Aneurysms: A Meta-Analytical Comparison of Comaneci-, Stent-, and Balloon-Coiling Assistance Techniques. *World Neurosurgery* (2023) 175:e1324–e1340. https://doi.org/10.1016/j.wneu.2023.05.008.

[19] Molina-Nuevo JD, et al. Comaneci device-assisted embolization of wide-necked carotid aneurysms with an unfavorable ratio. *BMC Neurology* (2020) 20 (1):384. https://doi.org/10.1186/s12883-020-01963-2.

[20] Sirakov A, et al. Comaneci-Assisted Coiling as a Treatment Option for Acutely Ruptured Wide Neck Cerebral Aneurysm: Case Series of 118 Patients. *Neurosurgery* (2020) 87 (6):1148–1156. https://doi.org/10.1093/neuros/nyaa200.

[21] Sirakov S, et al. Early experience with a temporary bridging device (Comaneci) in the endovascular treatment of ruptured wide neck aneurysms. *Journal of NeuroInterventional Surgery* (2018) 10 (10):978–982. https://doi.org/10.1136/neurintsurg-2017-013641.

[22] Sirakov S, et al. Early clinical experience with Cascade: A novel temporary neck bridging device for embolization of intracranial aneurysms. *Journal of NeuroInterventional Surgery* (2020) 12 (3):303–307. https://doi.org/10.1136/neurintsurg-2019-015338.

[23] Taqi MA, et al. Early Experience with Comaneci, a Newly FDA-Approved Controllable Assist Device for Wide-Necked Intracranial Aneurysm Coiling. *Cerebrovascular Diseases* (2021) 50 (4):464–471. https://doi.org/10.1159/000514371.

[24] Tomasello A, et al. Early experience with a novel net temporary bridging device (Cascade) to assist endovascular coil embolization of intracranial aneurysms. *Journal of Neurosurgery* (2021) 134 (2):591–599. https://doi.org/10.3171/2019.11.JNS192477.

[25] Vinacci G, et al. Comaneci-Assisted Coiling of Wide-Necked Intracranial Aneurysm: A Single-Center Preliminary Experience. *Journal of Clinical Medicine* (2022) 11 (22):6650. https://doi.org/10.3390/jcm11226650.

[26] Sirakov SS, Sirakov A, Hristov H, Raychev R. Coiling of ruptured, wide-necked basilar tip aneurysm using double Comaneci technique. *BMJ Case Reports* (2018) bcr2017222703. https://doi.org/10.1136/bcr-2017-222703.

[27] Sun B, et al. A systematic review and meta-analysis of Comaneci/Cascade temporary neck bridging devices for the treatment of intracranial aneurysms. *Frontiers in Human Neuroscience* (2023) 17:1276681. https://doi.org/10.3389/fnhum.2023.1276681.

[28] Bhogal P, et al. The Cascade device – In vitro tests to assess coil protrusion into the parent vessel. *Interventional Neuroradiology* (2020) 26 (4):494–500. https://doi.org/10.1177/1591019920925708.

[29] Bhogal P, et al. Use of the Cascade expandable net to treat cerebral vasospasm – initial clinical experience from a single centre with in vitro benchside tests. *CVIR Endovascular* (2021) 4 (1):82. https://doi.org/10.1186/s42155-021-00275-x.

[30] Wessels L, De Vries J, Boogaarts HD. The Comaneci Device for Entering an Acute-Angled Small Feeder during Cerebral Arteriovenous Malformation Embolization: A Novel Technique to Support Microcatheterization. *Neurointervention* (2020) 15 (2):79–83. https://doi.org/10.5469/neuroint.2020.00122.

[31] Salem MM, et al. COManeci MechANical Dilation for vasospasm (COMMAND): Multicenter experience. *Journal of NeuroInterventional Surgery* (2023) 15 (9):864–870. https://doi.org/10.1136/jnis-2022-019272.

[32] Ikezawa M, et al. Evaluation of the differences in pressure applied to the vessel wall by different types of balloon remodeling microcatheters in an experimental model. *Interventional Neuroradiology* (2022) 28 (3):323–331. https://doi.org/10.1177/15910199211031765.

[33] Sirakova K, Sirakov A, Ninov K, Minkin K, Sirakov S. Comaneci stent-angioplasty for the optimization of inadequately deployed flow diverter stents. *Interventional Neuroradiology* (2023).

[34] Vladev G, Sirakov A, Sirakova K, Sirakov SS. Mechanical Comaneci 17-stent angioplasty for a sub-optimally deployed flow-diverter stent. *Interventional Neuroradiology* (2025) 31 (1):143.

Chapter 10

The History and Development of Stent Retrieval

Maliya Delawan[1,*]
Ali Al-Jabri[2,†]
Ahmed Muthana[3,‡], MD
and Samer S. Hoz[4,§], MD
[1]College of Medicine, Gulf Medical University, Ajman, UAE
[2]Faculty of Medicine, University of Oslo, Oslo, Norway
[3]Department of Neurosurgery, University of Baghdad, Baghdad, Iraq
[4]Department of Neurosurgery, University of Cincinnati Medical Center, Cincinnati, OH, USA

Abstract

The chapter explores the history and development of stent retrieval in endovascular stroke intervention. Beginning in the late 1990s, the landscape of stroke intervention changed significantly with the emergence of stent retrievers such as Solitaire and Trevo. The chapter highlights a significant breakthrough in 2012 with the two landmark trials SWIFT and TREVO. Since then, stent retrievers have become widely adopted worldwide, and several newer models have been developed with enhanced navigability, clot engagement, and retrieval success rates. Techniques have been refined over time, integrating the use of stent retrievers with other techniques and devices. The chapter concludes with an overview of how the ongoing efforts to improve device design and technique may shape the trajectory of future research in stent retrieval.

Keywords: stent retrieval, mechanical thrombectomy, neurointerventional surgery, endovascular stroke intervention, recanalization

[*] Corresponding Author's Email: maliya.delawan@gmail.com
[†] Corresponding Author's Email: ali.al-jabri@medisin.uio.no
[‡] Corresponding Author's Email: ahmed.m.najm@gmail.com
[§] Corresponding Author's Email: hozsamer2055@gmail.com

In: World History of Neurointerventional Surgery
Editors: Xianli Lv and Zhongxue Wu
ISBN: 979-8-89530-792-2

Introduction

Over the last twenty years, the management of acute ischemic stroke resulting from large vessel occlusion (LVO) has undergone transformative changes. Beginning in the 1990s with intra-arterial (IA) thrombolysis, the field of endovascular stroke intervention (ESI) has rapidly progressed with the development of mechanical thrombectomy devices, eventually giving rise to the stent retriever. Through various trials, the stent retriever quickly gained traction as the standard of care in select patients with acute LVO stroke. This chapter seeks to trace the development of stent retrievers, emphasizing how each technological breakthrough has built on the last and shaped the criteria for evaluating new approaches.

Stent Retrieval History in Neurointerventional Surgery

The 1990s: Dawn of the Device Era in Stroke Treatment

The late 1990s marked a turning point in the treatment of acute ischemic stroke with the introduction of intra-arterial recombinant pro-urokinase (r-proUK), a direct thrombolytic agent. This development represented one of the initial forays into what would eventually become known as mechanical thrombectomy. Though not a mechanical device in the traditional sense, the application of r-proUK directly within the cerebral arteries to dissolve clots signified a significant shift toward more aggressive and targeted interventions.

At the time, intravenous tissue-type plasminogen activator (tPA) had been established as beneficial for some stroke patients, but only if administered within three hours of stroke onset. However, many patients arrived for treatment later than this window, underscoring a pressing need for alternative treatment options. In this milieu, the PROACT II (Prolyse in Acute Cerebral Thromboembolism II) randomized controlled trial (RCT) emerged, involving 180 patients who had experienced an acute ischemic stroke within the past 6 hours due to angiographically proven MCA occlusion, without hemorrhage or major early infarction signs on CT scans. Compared to the control group that received heparin alone, a higher percentage of patients treated with r-proUK achieved a favorable outcome and recanalization rate. However, the frequency of early intracranial hemorrhage with neurological deterioration remained high among patients treated with IA r-proUK [1].

This method was later eclipsed by the advent of mechanical devices, which promised direct and immediate clot retrieval without the systemic dispersion of thrombolytic agents. The Merci Retrieval System^{TM} (Concentric Medical, Mountain View, CA, USA), approved by the Food and Drug Administration (FDA) in 2004, was one of the first devices designed specifically for mechanical thrombectomy in ischemic stroke. It features a corkscrew-like design and is deployed distally to the clot to ensnare and remove the thrombus. Two pivotal trials assessed their use: the Merci trial (2005) and the subsequent Multi MERCI trial (2008) [2, 3].

The first trial investigated the safety and efficacy of the Merci Retriever in opening occluded intracranial large vessels within 8 hours of stroke symptom onset in a single-arm, prospective, nonrandomized setting. Results were promising; recanalization was achieved in 46% of patients on an intention-to-treat analysis, a significant increase compared to the 18% historical control rate from the control arm of PROACT-II [3]. Building on the findings of the initial Merci trial, the Multi-MERCI trial aimed to evaluate enhancements in embolectomy device design, particularly with the introduction of the newer generation L5 Retriever. In comparison to the initial MERCI Trial, the Multi-MERCI trial demonstrated superior results, including a higher recanalization rate, enhanced 90-day modified Rankin Scale (mRS) scores, fewer complications, and reduced 90-day mortality [2]. The success of these two studies significantly contributed to the widespread adoption of the Merci thrombectomy, leading to over 10,000 procedures being performed globally by 2010 [4]. However, its rapid adoption raised concerns in the setting of absent randomized data. Years would pass before randomized studies would be funded to evaluate the true efficacy of mechanical thrombectomy.

Year 2012: The Emergence of Stent Retrievers

During this period, the need for improved outcomes and recanalization rates highlighted by the Merci and Penumbra trials spurred a call for the development of more effective clot retrieval devices. The emergence of the two stent retrievers, Solitaire and Trevo, marked a new beginning in endovascular therapy for stroke. These devices are engineered with push-wires that allow for full deployment and subsequent retraction, enabling the stent to be removed after achieving clot retrieval. They demonstrated superior efficacy in recanalizing occluded vessels compared to earlier technologies [5] (Figure 1).

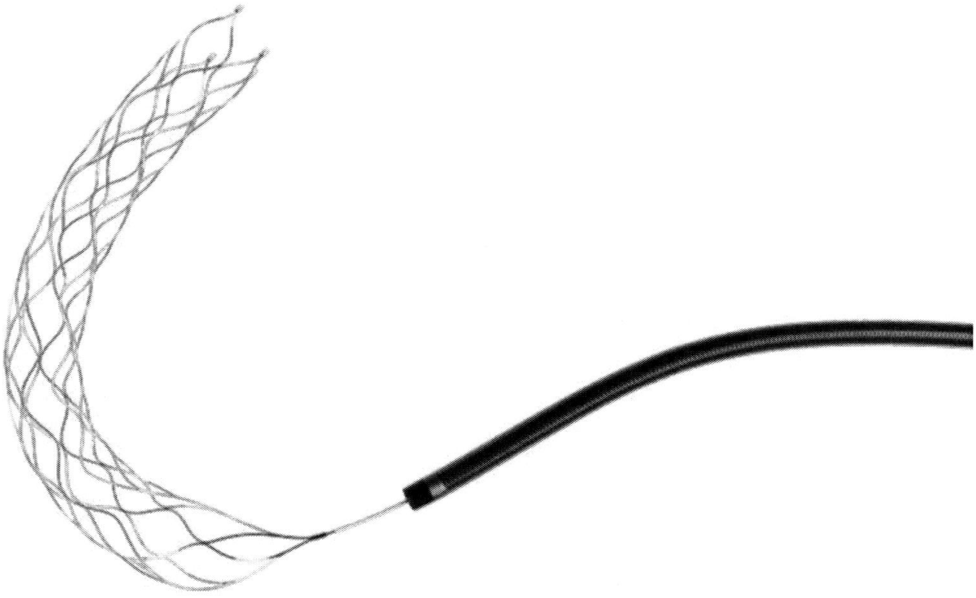

Figure 1. Stent-retrieval device.

It is worth noting that, although the invention of retrievable stents dates back to 2003, it was initially developed for the treatment of wide-necked aneurysms (Figure 2). The company behind its innovation was Dendron, a company based in Bochum, Germany, which was acquired by MTI (Irvine, California, USA) in 2002. The design of the stent retriever featured a nitinol stent with radiopaque markers at both ends, offered in a variety of sizes, and matched the flexibility of a micro-guidewire. The aim was to overcome the limitations of existing over-the-wire intracranial stents, particularly offering the unique capability to be retrieved and repositioned after full deployment if its placement was deemed suboptimal or the stent was found to be unnecessary [6]. The stent received the CE mark in 2004 and rapidly gained prominence as the Solitaire stent. By December 2007, it was introduced in the European market, specifically targeting the treatment of wide-necked aneurysms. Today, the Solitaire stent is manufactured and distributed by ev3 (Irvine, California, USA) [7].

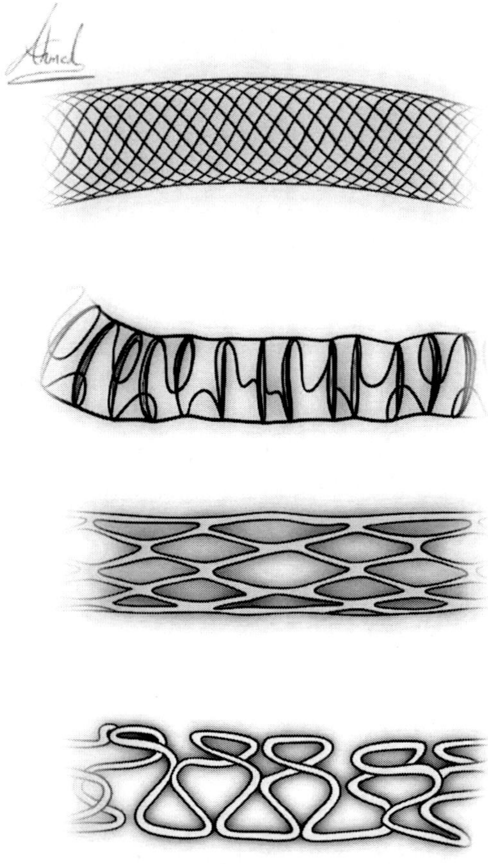

Figure 2. Schematic illustration showing different types of stents used for intracranial aneurysm procedures. Illustration prepared by Ahmed Muthana and courtesy of Samer Hoz.

It wasn't until 2011 that Pérez et al. published a report of the first successful human clinical use of a Solitaire stent for intracranial thrombectomy. The case was a 67-year-old woman who presented with a right hemispheric stroke 3.5 hours post-onset. Initial attempts at mechanical thrombectomy using a microbrush failed to achieve recanalization. With no other options available, a Solitaire stent was deployed in the occluded middle cerebral artery (MCA) and was successful in the complete removal of the thrombus, leading to complete recovery with an NIHSS score of 0 at the 30-day follow-up [7].

During the time between the development of stent retrievers in 2003 and their first recorded use for treating acute ischemic stroke in 2011, other neurointerventionalists experimented with using traditional self-expanding stents (not specifically designed for retrieval like Solitaire) in a manner that resembled the mechanism of stent retrievers. In a case report published in 2008 by Kelly et al. they describe a technique where a stent was partially deployed across the occlusion site, aiming to displace the clot circumferentially and temporarily restore blood flow. This approach enabled the localized infusion of antiplatelet medication directly through the guide catheter. After maintaining the bypass for approximately 20 minutes, the stent was then resheathed and removed [5, 8].

This innovative technique was thought to aid thrombolysis by facilitating the dispersal of prothrombotic factors within the clot with flow restoration and enhancing the penetration of thrombolytic or antiplatelet medications. However, tests in animal models revealed a crucial insight: while flow restoration alone was insufficient for dissolving thrombi, the mechanical clot retrieval capability of these new stents was highly effective [5, 9].

The aim of this "temporary endovascular bypass" technique was to circumvent the need for permanent implantation and long-term antiplatelet therapy required with permanent stent implantation, which was approved in the SARIS trial in 2009 for the treatment of acute ischemic stroke [10].

The demonstrations of the stent retrieval concept paved the way for two landmark trials, both published in 2012, which initiated their rapid adoption: the SWIFT (Solitaire with the Intention for Thrombectomy) trial, as well as the TREVO 2 trial that followed soon after. The SWIFT trial employed a randomized, parallel-group, non-inferiority approach, assigning 113 eligible stroke patients to receive thrombectomy treatment with either the Solitaire or Merci devices. Eligibility criteria included those with angiographically confirmed occlusions who presented within 8 hours of symptom onset, with moderate to severe neurological deficits. The primary endpoint was achieving TIMI scale 2 or 3 flow in all treatable vessels without symptomatic intracranial hemorrhage, which was assessed by a masked independent core lab. A case was classified as a failure if the primary endpoint was not reached after three attempts with the assigned device [11, 12].

During an interim analysis conducted by the Data Safety and Monitoring Board, the Solitaire device significantly outperformed the Merci Retriever, leading to the early termination of the trial. The primary efficacy outcome favored the Solitaire group significantly, with 61% achieving the desired flow compared to 24% in the Merci group ($p = 0.0001$). Furthermore, the Solitaire group exhibited more favorable 3-month neurological outcomes (58% vs. 33%; $p = 0.02$) and lower 90-day mortality rates (17% vs. 38%; $p = 0.02$). A "good neurological outcome" was defined as meeting any of the following criteria: i) achieving an mRS score of less than 2 at 90 days, ii) maintaining an unchanged mRS score if the patient's pre-stroke mRS score was greater than 2, or iii) experiencing an improvement of 10 points or more in NIHSS score [11, 12].

Following closely after the SWIFT trial, the TREVO 2 trial further solidified the position of stent retrievers in the treatment of acute ischemic stroke. The TREVO 2 trial compared the Trevo stent retriever developed by Stryker to the Merci Retriever, and unlike the SWIFT trial, only patients with no significant pre-stroke deficits (mRS ≤ 1) were enrolled. The trial also differed in the following areas: its primary endpoint focus (TREVO 2 used reperfusion, versus SWIFT which emphasized reperfusion without hemorrhage); the allowance of up to 6 passes with the assigned device before treatment was deemed unsuccessful (as opposed to 3 passes in SWIFT); and an unmasked core lab responsible for assessing angiographic outcomes. In the final analysis of the 178 included patients, the primary endpoint was reached in 86% of cases in the Trevo group compared to 60% in the Merci group ($p < 0.0001$), demonstrating once again that the stent retriever group outperformed the Merci group [13].

With the introduction of Solitaire and Trevo, stroke physicians were now able to attain impressive rates of recanalization, with partial reperfusion achieved in 80% to 90% of cases and complete reperfusion in over 50% (Figure 3). However, it later becomes apparent that this type of technological leap may pose a challenge in research. Trials that were being conducted over the previous several years testing first-generation interventions against medical therapy, either did not include these newer ESI devices or grouped them with older technologies. This oversight resulted in a diminished reflection of the potential of ESI compared to medical therapy, with far-reaching consequences for the reputation of ESI as a whole [11].

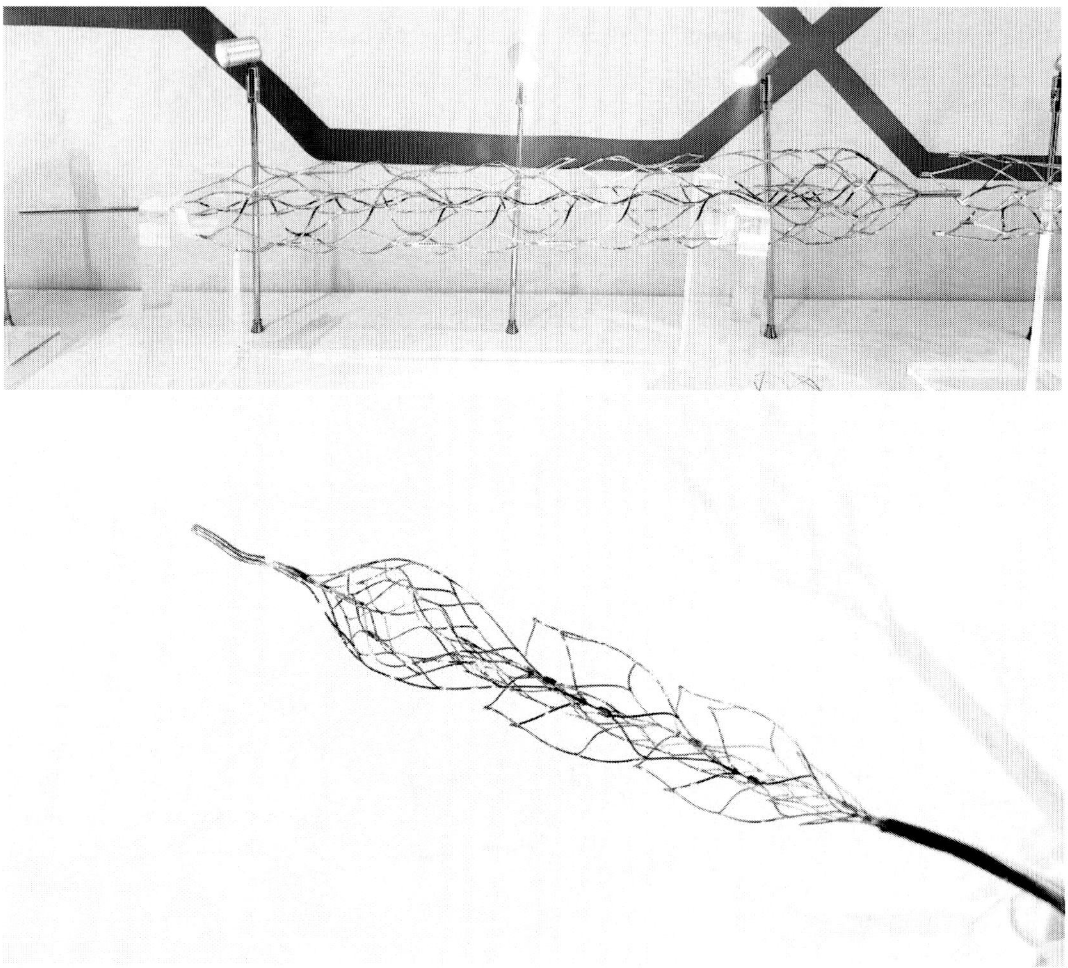

Figure 1. Different types of stent retrieval devices.

Year 2013: The Flaws of the ESI Trials

In the early period of ESI adoption with the first generation of thrombectomy technology (e.g., Merci), the field of ESI progressed for more than a decade without undergoing a large RCT comparing it to standard medical management. This was partly due to the lenient criteria for device clearance. However, this trajectory shifted in 2013 with the simultaneous release of IMS III, SYNTHESIS Expansion, and MR RESCUE, all of which failed to demonstrate the benefit of ESI.

While these three trials were the first to provide randomized data for ESI, they were critically flawed due to the heterogeneity in ESI methodologies employed. For instance, the ESI group in the IMS III trial comprised a range of techniques, from thrombectomy using devices like the Merci Retriever, Penumbra System, Solitaire, to endovascular t-PA. The SYNTHESIS Expansion trial also allowed both mechanical thrombectomy devices and endovascular t-PA, with stent retrievers used in only 13% of cases. In both these trials, ESI groups were compared to patients receiving IVT only. The MR RESCUE trial, which spanned eight years, entirely excluded stent retrievers; it included only patients treated with the Merci Retriever or Penumbra System [14-16].

In all three trials, no clinical benefit of ESI was observed, dealing a significant blow to the field's reputation. Despite these setbacks, these early trials provided invaluable insights into study design and played an important role in shaping future stroke trials.

Year 2015: The Landmark Trials

In a turn of events following the disappointing trials in 2013, subsequent studies conducted two years later demonstrated the superior effectiveness of stent retrievers over medical therapy alone for treating acute ischemic stroke caused by LVO. The MR CLEAN trial, published in January 2015 and originating from the Netherlands, was the first to show positive results. It involved 500 patients with anterior circulation LVOs, confirmed via angiography, who presented within six hours of symptom onset. In this trial, stent retrievers were used in 81.5% of cases in the ESI group, a rate higher than those included in previous trials. The final results demonstrated a significant 13.5% absolute difference in achieving functional independence (modified Rankin score of 0 to 2), favoring the ESI group, with rates of 32.6% compared to 19.1% in the standard therapy group [17].

The positive results of the MR CLEAN trial prompted early interim analyses and the early termination of seven other ongoing ESI trials due to positive results or loss of clinical equipoise [5]. By the end of 2015, four additional trials—ESCAPE, EXTEND-IA, SWIFT PRIME, and REVASCAT—further confirmed the benefits of ESI over standard therapy [18-21]. These trials collectively shifted the standard of care towards the use of mechanical thrombectomy with stent retrievers in eligible patients.

Technique and Technological Improvements

Subsequent research following the initial stent retriever trials has expanded the treatment window for certain patients to as much as 24 hours after symptom onset [22]. Additionally, the combination of stent retrievers with other advanced techniques and devices has become an area of focus, aiming to enhance the efficacy of ESI. One notable development in this area is the use of balloon guide catheters (BGCs) instead of conventional guide catheters. In 2019, a large multicenter registry from Korea demonstrated that the use of BGCs in ESI led to improved recanalization success rates and better functional outcomes, although ESI treatments were not exclusively performed with stent retrievers —44.9% of the cases employed the Direct Aspiration First Pass Technique (ADAPT), while stent retrievers were used in 55.1% of the patients.

Another innovative method is the Solumbra technique, first described in 2013, which involves the use of a stent retriever through an aspiration catheter that simultaneously applies suction to the clot [23]. To further refine the Solumbra technique, a series of small studies have led to the development of techniques such as CAPTIVE (Continuous Aspiration Prior to Intracranial Vascular Embolectomy), SAVE (Stent retriever Assisted Vacuum-locked Extraction), and ARTS (Aspiration (catheter)- (stent) Retriever Technique for Stroke) [24-26]. However, these innovations have not yet been tested in RCTs, and thus, their effectiveness and safety at a larger scale remain unverified. Currently, ADAPT is the only alternative thrombectomy technique to stent retrievers that has been evaluated within an RCT setting.

The design and capabilities of stent retriever devices have continuously evolved, with a focus on improving efficacy and safety. As of 2024, the latest advancements include the Solitaire™ X Revascularization Device from Medtronic, which offers a higher rate of first-pass recanalization, reduced post-procedural bleeding volumes, and shorter hospital stays compared to its predecessors [27]. Stryker's Trevo NXT ProVue Retriever has advanced visibility and builds on its predecessor by optimizing for use with aspiration catheters. It features a new hydrophilic-coated polymer jacket that facilitates smoother delivery and improved retraction into the aspiration catheter [28]. The market includes many other models, and the examples mentioned here are by no means exhaustive.

Future trends in stent retriever development will continue to focus on improving first-pass recanalization rates and reducing distal embolization. There is also growing interest in broadening the indications of thrombectomy to include distal or medium vessel occlusions, which would require the development of stents with smaller diameters. These stents are likely to feature an open-cell design, which can better navigate around anatomically complex areas such as the middle cerebral artery (MCA) genu and the smaller, more tortuous M2 and M3 segments [29].

Furthermore, the integration of multi-modal therapies holds significant potential for improving clinical outcomes. Randomized studies into the Solumbra technique and the combination of thrombectomy with other locally delivered therapies, such as the use of shear-driven release of thrombolytics alongside stent retrievers, periprocedural local hypothermia, and the administration of neuroprotective agents, are likely to become key areas of focus [30].

Conclusion

Beginning in the late 1990s, there was rapid progression in the field of ESI over a decade from intra-arterial thrombolysis to mechanical thrombectomy devices, and eventually to the stent retriever. Despite these rapid technological breakthroughs, early device development lacked rigorous regulatory scrutiny. Initial attempts at RCTs to evaluate the efficacy of ESI were flawed in methodology and trial design, leading to an underestimation of the efficacy of stent retrieval. Learning from these experiences, numerous landmark RCTs have since successfully established stent retrieval as the standard of care for select patients with acute LVO stroke. This narrative underscores the importance of rigorous assessment as research continues to build on past models and techniques to improve device navigability, clot engagement, and retrieval success rates.

References

[1] Furlan A, et al. Intra-arterial prourokinase for acute ischemic stroke: the PROACT II study: a randomized controlled trial. *JAMA* (1999) 282 (21):2003–2011.

[2] Smith WS, et al. Mechanical thrombectomy for acute ischemic stroke: final results of the Multi MERCI trial. *Stroke* (2008) 39 (4):1205–1212.

[3] Smith WS, et al. Safety and efficacy of mechanical embolectomy in acute ischemic stroke: results of the MERCI trial. *Stroke* (2005) 36 (7):1432–1438.

[4] Smith WS, Furlan AJ. Brief history of endovascular acute ischemic stroke treatment. *Stroke* (2016) 47 (2):e23–e26.

[5] Bageac DV, Gershon BS, De Leacy RA. The evolution of devices and techniques in endovascular stroke therapy. *Exon Publications* (2021):149–170.

[6] Henkes H, et al. A novel microcatheter-delivered, highly-flexible and fully-retrievable stent, specifically designed for intracranial use. *Interventional Neuroradiology* (2003) 9 (4):391–393.

[7] Pérez MA, et al. Intracranial thrombectomy using the Solitaire stent: a historical vignette. *Journal of NeuroInterventional Surgery* (2012) 4 (6):e32.

[8] Kelly ME, Furlan AJ, Fiorella D. Recanalization of an acute middle cerebral artery occlusion using a self-expanding, reconstrainable, intracranial microstent as a temporary endovascular bypass. *Stroke* (2008) 39 (6):1770–1773.

[9] Shrivastava S, Cam A, Slee E. A novel device for the revascularization in acute ischemic stroke patients. *Interventional Neuroradiology* (2010) 16 (3):306–308.

[10] Levy EI, et al. First Food and Drug Administration-approved prospective trial of primary intracranial stenting for acute stroke: SARIS (stent-assisted recanalization in acute ischemic stroke). *Stroke* (2009) 40 (11):3552–3556.

[11] Saver JL. The evolution of technology. *Stroke* (2013) 44 (6_suppl_1):S13–S15.

[12] Saver JL, et al. Solitaire flow restoration device versus the Merci Retriever in patients with acute ischaemic stroke (SWIFT): a randomised, parallel-group, non-inferiority trial. *The Lancet* (2012) 380 (9849):1241–1249.

[13] Nogueira RG, et al. Trevo versus Merci retrievers for thrombectomy revascularisation of large vessel occlusions in acute ischaemic stroke (TREVO 2): a randomised trial. *The Lancet* (2012) 380 (9849):1231–1240.

[14] Broderick JP, et al. Endovascular therapy after intravenous t-PA versus t-PA alone for stroke. *New England Journal of Medicine* (2013) 368 (10):893–903.

[15] Ciccone A, et al. Endovascular treatment for acute ischemic stroke. *New England Journal of Medicine* (2013) 368 (10):904–913.

[16] Kidwell CS, et al. A trial of imaging selection and endovascular treatment for ischemic stroke. *New England Journal of Medicine* (2013) 368 (10):914–923.

[17] Berkhemer OA, et al. A randomized trial of intraarterial treatment for acute ischemic stroke. *New England Journal of Medicine* (2015) 372 (1):11–20.

[18] Campbell BC, et al. Endovascular therapy for ischemic stroke with perfusion-imaging selection. *New England Journal of Medicine* (2015) 372 (11):1009–1018.

[19] Goyal M, et al. Randomized assessment of rapid endovascular treatment of ischemic stroke. *New England Journal of Medicine* (2015) 372 (11):1019–1030.

[20] Jovin TG, et al. Thrombectomy within 8 hours after symptom onset in ischemic stroke. *New England Journal of Medicine* (2015) 372 (24):2296–2306.

[21] Saver JL, et al. Stent-retriever thrombectomy after intravenous t-PA vs. t-PA alone in stroke. *New England Journal of Medicine* (2015) 372 (24):2285–2295.

[22] Nogueira RG, et al. Thrombectomy 6 to 24 hours after stroke with a mismatch between deficit and infarct. *New England Journal of Medicine* (2018) 378 (1):11–21.

[23] Deshaies EM. Tri-axial system using the Solitaire-FR and Penumbra Aspiration Microcatheter for acute mechanical thrombectomy. *Journal of Clinical Neuroscience* (2013) 20 (9):1303–1305.

[24] Massari F, et al. ARTS (aspiration–retriever technique for stroke): initial clinical experience. *Interventional Neuroradiology* (2016) 22 (3):325–332.

[25] Maus V, et al. Maximizing first-pass complete reperfusion with SAVE. *Clinical Neuroradiology* (2018) 28:327–338.

[26] McTaggart RA, et al. Continuous aspiration prior to intracranial vascular embolectomy (CAPTIVE): a technique which improves outcomes. *Journal of NeuroInterventional Surgery* (2017) 9 (12):1154–1159.

[27] Biederko R, et al. Improved first-pass effect in acute stroke thrombectomy using Solitaire-X compared to Solitaire-FR. *Frontiers in Neurology* (2023) 14:1215349.

[28] Etter MM, et al. Initial experience with the Trevo NXT stent retriever. *Frontiers in Neurology* (2021) 12:704329.

[29] Ahmed SU, et al. Stentrievers: An engineering review. *Interventional Neuroradiology* (2023) 29 (2):125–133.

[30] Kühn AL, et al. Biomechanics and hemodynamics of stent-retrievers. *Journal of Cerebral Blood Flow & Metabolism* (2020) 40 (12):2350–2365.

Chapter 11

The History and Development of Femoral Access

Minaam Farooq[1,*]**, MBBS**
Amna Khalid[1,†]**, MBBS**
Ahmed Muthana[2,‡]**, MD**
and Samer S. Hoz[3,§]**, MD**

[1]Department of Neurosurgery, King Edward Medical University, Mayo Hospital Lahore, Pakistan
[2]Department of Neurosurgery, University of Baghdad, Baghdad, Iraq
[3]Department of Neurosurgery, University of Cincinnati Medical Center, Cincinnati, OH, USA

Abstract

This chapter explores the beginnings of transfemoral access in the mid-18th century, with its use for invasive hemodynamic assessment in animals, and later progress to the 1960s, when transfemoral access was used for coronary angiography in humans and then to its use in neurointervention. It examines the anatomical aspects and obstacles encountered in the widespread use of femoral access in neurointerventional surgery. We discuss the advantages of femoral access, including the ones due to its anatomic location and large size, such as ease in hemostasis, decreased limb ischemia, easier repeated approach, and shorter learning curve. The current clinical evidence-supported applications of femoral access in various neurointerventional procedures highlight its efficacy and safety. Some complications have also been associated with femoral access, such as access site hemorrhage, groin hematoma, retroperitoneal hematoma, and arterial occlusion. Still, ongoing efforts are to address these challenges through procedural refinements and technological innovations. There has been a rise in the popularity of trans-radial access in cardiology to replace transfemoral access; however, it is still the gold standard in neurointerventional surgery. Moreover, we summarize insights into future directions and emerging trends in femoral access for neurointerventional surgery.

Keywords: femoral access, transfemoral, neurointerventional surgery

* Corresponding Author's Email: minaamkemu2018@gmail.com
† Corresponding Author's Email: amnakhalidiqbal@gmail.com
‡ Corresponding Author's Email: ahmed.m.najm@gmail.com
§ Corresponding Author's Email: hozsamer2055@gmail.com

In: World History of Neurointerventional Surgery
Editors: Xianli Lv and Zhongxue Wu
ISBN: 979-8-89530-792-2

Introduction

Femoral access refers to the technique of accessing the femoral artery, typically through a percutaneous puncture in the groin area, to facilitate various medical procedures, including diagnostic and interventional operations. This method allows inserting catheters and other instruments necessary for conducting procedures within the vascular system, particularly within the heart and brain [1].

Femoral access is crucial in neurointerventional surgery due to its direct and relatively straightforward route to the cerebral vasculature. The large diameter and superficial location of the femoral artery make it an ideal entry point for introducing catheters and other devices necessary for intricate neurointerventional procedures (Figure 1). Its use is limited to neuro interventions, cardiology, vascular surgery, and emergency medicine, demonstrating its versatility and essential role in modern medical practice [2].

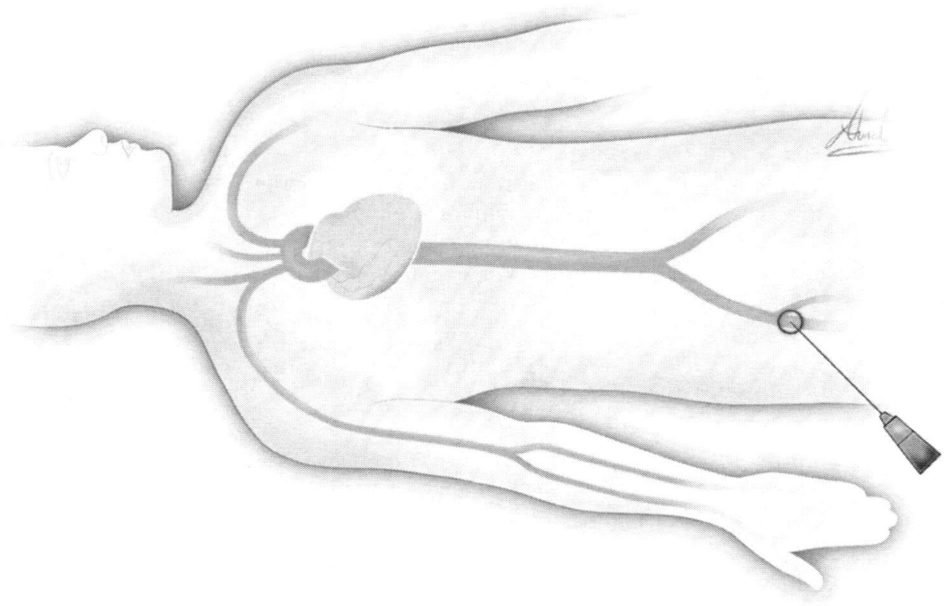

Figure 1. Schematic illustration depicts the femoral access route in the setting of neurointerventional procedures—illustration prepared by Ahmed Muthana and courtesy of Samer Hoz.

Femoral Access History in Neurointerventional Surgery

Early Beginnings in the Mid-18th Century

The origins of femoral access can be traced back to the mid-18th century. During this period, researchers began experimenting with invasive techniques to understand the dynamics of the vascular system in animals. One of the earliest documented uses of catheterization was performed by Claude Bernard, a French physiologist, who utilized the technique to measure blood pressure in animals, laying the groundwork for future applications in humans. This work by Bernard was foundational in understanding hemodynamics and vascular physiology.

In 1929, Werner Forssmann, a German physician, performed the first human cardiac catheterization by inserting a catheter into his antecubital vein and advancing it to the right atrium [3]. This daring experiment demonstrated the potential for using catheter-based techniques in humans, although it was not initially performed via the femoral route [4].

Advancements in the 1960s

The 1960s saw the introduction of femoral access for coronary angiography, revolutionizing the cardiology field. An American pediatric cardiologist, Dr. Mason Sones, inadvertently discovered the technique while performing aortic root angiography. His subsequent refinements led to the development of selective coronary angiography, allowing for detailed visualization of the coronary arteries. Sones' work marked a significant advancement in cardiovascular diagnostics [4].

The technique of femoral access was further refined by Dr. Sven-Ivar Seldinger in 1953, who introduced the Seldinger technique, a method for percutaneous vascular access that remains in use today (Figure 2). This technique involves puncturing the vessel with a needle, inserting a guidewire, and then threading a catheter over the guidewire. Dr. Melvin Judkins later adapted this technique for coronary angiography, developing pre-shaped catheters that facilitated the selective catheterization of coronary arteries. The Seldinger technique and Judkins' innovations significantly enhanced the safety and efficacy of vascular access.

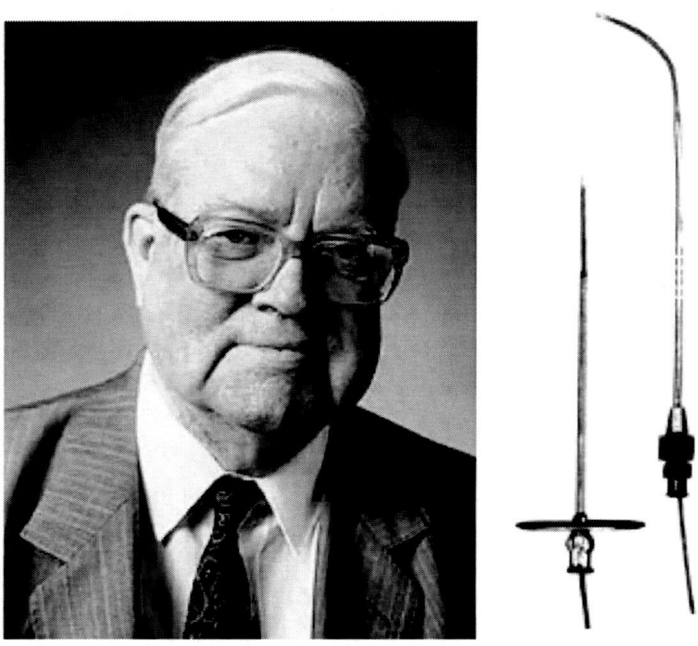

Figure 2. Dr. Sven-Ivar Seldinger introduced the Seldinger technique in 1953.

Femoral access was adopted in neurointerventional surgery as practitioners recognized the benefits of using a large, easily accessible artery to introduce catheters and other devices into the cerebral circulation. The ability to perform detailed diagnostic imaging and therapeutic interventions via the femoral artery has significantly advanced the field of neurointerventional surgery [5].

Anatomical and Technical Considerations

Anatomical Aspects

Suitability of the Femoral Artery

The femoral artery is favored for vascular access due to its large diameter and superficial location in the groin area, making it easily accessible for percutaneous interventions. Its size accommodates various catheter sizes and allows for the insertion of multiple devices necessary for complex neurointerventional procedures. The artery's straight course also facilitates the advancement of catheters and guidewires into the aorta and cerebral vasculature, which is crucial for neurointerventional surgery.

Anatomical Location and Accessibility

The femoral artery is located within the femoral triangle, bordered by the inguinal ligament superiorly, the adductor longus muscle medially, and the sartorius muscle laterally. This anatomical positioning makes it relatively easy to palpate and access, even in emergencies. The superficial nature of the artery at this location reduces the risk of complications such as accidental puncture of adjacent structures, enhancing the safety profile of the femoral approach [6].

Common Obstacles in Femoral Access

Groin Hematoma

Groin hematoma, a localized blood collection at the puncture site, is another frequent complication. It is usually self-limiting but can sometimes require intervention if it leads to significant discomfort or pressure effects. Hematomas can be minimized by meticulous technique and closure devices [7].

Retroperitoneal Hematoma

Retroperitoneal hematoma is a serious complication when the puncture site is too high, leading to bleeding into the retroperitoneal space. This condition is potentially life-threatening and requires prompt diagnosis and management, often necessitating imaging studies and surgical intervention [8].

Arterial Occlusion

Arterial occlusion can occur due to thrombosis at the puncture site or dissection of the femoral artery. It can lead to limb ischemia and requires immediate attention, often involving thrombectomy or surgical repair [9].

Innovations and Best Practices

Ultrasound-Guided Access

Using ultrasound guidance for femoral artery cannulation has become a standard practice to enhance the accuracy of vessel puncture and minimize complications. Studies have demonstrated that ultrasound guidance significantly reduces the incidence of failed punctures, hematomas, and arterial complications compared to the traditional landmark-based technique [10].

Hemostasis Management

Achieving effective hemostasis after femoral artery access is critical to preventing complications such as bleeding and pseudoaneurysms. Vascular closure devices (VCDs) have been developed to provide reliable closure of the femoral puncture site (Figure 3). These devices include collagen plugs, suture-mediated closure systems, and stapling devices, each offering distinct advantages in ease of use and hemostatic efficacy [11].

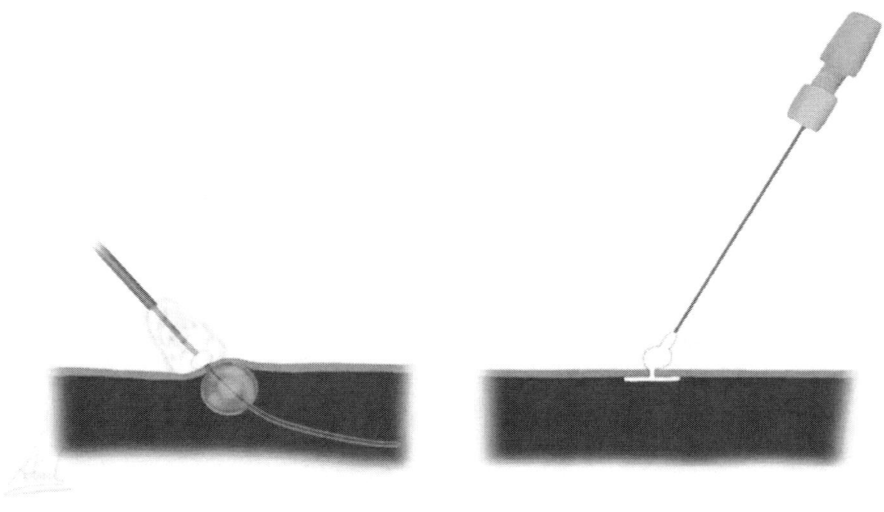

Figure 3. Examples of closure devices for femoral access. Right: Angio-Seal. Left: Mynx—illustration prepared by Ahmed Muthana and courtesy of Samer Hoz.

Training and Skill Development

The learning curve for femoral access can be steep, particularly for complex neurointerventional procedures. Training programs incorporating simulation-based learning and hands-on workshops have been shown to enhance practitioners' proficiency in femoral access techniques. These programs emphasize the importance of anatomical knowledge, technical skills, and complication management to ensure high standards of patient care [12].

Advantages of Femoral Access

Advantages of the Femoral Artery for Hemostasis

The femoral artery's anatomical location and size significantly facilitate hemostasis after procedures. The artery is easily compressible against the femoral head, allowing effective manual compression to stop bleeding. This makes achieving hemostasis more straightforward compared to other vascular access points, such as the radial artery, where bone support is less favorable [1]. Additionally, the larger diameter of the femoral artery permits closure devices, which further aids in rapid and effective hemostasis.

Lower Risk of Limb Ischemia

Femoral access is associated with a lower risk of limb ischemia than other access routes, particularly the radial artery. The femoral artery's size and robust collateral circulation contribute to this advantage [13].

Learning Curve for Clinicians

The learning curve for femoral access is shorter than that of other vascular access methods. This is partly due to the straightforward anatomical landmarks and the larger size of the femoral artery, which make puncture and catheterization easier to master [10]. Training programs often emphasize femoral access as a foundational skill, providing clinicians with the competence to perform various vascular interventions [14]. The shorter learning curve translates to quicker proficiency, enhancing patient safety and procedural efficiency [15].

Advantages over Other Access Points

While the trans-radial approach is gaining popularity in cardiology due to its lower complication rates at the access site, femoral access remains superior for neurointerventional procedures. This is due to the ability to navigate larger catheters necessary for treating cerebrovascular diseases [16].

Clinical Applications of Femoral Access

Cerebral Angiography

Cerebral angiography, a critical diagnostic tool in neurointerventional surgery, relies heavily on femoral access. This procedure involves injecting contrast dye into the cerebral arteries via a catheter introduced through the femoral artery, allowing for detailed visualization of the vascular anatomy and detecting abnormalities such as aneurysms, arteriovenous malformations, and stenosis [17]. The femoral artery's large diameter and direct route to the aorta make it an ideal access point for this procedure [18].

Mechanical Thrombectomy

Mechanical thrombectomy for acute ischemic stroke is another key application of femoral access. This procedure involves removing a clot from a blocked cerebral artery to restore blood flow to the brain. Studies have shown that femoral access provides the necessary support and stability for deploying large-bore catheters and stent retrievers in thrombectomy [19]. The success of mechanical thrombectomy procedures has significantly improved patient outcomes, reducing the disability associated with acute stroke.

Aneurysm Coiling

Femoral access is also used in the endovascular treatment of cerebral aneurysms through coil embolization. This procedure involves inserting coils into the aneurysm via a catheter to induce thrombosis and prevent rupture. The femoral artery's size allows for various coil delivery systems, contributing to the effectiveness of this minimally invasive technique [20].

Efficacy and Safety of Femoral Access

Clinical Evidence Supporting Femoral Access

Numerous studies have demonstrated the efficacy and safety of femoral access in neurointerventional procedures. For instance, a comprehensive review of endovascular treatments for ischemic stroke reported high rates of successful revascularization and favorable outcomes associated with femoral access [21].

Comparison with Radial Access

While the trans-radial approach is gaining traction in cardiology, femoral access remains the preferred method for neurointerventional procedures. This preference is due to the larger catheter sizes required for cerebrovascular interventions, which are more easily accommodated by the femoral artery [13]. Additionally, the femoral route provides a more direct path to the cerebral arteries, reducing procedure time and increasing the efficiency of interventions (Table 1).

Advantages of Trans-Radial Access

Trans-radial access has gained significant popularity in cardiology due to several key advantages over transfemoral access, including a lower risk of access site complications, such as bleeding and hematoma, and increased patient comfort. The radial artery is smaller and more superficial, contributing to faster patient mobilization and shorter hospital stays [22]. Additionally, the use of trans-radial access has been associated with reduced mortality and morbidity rates in coronary interventions, making it a preferred choice for many cardiologists [23]. Studies have shown that trans-radial access reduces the incidence of major bleeding complications, which is a significant advantage for patients undergoing percutaneous coronary interventions [24].

Table 1. Comparison of femoral and radial access

	Femoral Access	Radial Access
Vessel Diameter	Large, accommodates larger catheters	Smaller, limited to smaller catheters
Ease of Hemostasis	Easier, due to compression against femoral head	More challenging
Procedural Time	Generally shorter	Potentially longer due to navigation challenges
Complication Rates	Higher risk of bleeding and hematoma	Lower risk of major bleeding, but risk of spasm
Patient Mobilization	Longer recovery time	Faster recovery and mobilization

Technical Considerations

Neurointerventional procedures often require larger-bore catheters to accommodate various devices for embolization, thrombectomy, and stenting. With its larger size and direct route to the aortic arch and cerebral vessels, the femoral artery is better suited for these requirements. Additionally, the anatomical course of the radial artery presents challenges in navigating to the cerebral circulation, which can increase procedural time and complexity [25].

Contradictory Findings

While some studies suggest that trans-radial access may be feasible for certain neurointerventional procedures, the evidence still needs to be conclusive. For example, a study comparing trans-radial and transfemoral access for mechanical thrombectomy in stroke patients found no significant difference in procedural success or patient outcomes [19]. However, other studies highlight the technical difficulties and increased procedural times associated with the radial approach, suggesting that more research is needed to determine its efficacy and safety in neurointerventional settings [26].

Need for Further Research

The ongoing debate over the optimal access route for neurointerventional procedures underscores the need for further research. Larger randomized controlled trials are necessary to compare the long-term outcomes and complication rates of trans-radial versus transfemoral access in neurointerventional surgery. Additionally, advancements in catheter technology and procedural techniques may eventually address some of the limitations of trans-radial access, making it a more viable option.

Future Directions and Emerging Trends

Imaging Enhancements

Enhanced imaging technologies, including three-dimensional rotational angiography and intravascular ultrasound (IVUS), have significantly improved the precision of femoral access procedures. These imaging modalities provide detailed views of the vascular anatomy, aiding in accurate catheter placement and reducing the risk of complications [27]. Integrating real-time imaging with femoral access procedures facilitates better decision-making and outcomes [28].

Robotic Assistance

Introducing robotic systems in femoral access-based procedures represents a promising frontier. Robotic-assisted catheter navigation offers greater precision and control, minimizing human error and enhancing procedural accuracy [29]. These systems can be particularly beneficial in complex cases requiring delicate maneuvers. Robotic assistance can improve the safety and efficacy of femoral access procedures, although further research is needed to establish its long-term benefits.

Enhanced Hemostasis Techniques

Advancements in hemostasis techniques have further improved the safety profile of femoral access. New vascular closure devices (VCDs), such as absorbable collagen plugs and suture-mediated closure systems, have shown efficacy in achieving rapid hemostasis and reducing complications like bleeding and pseudoaneurysm formation. These devices have been increasingly adopted in clinical practice, improving patient outcomes [30].

Improved Patient Safety

The continuous evolution of femoral access techniques and technologies is poised to enhance patient safety. By reducing procedural complications and improving the accuracy of interventions, these advancements are expected to lower the overall risk associated with neurointerventional procedures. This, in turn, will lead to better patient outcomes and higher satisfaction rates [21].

Reduced Procedure Times and Costs

Technological and procedural innovations are likely to reduce procedure times, which can decrease the length of hospital stays and associated healthcare costs. Efficient procedures with fewer complications translate to lower resource utilization and better allocation of medical services. The economic benefits of these advancements are significant, particularly in resource-constrained healthcare settings [31].

Expanding Indications

As femoral access techniques evolve, their indications are expected to expand. These advancements will likely benefit emerging therapies for cerebrovascular diseases, such as endovascular treatments for intracranial atherosclerotic disease and complex aneurysms. This expansion will provide more patients access to minimally invasive treatment options, improving overall care [32].

Conclusion

Femoral access began in the mid-18th century with animal studies and was first applied in humans by Werner Forssmann in 1929. Major advancements occurred in the 1960s with the development of coronary angiography and the Seldinger technique.

The femoral artery's large diameter and superficial location make it ideal for accessing the vascular system, allowing the use of larger catheters necessary for complex neurointerventional procedures.

Femoral access is essential for cerebral angiography, mechanical thrombectomy, and aneurysm coiling. It offers high success rates and better patient outcomes than other access methods.

Common complications include access site hemorrhage, groin hematoma, and retroperitoneal hematoma. Strategies such as ultrasound-guided puncture and advanced hemostasis techniques with vascular closure devices help mitigate these risks.

Advancements in catheter technology, enhanced imaging, and robotic assistance are expected to improve the safety and efficacy of femoral access. Personalized approaches based on patient-specific anatomy and risk factors also enhance procedural outcomes.

References

[1] Kandarpa K, Machan L. *Handbook of Interventional Radiologic Procedures*. 2011: Lippincott Williams & Wilkins.

[2] Patton KT, et al. *Anatomy & Physiology with Brief Atlas of the Human Body and Quick Guide to the Language of Science and Medicine-E-Book*. 2022: Elsevier Health Sciences.

[3] Forssmann W. Die sondierung des rechten herzens. 1929.

[4] Proudfit WL, Shirey EK, Sones FM Jr. Selective cine coronary arteriography: correlation with clinical findings in 1,000 patients. *Circulation* (1966) 33 (6):901–910.

[5] Berenstein A, Kricheff II. Catheter and material selection for transarterial embolization: Technical considerations: I. Catheters. *Radiology* (1979) 132 (3):619–630.

[6] Bangalore S, Bhatt DL. Femoral arterial access and closure. *Circulation* (2011) 124 (5):e147–e156.

[7] Carrozza JP. Complications of diagnostic cardiac catheterization. *Circulation: Cardiovascular Interventions* (2012) 5:127.

[8] Kumar AR, Rajiv A. Percutaneous treatment of severe retroperitoneal hematoma after percutaneous coronary intervention. *Journal of Cardiology and Cardiovascular Medicine* (2021) 6 (3):055–058.

[9] McCann RL, Schwartz LB, Pieper KS. Vascular complications of cardiac catheterization. *Journal of Vascular Surgery* (1991) 14 (3):375–381.

[10] Li J, et al. Meta-analysis of ultrasound-guided and traditional femoral artery puncture. *Frontiers in Cardiovascular Medicine* (2023) 10:1161834.

[11] Castillo-Sang M, et al. Femoral artery complications after cardiac catheterization: a study of patient profile. *Annals of Vascular Surgery* (2010) 24 (3):328–335.

[12] Siegl G, Ott T, Cohnert T. Simulation-based training as a continuous means of vascular surgical education—a roadmap. *European Surgery* (2022) 54 (3):176–180.

[13] Phillips TJ, et al. Transradial versus transfemoral access for anterior circulation mechanical thrombectomy: analysis of 375 consecutive cases. *Stroke and Vascular Neurology* (2021) 6 (2).

[14] Qureshi AM, Mullins CE, Latson LA. Recent advances in managing vascular occlusions in the cardiac catheterization laboratory. *F1000Research* (2018) 7.

[15] Noori VJ, Eldrup-Jørgensen J. A systematic review of vascular closure devices for femoral artery puncture sites. *Journal of Vascular Surgery* (2018) 68 (3):887–899.

[16] Seldinger SI. Catheter replacement of the needle in percutaneous arteriography: a new technique. *Acta Radiologica* (1953) 39 (5):368–376.

[17] Wolpert S, Caplan L. Current role of cerebral angiography in the diagnosis of cerebrovascular diseases. *American Journal of Roentgenology* (1992) 159 (1):191–197.

[18] Willinsky RA, et al. Neurologic complications of cerebral angiography: prospective analysis of 2,899 procedures and review of the literature. *Radiology* (2003) 227 (2):522–528.

[19] Raha O, et al. Advances in mechanical thrombectomy for acute ischaemic stroke. *BMJ Medicine* (2023) 2 (1).

[20] Molyneux A. International Subarachnoid Aneurysm Trial (ISAT) of neurosurgical clipping versus endovascular coiling in 2143 patients with ruptured intracranial aneurysms: a randomised trial. *The Lancet* (2002) 360 (9342):1267–1274.

[21] Saver JL, et al. Stent-retriever thrombectomy after intravenous t-PA vs. t-PA alone in stroke. *New England Journal of Medicine* (2015) 372 (24):2285–2295.

[22] Jolly SS, et al. Radial versus femoral access for coronary angiography or intervention and the impact on major bleeding and ischemic events: a systematic review and meta-analysis of randomized trials. *American Heart Journal* (2009) 157 (1):132–140.

[23] Jolly SS, et al. Outcomes after thrombus aspiration for ST elevation myocardial infarction: 1-year follow-up of the prospective randomised TOTAL trial. *The Lancet* (2016) 387 (10014):127–135.

[24] Agostoni P, et al. Radial versus femoral approach for percutaneous coronary diagnostic and interventional procedures: systematic overview and meta-analysis of randomized trials. *Journal of the American College of Cardiology* (2004) 44 (2):349–356.

[25] Shaban S, et al. The association of transradial access and transfemoral access with procedural outcomes in acute ischemic stroke patients receiving endovascular thrombectomy: a meta-analysis. *Clinical Neurology and Neurosurgery* (2022) 215:107209.

[26] Nohara AM, Kallmes DF. Transradial cerebral angiography: technique and outcomes. *American Journal of Neuroradiology* (2003) 24 (6):1247–1250.

[27] Combaz X, et al. Three-dimensional rotational angiography in the assessment of the angioarchitecture of brain arteriovenous malformations. *Journal of Neuroradiology* (2011) 38 (3):167–174.

[28] Janardhan V, Qureshi AI. Advances in interventional neuroimaging. *Neurotherapeutics* (2007) 4:414–419.

[29] Crinnion W, et al. Robotics in neurointerventional surgery: a systematic review of the literature. *Journal of NeuroInterventional Surgery* (2022) 14 (6):539–545.

[30] Biancari F, et al. Meta-analysis of randomized trials on the efficacy of vascular closure devices after diagnostic angiography and angioplasty. *American Heart Journal* (2010) 159 (4):518–531.

[31] Brunet M-C, Chen SH, Peterson EC. Transradial access for neurointerventions: management of access challenges and complications. *Journal of NeuroInterventional Surgery* (2020) 12 (1):82–86.

[32] Goyal M, et al. Endovascular thrombectomy after large-vessel ischaemic stroke: a meta-analysis of individual patient data from five randomised trials. *The Lancet* (2016) 387 (10029):1723–1731.

Chapter 12

The History and Development of Radial Access

Muhammad Kashif[1,*]
Ahmed Muthana[2,†], MD
and Samer S. Hoz[3,‡], MD
[1]Midwesterner University, Glendale, AZ, USA
[2]Department of Neurosurgery, University of Baghdad, Baghdad, Iraq
[3]Department of Neurosurgery, University of Cincinnati Medical Center, Cincinnati, OH, USA

Abstract

The chapter titled "History and Development of Radial Access" provides a comprehensive overview of the evolution and advancements in the utilization of radial access in neurointerventional procedures. Beginning with the origins of radial access in the early 20th century, the chapter traces the challenges and milestones encountered in integrating this approach into neurointerventional surgery. Key topics include the anatomical considerations, early challenges, and technological innovations that have shaped the development of radial access techniques. Furthermore, the chapter explores the advantages and limitations of radial access compared to traditional femoral approaches, highlighting its potential to enhance patient outcomes and minimize procedural risks. Current applications of radial access in various neurointerventional procedures, supported by clinical evidence, are also discussed. Finally, the chapter offers insights into future directions and technological innovations that hold promise for further advancing the field of radial access in neurointerventional surgery.

Keywords: radial access, transradial, neurointerventional surgery

Introduction

In recent years, the field of neurointerventional surgery has witnessed significant changes and developments, with the emergence of new methods and strategies targeted at improving patient

* Corresponding Author's Email: kashiforakzai2500@gmail.com
† Corresponding Author's Email: ahmed.m.najm@gmail.com
‡ Corresponding Author's Email: hozsamer2055@gmail.com

In: World History of Neurointerventional Surgery
Editors: Xianli Lv and Zhongxue Wu
ISBN: 979-8-89530-792-2

outcomes and reducing procedure risks [1]. One of these innovations is radial access, which has gained a lot of attention due to its potential to revolutionize the subfield. Radial access has become a viable option for safer and more efficient procedures, with possible benefits over conventional femoral methods [2]. It involves gaining access to the vascular system via the wrist's radial artery, allowing for neurointerventional surgery (Figure 1). The radial artery, with its average diameter of 2 to 3 millimeters, is more accessible than the conventional femoral or carotid access points. Different shapes in the radial arteries, like hypoplasia, occlusion, loops, and tortuosity, can make things harder, such as by making cannulation harder or increasing the risk of complications during and after surgery. Despite these challenges, radiation access has proven to be a valid substitute in neurointerventional surgery, providing better patient outcomes and procedural efficacy [3].

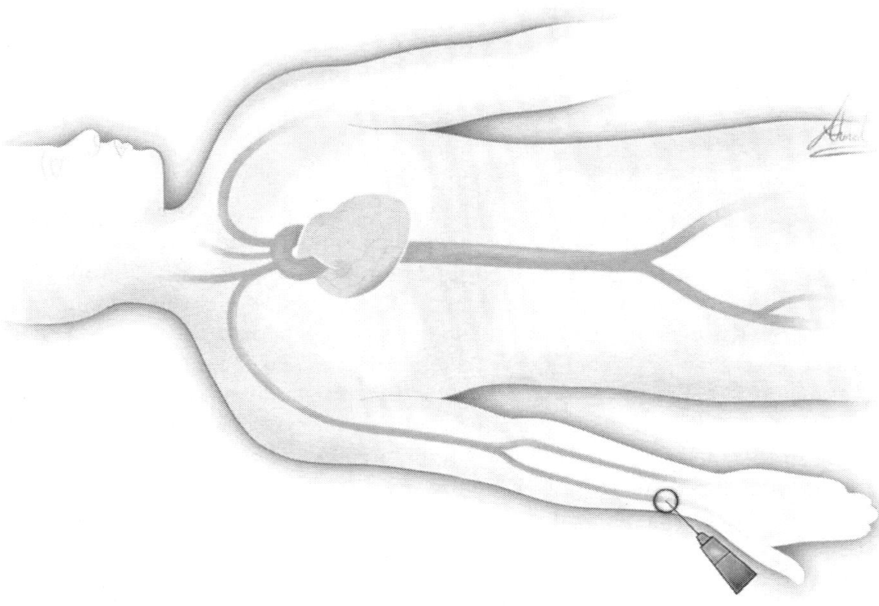

Figure 1. Schematic illustration depicts the radial access route in the setting of neurointerventional procedures—illustration prepared by Ahmed Muthana and courtesy of Samer Hoz.

Radial Access's History in Neurointerventional Surgery

Radial access for vascular procedures first emerged as an alternative to femoral access in the early 20th century. Although initially limited to diagnostic procedures like coronary angiography, it became apparent that radial access had therapeutic potential [4, 5]. However, adapting it for neurointerventional purposes posed significant challenges due to the cerebral vasculature's complex anatomical structure and advanced technology.

Initial Challenges and Milestones

Radial access for neurointerventional treatments faced several obstacles in its early years, including technological and anatomical limitations. Vascular tortuosity, poor catheter support, and limited device compatibility were some of the problems that made it harder to get into the radial artery for neurointerventional purposes at first [6]. Despite these difficulties, medical professionals continued to improve methods and overcome obstacles, resulting in significant advancements in the field [7]. The development of guidewires and specialized microcatheters for radial access marked a milestone in the late 1990s. These improvements made it easier to get through complicated artery paths and improved the distribution of devices, leading to more use of radial methods in neurointerventional treatments.

The shift from the traditional femoral access method initially presented significant challenges for neurointerventionalists. They had to learn new radial access procedures, such as hemostasis and radial artery cannulation. It was difficult to use larger tools or navigate through narrow channels due to the narrower diameter of the radial artery. However, as practitioners became more proficient with radial access, they developed new instruments and equipment tailored to radial access techniques. These included reduced-caliber guide catheters, hydrophilic-coated wires, and low-profile microcatheters. These advancements successfully addressed the technical difficulties of radial access and expanded its suitability for a wider range of neurointerventional treatments.

Another notable achievement was the creation of standardized protocols and optimal methods for radial access in neurointerventional surgery. These protocols included criteria for selecting patients, treatment methodologies, and strategies for managing patients after the procedure. They are designed to optimize safety and effectiveness while reducing potential risks, such as radial artery perforation or thrombosis during the procedure.

Collecting clinical data demonstrating the safety and effectiveness of radial access in neurointerventional surgery has been crucial to making it widely used. Comparative clinical investigations consistently show that radial access is equal to or better than femoral access in terms of access site problems, surgery success rates, and patient satisfaction. The growing body of evidence has given neurointerventionalists confidence in the practicality and advantages of radial access, resulting in greater acceptance and adoption of this method.

Educational activities and training programs have also been critical in overcoming initial obstacles and facilitating the acceptance of radial access for neurointerventional surgery. Several facilities were offered to neurointerventionalists such as hands-on workshops, simulation training, and proctoring programs to enhance their skills and knowledge of radial access methods.

By overcoming its early challenges, there are notable advancements that have made radial access for neurointerventional surgery easier. Radial access has become a viable alternative to traditional femoral access due to technical improvements, established procedures, clinical data, and educational initiatives. It offers crucial advantages regarding patient safety, procedural efficacy, and operator convenience. It is predicted that the role of radial access in neurointerventional surgery will continue to develop and expand as neurointerventionalists perfect their skills and gain more experience.

Current Applications and Clinical Evidence

Radial access is becoming more common for neurointerventional procedures. These include cerebral angiography, endovascular thrombectomy, and embolization of arteriovenous malformations and intracranial aneurysms [8, 9]. Clinical studies assessing the safety and efficacy of radial methods have shown comparable or better outcomes than femoral access in terms of procedural success rates and complication rates. Ferrante in his meta-analysis compares radial access to femoral access for endovascular treatment of acute ischemic stroke [10]. The study linked radial access to better functional outcomes at follow-up and a lower incidence of access-site problems. Similarly, Patel et al.'s prospective study found that radial access for cerebral aneurysm embolization had better results than femoral access, including fewer access site problems and shorter hospital stays [11].

The future looks promising with advancements in technology, and radial access offers a bright future in neurointerventional surgery. The continuous improvements in technology and procedural advancements have made radial methods more effective and viable. The development of robotic-assisted navigation technologies, along with better catheter and micro-catheter design, will further enhance the effectiveness of radial methods [12]. The focus on personalized care and minimally invasive procedures will encourage people to take an interest in radial access for neurointerventional procedures, which can help with funding. We need more research to select patients, enhance procedures, and expand the scope of radial interventions. This can improve patient outcomes and change the field of neurointerventional surgery.

Diagnostic Cerebral Angiography

In diagnostic cerebral angiography, radial access has become a viable alternative to femoral access, providing improved patient comfort, reduced access site problems, and faster recovery periods [9]. Clinical investigations have demonstrated that radial access is comparable to femoral access in terms of diagnostic image quality and procedural success rates. Ruzsa et al. found no significant differences in picture quality or procedural outcomes between radial and femoral access for diagnostic cerebral angiography [13]. Additionally, studies have linked radial access to shorter hospitalization durations and lower healthcare expenses than femoral access, further demonstrating its usefulness in this setting.

Coil Embolization

Coil embolization is a technique that can treat cerebral aneurysms. Radial access has shown promise in coil embolization treatments for cerebral aneurysms, providing benefits such as excellent patient safety, fewer problems at the access site, and improved operator ergonomics. Clinical studies have shown that radial access gives the same or better results in coil embolization procedures than femoral access. For example, Goktekin et al. conducted a meta-analysis that found comparable rates of procedural success and complication rates when comparing the radial and femoral routes for coil embolization of cerebral aneurysms [14]. Researchers have also found that radial access leads to shorter procedure times and reduced radiation exposure for patients and operators. This emphasizes its potential to make procedures safer and more efficient in this setting.

Mechanical Thrombectomy for Acute Stroke

Radial access has become increasingly popular in mechanical thrombectomy treatments for acute stroke due to its benefits, including quicker groin hemostasis, decreased access site problems, and enhanced patient comfort [15]. Clinical investigations show that radial access produces similar or better results than femoral access in mechanical thrombectomy operations. A study by Snelling et al. compared the radial and femoral routes for mechanical thrombectomy in people who had recently had a stroke [16]. They found no significant differences in the rates of procedure success, functional outcomes, or complications. Researchers have also found a link between radial access and shorter times between door-to-groin puncture and door-to-reperfusion. This could mean that people who have had an acute stroke get treatment faster and have better outcomes.

Embolization of Arteriovenous Malformation

Radial access has proven beneficial in embolization operations for arteriovenous malformations (AVMs), providing advantages such as greater patient comfort, fewer problems at the access site, and improved ergonomics for the operator. Empirical research has demonstrated that radial access yields equivalent or better results than femoral access in AVM embolization operations. A study by Kumar et al. found comparable procedural success and complication rates for AVM embolization using both radial and femoral routes [6]. Furthermore, studies have linked radial access to shorter recovery periods and hospital stays, highlighting its potential to improve patient outcomes and optimize healthcare resource utilization in this scenario.

Flow Diversion for Intracranial Aneurysms

Radial access has become a viable choice for flow diversion treatments in cerebral aneurysms, with benefits like increased patient safety, decreased problems at the access site, and improved ergonomics for the operator. Clinical investigations have demonstrated that radial access produces equivalent or better results than femoral access in flow diversion treatments. For example, a study by Tiseo et al. compared radial and femoral methods for flow diversion in cerebral aneurysms and found that both had similar success rates and complications [17]. Additionally, using radial access has been associated with shorter procedure times and reduced radiation exposure, potentially enhancing procedure efficiency and safety.

Advantages and Limitations of Radial Access

Radial access has several benefits and drawbacks for neurointerventional surgery, which are summarized in Table 1.

Advantages

Radial access has proven to be a promising method for neurointerventional procedures, with increasing clinical data demonstrating its safety and effectiveness in various clinical situations. In many ways, it is superior to traditional femoral access [18]. It can significantly benefit procedures such as diagnostic cerebral angiography, coil embolization of cerebral aneurysms, and mechanical thrombectomy for acute stroke. Radial access has several advantages, including increased patient comfort, reduced access site complications, and improved procedural efficiency. As neurointerventionalists refine their procedures and gain more clinical experience with radial access, we expect to see an increase in its use in neurointerventional surgery, resulting in better outcomes and a higher quality of care for patients.

Table 1. Advantages and limitations of radial access

ADVANTAGES	LIMITATIONS
a) Enhanced patient comfort	a) Anatomical constraints in certain patients
b) Reduced risk of access site complications	b) Technical challenges in complex procedures
c) Shorter recovery time	c) Learning curve for operators
d) Lower radiation exposure	d) Feasibility in patients with radial artery anomalies
e) Improved operator ergonomics	e) Increased risk of radial artery occlusion
f) Reduced risk of access site infection	f) Limited rapid and large-volume contrast injections
g) Lower rates of thromboembolic events	g) Discomfort due to prolonged wrist compression

Compared to femoral access, commonly used for brain-related surgical treatments, radial access offers several advantages. Unlike femoral access, it allows patients to sit up and move around soon after the procedure, significantly reducing the likelihood of complications such as bleeding and damage to blood vessels at the point of access. Besides, radial access eliminates the need for groin compression, which can cause discomfort and pain for patients.

Furthermore, compared to femoral access, radial access reduces the likelihood of access site problems. The radial artery is closer to the surface and has a smaller diameter, making it easier to apply pressure and reducing the risk of substantial bleeding or creating a pseudoaneurysm. The hand's collateral circulation ensures adequate blood flow even when the radial artery temporarily blocks, thus reducing the risk of ischemic effects. These advantages result in a lower risk of access site problems and an enhanced safety profile for neurointerventional operations.

Radial access also reduces radiation exposure and procedure duration for patients and operators. It eliminates the need for long arterial sheaths to navigate the iliac arteries, reducing contrast dye usage and limiting radiation exposure during the procedure. This feature is particularly beneficial for complex neurointerventional situations that require precise catheter manipulation and fluoroscopic supervision.

Finally, radial access provides greater procedural efficiency and less operator fatigue due to its superior ergonomics for the operator. The operator can sit comfortably beside the patient, maintaining a more ergonomic posture, unlike femoral access, which requires the operator to position themselves at the patient's groin level during the procedure. This feature is crucial during long neurointerventional operations, where the operator's comfort and focus play a significant role in achieving optimal results.

There are several advantages of radial and femoral access in reducing access site infections and thromboembolic events. The radial artery's superficial location allows easier bleeding control and reduces the risk of transferring pathogens into deeper tissues (Figure 2). Additionally, its smaller diameter makes it less likely to cause thromboembolic problems, such as distal embolization, which can occur at larger arterial access points. These benefits lead to better outcomes after procedures, as well as lower healthcare costs for managing access site problems.

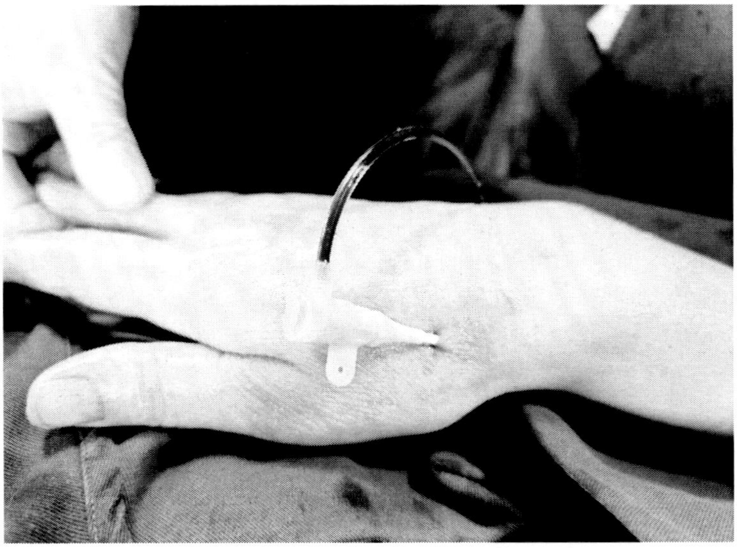

Figure 2. Radial artery puncture and implantation of arterial sheath.

Furthermore, radial access is particularly beneficial for certain patient groups, such as those with peripheral vascular disease or obesity, who may face technical difficulties or higher risks of complications with femoral access. In these individuals, the radial artery has less atherosclerotic buildup and is less prone to vascular damage, making it a safer and more practical site for neurointerventional treatments.

Radial access offers several benefits for neurointerventional surgery, including improved patient safety and comfort, fewer problems at the access site, shorter procedure times, less radiation exposure, better operator ergonomics, and lower infection and thromboembolic event rates. We anticipate its continued pivotal role in the advancement of neurointerventional surgery.

Limitations

Despite the many advantages, radial access also has some limitations and disadvantages that need to be considered. One significant drawback is that certain neurointerventional techniques have anatomical limitations. The radial artery's smaller diameter makes it impossible to perform complex procedures such as coil embolization of wide-necked aneurysms or mechanical thrombectomy for occlusions in large blood vessels. In these situations, femoral or carotid access may be more advantageous because they allow for larger and more durable devices, resulting in better procedural results.

Radial access may also present technical difficulties or become unfeasible for individuals with radial artery malformations or anatomical abnormalities. Radial loops, tortuosity, or blockage can make radial access difficult or dangerous. Furthermore, individuals with radial artery hypoplasia or radial artery spasm may not be suitable candidates for radial access, necessitating alternative access methods [19].

The learning curve required to become proficient in the approach is another limitation of radial access. Neurointerventionalists who have previously used the femoral artery as an access point may need more training and practice to become skilled at performing procedures using the radial artery as an access point. Proficiency in radial access entails acquiring expertise in accessing and cannulating the radial artery, navigating through complex radial loops, and ensuring proper bleeding control after the procedure. Consequently, there is an increased likelihood of experiencing procedural problems, such as radial artery perforation or thrombosis, while first learning the procedure.

Moreover, in many clinical situations, radial access may not be viable or ideal, especially for patients with pre-existing illnesses or comorbidities. Patients with significant peripheral arterial disease or radial artery blockage may experience restricted radial artery patency, making radial access technically tricky or not recommended. Patients with Raynaud's phenomenon or other vasospastic illnesses may have a higher likelihood of experiencing radial artery spasms. This could limit the effectiveness of radial access and cause complications during medical procedures.

Radial access is a commonly used arterial access route for neurointerventional surgery, but it has advantages and disadvantages. One drawback is that it can cause radial artery obstruction, limiting the use of the radial artery for future surgeries and procedures. Using smaller sheath diameters and minimizing the compression time can reduce this issue. However, it is still a potential disadvantage that needs to be considered, especially for patients who require multiple procedures.

Another disadvantage of radial access is that it may not be suitable for specific neurointerventional treatments that require large doses of contrast material. This is because the radial artery's smaller diameter can restrict the safe delivery rate and amount of contrast, which can impact the imaging quality and effectiveness of the procedure. In such cases, femoral or carotid access may be more beneficial, as they can accommodate larger catheters and provide better flow rates [20]. Choosing the right access route can help improve imaging quality and facilitate the supply of medical devices.

It is also important to consider the patient's comfort and preferences when selecting an access route for neurointerventional surgery. Although radial access has numerous benefits, some patients may prefer femoral access due to their familiarity with or discomfort with radial artery cannulation. Therefore, involving patients in decision-making and providing them with the necessary knowledge is crucial to ensuring that the selected access route aligns with their choices and priorities.

Generally, radial access has several advantages for neurointerventional surgery, including enhanced safety, patient comfort, and procedural efficiency. However, it also has specific limitations and disadvantages that require careful consideration. Factors such as anatomical limits, technical difficulties, the patient's existing health conditions, and limitations in using contrast can all impact the choice of access route for neurointerventional treatments. By carefully weighing the advantages and disadvantages of radial access compared to other methods, neurointerventionalists can improve patient outcomes and procedural success [20].

Future Directions

Radial access operations have promising opportunities for growth in the design and development of specialized tools and equipment [21]. This includes smaller catheters, advanced guide wire technology, and microcatheters that can accurately navigate challenging arterial structures and deliver therapeutic medicines. Incorporating robotics and artificial intelligence could also improve the precision, efficiency, and safety of radial access techniques. Robotic-assisted radial access systems can enable more precise catheter navigation, thereby reducing procedural complications and improving outcomes. Also, improvements in imaging technology like high-resolution fluoroscopy and three-dimensional rotational angiography can make it easier to view and move around during radial access procedures, which can lead to better planning and execution of the procedure. These future developments and technical advancements can further improve the safety, effectiveness, and adaptability of radial access in neurointerventional surgery, ultimately resulting in better patient outcomes.

Conclusion

Radial access in neurointerventional surgery has shown great promise for improving procedural results and patient satisfaction. It is becoming a competitive option for femoral access. With continued technological advancements and clinical research, radial access will be at the forefront of neurointerventional therapy. A radial-first approach for both diagnostic and interventional procedures is becoming more common and safer. It uses transradial access (TRA) for better patient outcomes, as well as tailored treatment strategies that supplement trans-femoral access (TFA) in certain situations. This approach aims to improve patient care through increased safety, with fewer crossovers and possible time disparities as the procedure becomes more well-known and new devices emerge.

References

[1] Kandarpa K, Machan L. *Handbook of Interventional Radiologic Procedures*. 2011: Lippincott Williams & Wilkins.

[2] Almallouhi E, et al. Fast-track incorporation of the transradial approach in endovascular neurointervention. *Journal of NeuroInterventional Surgery* (2020) 12 (2):176–180.

[3] Joshi KC, et al. Transradial approach for neurointerventions: a systematic review of the literature. *Journal of NeuroInterventional Surgery* (2020) 12 (9):886–892.

[4] Chivot C, Bouzerar R, Yzet T. Transitioning to transradial access for cerebral aneurysm embolization. *American Journal of Neuroradiology* (2019) 40 (11):1947–1953.

[5] Agostoni P, et al. Radial versus femoral approach for percutaneous coronary diagnostic and interventional procedures: systematic overview and meta-analysis of randomized trials. *Journal of the American College of Cardiology* (2004) 44 (2):349–356.

[6] Kumar A, Shukla D, Singh S. A comparative study of radial and femoral approaches for embolization of intracranial arteriovenous malformations. *Interventional Neuroradiology* (2019).

[7] Jolly SS, et al. Radial versus femoral access for coronary angiography and intervention in patients with acute coronary syndromes (RIVAL): a randomised, parallel group, multicentre trial. *The Lancet* (2011) 377 (9775):1409–1420.

[8] Khanna O, et al. A comparison of radial versus femoral artery access for acute stroke interventions. *Journal of Neurosurgery* (2020) 135 (3):727–732.

[9] Zussman BM, et al. Maturing institutional experience with the transradial approach for diagnostic cerebral arteriography: overcoming the learning curve. *Journal of NeuroInterventional Surgery* (2019) 11 (12):1235–1238.

[10] Ferrante G, et al. Radial versus femoral access for coronary interventions across the entire spectrum of patients with coronary artery disease: a meta-analysis of randomized trials. *JACC: Cardiovascular Interventions* (2016) 9 (14):1419–1434.

[11] Patel N, Shah CS, Kim W. Radial artery access for intracranial neuroendovascular procedures: A single center's initial experience and technical considerations. *Journal of NeuroInterventional Surgery* (2020).

[12] Li Y, et al. Lower complication rates associated with transradial versus transfemoral flow diverting stent placement. *Journal of NeuroInterventional Surgery* (2021) 13 (1):91–95.

[13] Ruzsa Z, et al. Radial vs femoral access for diagnostic cerebral angiography: a single-centre retrospective analysis. *Interventional Neuroradiology* (2017).

[14] Goktekin O, et al. Radial versus femoral access in coil embolization of cerebral aneurysms: a systematic review and meta-analysis. *Interventional Neuroradiology* (2020).

[15] Shaban S, et al. The association of transradial access and transfemoral access with procedural outcomes in acute ischemic stroke patients receiving endovascular thrombectomy: a meta-analysis. *Clinical Neurology and Neurosurgery* (2022) 215:107209.

[16] Snelling BM, et al. Radial versus femoral access for mechanical thrombectomy in acute ischemic stroke: a systematic review and meta-analysis. *Journal of NeuroInterventional Surgery* (2021).

[17] Tiseo B, et al. Transradial approach for flow diversion of cerebral aneurysms: a multicenter study. *Journal of NeuroInterventional Surgery* (2020).

[18] Valgimigli M, et al. Radial versus femoral access and bivalirudin versus unfractionated heparin in invasively managed patients with acute coronary syndrome (MATRIX): final 1-year results of a multicentre, randomised controlled trial. *The Lancet* (2018) 392 (10150):835–848.

[19] Brunet M-C, Chen SH, Peterson EC. Transradial access for neurointerventions: management of access challenges and complications. *Journal of NeuroInterventional Surgery* (2020) 12 (1):82–86.

[20] Phillips TJ, et al. Transradial versus transfemoral access for anterior circulation mechanical thrombectomy: analysis of 375 consecutive cases. *Stroke and Vascular Neurology* (2021) 6 (2).

[21] Nohara AM, Kallmes DF. Transradial cerebral angiography: technique and outcomes. *American Journal of Neuroradiology* (2003) 24 (6):1247–1250.

Chapter 13

The History and Development of Atypical (Non-Radio-Femoral) Access

Oday Atallah[1,*], MD
Amr Badary[2,†], MD
Zaid Aljuboori[3,‡], MD
Ahmed Muthana[4,§], MD
and Samer S. Hoz[5,‖], MD

[1]Department of Neurosurgery, Hannover Medical School, Hannover, Germany
[2]Department of Neurortraumatology, Gera Clinical Center, Gera, Germany
[3]Department of Neurosurgery, Geisinger Commonwealth School of Medicine, Department of Neurosurgery, Geisinger, Scranton, PA, USA
[4]Department of Neurosurgery, University of Baghdad, Baghdad, Iraq
[5]Department of Neurosurgery, University of Cincinnati Medical Center, Cincinnati, OH, USA

Abstract

The evolution of neurointerventional surgery has necessitated the development of diverse vascular access routes to address complex intracranial pathologies. Historically, the femoral and radial arteries have been the standard conduit for endovascular procedures, permitting the traversal of instruments to the cerebrovascular system. However, as the field advanced, certain patient anatomies and lesion locations revealed the limitations of the transfemoral approach, leading to the exploration of atypical access points. Advancement of non-radio-femoral approaches, including transcarotid, transcervical, and transbrachial approaches have gained prominence for their reduction in complication rates, patient comfort, and suitability in specific clinical scenarios such as aortic arch atherosclerosis or tortuous vascular anatomy. Advantages and limitations are elucidated after conduction comparative analyses between traditional and atypical access routes. Deciding the approach depends on patient criteria, anatomical considerations, and technical nuances associated with non-radio-femoral access. Special emphasis is placed on the role of

[*] Corresponding Author's Email: oday.atallah@yahoo.de
[†] Corresponding Author's Email: amr.badary@hot
[‡] Corresponding Author's Email: zaljuboori1@geisinger.edu
[§] Corresponding Author's Email: ahmed.m.najm@gmail.com
[‖] Corresponding Author's Email: hozsamer2055@gmail.com

In: World History of Neurointerventional Surgery
Editors: Xianli Lv and Zhongxue Wu
ISBN: 979-8-89530-792-2

imaging modalities such as ultrasound, fluoroscopy, and angiography in guiding and optimizing atypical access procedures.
This chapter delves into the historical milestones and technological innovations that have sculpted the contemporary landscape of neurointerventional surgery, illuminating how atypical approaches have broadened the arsenal of neurointerventionalists while driving the evolution of novel devices and techniques, thereby advancing the field and enhancing patient outcomes. Emphasizing the burgeoning importance of atypical access approaches, it offers insights into their clinical utility, technical nuances, and future trajectories, with the aim of empowering informed decision-making among neurointerventionalists and stimulating ongoing research endeavors aimed at optimizing patient care within this dynamic realm.

Keywords: neurointerventional surgery, femoral access, radial access, transcarotid, atypical approach

Introduction

Neurointerventional surgery stands at the forefront of innovation, continually pushing the boundaries of what is possible in the treatment of complex intracranial pathologies. Central to this evolution is the development of diverse vascular access routes, catering to the unique anatomical considerations and clinical needs of individual patients. While traditional femoral and radial arteries have long been the cornerstone of endovascular procedures, the emergence of atypical access approaches represents a transformative shift in the field.

Historical Context and Evolution

Early neurointerventional procedures predominantly relied on femoral access, with catheters navigated through the iliofemoral system to reach intracranial vessels. However, as the field progressed and the complexity of intracranial pathologies became apparent, neurointerventionalists encountered limitations inherent to femoral access. Challenges such as tortuous iliofemoral anatomy, groin complications, and restricted maneuverability in certain anatomical configurations prompted a quest for novel access routes [1, 2].

The emergence of radial access in the late 20th century marked a significant milestone in neurointerventional surgery. Offering advantages such as reduced access site complications and enhanced patient comfort, radial access quickly gained traction and became a viable alternative to femoral access for selective procedures. However, as neurointerventionalists ventured into more intricate cases, it became evident that even radial access had its occasional limitations, particularly in cases of radial artery tortuosity or hypoplasia [3].

In response to the intricate challenges encountered in neurointerventional surgery, the concept of atypical access approaches began to evolve. This transformative journey was fueled by the ingenuity of neurointerventionalists, who explored alternative pathways to intracranial targets. Among these pioneering approaches, the transcarotid method emerged as a breakthrough, offering a direct route to the cerebral vasculature while circumventing the conventional femoral and radial arteries. Subsequent advancements in atypical access strategies introduced the transcervical, transbrachial, and transorbital approaches; each tailored to specific clinical scenarios and presenting distinct advantages. The transcervical approach utilized the cervical vasculature to facilitate catheterization, whereas the transbrachial approach provided an alternative avenue through the brachial artery [4] (Figure 1). Although still in its nascent stages, the transophthalmic approach demonstrated promise in accessing intracranial targets, presenting a minimally invasive option with potential applications in select neurointerventional procedures [5]. Additionally, innovative solutions such as the umbilical and transvenous approaches emerged to address challenges in neonatal and pediatric cases, where traditional access routes posed limitations, grappling with complex intracranial pathologies [6].

As technology continues to advance and our understanding of vascular anatomy deepens, the journey of exploration and discovery in atypical access methods is poised to continue, offering new horizons in the treatment of neurovascular diseases.

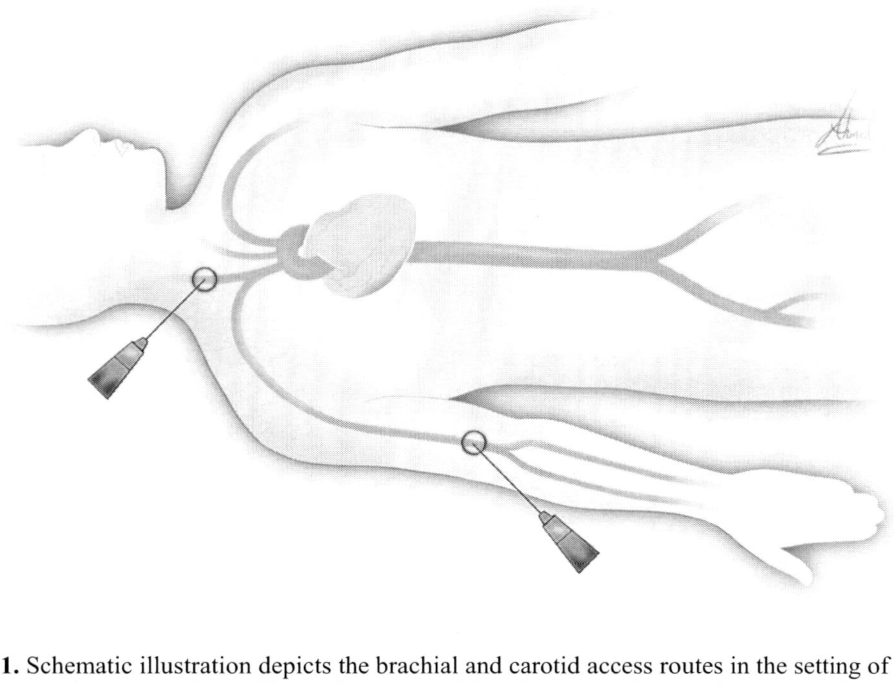

Figure 1. Schematic illustration depicts the brachial and carotid access routes in the setting of neurointerventional procedures. Illustration prepared by Ahmed Muthana and courtesy of Samer Hoz.

Atypical Access Approaches

Table 1 summarizes the atypical non-radio-femoral approaches.

Transbrachial Approach (TBA)

The brachial artery originates at the lower margin of the teres major muscle as a continuation of the axillary artery. It travels along the humerus and passes through the antecubital fossa beneath the lacertus fibrosus, alongside the median nerve. This fibrous structure originates from the biceps tendon and the fascia of the flexor-pronator mass. Approximately 1 cm distal to the elbow, the brachial artery bifurcates into the radial and ulnar arteries [7].

Equipment and Technique

The equipment used for TBA is the same as the radial artery access, except for the antispasmodic cocktail, which is typically unnecessary due to the larger caliber of the brachial artery. Basically, it includes a micropuncture set with a 4-French introducer sheath, dilators ranging from 5–8 Fr, depending on the size of the sheath, and a vascular sheath. To access the brachial artery, position the arm straight and externally rotated on an adjustable extension to facilitate palpation of the artery (Figure 1). Maximal pulsation should be identified by palpation, and ultrasound guidance may be used, especially in obese patients. Perform a percutaneous arterial puncture 1 cm above the antecubital fossa at a 60-degree angle using a micropuncture kit. Introduce a 7-French Short Sheath for therapeutic procedures or a 5-French Short Sheath for diagnostic procedures using the Seldinger technique and secure the sheath to the skin with two stitches. A guiding catheter is then introduced over a 4-French or 5-French Simmons catheter with a Terumo Glidewire [8, 9]. At the end of the procedure, remove the sheath and achieve hemostasis with 5–10 minutes of manual compression. Apply a pressure dressing, and ensure the patient keeps the arm straight for up to 6 hours. Vascular closure devices are contraindicated due to the small vessel size and high risk of arterial occlusion [8].

Advantages and Complications

TBA shares many advantages with the transradial approach (TRA), including a lower incidence of hemorrhage and avoidance of anatomical variations that complicate the transfemoral approach (TFA). Both the TRA and TBA provide increased stability and support to guide catheters due to the catheterization angles of the vertebral and carotid arteries. A significant advantage of the TBA is the larger caliber of the brachial artery, allowing for the use of larger guide catheters. However, the brachial artery's poor collateral circulation increases the risk of ischemic events. Complications from the TBA can include arm hematoma, arterial spasm, upper extremity ischemia, median nerve palsy, arterial dissection, and pseudoaneurysm, with complication rates ranging from 1.28% to 36% in the cardiac literature during coronary artery catheterization [8, 10].

Transcervical Approach (TCA)

TCA is an alternative method used to bypass anatomical challenges such as aortic arch anomalies, common carotid artery loops, severe ostial stenosis, and bilateral femoral occlusions. This approach is advantageous for accessing both the anterior and posterior circulations and is employed for diagnostic and therapeutic intracranial procedures, as well as carotid angioplasty and stenting [11, 12].

Table 1. Summary of the non-radio-femoral approaches

Approach	Anatomy & Exposure	Equipment	Technique	Advantages	Complications
Trans-brachial A.	Brachial artery begins at teres major, travels along humerus, and divides into radial and ulnar arteries.	Micropuncture set Vascular sheath	Puncture 1 cm above antecubital fossa, micropuncture, sheath placement, manual compression.	Larger caliber for larger catheters, increased stability and support.	Arm hematoma Arterial spasm, Ischemia Nerve palsy Dissection.
Trans-carotid A.	Access to anterior/posterior circulations, useful for overcoming anatomical anomalies.	Micropuncture kit Prolene stitch	Direct carotid puncture, micropuncture, Seldinger technique, purse-string suture.	Bypasses complex anatomy, direct access for diagnostic/therapeutic.	Thromboembolic events Dissection Pseudoaneurysm Neck hematoma.
Trans-ophthalmic V.	SOV drains into cavernous sinus, accessed through medial upper eyelid incision.	Micropuncture kit Prolene stitch	Incision above upper eyelid, orbital septum opened, SOV exposed, vascular sheath placed.	Alternative route to cavernous sinus, avoids arterial complications.	Intraocular pressure Orbital hemorrhage New-onset fistulas.
Trans-vertebral A.	Vertebral artery at lateral foramen magnum, exposed via vertical incision near mastoid process.	Micropuncture kit Prolene stitch	Vertical incision, dissection to vertebral artery, puncture, sheath placement.	Direct access for severe tortuosity cases.	Infection Arterial damage Ccomplications from advanced wires
Trans-femoral V.	Femoral vein runs medial to femoral artery, transitions into external iliac vein at inguinal ligament.	Same as femoral artery access	Puncture over femoral head, navigate through venous system to intracranial targets.	Familiar route, straightforward navigation to target areas.	DVT Puncture site hematoma Vessel damage
Trans-jugular V.	Drains brain, face, and neck, runs laterally by carotid artery, joins subclavian vein to form brachiocephalic vein.	Same as femoral artery access	Direct puncture in carotid triangle, lateral to carotid artery with 4 Fr micropuncture kit.	Direct route to central venous structures, alternative to femoral vein.	Puncture site complications including hematoma and vessel injury.

Direct Carotid Access Technique

The procedure is usually performed under general anesthesia or conscious sedation [11, 12]. The patient is positioned with slight neck extension and head rotation to the contralateral side (Figure 1). Puncturing is done using a 21-gauge needle under ultrasound guidance at a 45-degree angle, avoiding the jugular vein. After confirming proper entry and vascular anatomy using angiography, Introduction of 0.018-inch soft-tip microwire is conducted under fluoroscopic guidance and park it in the external carotid artery. The surgeon advances a 5-French dilator over the microwire, then replaces the microwire with a 0.035-inch Glidewire and introduces a 6-French sheath. Finally, the surgeon secures the sheath with sutures and administers heparin to achieve therapeutic anticoagulation. Perform the endovascular procedure using an intermediate catheter.

Possible complications include thromboembolic events, arterial dissection, transient vasospasm, pseudoaneurysm, thrombus formation, arteriovenous fistulas, and neck hematoma. Neck hematoma, particularly in patients on full anticoagulation or antiplatelet therapy, can result in cranial nerve neuropathies and airway compromise [11, 12].

Surgical Cutdown for Transcarotid Approach

In some cases, catheter navigation into the carotid artery via standard routes is not feasible due to anatomical anomalies. For these situations, a neurosurgeon or vascular surgeon can expose the common carotid artery (CCA) surgically for direct catheterization. This procedure involves making a small transverse incision at the level of the thyroid cartilage to expose the CCA, which lies medial to the internal jugular vein. The external, internal, and common carotid arteries are then dissected free and marked with vessel loops for identification [13].

Vertebral Artery Access

In cases of severe vertebrobasilar tortuosity, direct exposure of the vertebral artery may be necessary, typically performed by a neurosurgeon. The vertebral artery is located at the lateral margin of the foramen magnum, where it enters the dura.

The equipment includes micropuncture kit, 5–0 or 6–0 Prolene stitch, and 4 Fr to 6 Fr short sheath. To expose the vertebral artery, a vertical skin incision several centimeters long is made approximately 2 cm medial to the mastoid process. The muscular layers are carefully dissected to localize the medial arch of C1, where the vertebral artery can be found laterally. At this point, the vertebral artery is carefully dissected and punctured with a 21-gauge needle [14].

Superior Ophthalmic Vein Access

The superior ophthalmic vein (SOV) is formed by the convergence of the medial angulus oculi vein and the superior orbital vein, enters the orbit through the orbital septum above the ligament of the medial angulus oculi and runs lateral to the superior rectus muscle. It connects to the cavernous sinus through the superior orbital fissure, situated medial to cranial nerves III, IV, and VI. Fistulous connections can cause arterialization of the SOV, resulting in it becoming thicker and more dilated. With an average diameter exceeding 9 mm on lateral angiograms, this straight, valveless vein serves as an ideal route to the cavernous sinus [15].

The cavernous sinus is a complex network of venous sinusoids enclosed by a double dural leaflet and traversed by critical vascular and neural structures. Its venous drainage is categorized into anterior, posterior, inferior, and mediolateral routes. The anterior drainage includes the superior and inferior ophthalmic veins, both of which drain into the angular vein and then into the facial venous system [16].

Indirect access to the SOV can be achieved from the internal jugular vein via the facial and angular veins. However, when catheterization through the femoral or jugular veins is not feasible, direct surgical cannulation of the SOV provides an excellent alternative, leveraging its accessibility and optimal connection to the cavernous sinus [17].

Equipment and Technique

The equipment is similar to vertebral artery access. The patient is placed under general anesthesia with neuromonitoring in a supine position. A 2-cm incision is made medially in the skin crease above the upper eyelid. Using an operating microscope, Exposure is made through dissection of the orbicularis oculi muscle and opening the orbital septum. The surgeon bluntly dissects the orbital fat with cotton-tipped applicators until a small arterialized venous branch is located, typically found superior to the ligament of the angulus oculi medialis. Then, the surgeon follows the venous branch proximally, in a posterolateral direction, to find the main trunk of the arterialized SOV. Under direct vision, the surgeon catheterizes the SOV with a 20-gauge Angiocath and inserts a microcatheter all the way to the cavernous sinus under fluoroscopy. Proper placement is secured using angiogram by visualizing the opacification of the SOV as it drains into the cavernous sinus. Once confirmed, the sheath is secured properly to the skin. At the end of the procedure, the surgeon removes the Angiocath, ligates the SOV, and closes the eyelid incision [13, 17, 18]. This approach ensures safe and effective access to the cavernous sinus, leveraging the anatomical characteristics of the SOV to facilitate the intervention.

Advantages and Complications

The SOV, a valveless and straight vein, offers a reliable route to the cavernous sinus, preserving the arterial blood supply and minimizing the risk of arterial vasospasm and occlusion. This approach provides an essential alternative for achieving effective and safe access to the cavernous sinus. It is particularly useful for accessing the cavernous sinus to embolize carotid-cavernous fistulae (CCFs). The SOV approach was first described by Peterson et al. in 1969 for treating CCFs through electrical induction of thrombosis. It has since become a valuable alternative for treating CCFs, especially when other transvenous routes are impeded by anatomical variations, intracavernous septations, or venous thrombosis [9, 17].

Potential complications of the superior ophthalmic vein approach include increased intraocular pressure from thrombosis of the ophthalmic veins, orbital hemorrhage, and retro-orbital hematoma, which can impair visual acuity. New fistulas are at a higher risk of hemorrhage due to insufficient arterialization, making veins more prone to perforation. The abducens nerve is particularly vulnerable to neuropathy because of its fixed position within the trabeculae of the sinus. Other risks include misidentifying the superior oblique tendon as the superior ophthalmic vein, infections, and overpacking of the cavernous sinus, leading to cranial nerve palsies, dissection, and perforations [13].

Umbilical Approach

The umbilical artery stems from the anterior division of the internal iliac artery. During fetal development, it runs through the umbilical cord, transporting oxygen-poor blood from the fetus to the placenta. Typically, the umbilical cord contains two umbilical arteries and one umbilical vein. However, in about 1% of pregnancies, one umbilical artery may not develop properly, leading to a single umbilical artery. This condition is usually isolated, but when combined with other fetal anomalies, it raises the risk of chromosomal abnormalities. The umbilical arteries are distinguished by their caudal position in the cord, thicker walls, and smaller lumen [19].

Equipment and Technique

The umbilical approach requires the following equipment [20]:

- Sterile gown, gloves, cap, mask, drapes, gauze sponges.
- Bactericidal solution.
- Umbilical tie, measuring tape, scissors, scalpel.
- Iris forceps (toothed and nontoothed), mosquito hemostats.
- Umbilical catheter (5-Fr for >1200 g, 3.5-Fr for <1500 g).
- Three-way stopcock, IV tubing, sterile saline flush.
- Needle driver, 3-0 silk suture.

Basically, access using the umbilical approach is made through the following steps:

Preparation [21-23]

- Prevent hypothermia using a radiant warmer and/or exothermic mattress.
- Flush catheter with 0.45% saline and attach a three-way stopcock.
- Measure catheter insertion length (Formula: (birthweightinkg x 3) + 9 x (birthweightinkg x 3) + 9 cm).
- Plan catheter tip position in the descending aorta (T6-T9).

Exposure [21]

- Restrain the infant.
- Clean the umbilical cord and surrounding skin.
- Drape the area and place an umbilical tie around the cord.
- Cut the cord 1-1.5 cm from the skin.

Cannulation [21]

- Identify and dilate the umbilical artery lumen.
- Insert the catheter into the dilated artery (Figure 2).

Confirmation and Securing [21]

- Secure the catheter with sutures.
- Confirm catheter tip position with radiology.

Closure [21]

- Start infusion of heparinized solution once the position is verified.

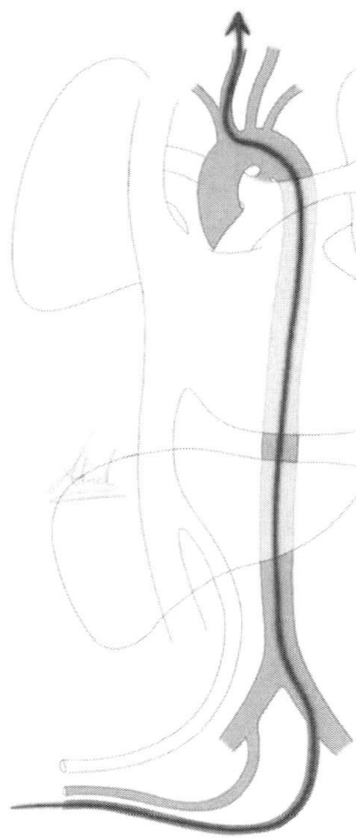

Figure 2. Transumbilical arterial approach is shown as a blue line with an arrowhead.

Possible Complications

Thromboembolism is a major concern with umbilical arterial catheters, potentially causing gut ischemia, bowel infarction, necrotizing enterocolitis, hypertension, or acute renal failure. Distal vascular accidents can lead to ischemic injuries to the back, buttocks, and lower extremities. Catheter removal should be considered at the first sign of vascular compromise. Other complications include vessel and peritoneal perforation, bladder injury, false aneurysm, infection, and bleeding. Refractory hypoglycemia is a rare complication with high-position catheters near the celiac and mesenteric arteries [24-27].

Although there is theoretical concern about necrotizing enterocolitis with enteral feeding in the presence of an umbilical arterial catheter, there is no supporting evidence, and withholding enteral feeds is not recommended.

Femoral Vein Access

The femoral vein is situated just medial to the common femoral artery. It continues from the popliteal vein and terminates at the inguinal ligament, where it becomes the external iliac vein. From the external iliac vein, one can navigate through the inferior vena cava, past the heart, into the superior vena cava, and then into the internal jugular vein. This path allows access to the sigmoid and transverse sinuses, the inferior petrosal sinus, the basilar plexus, and the facial vein. Similar to arterial access, the vein should be punctured over the femoral head to allow for effective post-procedural compression, but care must be taken to puncture below the inguinal ligament to prevent retroperitoneal hematoma [28, 29].

The same equipment for femoral artery access is used for femoral vein access. Similarly, the technique for femoral vein access mirrors that of femoral artery access [28]. Ensure proper puncture over the femoral head while avoiding the inguinal ligament area to prevent complications.

Internal Jugular Vein Access

The internal jugular vein drains blood from the brain, superficial parts of the face, and neck. At its origin near the sigmoid sinus, it is somewhat dilated and often referred to as the jugular bulb. It receives a common trunk that drains the anterior branch of the retromandibular vein, the facial vein, and the lingual vein. The internal jugular vein travels laterally by the carotid artery and unites with the subclavian vein to form the brachiocephalic (innominate) vein [30].

The same equipment for femoral artery access is used for internal jugular vein access. The internal jugular vein can be punctured directly in the carotid triangle, lateral to the carotid artery, using a 4 Fr micropuncture kit. This technique is particularly useful if navigation from the femoral vein is impeded by stenosis, although such cases are rare.

Patient Selection Criteria

Vascular Anatomy

Understanding patient-specific vascular anatomy is paramount in guiding atypical access route selection [34]. Variations in vessel tortuosity, diameter, and accessibility influence the feasibility and safety of atypical access approaches [31, 32]. Vascular imaging modalities, including computed tomography angiography (CTA) and magnetic resonance angiography (MRA), facilitate comprehensive pre-procedural assessment of vascular anatomy to inform access route selection [33].

Lesion Characteristics

The location, size, and complexity of the target lesion play a pivotal role in determining the appropriateness of atypical access routes. Lesions located in challenging anatomical locations or associated with complex vascular configurations may necessitate alternative access routes to optimize procedural success and mitigate procedural risks like the promising cavernous sinus catheterization [17].

Contraindications to Traditional Routes

Patient factors, such as peripheral vascular disease, obesity, and previous access site complications, may preclude the use of traditional femoral or radial access routes, necessitating consideration of atypical approaches [1, 2]. Atypical access routes offer alternative solutions for patients with contraindications to traditional routes, thereby expanding the scope of neurointerventional therapy [4-6].

Technical Considerations

Access Site Preparation

Optimal access site preparation is essential to mitigate procedural risks and ensure patient comfort. Factors like aseptic technique, vessel palpation, and local anesthesia administration facilitate safe and effective access site establishment [34]. Atypical access routes require specialized access site preparation techniques tailored to the unique anatomical considerations of each approach.

Device Selection and Compatibility

Device selection is guided by the anatomical characteristics of the target lesion, vessel size, and procedural objectives [35]. Atypical access routes necessitate the use of specialized catheters, guidewires, and microcatheters compatible with the unique anatomical constraints of each approach. Customized device selection enhances procedural efficacy and optimizes patient outcomes [36].

Navigational Techniques, Hemostasis, and Closure Techniques

Proficiency in navigational techniques is essential for precise catheter manipulation and accurate lesion targeting [37]. Advanced navigational tools, such as roadmap guidance and three-dimensional rotational angiography, augment procedural precision and facilitate complex interventions via atypical access routes [38]. Operator proficiency in navigational techniques enhances procedural efficiency and mitigates technical challenges associated with atypical access approaches.

Atypical access routes require specialized hemostasis and closure techniques tailored to the unique anatomical considerations of each approach. Proactive management of access site complications, including vascular perforation and hemorrhage, mitigates procedural risks and enhances patient outcomes [39].

Future Directions

Continued advancements in imaging modalities, navigational tools, and catheter-based technologies will drive innovation in atypical access approaches. Emerging technologies, such as robotic-assisted navigation systems and artificial intelligence algorithms, have the potential to enhance procedural precision, streamline workflow, and optimize patient outcomes in atypical access procedures [40].

The development and refinement of tailored devices will enhance procedural efficacy and broaden the applicability of atypical access approaches. Creating specialized catheters, guidewires, and microcatheters specifically designed for these unique access routes will improve device compatibility, navigational capabilities, and procedural success rates. This mirrors the significant advancements already achieved in coronary artery catheterization [41].

The advent of personalized medicine and precision-guided interventions will revolutionize treatment paradigms in neurointerventional surgery. Patient-specific anatomical considerations, lesion characteristics, and clinical indications will inform individualized treatment strategies, driving the adoption of atypical access approaches tailored to the unique needs of each patient.

Conclusion

Neurointerventional surgery is undergoing a significant transformation, driven by the continuous development of diverse vascular access routes tailored to address the unique anatomical and clinical needs of patients. Historically anchored in femoral and radial artery access, the field is now embracing a wider array of atypical approaches to overcome the limitations and complications associated with traditional methods.

The transradial and transcarotid approaches have marked significant advancements, providing viable alternatives to the femoral route and offering enhanced patient comfort and reduced complication rates. However, as neurointerventionalists encounter increasingly complex intracranial pathologies, the need for innovative access routes has become paramount. The evolution of techniques such as the transbrachial, transcervical, and superior ophthalmic vein approaches demonstrates the field's commitment to expanding the neurointerventional toolkit. These methods offer direct, minimally invasive pathways to cerebral targets, catering to specific clinical scenarios and anatomical challenges.

Each non-radio-femoral approach discussed in this chapter has its own personality and specific advantages. TBA is preferred for its larger caliber and stability, allowing for the use of larger catheters. However, it carries risks of hematoma, arterial spasm, and nerve damage. TCA offers direct access to the carotid artery, bypassing complex anatomical challenges, and providing a streamlined pathway for interventions in the anterior circulation, but poses significant risks such as thromboembolic events and neck hematoma. The SOV Approach is particularly useful for accessing the cavernous sinus without risking arterial complications, though it comes with the risk of elevated intraocular pressure and orbital hemorrhage. For cases involving severe vertebrobasilar tortuosity, Vertebral Artery Access provides direct access but is technically demanding and carries risks of infection and arterial damage. Femoral Vein Access is a familiar and straightforward route for many clinicians, offering extensive experience and ease of navigation, though it is not without the risk of deep vein thrombosis and puncture site complications. Finally, the Internal Jugular Vein Access serves as an alternative when femoral vein access is compromised, providing a direct route to central venous structures but with potential for puncture site complications.

Each approach must be carefully considered based on the specific anatomical and procedural requirements, weighing the benefits of direct access and stability against the risks of complications associated with each technique. In addition, the decision hinges on several key factors, including procedural efficacy, patient safety, operator comfort, and anatomical considerations.

References

[1] Lux A, et al. Iliofemoral tortuosity increases the risk of access-site-related complications after aortic valve implantation and plug-based access-site closure. *CJC Open* (2022) 4 (7):609–616.

[2] Mach M, et al. The Iliofemoral tortuosity score predicts access and bleeding complications during transfemoral transcatheter aortic valve replacement: Data from the VIenna Cardio Thoracic aOrtic valve registrY (VICTORY). *European Journal of Clinical Investigation* (2021) 51 (6):e13491.

[3] Joshi KC, et al. Transradial approach for neurointerventions: a systematic review of the literature. *Journal of NeuroInterventional Surgery* (2020) 12 (9):886–892.

[4] Matsuda Y, et al. The clinical results of transcervical carotid artery stenting and frequency chosen as the approach route of carotid artery stenting in 1,067 consecutive cases. *Acta Neurochirurgica* (2013) 155:1575–1581.

[5] Iglesias B, et al. Approach to the superior ophthalmic vein for endovascular treatment of cavernous dural fistula. *World Neurosurgery* (2021) 151:1.

[6] Kappel AD, Orbach DB. Standard umbilical artery catheters used as diagnostic and neurointerventional guide catheters in the treatment of neonatal cerebrovascular malformations. *Journal of NeuroInterventional Surgery* (2023) 15 (4):375–379.

[7] Epperson TN, Varacallo M. Anatomy, shoulder and upper limb, brachial artery. In: *StatPearls [Internet]*. 2023: StatPearls Publishing.

[8] Heenan S, et al. Transbrachial arteriography: indications and complications. *Clinical Radiology* (1996) 51 (3):205–209.

[9] Winn HR. *Youmans and Winn Neurological Surgery E-Book: 4-Volume Set*. 2022: Elsevier Health Sciences.

[10] Hildick-Smith DJ, et al. Coronary angiography in the presence of peripheral vascular disease: femoral or brachial/radial approach? *Catheterization and Cardiovascular Interventions* (2000) 49 (1):32–37.

[11] Colombo E, Rinaldo L, Lanzino G. Direct carotid puncture in acute ischaemic stroke intervention. *Stroke and Vascular Neurology* (2020) 5 (1).

[12] Miszczuk M, et al. Direct puncture of the carotid artery as a bailout vascular access technique for mechanical thrombectomy in acute ischemic stroke—the revival of an old technique in a modern setting. *Neuroradiology* (2021) 63:275–283.

[13] Takano I, et al. Carotid surgical cut-down technique for neuroendovascular therapy. *Interventional Neuroradiology* (2019) 25 (3):348–352.

[14] Jabre R. Applied anatomy of the vertebral arteries for endovascular neurointerventions. *Neurochirurgie* (2024) 70 (3):101531.

[15] Azzam D, Cypen S, Tao J. Anatomy, head and neck, eye ophthalmic vein. In: *StatPearls [Internet]*. 2020.

[16] Massa RN, Minutello K, Mesfin FB. Neuroanatomy, cavernous sinus. In: *StatPearls [Internet]*. 2023.

[17] Haider AS, et al. Superior ophthalmic vein access for embolization of an indirect carotid cavernous fistula. *Cureus* (2017) 9 (9).

[18] Ross IB, Luzardo GD. Direct access to the carotid circulation by cut down for endovascular neuro-interventions. *Surgical Neurology* (2006) 65 (2):207–211.

[19] DeFreitas M, et al. Umbilical artery histomorphometry: a link between the intrauterine environment and kidney development. *Journal of Developmental Origins of Health and Disease* (2017) 8 (3):349–356.

[20] Elser HE. Options for securing umbilical catheters. *Advances in Neonatal Care* (2013) 13 (6):426–429.

[21] Barrington KJ, Group CN. Umbilical artery catheters in the newborn: effects of position of the catheter tip. *Cochrane Database of Systematic Reviews* (1996) 2010 (1).

[22] Rosenfeld W, et al. Evaluation of graphs for insertion of umbilical artery catheters below the diaphragm. *The Journal of Pediatrics* (1981) 98 (4):627–628.

[23] Shukla H, Ferrara A. Rapid estimation of insertional length of umbilical catheters in newborns. *American Journal of Diseases of Children* (1986) 140 (8):786–788.

[24] McAdams RM, et al. Complications of umbilical artery catheterization in a model of extreme prematurity. *Journal of Perinatology* (2009) 29 (10):685–692.

[25] Ramasethu J. Complications of vascular catheters in the neonatal intensive care unit. *Clinics in Perinatology* (2008) 35 (1):199–222.

[26] Malik M, Wilson DP. Umbilical artery catheterization: a potential cause of refractory hypoglycemia. *Clinical Pediatrics* (1987) 26 (4):181–182.

[27] Sobczak A, et al. Umbilical catheters as vectors for generalized bacterial infection in premature infants regardless of antibiotic use. *Journal of Medical Microbiology* (2019) 68 (9):1306–1313.

[28] Castro D, LM ML, Bhutta BS. Femoral vein central venous access. In: *StatPearls [Internet]*. 2017.

[29] Saugel B, Scheeren TW, Teboul J-L. Ultrasound-guided central venous catheter placement: a structured review and recommendations for clinical practice. *Critical Care* (2017) 21 (1):225.

[30] Rivard AB, Kortz MW, Burns B. Anatomy, head and neck, internal jugular vein. In: *StatPearls [Internet]*. 2018.

[31] Yoo B-S, et al. Anatomical consideration of the radial artery for transradial coronary procedures: arterial diameter, branching anomaly and vessel tortuosity. *International Journal of Cardiology* (2005) 101 (3):421–427.

[32] MontAlverne FJA, et al. Unfavorable vascular anatomy during endovascular treatment of stroke: challenges and bailout strategies. *Journal of Stroke* (2020) 22 (2):185–200.

[33] Stalcup S, Johnson J, Romero J. Neurovascular Imaging (CTA and MRA). In: *PanVascular Medicine*. 2013. Springer Berlin Heidelberg: Berlin, Heidelberg. p. 1–25.

[34] O'Grady NP, et al. Guidelines for the prevention of intravascular catheter-related infections. *Clinical Infectious Diseases* (2011) 52 (9):e162–e193.

[35] Hassan AE, et al. Utilization of the ballast long guiding sheath for neuroendovascular procedures: institutional experience in 68 cases. *Frontiers in Neurology* (2021) 12:578446.

[36] von Hessling A, et al. The Columbus steerable guidewire in neurointerventions: early clinical experience and applications. *Journal of NeuroInterventional Surgery* (2022) 14 (3):291–296.

[37] Cotin S, et al. New approaches to catheter navigation for interventional radiology simulation. In: *International Conference on Medical Image Computing and Computer-Assisted Intervention*. 2005. Springer.

[38] Raabe A, et al. Three-dimensional rotational angiography guidance for aneurysm surgery. *Journal of Neurosurgery* (2006) 105 (3):406–411.

[39] Ciprian Cacuci A, et al. Access site complications of peripheral endovascular procedures: a large, prospective registry on predictors and consequences. *Journal of Endovascular Therapy* (2021) 28 (5):746–754.

[40] Beyar R, et al. Robotics, imaging, and artificial intelligence in the catheterisation laboratory: Cath lab robotics, imaging, and AI. *EuroIntervention* (2021) 17 (7):537–544.

[41] Vemmou E, et al. Recent advances in microcatheter technology for the treatment of chronic total occlusions. *Expert Review of Medical Devices* (2019) 16 (4):267–273.

Chapter 14

The History of Cerebral Aneurysm: Endovascular Surgery

Romeo Eleni[1], MD, MSc
Alexiou A. George[1,2,*], MD, PhD
and Spyridon Voulgaris[1]

[1]Department of Neurosurgery, University Hospital of Ioannina, Ioannina, Greece
[2]Corresponding author: Department of Neurosurgery, University of Ioannina, School of Medicine, Ioannina, Greece

Abstract

Cerebral aneurysms comprised a pathology that was first described in ancient times in the Ebers Papyrus and eventually got its name from Galen in the 2nd century AD. The ligation of the proximal portion of cerebral aneurysms constituted the first attempt at comprehensive treatment in 1928. For many years, therefore, microsurgery dominated as the primary approach to managing aneurysms until 1989, when endovascular treatment with coils began to be implemented. Just a decade later, efforts to manage aneurysms by altering their hemodynamic circulation commenced, leading to the introduction of the first intraluminal flow diverter device in 2007. Pilot use of the Woven EndoBridge device (WEB) for treating wide-neck bifurcation aneurysms began in 2010, and five years ago, it received Food and Drug Administration (FDA) approval and started being widely used. Since then, several devices have been reported in the literature based on the principles of flow divertors, and some of them combine the application of coils. The aim of this review was to present the development of endovascular surgery for brain aneurysms and highlight the landmark techniques that made this technique dominant. It's evident that endovascular neurosurgery has largely replaced traditional neurosurgery in treating cerebral aneurysms, especially in certain locations of aneurysms, and continues to evolve. However, there are still cases where endovascular repair cannot be applied, underscoring the need for ongoing advancement and development.

Keywords: endovascular treatment, intracranial aneurysms, lip occlusion, flow divertors, coils, Woven EndoBridge device

---

* Corresponding Author's Email: galexiou@uoi.gr, alexiougrg@yahoo.gr

In: World History of Neurointerventional Surgery
Editors: Xianli Lv and Zhongxue Wu
ISBN: 979-8-89530-792-2

Abbreviations

DSA	Digital Subtraction Angiography
EV	enhanced visualization
FDA	Food and Drug Administration
ISAT	International Subarachnoid Aneurysm Trial
LVIS	Low-Profile Visualized Intraluminal Support
PED	Pipeline Embolization Device
WEB	Woven EndoBridge device
WEB-DL	Double layer WEB
WEB-SL	Single layer
WEB-SSL	Spheroid Single layer WEB.

Introduction

The first attempt to describe cerebral aneurysms dates back to pre-Christian times in the Ebers papyrus. However, the first to describe the dilation of arteries as a pathology and give them the name "aneurysms" was Galen in 200 AD [1]. Aneurysms of the brain can occur due to abnormal dilation or weakening of the walls of the intracranial arteries [2]. The foundations for the surgical treatment of aneurysms were laid by John Hunter in the 18th century, who introduced the ligation of peripheral arteries during surgical procedures, a technique established as the "Hunterian Principle or Hunterian Ligation" [3, 4]. The first neurosurgical intervention for the ligation of a giant cerebral aneurysm was performed by Victor Horsley during the surgical removal of a tumor in the middle cranial fossa in 1855 [03]. In the early next century, Dandy was among the first to perform planned surgical treatment of an intracranial aneurysm using microsurgery techniques and clips and for this reason, he is considered the father of endovascular neurosurgery [5]. Until the late 19th century, microsurgical placement of clips for the management of this entity was the only approved therapeutic option, and it predominated. Before the advent of detachable coil systems in 1990, several neurosurgeons and neuroradiologists attempted to develop techniques and use catheters and intravascular balloons to occlude intracranial aneurysms [6]. All these efforts and techniques laid the groundwork for the emergence of the era of endovascular treatment of cerebral aneurysms. Coils were just the beginning of this era, and to this day, endovascular techniques are constantly evolving, with gradually emerging new devices designed for use even in the most challenging and accessible areas.

Endovascular treatment of cerebral aneurysms now stands as a powerful tool in combating the disease, offering patients a smaller and smoother postoperative course, and reducing mortality and morbidity rates [7]. However, it is not a panacea and cannot be applied to all patients or all types of aneurysms. With technological advancements, endovascular therapy has progressed and continues to evolve, possibly leading to the future restoration of open surgery. Until then, the choice between endovascular and conventional surgical repair of a cerebral aneurysm should be based on each patient's individual characteristics and clinical presentation [7]. This chapter will present the history and technological evolution of endovascular treatment of brain aneurysms.

The Beginning of Endovascular Treatment of Cerebral Aneurysms

Endovascular surgical management of brain aneurysms would not exist today without the discovery of cerebral angiography. Egas Moniz, also known as Antonio Caetano de Abreu Freire, is considered the father of cerebral angiography as he was the first to apply diagnostic angiography of the brain's vessels in 1927 [8]. He argued that brain tumors have the capability to distort the normal structure of blood vessels, thus believing that imaging of the vessels was necessary for better localization of these tumors radiologically [8]. In 1937, Moniz succeeded in visualizing and describing the first successful occlusion of the internal carotid artery through angiography [9]. Later, he and his collaborators conducted a series of experiments in animals where they catheterized the internal carotid artery and injected various contrast agents to visualize the brain's vessels. A few years later, they published an extensive series of cases presenting brain angiograms in patients, which laid the foundation for the development of today's Digital Subtraction Angiography (DSA) [10]. Luessnhop and Velasquez, 30 years later, were the first neurosurgeons to describe the embolization of a ruptured saccular aneurysm of the internal carotid artery using a spherical silastic embolus. In the same publication, they presented the use of the same embolus for certain arteriovenous malformations, suggesting that this technique could be used for the treatment of both of these vascular pathologies [11]. The experiments of these physicians inspired others, gradually giving rise to neurointervention.

Before the creation of the detachable coil systems, the largest series of endovascular balloon occlusion of cerebral aneurysms was published by Serbinenko. He described 304 cases, among which, 187 concerned the embolization of the internal carotid artery, 49 involved the middle cerebral artery and its branches, and 23 involved the anterior cerebral artery [12]. Additionally, he described angiography of the external carotid artery and selective angiography of its branches. This publication by Serbinenko demonstrated the effective use of detachable balloons and laid the necessary groundwork for the gradual establishment of endovascular treatment of cerebral aneurysms. Subsequent studies followed, which utilized this technique for the treatment of other vascular pathologies such as traumatic carotid cavernous fistulas and arteriovenous malformations, the largest of which was that of Picard et al. [13]. For several years, many centers utilized the use of balloon embolization for brain aneurysms; however, this technique was associated with high rates of recurrence and complications. Until 1989, the treatment of this condition was impossible and could not be done without the development of coils.

The Era of Coils

The evolution of endovascular treatment of cerebral aneurysms as we know it today would not have been possible without the advent of coils. Although the principles and concept of endovascular occlusion of an aneurysm existed since the advent of microcatheters and detachable balloons, the first attempt to occlude an aneurysm using coil-type spirals dates back to 1988 by Hilal [14]. Hilal placed a short platinum coil at the tip of a microcatheter and then advanced the coil through it into the neck of the aneurysm with the aim of occluding it. The advancement of the material through the microcatheter was based on the principles of electrothrombosis, which allowed the coil to detach from the microcatheter. Unfortunately, this attempt was not successful because the coil material was too rigid, preventing it from fully occluding the aneurysmal vessel [14]. Just one year later, Guglielmi et al. building on Hilal's work, developed softer platinum coils that could conform to the shape of the aneurysmal sac. This innovation allowed them to achieve either complete or partial occlusion of aneurysms in a large series of patients. Thus, 1989 became a landmark year for the initiation of endovascular treatment of cerebral aneurysms, even permitting their management during the acute phase of rupture. Researchers initially believed that the therapeutic benefit of coils in endovascular aneurysm occlusion was due to electrothrombosis, as they thought the coil was positively charged in contrast to blood products, thus creating a thrombus. In 2004, a study by Henkes et al. compared the effectiveness of non-electrolytic coils with electrolytically detachable coils and demonstrated that the action of the coils relied on their space-occupying effect within the aneurysmal sac, because in both cases, the results were equally successful [15].

The introduction of coils and the increase in the number of cases with successful endovascular treatment of ruptured aneurysms led to the publication of the landmark clinical trial, the International Subarachnoid Aneurysm Trial (ISAT) in 2002, which established endovascular treatment as a standard practice for ruptured cerebral aneurysms [16]. The results of this study showed that patients treated endovascularly had higher survival rates, less morbidity, and lower rates of disability compared to those treated with traditional open surgery [16]. The findings generated a great deal of controversy, as they challenged the prevailing method of aneurysm management at the time [17]. Ultimately, however, it marked the beginning of the dominance of endovascular neurosurgery in the treatment of this condition. Another equally important study for the establishment of endovascular treatment of cerebral aneurysms was the International Study of Unruptured Intracranial Aneurysms 2 (ISUIA), published one year later [18]. This study highlighted the benefits of endovascular treatment for unruptured aneurysms and identified risk factors for their rupture, thereby defining the indications for their treatment [18].

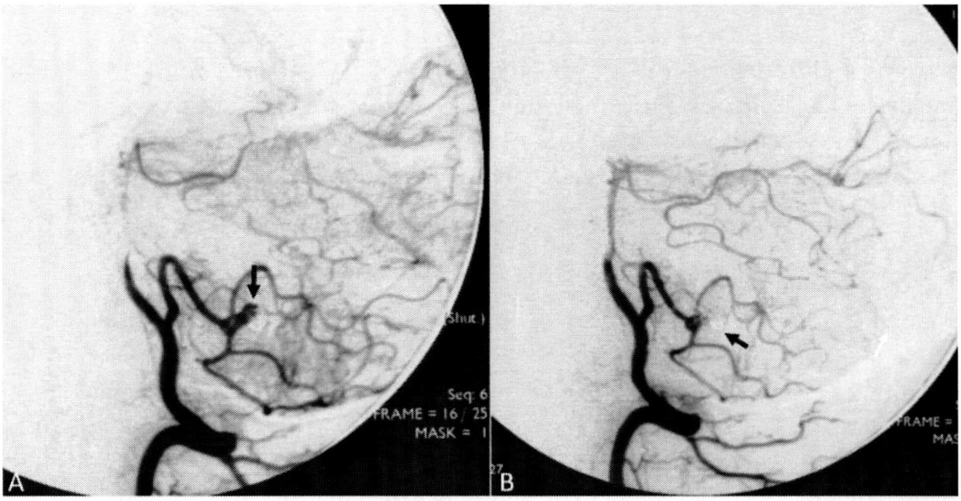

Figure 1. A 31-year-old man with a recurrent distal posterior inferior cerebellar artery aneurysm was coiled. A, lateral view of the right vertebral artery injection showing the recurrent aneurysm of the distal posterior inferior cerebellar artery (arrow). B, lateral view of the right vertebral artery injection showing the aneurysm was occluded with coils (Microplex, 3mm×6cm, 2mm×4cm; Microvention, USA) (arrow).

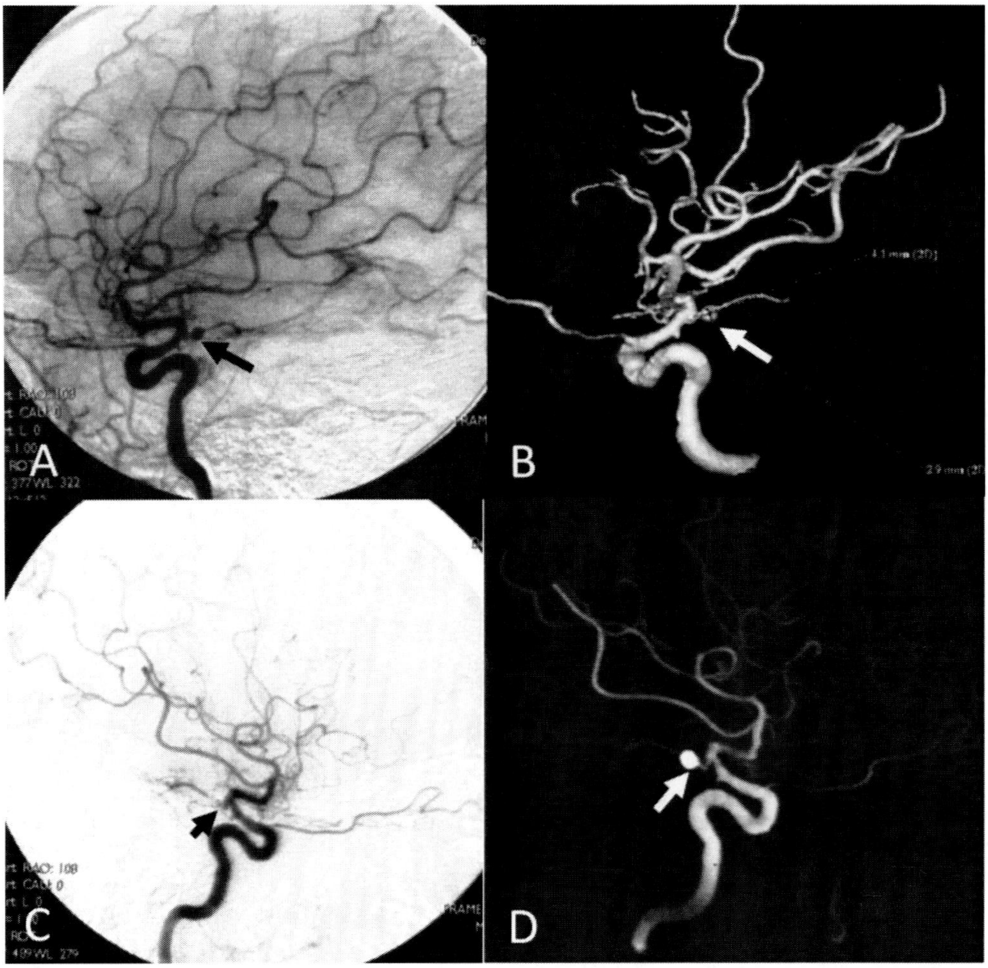

Figure 2. A 37-year-old man with a ruptured anterior choroidal artery aneurysm was coiled. A, lateral view of the right internal carotid artery injection. B, 3-D reconstruction of the right internal carotid artery injection. Showing the 3mm×4mm aneurysm of the origin of the anterior choroidal artery (arrows). C, lateral view of the right internal carotid artery injection showing the disappearance of the aneurysm (arrow). D, 3-D reconstruction of the right internal carotid artery injection showing the coil mass after treatment (arrow).

From 1989 to the present day, various materials have been proposed for the construction of coils. However, most of them remain made of bare platinum, like those developed by Gugliemi (Figure 1 and 2). Some examples include the HydroCoil Embolic System, which consists of hydrogel-coated bare platinum coils, the Matrix Bioactive Coils, which are bare platinum coils coated with polyglycolic acid, and the Cerecyte Coil, which features platinum coils with polyglycolic acid running through the lumen of the primary platinum wind [10]. Bioactive coils, in contrast to hydrogel coils and bare platinum coils, have been found to present certain drawbacks [10]. They are not as flexible as bare platinum and hydrogel coils, do not conform as well, and have a significantly higher manufacturing cost [10, 19]. On the other hand, hydrogel coil systems appear to have lower rates of recurrence and fill the aneurysmal sac with greater density than bare platinum coils [20]. Today, manufacturers focus on the mechanisms of detachment and filling of the aneurysmal vessel. Various detachment methods are employed, including electrical, hydraulic, thermal, and mechanical, but most manufacturers recommend mechanical detachment of coils with the aid of supporting tools [10, 21]. A notable category of coils is the Avenir® coil system (Wallaby Medical, Shanghai, China), which is a passive mechanically-detachable system that requires no detachment tools and appears to be as effective as other systems [21].

Endovascular treatment of intracranial aneurysms with coils is widely used for managing ruptured aneurysms, but it presents certain drawbacks and limitations. These challenges include the difficulty in effectively using coils for wide-neck and bifurcation aneurysms, issues with recanalization and recurrence of aneurysms, coil migration and displacement, failure to achieve optimal packing density within the aneurysm sac, and difficulties in advancing coils into aneurysms located far from the catheter entry point [22-24]. For these reasons, new techniques have been proposed that combine coils with other materials to achieve better outcomes and address aneurysms for which coils alone are insufficient, such as those with wide necks.

The Integration of Coils with Other Materials

One of the major limitations of using coils for aneurysm treatment was incomplete filling of the aneurysmal sac, which often led to frequent recurrences. The first device proposed to improve sac filling was the balloon-assisted coiling technique [25]. Moret et al. were the first to introduce this technique, where a balloon is placed across the neck of the aneurysm, keeping it open until a sufficient mass of coils is deployed to fully fill the sac. Additionally, the balloon can stabilize the branches of the aneurysmal vessel near the neck, thereby preventing their rupture [25]. This technique is more complex than simple coiling of the aneurysm and requires more tools and equipment, but it can successfully treat aneurysms with a broad neck [26].

Another technique developed during the same period for managing large wide-neck and bifurcation aneurysms is stent-assisted coiling. It's worth noting that an aneurysm is considered to have a wide neck if it has a neck diameter exceeding 4 mm and a dome-to-neck ratio of less than 2 [27]. The stent-assisted coiling technique provides greater support and better management of the aneurysm as it promotes re-epithelialization and additionally diverts blood flow away from the point of attachment [27, 28]. Unlike the balloon-assisted technique, the stent remains in place, ensuring greater tightness and better anchoring of the coil [28]. The father of this technique can be considered to be Higashida, as he and his colleagues were the first to successfully use a rigid cardiac stent along with coils to embolize an aneurysm in the basilar artery in 1997 [29]. The use of these stents had disadvantages and could not be utilized effectively in cerebral circulation, leading to their abandonment [10]. Since then, significant progress has been made in endoluminal support devices and in the techniques that combine the use of stents and coils.

The classic stent-assisted coiling technique involves first placing the stent and then advancing a microcatheter through it into the lumen of the aneurysm to deploy the coil. The first stent that enabled the application of this technique was the Neuroform stent (Boston Scientific/Target, Fremont, CA, USA) in 2002 (Figure 3 and 4). It is a self-expandable nitinol intracranial stent made of a flexible and wide mesh that allows the advancement of the coil through it, using a relatively large microcatheter [30]. This restricts its use in small, tortuous, or acutely angled vessels. Just three years later, in addition to the open-cell design of the Neuroform stent, the closed-cell Enterprise stent (Cordis Neurovascular, Miami Lakes, FL,

USA) emerged, offering better conformability and more secure support for the coils [31]. This stent is introduced using a smaller microcatheter compared to the Neuroform and allows for repositioning in case of proce dural errors, thanks to its closed-cell design, in contrast to the open-cell stents [31].

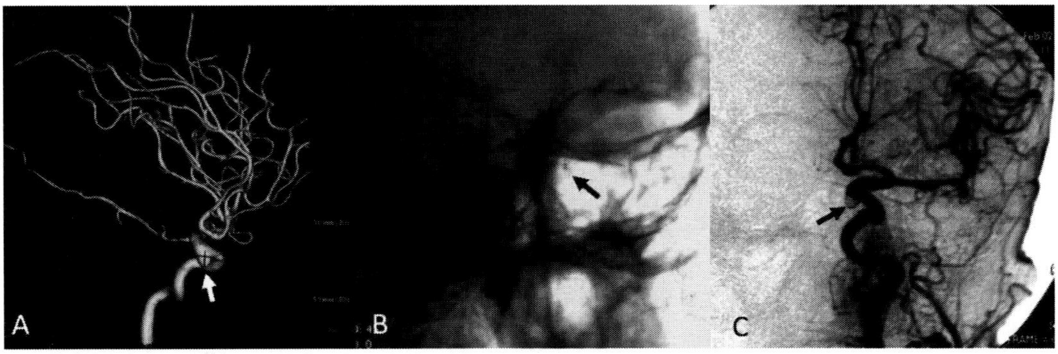

Figure 3. A 58-year-old woman presented with an incidental paraclinoid aneurysm of the internal carotid artery. A, 3-D reconstruction of the left internal carotid artery injection showing the 5mm×5mm paraclinoid aneurysm of the internal carotid artery (arrow), which was treated with 4mm×20mm Neuroform stent and coils. B, the unsubtracted image showing the Neuroform stent (black arrow). D, oblique view of the left internal carotid artery injection after treatment showing the aneurysm was occluded completely (arrow).

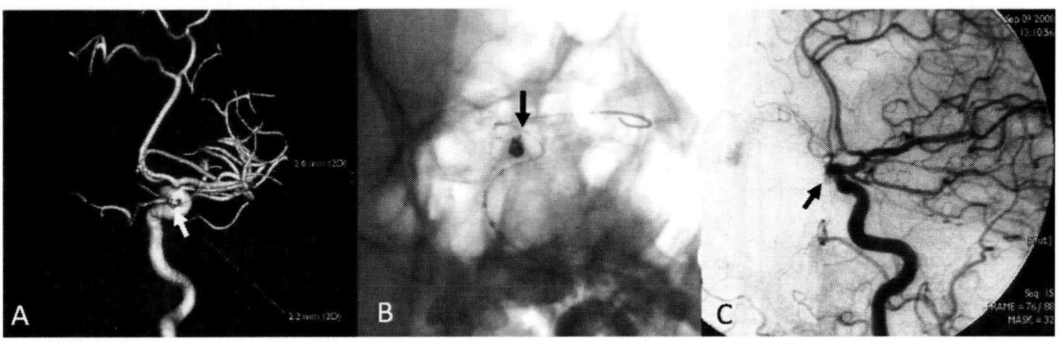

Figure 4. A 55-year-old man presented with subarachnoid hemorrhage. A, 3-D reconstruction of the left internal carotid artery injection showing a 2mm×3mm paraclinoid aneurysm (arrow) of the internal carotid artery. B, oblique view of the unsubtracted image showing the aneurysm was treated with 4mm×20mm Neuroform stent and coils (Microplex, 3mm×4cm, 2mm×2cm, 2mm×2cm, 2mm×1cm, Microvention, USA) (arrow). C, oblique view of the left internal carotid artery injection after treatment showing the complete occlusion of the aneurysm (arrow).

For years, the Neuroform and Enterprise stents were the only devices approved by the FDA for stent-assisted coiling technique. In 2018, two new self-expanding devices, the Low-Profile Visualized Intraluminal Support (LVIS) stent and the LVIS Jr. stent (Microvention, Aliso Viejo, CA, USA), emerged, offering new possibilities in the endovascular treatment of cerebral aneurysms [10]. These devices feature a closed-cell design and an automatic fixation mechanism to the vessel, allowing for catheterization of smaller and more tortuous vessels while also enabling the use of dual-lumen microcatheters [10, 27]. Additionally, it has been shown that, compared to previous stents, they have lower aneurysm recurrence rates and allow for better vessel occlusion. However, due to their ability to cover a large surface area despite their initially small size, it has been observed that in-stent stenosis may occur, potentially leading to long-term ischemic changes postoperatively [32].

The use of LVIS stents allowed the development of an alternative technique to the classic stent-assisted coiling technique, which involves jailing the coiling microcatheter. In this method, the microcatheter is placed first and "jailed" between the vessel wall and the stent, which is deployed second. Unlike the classic technique, in this approach, the coiling microcatheter does not need to pass through the stent mesh to release the coils, making it a relatively easier technique. However, this method has drawbacks as well, since the stent may not fully conform to the coils and the microcatheter may not be able to move easily, making it challenging to safely withdraw from the vessel [27].

In 2019, an improved version of the Neuroform, the Neuroform Atlas (Stryker Neurovascular, Fremont, CA, USA), received approval for endovascular treatment of cerebral aneurysms. This stent offers the advantage of being used in more remote locations due to its compatibility with much smaller diameter microcatheters, and additionally, its design allows for a more secure placement against the vessel walls [33]. Besides the development of stents and devices that allow embolization of a wider variety of vessels, various techniques have also been developed, such as the placement of two stents in a Y-configuration for bifurcation aneurysms. In this method, the two stents overlap in the main trunk while each one covers the two branches of the bifurcation of the main vessel [34]. Other variations of this technique include placing the stents in parallel, the waffle-cone stenting, the rescue-stent, the X-stenting, and the H-stenting for aneurysms in the anterior communicating artery [27]. These techniques are significantly more complex than the classic stent-assisted coiling, and the aneurysmal vessels selected for their application must be at bifurcation points that allow for the placement of the stents.

The stent-assisted coiling technique expanded the range of treatable aneurysms. However, wide-neck aneurysms located in distal sites and branches of the circle of Willis are not easily managed with this technique. Additionally, this technique requires the use of dual antiplatelet therapy, which increases the risk of bleeding. Moreover, the overall risk of complications appears to be higher compared to the use of coils alone, primarily due to the technical challenges involved [35].

Flow Diverters

The limitations of traditional embolization techniques, with or without the aid of stents, led to the development of devices that divert blood flow away from the aneurysmal vessel. These devices first appeared in the field of endovascular aneurysm treatment under the name "flow-disrupting" devices in 2007, and shortly thereafter they were renamed flow diverters [36]. These devices have the ability to divert blood flow away from the aneurysmal vessel, promoting thrombosis within it due to blood stasis inside, and ultimately leading to vessel remodeling through the re-epithelialization of the vessel neck [37].

In 2011, the first flow diverter known as the Pipeline Embolization Device (PED) (Medtronic Neurovascular, Irvine, CA, USA) received FDA approval for the endovascular treatment of cerebral aneurysms, as it was shown to be as safe as the stent-assisted coiling technique [38]. These devices enabled the treatment of large-diameter, wide-neck, fusiform, dissecting, and bifurcation with side branches aneurysms that were difficult to address with traditional coiling techniques [38]. The PED is made of metal, which necessitates dual antiplatelet therapy, thereby increasing the risk of hemorrhage [39]. Additionally, the PED did not allow for easy repositioning in case of movement or misplacement. For this reason, efforts were made to create new devices that would present a lower risk of thrombosis and provide the option for repositioning. In 2014, the Pipeline Flex device was introduced, which, thanks to its design and materials, allowed for placement with a smaller microcatheter and offered the ability for repositioning [40]. Just three years ago, following the completion of the SHIELD study (Periprocedural to 1-year safety and efficacy outcomes with the Pipeline Embolization Device with Shield technology for intracranial aneurysms: a prospective, post-market, multi-center study), an even more advanced version, the Pipeline Flex-Shield, received FDA approval [10, 41]. This device features a synthetic surface of phosphorylcholine, which covers the metal components to reduce the risk of stenosis and thrombus formation [41].

In addition to the three generations of Pipeline devices, five other types of flow diverters have received FDA approval and are currently in use: the Silk flow diverter and Silk Vista Baby (Balt Extrusion, Montmorency, Fr), the Flow Re-Direction Endoluminal Device (FRED) (Microvention, Aliso Viejo, CA, USA), the FRED Jr., and the Surpass Streamline and Surpass Evolve stents (Stryker Neurovascular, Fremont, CA, USA) [38]. Each of these devices has its own characteristics and can be combined with various sizes of microcatheters, making flow diverters a good choice for endovascular treatment of complex aneurysms [42]. Despite of these devices, many others have been proposed and utilized for the endovascular treatment of cerebral aneurysms. However, research into the evolution of these devices continues, as there is a need for the development of new materials that offer enhanced biocompatibility and reduced thrombogenicity, as well as complementary techniques to support flow diversion.

Woven EndoBridge Device

Flow diverters have been able to address complex and large cerebral aneurysms with considerable success, overcoming the limitations of the coiling technique [38]. Although, these devices have not provided a comprehensive and successful solution for treating large bifurcation aneurysms. The only technique that could be utilized for these aneurysms was coiling with adjunctive devices, primarily stent-assisted coiling [42]. However, this technique also has its drawbacks, as it is more complex and requires dual antiplatelet therapy [39]. These limitations led to the development of a different device that could more safely address large bifurcation aneurysm. This device, called the Woven EndoBridge (WEB), began pilot use in 2010 and is designed for intrasaccular flow disruption [43].

The WEB device is a self-expanding ellipsoidal structure made of nitinol wires with a platinum core. It reduces blood flow within the aneurysmal sac, promoting thrombosis and simultaneously inducing re-epithelialization [44]. From its initial experimental use, the WEB device has demonstrated considerable effectiveness for this category of aneurysms and has shown potential for providing long-term treatment [43]. By 2018, when it received FDA approval for the treatment of wide-neck bifurcation aneurysms, there were various clinical studies assessing its safety and efficacy, with the most well-known being the WEB Clinical Assessment of Intrasaccular Aneurysm Therapy [(WEBCAST) and (WEBCAST-2), the French Observatory and the WEB Intrasaccular Therapy study (WEB-IT) [44-47].

The first device developed was the WEB-I, featuring a single layer of 144 braided nitinol wires. This was followed by the dual-layer version (WEB-DL), which was eventually replaced by the single-layer WEB (WEB-SL) and the single-layer spherical WEB (WEB-SLS). The WEB device was subsequently developed into enhanced visualization (EV) models, including the dual-layer (WEB-DL EV), single-layer cylindrical (WEB-SL EV), and single-layer spherical (WEB-SLS EV) versions [48, 49]. In addition to the device itself, the catheters used to deploy the WEB have also evolved. Specialized VIA microcatheters (MicroVention) are now used, each designed specifically for the different available WEB devices. It's worth mentioning that, regardless of the model, all devices use the same detachment method via an electrothermal mechanism [49].

All WEB models, depending on their shape and diameter, are specifically designed for placement in certain types of aneurysms [49]. Specifically, the WEB-SL is better suited for cylindrical bifurcation aneurysms, while the WEB-SLS is ideal for more spherical or oval-shaped aneurysms. Additionally, it has been observed that single-layer devices, such as the WEB-SL and WEB-SLS, have better outcomes in terms of complete vessel occlusion compared to the dual-layer devices like the WEB-DL, as they allow for better navigation and placement in more distal locations. This advantage is due to the smaller diameter of the WEB-SL and WEB-SLS compared to the WEB-DL, which facilitates their deployment with smaller diameter microcatheters [50].

Compared to other techniques, the use of WEB devices does not require dual antiplatelet therapy, which reduces the risk of thromboembolic complications. It has been shown that WEB devices have a similar risk of complications to other endovascular techniques for aneurysm treatment [49]. In comparison, the stent-assisted coiling technique, which can be used as effectively as WEB for wide-neck bifurcation aneurysms, appears to have a lower rate of complications [51]. For the reasons mentioned above, the use of WEB devices for this specific category of aneurysms appears to be the prevailing choice today.

In recent years, efforts have been made to combine these devices with other endovascular tools to achieve better therapeutic outcomes. This is primarily done using remodeling balloons and stents when there is a remnant or difficulty in placing the WEB device. The combined use of WEB devices with coils has been proposed only in cases where complete occlusion is not achieved. However, their combination with flow diverters has not been utilized due to their similar mechanisms of action [49].

Conclusion

The history of intravascular treatment of cerebral aneurysms is very long and its evolution even greater as from the first use of catheter balls to the devices used today the technological progress is rapid. The available devices are constantly evolving, and the techniques of catheterization are also leading to the gradual prevalence of intra-vascular surgery to treat cerebral aneurysms. However, there are still some cases where intravenous therapy cannot provide a solution and open surgery prevails.

References

[1] Polevaya NV, Kalani MYS, Steinberg GK, Tse VCK. The Transition from Hunterian Ligation to Intracranial Aneurysm Clips: A Historical Perspective. *Neurosurgical Focus* (2006) 20 (6):E3. https://doi.org/10.3171/foc.2006.20.6.3.

[2] Reddy A, Masoud H. Endovascular and Medical Management of Unruptured Intracranial Aneurysms. *Seminars in Neurology* (2023) 43 (03):480–492. https://doi.org/10.1055/s-0043-1771299.

[3] Lai LT, O'Neill AH. History, Evolution, and Continuing Innovations of Intracranial Aneurysm Surgery. *World Neurosurgery* (2017) 102:673–681. https://doi.org/10.1016/j.wneu.2017.02.006.

[4] Ramadan OMA, Lv X. History of Endovascular Surgery of Cerebral Aneurysms. In: *Endovascular Surgery of Cerebral Aneurysms*, edited by Lv X. 2022:29–40. Singapore: Springer Nature Singapore. https://doi.org/10.1007/978-981-16-7102-9_3.

[5] Dandy WE. Intracranial Aneurysm of the Internal Carotid Artery Cured by Operation. *Annals of Surgery* (1938) 107 (5):654.

[6] Laurent D, Lucke-Wold B, Leary O, Randall MH, Porche K, Koch M, Chalouhi N, Polifka A, Hoh BL. The Evolution of Endovascular Therapy for Intracranial Aneurysms: Historical Perspective and Next Frontiers. *Neuroscience Insights* (2022) 17:26331055221175. https://doi.org/10.1177/26331055221 117560.

[7] Belavadi R, Gudigopuram S, Raguthu CC, Gajjela H, Kela I, Kakarala CL, Hassan M, Sange I. Surgical Clipping Versus Endovascular Coiling in the Management of Intracranial Aneurysms. *Cureus* (2021). https://doi.org/10.7759/cureus.20478.

[8] Tondreau RL. The Retrospectoscope: Egas Moniz 1874-1955. *RadioGraphics* (1985) 5 (6):994–997. https://doi.org/10.1148/radiographics.5.6.3916824.

[9] Ferro JM. Egas Moniz and Internal Carotid Occlusion. *Archives of Neurology* (1988) 45 (5):563–564. https://doi.org/10.1001/archneur.1988.00520290099021.

[10] Lauzier DC, Huguenard AL, Srienc AI, Cler SJ, Osbun JW, Chatterjee AR, Vellimana AK, et al. A Review of Technological Innovations Leading to Modern Endovascular Brain Aneurysm Treatment. *Frontiers in Neurology* (2023) 14:1156887. https://doi.org/10.3389/fneur.2023.1156887.

[11] Luessenhop AJ, Velasquez AC. Observations on the Tolerance of the Intracranial Arteries to Catheterization. *Journal of Neurosurgery* (1964) 21 (2):85–91. https://doi.org/10.3171/jns.1964. 21.2.0085.

[12] Serbinenko FA. Balloon Catheterization and Occlusion of Major Cerebral Vessels. *Journal of Neurosurgery* (1974) 41 (2):125–145. https://doi.org/10.3171/jns.1974.41.2.0125.

[13] Picard L, Manelfe C, Roland J, Treil J, André JM, Morel C. Embolisation et Occlusions par Ballonnets dans les Lésions Vasculaires Crânio-Faciales: Sept Années d'Expérience. *Neuroradiology* (1978) 16 (1):393–394. https://doi.org/10.1007/BF00395314.

[14] Hilal SK, Khandji A, Solomon RW, Chi L. Obliteration of Intracranial Aneurysms with Pre-Shaped Highly Thrombogenic Coils. *Radiology* (1989) 173 (1):250–257.

[15] Henkes H, Brew S, Felber S, Miloslavski E, Mogilevski G, Tavrovski I, Kühne D. In Vitro and In Vivo Studies of the Extent of Electrothrombotic Deposition of Blood Elements on the Surface of Electrolytically Detachable Coils. *Interventional Neuroradiology* (2004) 10 (3):189–201. https://doi.org/10.1177/159101990401000301.

[16] Molyneux AJ, Kerr RS, Yu LM, Clarke M, Sneade M, Yarnold JA, Sandercock P. International Subarachnoid Aneurysm Trial (ISAT) of Neurosurgical Clipping versus Endovascular Coiling in 2143 Patients with Ruptured Intracranial Aneurysms: A Randomised Comparison. *The Lancet* (2005) 366 (9488):809–817. https://doi.org/10.1016/S0140-6736 (05)67214-5.

[17] Murphy K. ISAT and ISUIA: The Impact on Informed Consent. *Techniques in Vascular and Interventional Radiology* (2005) 8 (3):106–107. https://doi.org/10.1053/j.tvir.2005.10.001.

[18] Wiebers DO. Unruptured Intracranial Aneurysms: Natural History, Clinical Outcome, and Risks of Surgical and Endovascular Treatment. *The Lancet* (2003) 362 (9378):103–110. https://doi.org/10. 1016/S0140-6736 (03)13860-3.

[19] Broeders JA, Ali UA, Molyneux AJ, Poncyljusz W, Raymond J, White PM, Steinfort B. Bioactive versus Bare Platinum Coils for the Endovascular Treatment of Intracranial Aneurysms: Systematic

Review and Meta-Analysis of Randomized Clinical Trials. *Journal of NeuroInterventional Surgery* (2016) 8 (9):898–908. https://doi.org/10.1136/neurintsurg-2015-011881.

[20] Abi-Aad KR, Rahme RJ, Patra DP, Turcotte EL, Richter KR, Merrill SA, Syal A, et al. Clinical Outcomes of First- and Second-Generation Hydrogel Coils Compared with Bare Platinum Coils: A Systematic Literature Review. *Neurosurgical Review* (2022) 45 (3):1873–1882. https://doi.org/10.1007/s10143-021-01632-z.

[21] Li W, Ye M, Cimpoca A, Henkes H, Wang H, Xu X, Gu Y, et al. Avenir® vs. Axium Coils for Intracranial Aneurysms: Results of a Multicenter Randomized Controlled Trial. *Frontiers in Neurology* (2022) 12:817989. https://doi.org/10.3389/fneur.2021.817989.

[22] Pierot L, Barbe C, Thierry A, Bala F, Eugene F, Cognard C, Herbreteau D, et al. Patient and Aneurysm Factors Associated with Aneurysm Recanalization after Coiling. *Journal of NeuroInterventional Surgery* (2022) 14 (11):1096–1101. https://doi.org/10.1136/neurintsurg-2021-017972.

[23] Webb M, Riina H, Mascitelli J. Wide-Neck and Bifurcation Aneurysms. *Neurosurgery Clinics of North America* (2022) 33 (4):359–369. https://doi.org/10.1016/j.nec.2022.05.002.

[24] Tosello RT, Batista UC, Pereira BJA, Piske RL. Packing Density Necessary to Reach a High Complete Occlusion Rate in Circumferential Unruptured Intracranial Aneurysms Treated with Stent-Assisted Coil Embolization. *American Journal of Neuroradiology* (2017) 38 (10):1973–1977. https://doi.org/10.3174/ajnr.A5303.

[25] Wallace AN, Samaniego E, Kayan Y, Derdeyn CP, Delgado Almandoz JE, Dandapat S, Fease JL, et al. Balloon-Assisted Coiling of Cerebral Aneurysms with the Dual-Lumen Scepter XC Balloon Catheter: Experience at Two High-Volume Centers. *Interventional Neuroradiology* (2019) 25 (4):414–418. https://doi.org/10.1177/1591019919828677.

[26] Nelson PK, Levy DI. Balloon-Assisted Coil Embolization of Wide-Necked Aneurysms of the Internal Carotid Artery: Medium-Term Angiographic and Clinical Follow-up in 22 Patients. *American Journal of Neuroradiology* (2001) 22 (1):19–26.

[27] Munich SA, Lopes DK, Crowley RW. Stent-Assisted Coil Embolization. In: *Management of Cerebrovascular Disorders*, edited by Spiotta AM, Turner RD, Chaudry MI, Turk AS. 2019:187–205. Cham: Springer. https://doi.org/10.1007/978-3-319-99016-3_12.

[28] Dandapat S, Mendez-Ruiz A, Martínez-Galdámez M, Macho J, Derakhshani S, Torres GF, et al. Review of Current Intracranial Aneurysm Flow Diversion Technology and Clinical Use. *Journal of NeuroInterventional Surgery* (2021) 13 (1):54–62. https://doi.org/10.1136/neurintsurg-2020-015877.

[29] Higashida RT, Smith W, Gress D, Urwin R, Dowd CF, Balousek PA, Halbach VV. Intravascular Stent and Endovascular Coil Placement for a Ruptured Fusiform Aneurysm of the Basilar Artery: Case Report and Review of the Literature. *Journal of Neurosurgery* (1997) 87 (6):944–949. https://doi.org/10.3171/jns.1997.87.6.0944.

[30] Henkes H, Bose A, Felber S, Miloslavski E, Berg-Dammer E, Kühne D. Endovascular Coil Occlusion of Intracranial Aneurysms Assisted by a Novel Self-Expandable Nitinol Microstent (Neuroform). *Interventional Neuroradiology* (2002) 8 (2):107–119. https://doi.org/10.1177/159101990200800202.

[31] Feng X, Qian Z, Liu P, Zhang B, Wang L, Guo E, Wen X, et al. Comparison of Recanalization and In-Stent Stenosis Between the Low-Profile Visualized Intraluminal Support Stent and Enterprise Stent-Assisted Coiling for 254 Intracranial Aneurysms. *World Neurosurgery* (2018) 109:e99–e104. https://doi.org/10.1016/j.wneu.2017.09.112.

[32] Jankowitz BT, Hanel R, Jadhav AP, Loy DN, Frei D, Siddiqui AH, Puri AS, et al. Neuroform Atlas Stent System for the Treatment of Intracranial Aneurysm: Primary Results of the Atlas Humanitarian Device Exemption Cohort. *Journal of NeuroInterventional Surgery* (2019) 11 (8):801–806. https://doi.org/10.1136/neurintsurg-2018-014455.

[33] Ko JK, Han IH, Cho WH, Choi BK, Cha SH, Choi CH, Lee SW, Lee TH. Crossing Y-Stent Technique with Dual Open-Cell Stents for Coiling of Wide-Necked Bifurcation Aneurysms. *Clinical Neurology and Neurosurgery* (2015) 132:54–60. https://doi.org/10.1016/j.clineuro.2015.02.002.

[34] Bsat S, Bsat A, Tamim H, Chanbour H, Alomari SO, El Houshiemy MN, Moussalem C, Omeis I. Safety of Stent-Assisted Coiling for Wide-Necked Ruptured Aneurysm: A Systematic Literature Review and Meta-Analysis of Prevalence. *Interventional Neuroradiology* (2020) 26 (5):547–556. https://doi.org/10.1177/1591019920945059.

[35] Kallmes DF, Ding YH, Dai D, Kadirvel R, Lewis DA, Cloft HJ. A New Endoluminal, Flow-Disrupting Device for Treatment of Saccular Aneurysms. *Stroke* (2007) 38 (8):2346–2352. https://doi.org/10.1161/STROKEAHA.106.479576.

[36] Kühn AL, Gounis MJ, Puri AS. Introduction: History and Development of Flow Diverter Technology and Evolution. *Neurosurgery* (2020) 86 (Supplement_1):S3–S10. https://doi.org/10.1093/neuros/nyz307.

[37] Briganti F, Leone G, Marseglia M, Mariniello G, Caranci F, Brunetti A, Maiuri F. Endovascular Treatment of Cerebral Aneurysms Using Flow-Diverter Devices: A Systematic Review. *Neuroradiology Journal* (2015) 28 (4):365–375. https://doi.org/10.1177/1971400915602803.

[38] Becske T, Kallmes DF, Saatci I, McDougall CG, Szikora I, Lanzino G, Moran CJ, et al. Pipeline for Uncoilable or Failed Aneurysms: Results from a Multicenter Clinical Trial. *Radiology* (2013) 267 (3):858–868. https://doi.org/10.1148/radiol.13120099.

[39] Pereira VM, Kelly M, Vega P, Murias E, Yilmaz H, Erceg G, Pellaton A, Lovblad KO, Krings T. New Pipeline Flex Device: Initial Experience and Technical Nuances. *Journal of NeuroInterventional Surgery* (2015) 7 (12):920–925. https://doi.org/10.1136/neurintsurg-2014-011347.

[40] Rice H, Martínez Galdámez M, Holtmannspötter M, Spelle L, Lagios K, Ruggiero M, Vega P, et al. Periprocedural to 1-Year Safety and Efficacy Outcomes with the Pipeline Embolization Device with Shield Technology for Intracranial Aneurysms: A Prospective, Post-Market, Multi-Center Study. *Journal of NeuroInterventional Surgery* (2020) 12 (11):1107–1112. https://doi.org/10.1136/neurintsurg-2020-015943.

[41] Jiang B, Colby GP, Coon AL, Lin LM. Cerebral Aneurysm Treatment: Modern Neurovascular Techniques. *Stroke and Vascular Neurology* (2016) 1 (3):93–100. https://doi.org/10.1136/svn-2016-000027.

[42] Ding YH, Lewis DA, Kadirvel R, Dai D, Kallmes DF. The Woven EndoBridge: A New Aneurysm Occlusion Device. *American Journal of Neuroradiology* (2011) 32 (3):607–611. https://doi.org/10.3174/ajnr.A2399.

[43] Pierot L, Costalat V, Moret J, Szikora I, Herbreteau D, Stockx L, Spelle L, et al. Safety and Efficacy of Aneurysm Treatment with WEB: Results of the WEBCAST Study. *Journal of Neurosurgery* (2016) 124 (5):1250–1256. https://doi.org/10.3171/2015.2.JNS142634.

[44] Pierot L, Gubucz I, Buhk JH, Holtmannspötter M, Herbreteau D, Stockx L, Spelle L, et al. Safety and Efficacy of Aneurysm Treatment with the WEB: Results of the WEBCAST 2 Study. *American Journal of Neuroradiology* (2017) 38 (6):1151–1155. https://doi.org/10.3174/ajnr.A5178.

[45] Pierot L, Moret J, Turjman F, Herbreteau D, Raoult H, Barreau X, Velasco S, et al. WEB Treatment of Intracranial Aneurysms: Feasibility, Complications, and 1-Month Safety Results with the WEB DL and WEB SL/SLS in the French Observatory. *American Journal of Neuroradiology* (2015) 36 (5):922–927. https://doi.org/10.3174/ajnr.A4230.

[46] Fiorella D, Molyneux A, Coon AL, Szikora I, Saatci I, Baltacioglu F, Sultan A, Arthur AS. Demographic, Procedural and 30-Day Safety Results from the WEB Intra-Saccular Therapy Study (WEB-IT). *Journal of NeuroInterventional Surgery* (2017) 9 (12):1191–1196. https://doi.org/10.1136/neurintsurg-2016-012841.

[47] Goyal N, Hoit D, DiNitto J, Elijovich L, Fiorella D, Pierot L, Lamin S, et al. How to WEB: A Practical Review of Methodology for the Use of the Woven EndoBridge. *Journal of NeuroInterventional Surgery* (2020) 12 (5):512–520. https://doi.org/10.1136/neurintsurg-2019-015506.

[48] Pierot L. Ten Years of Clinical Evaluation of the Woven EndoBridge: A Safe and Effective Treatment for Wide-Neck Bifurcation Aneurysms. *Neurointervention* (2021) 16 (3):211–221. https://doi.org/10.5469/neuroint.2021.00395.

[49] Mine B, Pierot L, Lubicz B. Intrasaccular Flow-Diversion for Treatment of Intracranial Aneurysms: The Woven EndoBridge. *Expert Review of Medical Devices* (2014) 11 (3):315–325. https://doi.org/10.1586/17434440.2014.907741.

[50] El Naamani KE, Chen CJ, Abbas R, Sweid A, Sioutas GS, Badih K, Ramesh S, et al. Woven EndoBridge versus Stent-Assisted Coil Embolization of Cerebral Bifurcation Aneurysms. *Journal of Neurosurgery* (2022) 137 (6):1786–1793. https://doi.org/10.3171/2022.3.JNS2217.

Chapter 15

The Historical Development of Embolization of Spinal Vascular Malformations and Classifications

Yigit Can Senol[1,2,*], MD
Halis Emre Cifci[2], MD
and Ergun Daglioglu[2], MD, PhD
[1]Department of Neurosurgery, University of California San Francisco, San Francisco, California, USA
[2]Department of Neurosurgery, Health Sciences University Bilkent City Hospital, Ankara, Türkiye

Abstract

Spinal vascular malformations (SVMs) are a diverse group of disorders characterized by abnormal blood vessel morphology, including spinal dural arteriovenous fistulas (DAVFs), spinal arteriovenous malformations (AVMs), cavernous malformations, and spinal artery aneurysms. This overview focuses on spinal AVFs and AVMs, which can lead to various forms of spinal cord dysfunction. Clinical presentations vary due to differences in pathophysiology, necessitating specific treatment approaches. The history of spinal vascular malformations reveals a challenging journey toward understanding their angioarchitecture and developing effective diagnostic and treatment methods. Initial recognition dates back to the late 19th century, with Dr. Charles Elsberg performing the first successful surgical intervention in 1914. Significant advancements were made with the introduction of spinal arteriography, enhancing the understanding of SVM pathophysiology. The development of endovascular embolization, pioneered by Doppman and colleagues, marked a significant milestone, offering a less invasive alternative to surgery. Endovascular embolization has evolved over the past 40 years, with advancements in microcatheters and embolic agents such as IBCA, NBCA, and Onyx. These innovations have improved the safety and efficacy of the procedure, allowing for better navigation of small, tortuous vasculature and controlled delivery of embolic agents. Despite these advancements, challenges remain, including the risk of spinal cord infarctions. Various classification systems for SVMs have been developed and are evolving alongside diagnostic and treatment advancements. A recent 2024 classification system emphasizes the presence or absence of retrograde flow in cortical veins, aiding in better patient management by identifying high-risk lesions. The literature on endovascular management of SVMs is limited, primarily consisting of case reports and small series, but the

* Corresponding Author's Email: ygtsenol@gmail.com

In: World History of Neurointerventional Surgery
Editors: Xianli Lv and Zhongxue Wu
ISBN: 979-8-89530-792-2

advancements in embolic agents and techniques hold promise for better treatment outcomes.

Keywords: spinal cord vascular malformation, arteriovenous malformation, history, embolization

Introduction

Spinal vascular malformations (SVMs) are characterized by abnormal blood vessel morphology and include spinal dural arteriovenous fistulas (DAVFs), spinal arteriovenous malformations (AVMs), cavernous malformations, and spinal artery aneurysms. These lesions, whether congenital or acquired, can lead to various forms of spinal cord dysfunction. The clinical presentation varies due to differences in pathophysiology, necessitating specific treatment approaches. The history of SVMs reveals a challenging journey towards understanding their angioarchitecture and developing effective diagnostic and treatment methods. Recognized in the late nineteenth century, early knowledge of SVMs was limited to case reports and surgical or autopsy findings. It was not until the advent of modern neuroradiological techniques in the late 1960s that the pathophysiology of these conditions became clearer. Collaborative efforts between neurosurgeons and neuroradiologists in Great Britain, France, and the United States have led to the current diagnostic and treatment methods.

Endovascular embolization, a significant milestone in the treatment of SVMs, has a rich history of development. Pioneered by Doppman and colleagues, this technique has evolved over the past 40 years, with major advancements in microcatheters and embolic agents such as IBCA, NBCA, and Onyx [1]. These innovations have improved the safety and efficacy of the procedure, allowing for better navigation of small, tortuous vasculature and controlled delivery of embolic agents. The introduction of these technologies has revolutionized the management of SVMs, offering a less invasive alternative to surgery. Despite challenges such as the risk of spinal cord infarctions, endovascular embolization has become a crucial component of SVM management, significantly improving treatment outcomes and expanding therapeutic options for patients.

First Cases

Despite their variability in pathophysiology and clinical presentation, spinal vascular malformations have been recognized for their significant morbidity since their initial description in the late 19th century by Hebold and Gaupp[2]. Due to the natural history of these lesions driving the need for intervention, surgical correction has been attempted since the early 1900s. Dr. Charles Elsberg reported the first successful operation in 1914 [2]. A 23-year-old man was admitted to Mount Sinai Hospital with severe pain, weakness, and spasticity in his lower extremities, rendering him unable to walk. During the surgery, T5-9 laminectomies were performed, revealing an enlarged left posterior spinal vein after durotomy. This vein was ligated at the dural opening, and a 2-cm segment was excised. The patient recovered without neurological dysfunction within three months.

Following this initial success, therapeutic efforts continued. Significant advancements were made possible by the introduction and refinement of spinal arteriography by Djindjian, Doppman, DiChiro, and others, which enhanced the understanding of the pathophysiology and treatment of these lesions [3]. Doppman and colleagues further advanced the field by introducing percutaneous embolization, successfully treating a 16-year-old boy by embolizing an arterial feeder with steel pellets[2]. Angiography has since become the gold standard for diagnosis and has evolved technically and technologically, increasing its utility in treating spinal vascular malformations, either alone or combined with surgical intervention.

Over the past 40 years, nearly every aspect of endovascular technology has advanced. Two principal components of therapeutic enhancement have been the advent of microcatheters and the continued innovation in related technologies. Newer microcatheters allow the neurointerventionalist to navigate small and tortuous vasculature with increased safety and to promote canalization of previously inaccessible vascular territories. Concerning the advancement in embolic agents, the use of liquid adhesives such as isobutyl 2-cyanoacrylate (IBCA) and, more recently, n-butyl 2-cyanoacrylate (NBCA) has resulted in substantial improvements compared to particles like organic fragments, silk, and polyvinyl alcohol (PVA) [4]. Additional benefits include adjustable polymerization time and superior vessel permeation. However, despite these advantages, liquid embolic agents are not without problems, including the risk of catheter adhesion, variability in physical behavior, and an increased risk of spinal cord infarctions. The recent application of Onyx (a liquid embolization agent consisting of ethylene vinyl alcohol; *Medtronic, Minneapolis, USA*), an innovative liquid embolic substance, offers further improvements. Onyx can be delivered in a more controlled fashion over several minutes, carries a lower risk of premature venous occlusion or occlusion of a large intradural portion of the draining vein, and poses a lower risk of retained catheter. Although the experience with spinal vascular malformations is still evolving, these advancements hold promise for better treatment outcomes.

Classification

Between 1967 and 2021, several major classification systems for spinal arteriovenous shunts were developed. These classifications evolved alongside advancements in diagnostic studies and treatment approaches (Figure 1).

The first classification system was introduced by Di Chiro G and colleagues in 1971, based on angiographic findings: single-coiled vessel type I, glomus type II, and juvenile type III [5]. In 1986, Hero RC and colleagues identified a new type of spinal arteriovenous shunt that did not fit the existing classification. They described a direct connection between the anterior spinal artery and vein located ventrally, termed as a direct spinal arteriovenous fistula type IV (Figure 2).

In 1987, Rosenblum B proposed another classification system, categorizing spinal arteriovenous shunts into four types (Table 1): type I as dural arteriovenous fistula, type II as intramedullary glomus arteriovenous malformation, type III as intramedullary juvenile arteriovenous malformation, and type IV as direct arteriovenous fistula [6]. By 1993, Mourier KL and Merland JJ reported a series of intradural direct arteriovenous fistulas, describing them as perimedullary arteriovenous fistulas and classifying them into three subtypes based on the number of feeding arteries and the size of the arteriovenous fistula: Type I with a single feeding artery and a small fistula, Type II with multiple feeding arteries and a medium fistula, and Type III with multiple feeding arteries and a giant fistula [7].

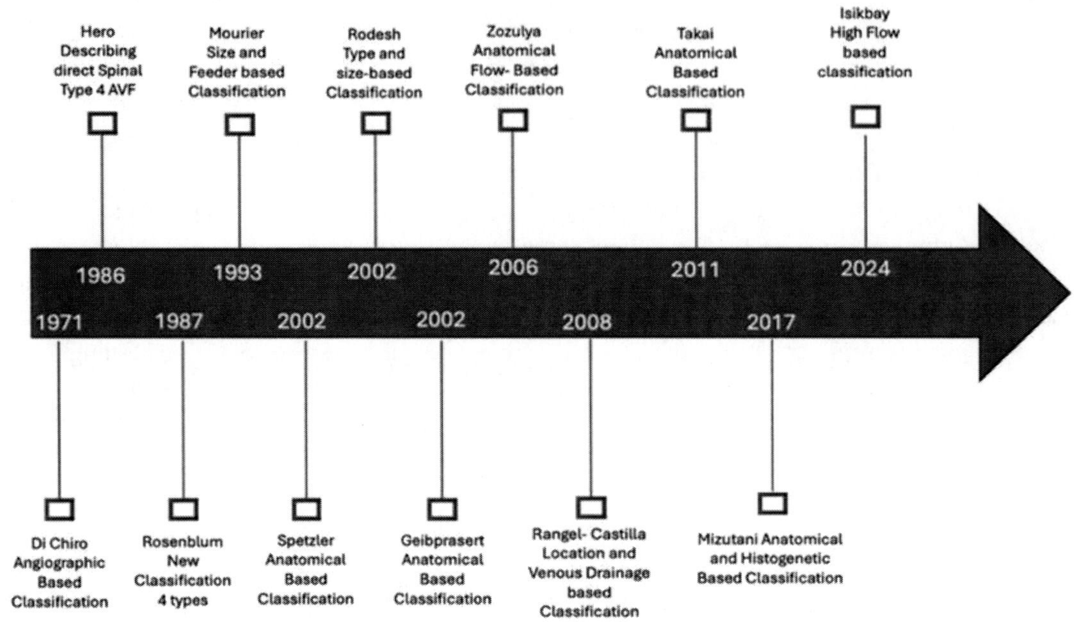

Figure 1. Historical Development of Spinal Vascular Malformations Classification.

Table 1. Rosenblum's classification system

Classification by Rosenblum et al	Type I	Dural AV fistula	
	Type II	Glomus-type intradural AV malformation	
	Type III	Juvenile-type intradural AV malformation	
	Type IV	Intradural AV fistula	simple extramedullary fistulas fed by a single arterial branch
			intermediate-sized fistulas with multiple, dilated arterial feeders
			giant multipediculated fistulas

In 2002, Spetzler RF introduced a classification system based on anatomical locations (Table 2). Dural arteriovenous fistulas were termed dorsal arteriovenous fistulas due to their common development at the dorsolateral aspect of the dura [8]. Perimedullary arteriovenous fistulas, typically developing at the ventral portion, were defined as ventral arteriovenous fistulas. Intramedullary glomus arteriovenous malformations were labeled compact arteriovenous malformations, and intramedullary juvenile arteriovenous malformations as extradural-intradural arteriovenous malformations. Additionally, three new types were defined: extradural arteriovenous fistulas, diffuse type arteriovenous malformations, and conus arteriovenous malformations.

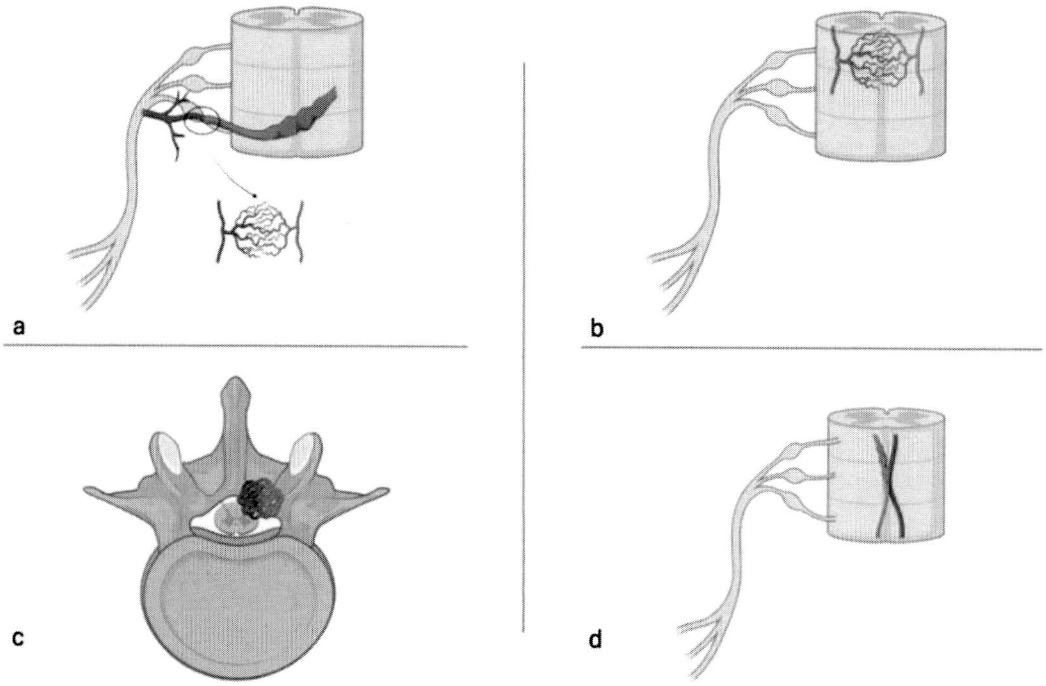

Figure 2. A: Type I spinal dural AVF, the typical presentation is an older (range, 55–60 years of age) man (male/female ratio 1⁄4 5:1) with a history of nonspecific progressive myelopathic symptoms. Symptoms are related to cord edema and ischemia resulting from arterialized intravenous pressure competing with cord drainage, though venous thrombosis has also been described. B: Type II spinal "glomus" arteriovenous malformations (SGAVMs) account for 19%–45% of all SVMs. SGAVMs are congenital, high-flow lesions that may be thoracic (51%), cervical (29%), or lumbar/conus (20%). This intramedullary and/or pial-based nidus of abnormal vascular channels may be supplied by ≥1 branch of the anterior or posterior spinal artery, vertebral arteries, dural arteries, and/or vasocorona. C: Type III spinal juvenile (metameric) arteriovenous malformations are the least common type of SVMs, with estimated frequencies between 5.4% and 9%. Most cases involve the thoracic spine, followed by the cervical spine. Besides the cord, these lesions may involve the bony spine, paraspinal tissues, and skin, sharing a common metameric tissue origin. D, Type IV Intradural perimedullary AVF are pial-based lesions supplied by the anterior or posterior spinal artery, sometimes with a small intervening nidus. This morphologically based SVM is limited in scope because some SVMs remain outside their descriptive criteria. Recent proposals to address this limitation include a location-based SVMs consisting of 6 lesion types proposed by Zozulya et al and a type V extradural AVF proposed by Takai[9]. Syndromic associations with IPAVFs have been reported, including Osler-Weber-Rendu, Proteus, Klippel-Trenaunay, and Down syndromes.

Table 2. Spetzler's classification system

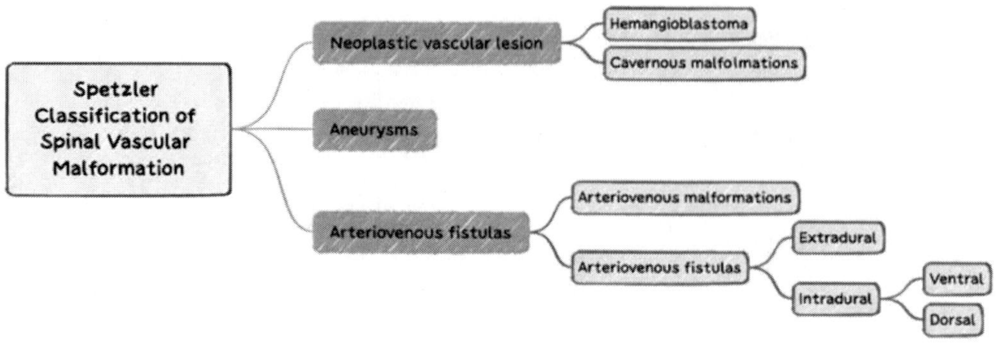

According to the Spetzler classification, spinal vascular lesions can be subdivided into neoplasms, aneurysms and arteriovenous lesions. Arteriovenous lesions are further classified as arteriovenous fistulas and AVMs. Arteriovenous fistulas can be extradural, intradural and a new categorization of "conus medullaris AV malformations." Intradural arteriovenous fistulas may be located ventrally or dorsally. Unfortunately, different pathologies are ascribed to the same group in this classification, which can create confusion. For example, spinal dural AV fistulas and fistulous spinal cord AV malformations on the dorsal surface of the spinal cord belong to the same category (intradural dorsal AV fistulas).

In 2002, Geibprasert classified cranio-spinal arteriovenous shunts into three types: ventral, dorsal, and lateral epidural groups. In 2011, Rangel-Castilla reported an endovascular case series of extradural arteriovenous fistulas, subdividing them into three types: type A (with intradural venous drainage), type B1 (without intradural venous drainage but with neurological deficits), and type B2 (without intradural venous drainage and without neurological deficits)[3].

In 2011, Takai K proposed a practical classification system based on the classic second classification, which has been widely used in the literature. Spinal dural arteriovenous fistulas were classified into five categories: type I (dural AVF), type II (intradural intramedullary glomus AVM), type III (intradural intramedullary juvenile AVM), type IV (perimedullary AVF), and type V (extradural AVF) [9]. The classification system further subdivided perimedullary and extradural AVFs based on the size of the AV shunts, drainage system, and feeding artery. This sub-classification aids in suggesting different treatment approaches depending on the subtypes. For example, type IVa perimedullary AVFs are more amenable to microsurgery, while type IVc perimedullary AVFs are suited to endovascular embolization. Similarly, type Vb extradural AVFs respond better to endovascular embolization than type Va extradural AVFs, which can be treated with both microsurgery and endovascular embolization. This system is appropriate for developing treatment strategies using microsurgical and/or endovascular treatments due to its basis in the microvascular anatomy and hemodynamics of AV shunts.

In 2021, Mizutani et al. proposed a novel classification system based on the anatomical disposition, angioarchitecture, and histogenetic location of spinal dural arteriovenous fistulas [10]. They identified five phenotypes: macro arteriovenous fistulas, micro arteriovenous fistulas, pial niduses, intramedullary lesions, and sulcal lesions.

In 2024, a new classification system was introduced focusing on the presence or absence of retrograde flow in the cortical veins of the brain or spinal cord medullary vein, labeling any shunting lesion with such retrograde flow as "high risk." This updated classification was derived from an analysis of cervical spine shunting lesions at a single center. The study reviewed electronic medical records to identify shunting lesions and evaluated craniospinal digital subtraction angiograms for shunt location, type (arteriovenous malformation (AVM) vs arteriovenous fistula (AVF)), and high-risk venous drainage [11].

Dural Arteriovenous Fistulas

Dural arteriovenous fistulas (DAVFs), also known as Type I lesions, are low-flow anomalies formed by an abnormal connection between a radicular artery and a medullary vein within the dural sleeve of a nerve root (Figure3). This results in retrograde flow into the coronal venous plexus surrounding the spinal cord, leading to venous hypertension, chronic venous congestion, and cord ischemia. Venous pressures in these fistulas average about 75% of systemic arterial circulation. DAVFs are the most common type of spinal vascular malformation, accounting for 80-85% of cases, typically occurring in older adults, with a male predominance and an acquired nature.

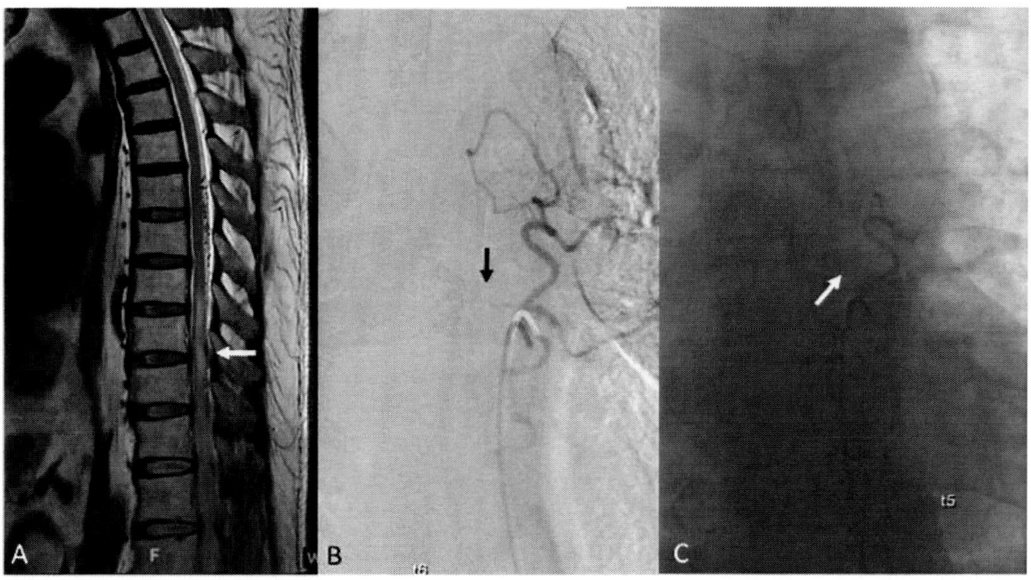

Figure 3. A 55-year-old male patient presented with back pain for 8 months and lower limb pain for 7 months. A, MR image, saggital view of T2-weighted, showing spinal cord edema and flow-void signals on the doral surface (arrow). B, the left T6 segmental artery angiography showing a dural arteriovenous fistula (TypeI) between a radioculomeningeal artery and a radicular vein (arrow). C, unsubtracted image showing the dural arteriovenous fistula is within the dural sleeve of a nerve root (arrow).

Patients often present with non-specific symptoms such as back or radicular pain, leading to diagnostic delays. This can progress to lower-extremity paresis, sphincter dysfunction, and eventually paraplegia. Early case series, including that by Morgan and Marsh, suffered from high recurrence rates due to the use of PVA particles for embolization. However, the introduction of liquid embolic materials improved success rates. Niimi et al. reported an 87% success rate in treating 38 out of 49 cases with microcatheter technology and liquid embolic agents [12]. Most patients experienced symptomatic improvement with no procedural complications.

Subsequent studies have supported the efficacy of liquid cyanoacrylate for DAVF embolization. Ushikoshi et al. achieved complete obliteration in 4 out of 6 patients using NBCA, with symptomatic improvement or stabilization in all patients. Song et al. reported a 90% angiographic occlusion rate in 27 patients, with a 15% recurrence rate over an average follow-up period of 3.1 years. Guillevin et al. emphasized the importance of NBCA penetration into the fistula and proximal vein for successful outcomes. Eskandar et al. achieved an 88% success rate with liquid acrylic-based embolization as the primary treatment, although 39% eventually required surgery due to recurrence [13].

However, not all studies have demonstrated equivalent success. Van Dijk et al. reported only a 25% angiographic cure rate over 15 years, and Steinmetz et al. found definitive treatment possible in only 46% of cases. Nonetheless, endovascular embolization with liquid acrylic agents is considered a safe initial treatment option for DAVFs, providing durable cure in 70-85% of cases when the agent penetrates the proximal draining vein. Despite this, surgery remains the gold standard due to its established efficacy and durability. With further advancements and long-term follow-up, endovascular therapy may become the first-line treatment, but surgical intervention will continue to provide definitive management when necessary.

Glomus AVMs

Glomus malformations, or Type II lesions, are characterized by a compact nidus located within the spinal cord, supplied by multiple feeding vessels from the ASA and posterior spinal artery (Figure4). These high-flow, low-resistance lesions often include associated arterial or venous aneurysms and frequently occur in children or young adults. Unlike DAVFs, glomus AVMs are prone to hemorrhage, leading to rapid deterioration of spinal cord function. Rehemorrhage rates are significant, with 10% within 30 days and 40% within the first year [14].

Therapeutic decisions for glomus AVMs depend on medical comorbidities, lesion location, and angioarchitecture, as both microsurgical excision and endovascular embolization carry significant neurological risks. Early series using PVA particles showed limited success, but modern technology has improved outcomes. Biondi et al. reported long-term improvement in 63% of patients with thoracic intramedullary AVMs treated over 15 years, with a low incidence of adverse effects.

Corkill et al. demonstrated the efficacy of Onyx for embolization of intramedullary AVMs, achieving complete obliteration in 45% of patients and subtotal occlusion in 36% [15]. Although 55% experienced acute neurological decline, all recovered to at least baseline status. Surgical intervention remains a viable option, with Spetzler et al. reporting a 68% improvement rate in 27 patients[8]. Endovascular management is justified as an initial attempt, particularly for deep or ventrally located lesions or patients unsuitable for surgery.

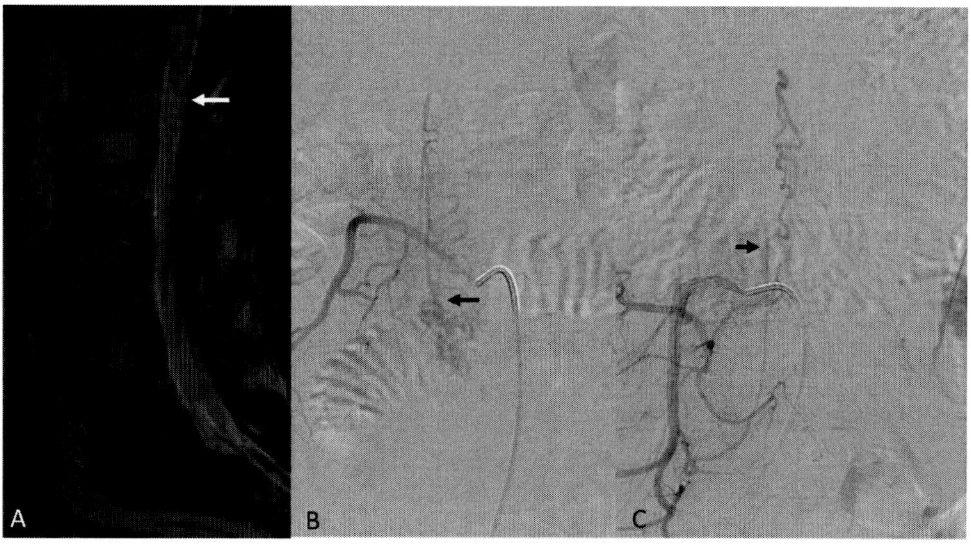

Figure 4. A 31-year-old male patient with cone arteriovenous malformation. A, MR image, saggital view of T2-weighted, showing spinal cord edema and perimedullary flow-void signals (arrow). B, the right T11 segmental artery angiography showing a glomus arteriovenous malformation of the cone (TypeII) between a radioculopial artery, posterior spinal artery and intramedullary veins (arrow). C, the right L1 segmental artery angiography showing a coexisting arteriovenous shunt between a radioculopial artery and a perimedullary vein (arrow).

Juvenile AVMs

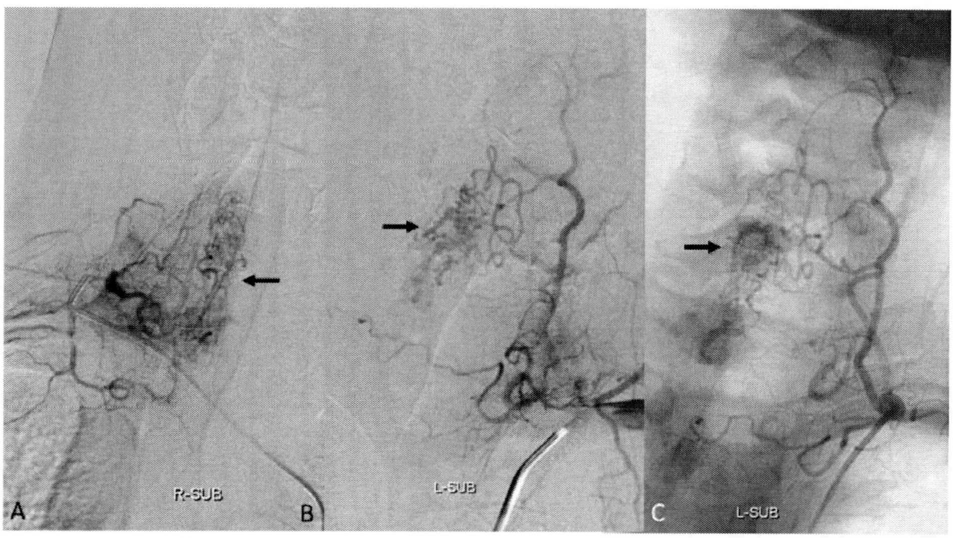

Figure 5. A 47-year-old male patient presented with numbness in the hip and left lower limb, loss of pain and temperature sensation, slightly abnormal walking posture, poor perineal perception, and occasional urinary and fecal incontinence. A, the angiography of the right subclavian artery, anteroposterior view. B, the angiography of the left subclavian artery, anteroposterior view. C, the unsubtracted image of the angiography of the left subclavian artery, anteroposterior view. Showing a juvenile AVM (TypeIII) involving two metameres of the neural tissue, dura, bone, muscle and skin.

Juvenile AVMs, or Type III lesions, are large, high-flow malformations involving paraspinal structures, presenting typically in children or adolescents with pain and progressive myelopathy (Figure5). These lesions cause neurological deficits due to spinal cord compression, venous congestion, vascular steal phenomenon, and hemorrhage.

Endovascular management of juvenile AVMs, often using PVA particles, can provide clinical stabilization or improvement. Corkill et al. reported complete or subtotal obliteration in two patients, with 50% showing improvement[15]. However, optimal management is best achieved through a multidisciplinary approach, with treatment often being palliative.

Perimedullary AVFs

Perimedullary AVFs, or Type IV lesions, involve a direct connection between spinal arteries and veins without an intervening network (Figure 6). These high-flow lesions are typically located near the conus medullaris and are often accompanied by aneurysms and ectatic venous malformations. They manifest clinically with progressive decline due to venous hypertension or acute neurological deterioration from aneurysm rupture. Merland et al. subclassified these lesions into Type I, II, and III based on size, length, and number of vessels[7].

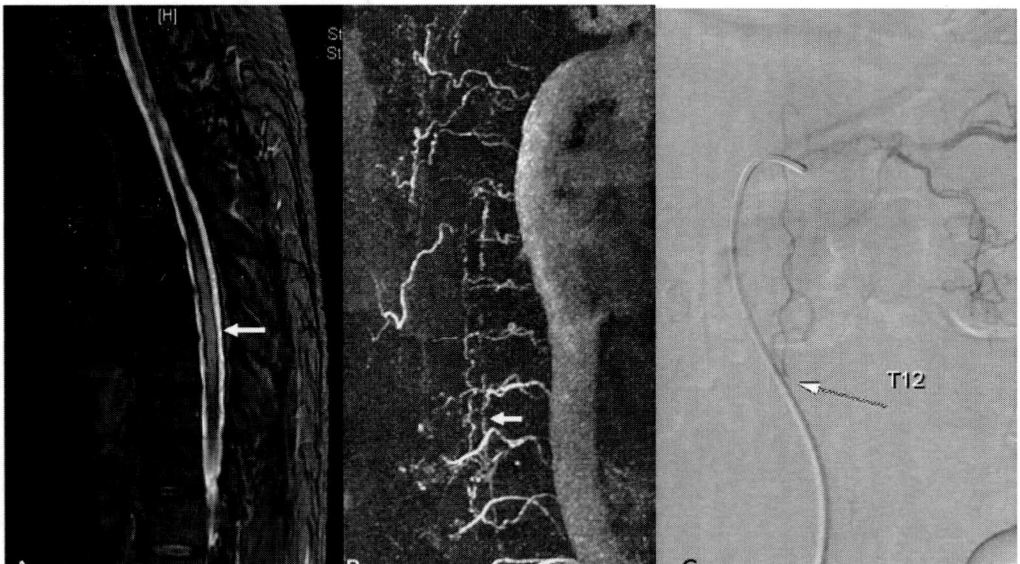

Figure 6. A 63-year-old male patient presented with weakness in both lower limbs for 3 months. A, MR image, saggital view of T2-weighted, showing spinal cord edema and flow-void signals on the doral surface (arrow). B, the MR angiography showing perimedullary veins, which suggesting a arteriovenous shunt (arrow). C, the right T12 segmental artery angiography showing an arteriovenous fistula (TypeIV) between a radioculomedullary artery, anterior spinal artery and a perimedullary vein (arrow).

Lv et al. reported on four patients (three males, one female, aged 17–35) with perimedullary arteriovenous fistulas (AVFs). Three AVFs were in the cervical region, and one in the thoracic. Symptoms included myelopathy in three patients and subarachnoid hemorrhage (SAH) in one.

Three patients were successfully treated with a single embolization, while one required two procedures. No complications occurred. Follow-up angiography at 9.6 months confirmed complete AVF resolution, and clinical follow-up at 15 months showed near-complete resolution of spinal cord abnormalities [16].

In conclusion, Type I lesions are best managed surgically, while Type II abnormalities, with multiple afferent pedicles, are difficult to cure endovascularly but remain an option for non-surgical candidates. Type III lesions generally benefit from initial embolization, with surgery reserved for cases where this fails.

Discussion

The history of endovascular embolization for spinal vascular malformations (SCVMs) reflects significant advancements in medical technology and techniques, transforming the management of these complex conditions. Initially, treatment options were limited to surgical interventions, which carried high risks and variable outcomes. The development of neuroradiological techniques in the late 1960s marked a turning point, providing a clearer understanding of the pathophysiology of SCVMs and paving the way for less invasive treatments.

Early attempts at embolization faced numerous challenges. In the 1970s, Djindjian, Di Chiro, and others began experimenting with spinal arteriography, which significantly enhanced the visualization of spinal vascular lesions. This improved understanding laid the groundwork for the first attempts at endovascular treatments. The introduction of particulate embolic agents such as polyvinyl alcohol (PVA) particles marked the beginning of endovascular therapy, but these early efforts were often plagued by high recurrence rates and incomplete obliteration of the malformations.

The evolution of endovascular embolization techniques has been driven by advancements in catheter technology, embolic materials, and imaging modalities. The development of microcatheters in the 1980s allowed for more precise navigation of the tortuous spinal vasculature, enabling better targeting of the feeding arteries and reducing the risk of non-target embolization. Concurrently, the introduction of liquid embolic agents like n-butyl cyanoacrylate (NBCA) and, more recently, Onyx, has significantly improved the effectiveness of the procedure. These agents offer the advantage of controlled, progressive embolization, allowing for complete obliteration of the malformations while minimizing the risk of complications such as spinal cord infarction.

Recent case studies and clinical trials have demonstrated the efficacy and safety of modern endovascular techniques in treating various types of SCVMs, including dural arteriovenous fistulas, intramedullary arteriovenous malformations, and perimedullary arteriovenous fistulas. The success rates have steadily improved, with many patients experiencing significant symptomatic relief and long-term stability following embolization. However, the risk of recurrence and the need for re-treatment remain challenges, particularly in complex or extensive lesions.

Overall, the advancements in endovascular embolization have significantly expanded the therapeutic options for patients with SCVMs, offering a less invasive alternative to surgery with comparable, if not superior, outcomes. The continuous evolution of this field, driven by technological innovations and clinical research, promises further improvements in the management of these challenging vascular lesions.

Conclusion

The history of spinal vascular malformations reveals a difficult journey to understand their vascular architecture and develop effective diagnostic and therapeutic approaches. Over the past 40 years, endovascular embolization techniques have evolved, as have advances in microcatheters and embolic agents such as IBCA, NBCA, and Onyx. These innovations have improved the safety and efficacy of the procedure, allowing for better guidance of small tortuous vessels and controlled delivery of embolic agents. Despite these advances, challenges remain, including the risk of spinal cord infarction. Various SVM classification systems have been developed and continue to evolve as diagnostic and therapeutic advances are made.

Disclaimer

None.

References

[1] Ducruet AF, Crowley RW, McDougall CG, Albuquerque FC. Endovascular management of spinal arteriovenous malformations. *Journal of NeuroInterventional Surgery* (2013) 5 (6):605-611. https://doi.org/10.1136/neurintsurg-2012-010487.

[2] Gailloud P. The contributions of Otto Hebold and Julius Gaupp to the study of spinal vascular malformations: Original documents and historical context. *Interventional Neuroradiology* (2019) 25 (6):604-612. https://doi.org/10.1177/1591019919845648.

[3] Medel R, Crowley RW, Dumont AS. Endovascular management of spinal vascular malformations: history and literature review. *Neurosurgical Focus* (2009) 26 (1):E7. https://doi.org/10.3171/FOC.2009.26.1.E7.

[4] Brothers MF, Kaufmann JC, Fox AJ, Deveikis JP. n-Butyl 2-cyanoacrylate—substitute for IBCA in interventional neuroradiology: histopathologic and polymerization time studies. *American Journal of Neuroradiology* (1989) 10 (4):777-786.

[5] Ommaya AK, Di Chiro G, Doppman J. Ligation of arterial supply in the treatment of spinal cord arteriovenous malformations. *Journal of Neurosurgery* (1969) 30 (6):679-692. https://doi.org/10.3171/jns.1969.30.6.0679.

[6] Rosenblum B, Oldfield EH, Doppman JL, Di Chiro G. Spinal arteriovenous malformations: a comparison of dural arteriovenous fistulas and intradural AVM's in 81 patients. *Journal of Neurosurgery* (1987) 67 (6):795-802. https://doi.org/10.3171/jns.1987.67.6.0795.

[7] Riché MC, Melki JP, Merland JJ. Embolization of spinal cord vascular malformations via the anterior spinal artery. *American Journal of Neuroradiology* (1983) 4 (3):378-381.

[8] Spetzler RF, Detwiler PW, Riina HA, Porter RW. Modified classification of spinal cord vascular lesions. *Journal of Neurosurgery: Spine* (2002) 96 (2 Suppl):145-156. https://doi.org/10.3171/spi.2002.96.2.0145.

[9] Takai K. Spinal Arteriovenous Shunts: Angioarchitecture and Historical Changes in Classification. *Neurologia Medico-Chirurgica* (2017) 57 (7):356-365. https://doi.org/10.2176/nmc.ra.2016-0316.

[10] Mizutani K, Consoli A, Maria FD, et al. Intradural spinal cord arteriovenous shunts in a personal series of 210 patients: novel classification with emphasis on anatomical disposition and angioarchitectonic distribution, related to spinal cord histogenetic units. *Journal of Neurosurgery: Spine* (2021) 34 (6):920-930. https://doi.org/10.3171/2020.9.SPINE201258.

[11] Isikbay M, Caton MT, Mattay R, et al. Arteriovenous shunts of the cervical spine: patient demographics, presentation, patterns of high-risk venous drainage, and updated classification. *Journal of Neuro Interventional Surgery* (2024). https://doi.org/10.1136/jnis-2023-021353.

[12] Niimi Y, Berenstein A, Setton A, Neophytides A. Embolization of Spinal Dural Arteriovenous Fistulae: Results and Follow-up. *Neurosurgery* (1997) 40 (4):675-682.

[13] Zanin L, Di Bonaventura R, Agosti E, et al. Surgery versus endovascular treatment for spinal dural arteriovenous fistulas: a multicenter experience and systematic literature review. *Neurosurgical Review* (2024) 47 (1):206. https://doi.org/10.1007/s10143-024-02443-8.

[14] Gross BA, Du R. Spinal glomus (type II) arteriovenous malformations: a pooled analysis of hemorrhage risk and results of intervention. *Neurosurgery* (2013) 72 (1):25-32. https://doi.org/10.1227/NEU.0b013e318276b5d3.

[15] Corkill RA, Mitsos AP, Molyneux AJ. Embolization of spinal intramedullary arteriovenous malformations using the liquid embolic agent, Onyx: a single-center experience in a series of 17 patients. *Journal of Neurosurgery: Spine* (2007) 7 (5):478-485. https://doi.org/10.3171/SPI-07/11/478.

[16] Lv X, Li Y, Yang X, Jiang C, Wu Z. Endovascular embolization for symptomatic perimedullary AVF and intramedullary AVM: a series and a literature review. *Neuroradiology* (2012) 54 (4):349-359. https://doi.org/10.1007/s00234-011-0880-0.

Chapter 16

The History of Endovascular Treatment for Spinal Vascular Diseases

Idan Levitan[1,*], MD
David Felzensztein[1], MD
Saeed Yassin[1], MD
Roozbeh Shafafy[2], MD
and Eyal Itshayek[1], MD
[1]Department of Neurosurgery, Rabin Medical Center, Petah Tikva, Israel
[2]Royal National Orthopaedic Center, London, England

Abstract

Spinal vascular malformations (SVM) are heterogenous group of vascular diseases often diagnosed after acute, subacute, and chronic neurological deterioration. This group consists of spinal dural arteriovenous fistula (sDAVF), which account for most of these lesions (about 70%), spinal arteriovenous malformations (sAVM) constitute the remainder of these lesions. These lesions are classified according to anatomic and pathophysiologic characteristics. Flow patterns (high-flow, low-flow, and no arteriovenous shunt) and location (intramedullary, peri-medullary radicular and extradural) are most helpful in further classifying these lesions. It emphasizes the importance of understanding the specific characteristics of each type to guide effective treatment. Neurological symptoms are caused by mass effect, hemorrhage, and hemodynamic disturbance. A small portion of these SVMs is discovered incidentally.

The history of SVM began with Julius Gaupp's early description in 1988 of what appears to be a perimedullary arteriovenous fistula, a type of SVM. Almost 20 years later, in 1916 Elsberg was the first to document the first surgical treatment of an sDAVF. Since then, surgical intervention has remained the most definitive treatment option to date. In 1968 Doppman et al. described the first endovascular treatment for sAVM. Since then the role of endovascular in diagnosing and treating of SVMs has constantly expanded alongside advancements in endovascular technology. This includes embolization techniques that feature advanced microcatheter navigability and detachable tips, and the advancement of liquid embolic agents such as n-butyl cyanoacrylate (n-BCA) and ethylene-vinyl alcohol

* Corresponding Author's Email: idan.levitan@mail.huji.ac.il

In: World History of Neurointerventional Surgery
Editors: Xianli Lv and Zhongxue Wu
ISBN: 979-8-89530-792-2

copolymer (Onyx). Indications for endovascular embolization of SVMs have greatly increased, serving both as adjunctive treatment prior to surgical resection as well as a standalone treatment. Currently the management of SVM includes multimodality strategies involving surgery, endovascular treatment, and, in selected cases, radiotherapy.

Keywords: literature review, spinal vascular malformations, endovascular treatment, spinal dural arteriovenous fistula, spinal arteriovenous malformations

Introduction

Otto Hebold and Julius Gaupp are often credited with the first descriptions of isolated spinal cord vascular malformation in 1885 and 1888, respectively [1-3]. A recent study by Philippe Gailloud, revisits the historical contributions of two German physicians to the understand spinal vascular malformations [4]. Hebold's work, originating from a lecture in 1885, described cases of intramedullary microaneurysms in the spinal cord, which he observed in a young girl with infectious symptoms, including brain abscesses and meningitis. Hebold's findings were later considered potentially linked to syphilis rather than true vascular malformations. In a case study involving a 45 years old woman published in 1888, Gaupp provided the first reliable description of a perimedullary arteriovenous fistula. These early descriptions predate the use of spinal angiography [4].

Almost 20 years later, in 1916, Elsberg was the first to document the first surgical treatment of an sDAVF [5]. Since then, surgical intervention has remained the most definitive treatment option [6].

The first successful treatment for sAVM using percutaneous embolization was performed in 1968 by a team of researchers at the National Institutes of Health (NIH). This groundbreaking procedure involved using stainless-steel pellets introduced through a catheter to occlude the main feeding artery of the malformation. The patient was a 16-year-old boy with a midthoracic spinal-cord AVM and a large angiomatous lesion on his back, which made traditional surgical approaches unfeasible. Using selective arteriography to identify the left 6th intercostal artery as the main feeder, the team successfully embolized the malformation with 3.0 mm pellets. Within a week, the patient showed objective signs of improved cord function. This minimally invasive technique proved to be less traumatic and as effective as previous surgical methods, marking a significant advancement in the treatment of spinal AVMs [7].

Epidemiology

Spinal dural arteriovenous fistulas (sDAVFs) are the most common type of spinal vascular malformation, accounting for approximately 70-85% of all spinal arteriovenous shunts. Despite this, they are still relatively rare lesions, with an estimated annual incidence of 5-10 cases per million population [8-10]. Spinal DAVFs predominantly affect males, with a male to female ratio of approximately 5:1. The typical age of onset is between 50-60 years old, with 80% of cases presenting between ages 20-60. These lesions most commonly occur in the thoracolumbar region, though they can be found at any spinal level [11, 12]. The true prevalence is difficult to determine precisely due to the rarity of these lesions and potential underdiagnosis. While most

SDAVFs are sporadic, some cases may be associated with genetic syndromes, such as hereditary hemorrhagic telangiectasia [13, 14]. The rarity and often nonspecific clinical presentation of SDAVFs can lead to delays in diagnosis, highlighting the importance of increased awareness among clinicians to facilitate earlier detection and treatment [15].

Clinical Manifestations

The clinical manifestations of SDAVFs are often progressive and insidious, developing over six months to 2 years. Common presenting symptoms include lower extremity weakness (seen in 52% of patients in one series), gait disturbance, sensory symptoms such as pain and paresthesia, and sphincter/bladder disturbances. Low back pain and mono- or poly-radiculopathy may also occur. As the disease progresses, patients may experience bowel and bladder incontinence, sexual dysfunction, and urinary retention. The symptoms are typically exacerbated by exercise due to increased venous pressure. If left untreated, about 50% of patients become severely disabled within three years of symptom onset. Abrupt deterioration can occur in some cases. Diagnosis is often delayed because similar symptoms can be caused by more common conditions in elderly patients, such as degenerative disk disease or spinal stenosis [15]. Rarely, SDAVFs can present with hemorrhage, mainly when located in the cervical region or foramen magnum. Subarachnoid hemorrhage is seen in 45% of patients with cervical DAVFs but is exceedingly rare in thoracolumbar lesions. The severity and duration of symptoms before treatment correlate strongly with prognosis after intervention, highlighting the importance of early diagnosis and management [16, 17].

Subacute ascending necrotizing myelitis a rare clinical syndrome, also known as Foix-Alajouanine syndrome, characterized by subacute congestive myelopathy due to DAVF, leading to progressive paraplegia primarily affecting the lower thoracic and lumbosacral regions. This syndrome results from increased venous pressure that reduces spinal cord perfusion, causing edema and necrosis. Early diagnosis is crucial, as misdiagnosis can lead to poor outcomes, while prompt treatment can significantly improve patient prognosis [18].

Classification

The classification of spinal vascular malformations has evolved over the years, with various systems developed to categorize these conditions based on anatomical and pathophysiological features. New classification systems have incorporated advancements in both diagnostic techniques and treatment options. The earliest classification system introduced by Di Chiro G in 1971, divided into three types based on angiographic findings: single-coiled vessel type I, glomus type II, and juvenile type III (Figures 1 to 3) [19]. In subsequent years, additional types were introduced to accommodate cases that did not fit the original classification, such as the direct AVF described by Heros RC et al. in 1986, which was later labeled as type IV (Figure 4) [20]. In 1987, Rosenblum and colleagues proposed a four-type classification, incorporating dural AVFs and intramedullary AVMs into the schema [21]. Further refinements in 1993 by Mourier et al. introduced subtypes for perimedullary AVFs based on the number of feeding arteries and fistula size [22]. These were known as the American/British/French connection (ABF) which has been widely accepted and utilized in neurosurgical literature ever since [23].

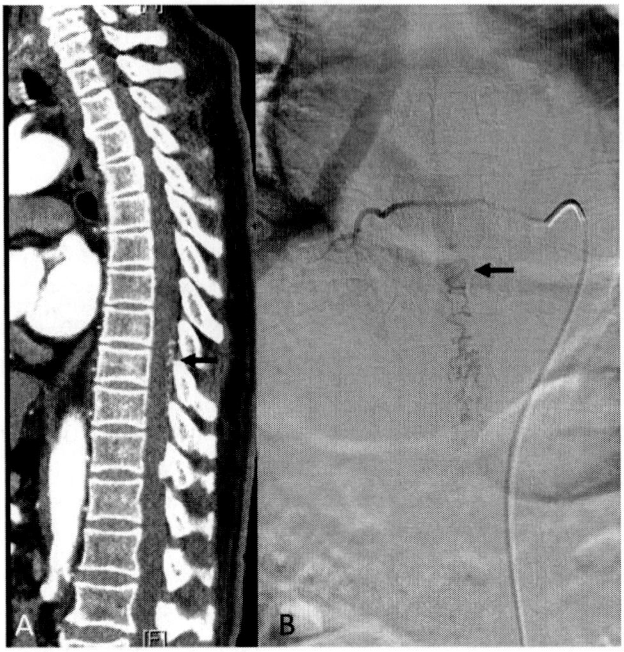

Figure 1. Is a type I sAVM, dural arteriovenous fistula, in a 68-year-old male patient presenting stiff lower limbs. A, enhanced CT scanning, sagittal view, showing an enhanced vascular lesion on the dorsal side of the spinal cord (arrow). B, the right intercostal segmental artery angiography showing a dural arteriovenous fistula causing venous drainage to the spinal cord surface (arrow).

By 2002, Spetzler introduced a classification based on anatomical location and pathophysiology. Extradural and intradural AVFs are distinguished, with further subdivisions into ventral and dorsal groups [24]. At the same time, Lasjaunias and his colleagues came up with a new classification for spinal vascular malformations based on their experience with 155 patients treated between 1981 and 1999 [25]. The authors distinguish between AVM and DAVF, with further categorizing the lesions into three main groups: genetic hereditary lesions, genetic non-hereditary lesions, and single lesions. Genetic hereditary lesions are associated with conditions like hereditary hemorrhagic telangiectasia (HHT) and always present as sporadic/single macro-fistulas (Table 1). Genetic non-hereditary lesions are always multiple, with potential metameric links (a lesion that extends beyond the spinal cord that might involve bone and paraspinal structures) and include conditions like Cobb syndrome and Klippel-Trenaunay syndrome. Focal, sporadic/single lesions may represent incomplete presentations of the other categories, which are further classified according to the location of the lesion (cord, nerve root, filum). This classification emphasizes the evolutive potential of lesions over time and incorporates genetic and biological understanding [25].

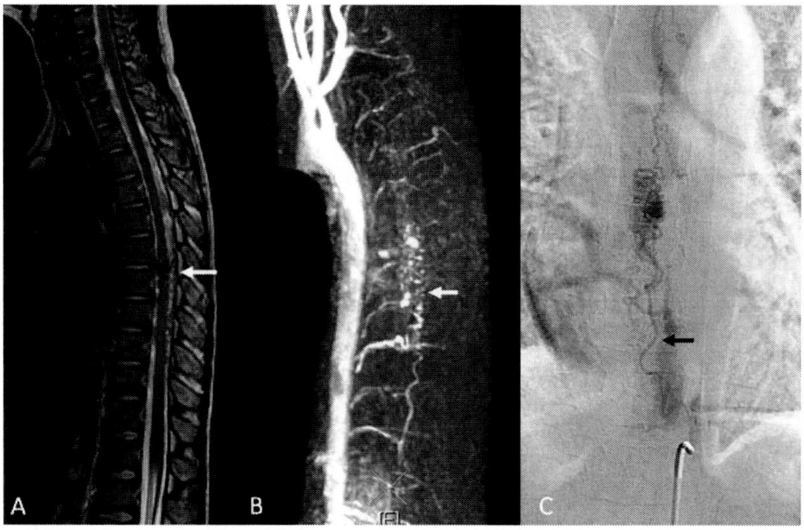

Figure 2. Is a type II sAVM, glomus AVM, in a 17-year-old male patient presenting weakness of the left lower limb and poor pain and temperature sensation in the right lower limb. A, spinal cord MR examination, T2-weighted, sagittal view, showing abnormal vascular signals around the thoracic spinal cord, and low signal within the spinal cord indicating a hemorrhagic lesion (arrow). B, spinal MRA examination showing abnormal vascular signals around the thoracic spinal cord (arrow). C, the left intercostal segmental angiography showing a intramedullary glomus arteriovenous malformation, with blood supply coming from the radiculopial artery and posterior spinal artery (arrow).

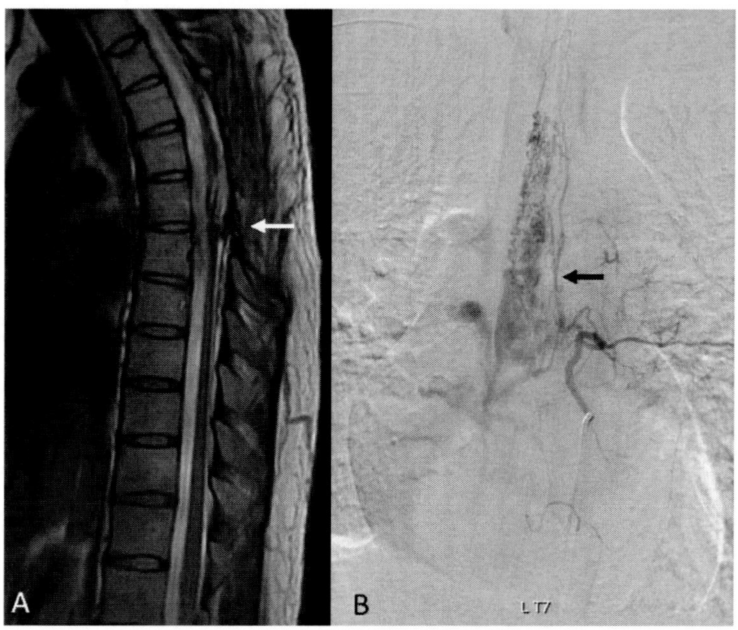

Figure 3. Is type III sAVM, juvenile AVM, in a 29-year-old female patient presenting weakness in both lower limbs and urinary incontinence for 5 years. On her back, adjacent to the thoracic vertebrae, there was a cavernous hemangioma of the skin. A, spinal cord MR examination, T2-weighted, sagittal view, showing postoperative changes in the spinal cord, thinning and edema of the spinal cord (arrow). B, the angiography of the left T7 intercostal segmental artery showing a multiple segmental arteriovenous malformation in the spinal cord, supplied by the radiculomedullary and radiculopial arteries (arrow).

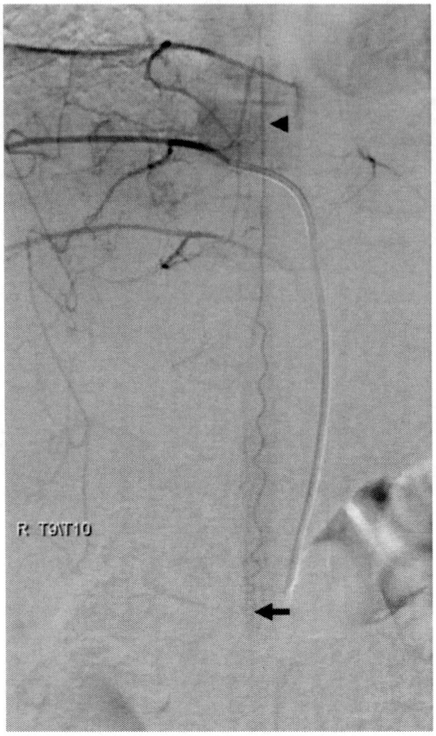

Figure 4. is type IV sAVM, perimedullary AVF, in a 4-year-old female patient presenting weakness in both lower limbs and urinary incontinence for 2 months. Angiography of the right T9 intercostal segmental artery showing that the intercostal arteries of T8 and T10 were visualized through vascular anastomosis. The perimedullary AVF was located at the cone of spinal cord and was supplied by the artery of Adamkiewicz and the anterior spinal artery, leading to the venous drainage on the surface of the spinal cord.

Table 1. Rodesch's classification of spinal AVMs

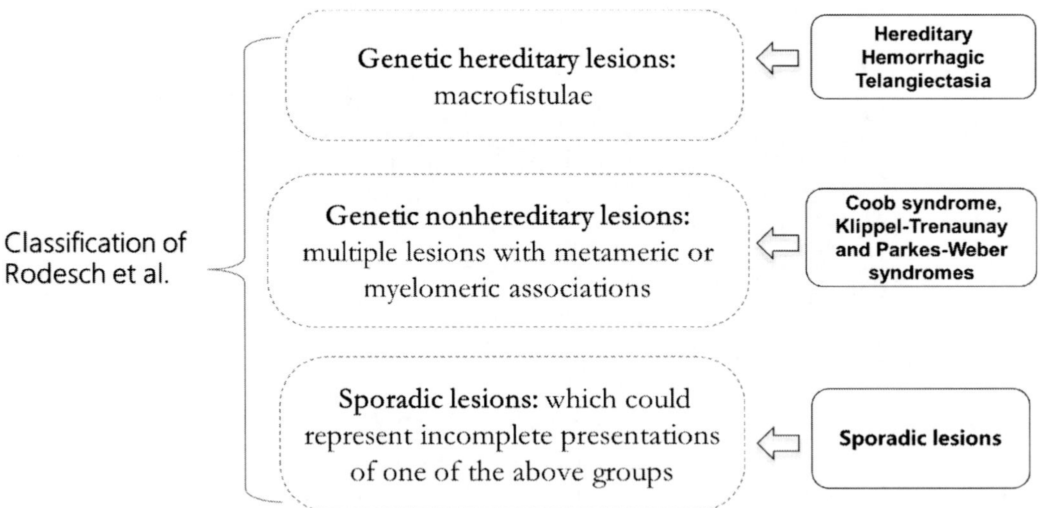

In 2008, Geibprasert and colleagues Classified cranio-spinal dural AV shunts into ventral, lateral, and dorsal epidural groups [26]. By 2011, Rangel-Castilla focused on extradural AVFs [27].

A more recent and widely adopted classification proposed by Takai in 2017, categorizes these malformations into five main categories: Type I is dural AVF; Type II is intradural intramedullary glomus AVM; Type III is intradural intramedullary juvenile AVM; Type IV is perimedullary AVF; and Type V is extradural AVF. The perimedullary AVFs (Type IV) are subdivided into three subtypes: IVa with a single feeder and small AVF, IVb with multiple feeders and medium AVFs, and IVc with multiple feeders and a giant AVF. The extradural AVFs (Type V) are subdivided into two subtypes: Va with intradural venous drainage and Vb without intradural venous drainage. This classification system maintains consistency with previously used type numbers (I-IV) while adding extradural AVFs as a new type. Types IV and V subclassifications are particularly useful for indicating appropriate treatment approaches, as type IVa perimedullary AVF are more amendable to microsurgery. In contrast, type IVc perimedullary AVFs and type Vb extradural AVFs are more suitable for endovascular embolization. Type Va extradural AVFs, on the other hand, can be effectively treated with either microsurgery and endovascular embolization [28].

Treatment

Endovascular treatment has significantly progressed in managing patients with spinal vascular malformations, particularly SDAVFs. Since the initial description of embolizing SDAVFs using stainless steel pellets in 1968 [7], endovascular treatment approaches have evolved significantly. While early particle embolization agents demonstrated high recanalization rates [29], the development of advanced liquid embolic materials and better catheter navigability has transformed endovascular techniques into a primary treatment option, alongside traditional surgical methods [15, 16]. Endovascular embolization has proven to be highly effective for SDAVFs when the anatomical conditions are favorable, achieving high rates of initial occlusion. For instance, the use of liquid embolic agents such as N-butyl cyanoacrylate (NBCA) and ethylene-vinyl alcohol copolymer (EVOH), commonly known as Onyx, has allowed for the accurate delivery of embolic material to the fistula and proximal draining vein. This precision reduces the likelihood of recanalization and enhances long-term treatment outcomes [15, 16, 30].

Endovascular treatment can provide symptomatic relief and halt disease progression of SDAVF, with reported success rates ranging from 69% to 90% for complete fistula and draining vein embolization [16]. Additionally, advancements in imaging technologies, such as digital subtraction angiography (DSA) and MR angiography, have significantly improved the diagnosis and planning of endovascular procedures. These improvements allow for more precise and effective treatment [15]. For specific lesions, surgical intervention remains the preferred treatment approach, mainly when the malformation's blood supply is closely associated with critical spinal arteries like the anterior spinal artery (ASA), posterior spinal artery (PSA), or artery of Adamkiewicz. In these cases, attempting curative embolization carries an increased risk of causing spinal cord ischemia and worsening neurological function [15, 16, 31].

Overall, endovascular management have expanded the therapeutic options for treatment of spinal vascular malformations, contributing to better patient outcomes and less invasive treatment alternatives [15].

The role of embolization in treating spinal cord AVMs has been extensively studied and is increasingly recognized as a preferred treatment option in several institutions [32-36].

The management hemorrhagic presentation in sAVM closely resembles that of cerebral AVM as in most institutions a delayed treatment approach to allow hematoma reabsorption would take place. However, unlike their cerebral AVMs partial treatment of spinal AVM may be enough to improve neurological outcome and prognosis [32]. For unruptured spinal AVMs that are asymptomatic, a more assertive approach may occur as those lesions become symptomatic in time due to venous congestion rather than hemorrhage; the primary goal of treatment is often to reduce the shunting volume. This approach is particularly relevant for managing complex AVMs such as metameric or juvenile AVMs, where complete surgical resection or endovascular obliteration is often impractical [32, 35].

Partial obliteration of spinal AVMs can be acceptable even in patients with high-risk features, such as associated nidal or prenidal aneurysms or large venous varices. Partial obliteration appears to offer a protective effect against future hemorrhage in glomus (type II) AVMs [36].

A paradigm shift has occurred, in modern SVM treatment, emphasizing a multidisciplinary approach that leverages the strengths of both endovascular techniques and microsurgery. Despite advancements in endovascular obliteration, the complexity of SVMs requires a well-rounded treatment plan. In many high-volume surgical centers, around half of SVM cases either involve preoperative embolization or are managed entirely through endovascular methods. This approach is key for addressing high-risk factors and targeting deep arterial feeders can be difficult to reach with microsurgery alone. Incorporating endovascular techniques into the treatment of SVMs has significantly improved perioperative blood loss, minimized dissection injury, and lowered the risk of postoperative neurological complications. Combining endovascular and microsurgical techniques has become a standard of care in modern SVMs treatment, offering patients the best possible outcomes by joining the expertise of multiple specialties and advanced technologies.

Conclusion

Spinal vascular malformations (SVM) are a heterogeneous group of vascular disorders usually diagnosed after acute, subacute, and chronic neurologic decline. Spinal vascular malformations include spinal dural arteriovenous fistulae (sDAVF), which account for the majority of these lesions (approximately 70%), and spinal arteriovenous malformations (sAVM), which account for the remainder of these lesions. The pattern of blood flow (high flow, low flow, and no arteriovenous shunt) and location (intramedullary, perimedullary radicular, and epidural) are most helpful in further categorizing these lesions. It emphasizes the importance of knowing the specific features of each type to guide effective treatment. Neurologic symptoms are caused by mass effect, bleeding and hemodynamic disturbances. The role of endovascular therapy in the diagnosis and treatment of SVM has expanded with advances in endovascular technology. This includes embolization techniques characterized by advanced microcatheter navigability and removable tips, as well as advances in liquid embolic agents such as n-butyl cyanoacrylate (n-

BCA) and ethylene vinyl alcohol copolymer (Onyx). The indications for endovascular embolization for the treatment of SVM have greatly increased, either as an adjunctive therapy prior to surgical resection or as a stand-alone treatment.

References

[1] Medel R, Crowley RW, Dumont AS. Endovascular management of spinal vascular malformations: History and literature review. *Neurosurg Focus*. 2009;26 (1). doi:10.3171/FOC.2009.26.1.E7.

[2] Cenzato M, Debernardi A, Stefini R, et al. Spinal dural arteriovenous fistulas: Outcome and prognostic factors. *Neurosurg Focus*. 2012;32 (5). doi:10.3171/2012.2.FOCUS1218.

[3] Akopov S, Schievink W. History of spinal cord vascular malformations and their treatment. *Semin Cerebrovasc Dis Stroke*. 2002;2 (3):178-185. doi:10.1053/scds.2002.128825.

[4] Gailloud P. The contributions of Otto Hebold and Julius Gaupp to the study of spinal vascular malformations: Original documents and historical context. *Interv Neuroradiol*. 2019;25 (6):604-612. doi:10.1177/1591019919845648.

[5] Diagnosis and treatment of surgical diseases of the spinal cord and its membranes. By Charles A. Elsberg, M. D., F. A. C. S., Professor of Clinical Surgery at New York University Pp. 330, with 153 illustrations, 3 in colours. 1916. Philadelphia and London W. B. Saunders Co. 21s. net. *Br J Surg*. 2006;4 (16):780-781. doi:10.1002/bjs.1800041613.

[6] Koch MJ, Stapleton CJ, Agarwalla PK, et al. Open and endovascular treatment of spinal dural arteriovenous fistulas: A 10-year experience. *J Neurosurg Spine*. 2017;26 (4):519-523. doi:10.3171/2016.9.SPINE16394.

[7] Doppman JL, Di Chiro G, Ommaya A. Obliteration of spinal-cord arteriovenous malformation by percutaneous embolisation. *Lancet*. 1968 Mar 2;1 (7540):477. doi:10.1016/s0140-6736 (68)92812-2. PMID:4170644.

[8] Aminoff MJ, Logue V. Clinical features of spinal vascular malformations. *Brain*. 1974 Mar;97 (1):197-210. doi:10.1093/brain/97.1.197. PMID:4373119.

[9] Clark S, Powell G, Kandasamy J, Lee M, Nahser H, Pigott T. Spinal dural arteriovenous fistulas – presentation, management and outcome in a single neurosurgical institution. *Br J Neurosurg*. 2013;27 (4):465-470. doi:10.3109/02688697.2012.752433.

[10] Cecchi PC, Musumeci A, Faccioli F, Bricolo A. Surgical treatment of spinal dural arterio-venous fistulae: long-term results and analysis of prognostic factors. *Acta Neurochir* (Wien). 2008;150 (6):563-570. doi:10.1007/s00701-008-1560-7.

[11] Krings T, Geibprasert S. Spinal dural arteriovenous fistulas. *Am J Neuroradiol*. 2009;30 (4):639-648. doi:10.3174/ajnr.A1485.

[12] Peng Y, Ren Y, Hou J, et al. Clinical outcomes and prognostic factors in the surgical treatment of spinal dural arteriovenous fistulas: a retrospective study of 118 patients. *Sci Rep*. 2023;13 (1):18266. doi:10.1038/s41598-023-45599-x.

[13] Krings T, Chng SM, Ozanne A, Alvarez H, Rodesch G, Lasjaunias PL. Hereditary hemorrhagic telangiectasia in children: endovascular treatment of neurovascular malformations. *Neuroradiology*. 2005;47 (12):946-954. doi:10.1007/s00234-005-1448-7.

[14] Krings T, Ozanne A, Chng SM, Alvarez H, Rodesch G, Lasjaunias PL. Neurovascular phenotypes in hereditary haemorrhagic telangiectasia patients according to age. *Neuroradiology*. 2005;47 (10):711-720. doi:10.1007/s00234-005-1390-8.

[15] Patsalides A, Santillan A, Knopman J, Tsiouris AJ, Riina HA, Gobin YP. Endovascular management of spinal dural arteriovenous fistulas. *J Neurointerv Surg*. 2011;3 (1):80-84. doi:10.1136/jnis.2010.003178.

[16] Ducruet AF, Crowley RW, McDougall CG, Albuquerque FC. Endovascular management of spinal arteriovenous malformations. *J Neurointerv Surg*. 2013;5 (6):605-611. doi:10.1136/NEURINTSURG-2012-010487.

[17] Guo L-M, Zhou H-Y, Xu J-W, et al. Dural arteriovenous fistula at the foramen magnum presenting with subarachnoid hemorrhage: case reports and literature review. *Eur J Neurol*. 2010;17 (5):684-691. doi:10.1111/j.1468-1331.2009.02895.x.

[18] Rathnam AS, Memon AB. Foix-Alajouanine Syndrome Mimicking Longitudinally Extensive Transverse Myelitis. *Eur J Case Rep Intern Med*. 2020; (LATEST ONLINE). doi:10.12890/2020_002063.

[19] Doppman JL, Di Chiro G, Ommaya AK. Percutaneous embolization of spinal cord arteriovenous malformations. J Neurosurg. 1971;34 (1):48-55. doi:10.3171/jns.1971.34.1.0048.

[20] Heros RC, Debrun GM, Ojemann RG, Lasjaunias PL, Naessens PJ. Direct spinal arteriovenous fistula: a new type of spinal AVM. Case report. *J Neurosurg*. 1986;64 (1):134-139. doi:10.3171/jns.1986.64.1.0134.

[21] Rosenblum B, Oldfield EH, Doppman JL, Di Chino G. Spinal Arteriovenous Malformations: A Comparison of Dural Arteriovenous Fistulas and Intradural AVM's in 81 Patients. Vol 67.; 1987.

[22] Mourier KL, Gobin YP, George B, Lot G, Merland JJ. Intradural perimedullary arteriovenous fistulae: results of surgical and endovascular treatment in a series of 35 cases. *Neurosurgery*. 1993;32 (6):885-891; discussion 891. doi:10.1227/00006123-199306000-00001.

[23] Black P. Spinal vascular malformations: an historical perspective. *Neurosurg Focus*. 2006;21 (6):1-7. doi:10.3171/foc.2006.21.6.2.

[24] Spetzler RF, Detwiler PW, Riina HA, Porter RW. Modified classification of spinal cord vascular lesions. *J Neurosurg*. 2002;96 (2 Suppl):145-156. doi:10.3171/spi.2002.96.2.0145.

[25] Rodesch G, Hurth M, Alvarez H, Tadié M, Lasjaunias P. Classification of spinal cord arteriovenous shunts: proposal for a reappraisal--the Bicêtre experience with 155 consecutive patients treated between 1981 and 1999. *Neurosurgery*. 2002;51 (2):374-379; discussion 379-80. Accessed May 4, 2024. http://www.ncbi.nlm.nih.gov/pubmed/12182775.

[26] Geibprasert S, Pereira V, Krings T, et al. Dural arteriovenous shunts: A new classification of craniospinal epidural venous anatomical bases and clinical correlations. *Stroke*. 2008;39 (10):2783-2794. doi:10.1161/STROKEAHA.108.516757.

[27] Rangel-Castilla L, Holman PJ, Krishna C, Trask TW, Klucznik RP, Diaz OM. Spinal extradural arteriovenous fistulas: a clinical and radiological description of different types and their novel treatment with Onyx. *J Neurosurg Spine*. 2011;15 (5):541-549. doi:10.3171/2011.6.SPINE10695.

[28] Takai K. Spinal arteriovenous shunts: Angioarchitecture and historical changes in classification. *Neurol Med Chir* (Tokyo). 2017;57 (7):356-365. doi:10.2176/nmc.ra.2016-0316.

[29] Hall WA, Oldfield EH, Doppman JL. Recanalization of spinal arteriovenous malformations following embolization. *J Neurosurg*. 1989;70 (5):714-720. doi:10.3171/jns.1989.70.5.0714.

[30] Jellema K, Sluzewski M, van Rooij WJ, Tijssen CC, Beute GN. Embolization of spinal dural arteriovenous fistulas: importance of occlusion of the draining vein. *J Neurosurg Spine*. 2005;2 (5):580-583. doi:10.3171/spi.2005.2.5.0580.

[31] Flores BC, Klinger DR, White JA, Batjer HH. Spinal vascular malformations: treatment strategies and outcome. Neurosurg Rev. 2017;40 (1):15-28. doi:10.1007/S10143-016-0713-Z.

[32] Veznedaroglu E, Nelson PK, Jabbour PM, Rosenwasser RH. Endovascular Treatment of Spinal Cord Arteriovenous Malformations. *Neurosurgery*. 2006;59 (suppl_5):S3-202-S3-209. doi:10.1227/01.NEU.0000237409.28906.96.

[33] Krings T, Thron AK, Geibprasert S, et al. Endovascular management of spinal vascular malformations. *Neurosurg Rev*. 2010;33 (1):1-9. doi:10.1007/s10143-009-0204-6.

[34] Casasco A, Guimaraens L, Senturk C, Cotroneo E, Gigli R, Theron J. Endovascular Treatment of Cervical Giant Perimedullary Arteriovenous Fistulas. *Neurosurgery*. 2012;70 (1):141-149. doi:10.1227/NEU.0b013e31822ec19e.

[35] Cho WS, Kim KJ, Kwon OK, et al. Clinical features and treatment outcomes of the spinal arteriovenous fistulas and malformations. *J Neurosurg Spine*. 2013;19 (2):207-216. doi:10.3171/2013.4.SPINE12732.

[36] Corkill RA, Mitsos AP, Molyneux AJ. Embolization of spinal intramedullary arteriovenous malformations using the liquid embolic agent, Onyx: a single-center experience in a series of 17 patients. *J Neurosurg Spine*. 2007;7 (5):478-485. doi:10.3171/SPI-07/11/478.

Chapter 17

The History and Development of Brain Arteriovenous Malformation Embolization

Jinlu Yu[1,*]
and Kun Zhang[2]
[1]Department of Neurosurgery, the First Hospital of Jilin University, Changchun, China
[2]Department of Cerebrovascular Disease, Henan Provincial People's Hospital of Zhengzhou University, Zhengzhou, China

Abstract

Brain arteriovenous malformation [BAVM] is a congenital abnormal arteriovenous nidus without an intervening capillary network. BAVMs have a variable natural history. They can remain silent for life or become symptomatic, presenting with intracranial hemorrhage, seizure, or headache. For BAVMs with a poor natural history, intervention can be attempted. The treatments include surgical resection, radiotherapy, endovascular treatment [EVT], or their combination. EVT has been used to treat BAVM since the 1960s. Since then, with the development of new materials, equipment and techniques, EVT for BAVMs has evolved and become popular in recent decades. However, the use of EVT in the context of the poor natural history of BAVM is uncertain. In addition, EVT has complication risks when treating BAVMs. These uncertainties and complications affect which cases are applicable and the clinical practice of BAVM embolization. Throughout the history of BAVM embolization, the growth of EVTs occur in a zigzag pattern. For inexperienced doctors, it is difficult to understand and learn history of this condition by reading sporadic literature in a short period. Therefore, a review of the literature concerning the history and development of BAVM embolization is needed. In this review, the following issues are discussed: the development of materials for BAVM embolization, EVT status in treating BAVM, the role of curative EVT in treating BAVM, the proposal and development of a grading scale for BAVM embolization, and the future of EVT for treating BAVM. This review revealed that the EVT of BAVMs has a complex zigzag growth history. Currently, BAVM embolization is being developed and has evolved. EVT plays an important role in curing BAVM or assisting in the treatment of BAVM. In the future, with the advancement of materials, equipment and techniques and the accumulation of clinical experience, EVT will be promising for BAVM embolization.

* Corresponding Author's Email: jlyu@jlu.edu.cn

In: World History of Neurointerventional Surgery
Editors: Xianli Lv and Zhongxue Wu
ISBN: 979-8-89530-792-2

Keywords: brain arteriovenous malformation, embolization, development, history

Introduction

In brain arteriovenous malformations [BAVMs], high-pressure direct shunting from artery to vein leads to blood flow overload in the feeding artery, nidus and draining vein [1]. In addition, the redistribution of blood flow can lead to the redirection of arterialized flow from eloquent cerebral regions [2, 3]. Owing to the above hemodynamics, BAVMs can present with hemorrhage, seizures, headache, and neurofunction deficits (Figure 1). Among these presentations, intracranial hemorrhage from BAVM rupture is the most severe [4]. For hemorrhagic and certain unruptured BAVMs with high-risk weak structures, interventions, including surgical resection, radiotherapy, endovascular treatment [EVT] or a combination, can be attempted [5]. In the 1960s, doctors started using EVT to treat BAVM [6].

Currently, EVT, including transarterial embolization [TAE] and transvenous embolization [TVE], is promising for the management of BAVM [7]. TAE has been used for more than 60 years in the treatment of BAVMs. In TAE, the practitioner uses a microcatheter in the feeding artery to access the nidus and then performs embolization. TVE is a more recent procedure and has been a popular method since 2010. In TVE, the practitioner uses a microcatheter in the draining vein to reach and fill the nidus with a liquid embolic agent in a retrograde fashion [8, 9]. Throughout the history of BAVM embolization, growth has exhibited a zigzag shape. For inexperienced doctors, it is difficult to understand the full history by reading sporadic literature. Therefore, a literature review on this topic is needed.

Development of Materials to Embolize BAVMs

1960s-1970s

On the basis of the technique of carotid angiography, in a 1960 report, Luessenhop et al. described the first case of BAVM embolization [5]. In this report, the authors used a flow-directed embolization technique in which spherical emboli of methyl methacrylate were injected via the extracranial internal carotid artery, after which these emboli floated into the feeding arteries to embolize the BAVM. Apparently, the procedure carried a risk because these emboli can float into normal vessels after the release of spherical emboli. However, this was an important pioneer work.

To overcome the embolization of normal vessels, catheterization of the feeding artery was presented as an idea. In a report in 1964, Luessenhop et al. used a catheter consisting of delicate flexible silastic tubing with an enlarged inflatable tip. The catheter had flow-direct ability and accessed the BAVM; then, spherical silastic emboli and silk sutures were used to embolize BAVMs via the catheter [10]. In a 1971 study in an animal model, Doppma et al. embolized kidney arteries through a catheter with silicone rubber elastomer by injecting diluted silicone fluid [11]. These reports suggested that BAVM embolization can be performed via an inert catheter into the feeding artery to avoid the embolization of normal vessels. Thus, the concept of catheterization of the feeding artery to embolize BAVMs was established.

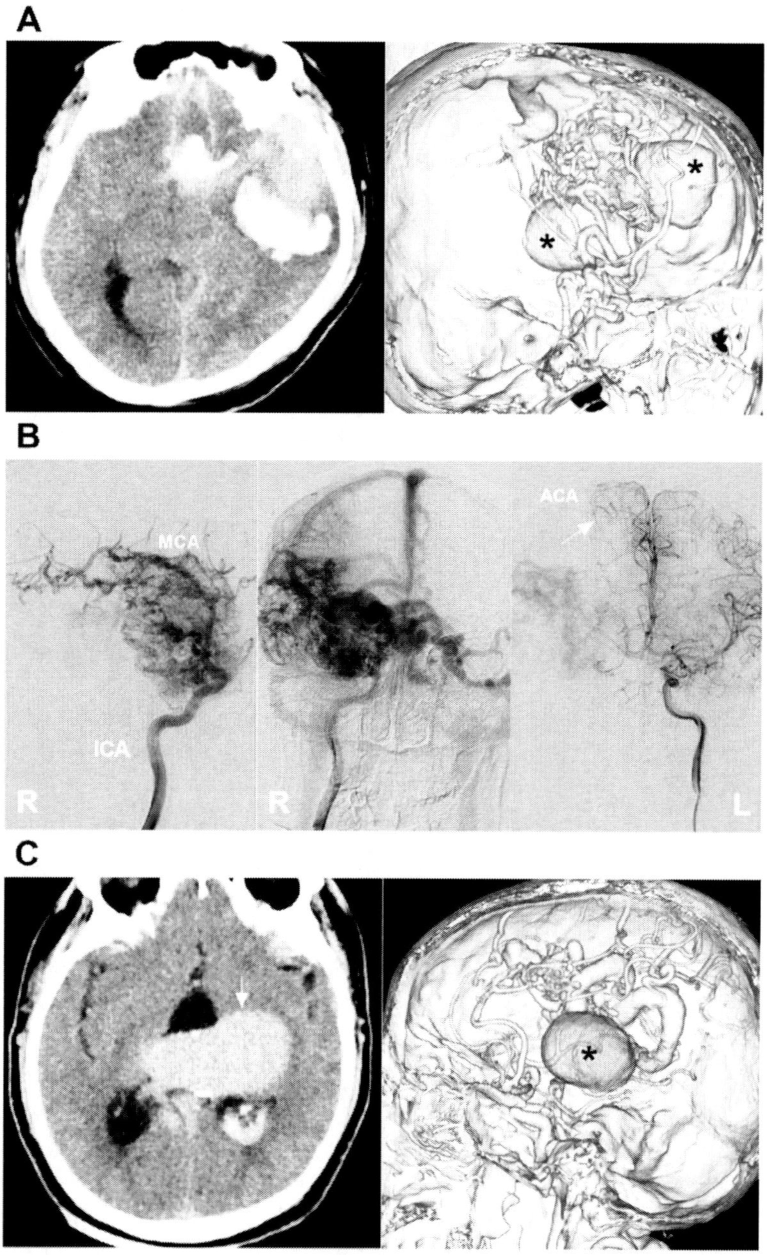

Abbreviations: ACA: anterior cerebral artery; BAVM: brain arteriovenous malformation; CT: computed tomography; DSA: digital subtraction angiography; ICA: internal carotid artery; L: left; MCA: middle cerebral artery; R: right.

Figure 1. BAVM images. A: Left panel: CT image showing left multiple intracranial hemorrhages; Right panel: CT angiography image showing a BAVM with two giant aneurysmal dilatations (asterisks). B: Left panel: Arterial-phase DSA of the right ICA showing a diffuse BAVM supplied by innumerable branches of the MCA; Middle panel: Venous-phase DSA showing extensive venous drainage of the BAVM; Right panel: DSA of the left ICA showing the compensation of blood flow in the right MCA region (arrow) from the ACA, indicating that the BAVM stole blood flow in the MCA region. C: Left panel: CT image showing a lesion (arrow) with an occupying effect. Right panel: CT image showing that the lesion was a large aneurysmal dilatation (asterisk) of the BAVM.

During the 1960s, owing to the absence of the availability of a long and thick supporting catheter, practitioners had to use direct puncture for the carotid artery approach to embolize BAVM [12]. The transfemoral approach became possible with the development of appropriate supporting catheters. In a report in 1972, Kricheff et al. embolized BAVMs via the transfemoral approach and reported the first embolization of posterior fossa BAVMs due to feasible catheterization of the vertebral artery [13]. In the transfemoral approach, a large catheter is placed in the external internal carotid artery or vertebral artery; then, a smaller catheter is inserted through the larger catheter to access BAVMs to perform embolization [14]. In the 1970s, the transfemoral approach was established and widely used, such as in the following reports by Fleischer et al. in 1972 [15], Djindjian et al. in 1973 [16, 17], Wolpert et al. in 1975 [18], Djindjian et al. in 1975 [19], Debrun et al. in 1978 [20], Romodanov et al. in 1979 [21] and Berenstein in 1979 [22].

From the 1960s-1970s, embolic agents enabled substantial progress in this field. In the early part of this period, the main embolic agents used were solid silastic spheres, Teflon beads and Gelfoam strips [23, 24]. In addition, detachable balloons were used and reported in 1974 by Serbinenko et al. [12], in 1978 by Debrun et al. [20] and in 1979 by Romodanov et al. [21]. It is difficult for solid embolic agents to penetrate the nidus. In the later part of this period, a liquid embolic agent was introduced that could enter the nidus to embolize the BAVM in its true sense. For example, in 1976, Kerber et al. used liquid isobutyl cyanoacrylate [IBCA] to embolize BAVMs [14]. In the 1960s-1970s, various flow-guided catheters, such as tapered/nontapered catheters, single/double-lumen catheters and detachable balloon catheters, were developed to facilitate TAE of BAVMs [22]. Solid embolic agents need larger catheters for delivery. IBCA can be cast via silastic microcatheters with lateral-leak holes.

On the basis of the achievements of EVT for BAVMs in the 1960s-1970s, in a report from 1980, criteria for BAVM embolization with IBCA were established. Cromwell et al. described the criteria as follows: 1] the catheterized vessel is a feeding artery and 2] the contrast material flows in the BAVM without the opacification of normal cortical vessels [25]. Although basic principles for BAVM embolization have been established, due to the limitations of embolic materials, optimal conditions for catheterization of the feeding artery to assess BAVM are difficult to obtain, which results in an unsatisfactory outcome for BAVM embolization.

1980s-1990s

Compared with the previous 20 years, in the 1980s-1990s, substantial developments occurred regarding microcatheters capable of navigating new embolic agents. In the early 1980s, a new calibrated-leak latex balloon was developed to inject IBCA [26]. This balloon can be used in vessels 1 to 4 mm in diameter [27]. To increase IBCA penetration, in 1986, ApSimon et al. used temporary balloon occlusion of other feeding arteries to improve IBCA embolization by providing insights into the dynamics of blood flow to the BAVM [28].

IBCA was no longer produced in the late 1980s. In 1989, n-butyl 2-cyanoacrylate (NBCA) was substituted for IBCA [29]. Because NBCA has adhesive properties, there is a risk of the microcatheter adhering to the vessel. In addition, the use of NBCA requires an experienced and skilled practitioner because its polymerization is quick and unpredictable [30]. Owing to the limitations of NBCA, other embolic agents are continuously being identified. In 1990, Taki et al. developed a mixture of ethylene vinyl alcohol copolymer (EVOH) and metrizamide that was dissolved in dimethyl sulfoxide [31]. EVOH is nonadhesive, polymerizes slowly and is easy to handle. In 1991, Terada et al. used EVOH to embolize BAVMs with flow-related aneurysms [32]. EVOH was the first of the nonadhesive liquid embolic agents. In the 1990s, polyvinyl alcohol particles were also used [27, 33-38]. Since the introduction of the detachable Guglielmi detachable coil in 1991, coils have been used to occlude fistulas within BAVMs or flow-related aneurysms [39, 40]. These coils can be used alone or in combination with a liquid embolic agent.

In the 1990s, a perfect transfemoral approach was developed, in which a thin-walled guiding catheter was placed as close as possible to the cranial base; then, guidewire steerable or flow-directed microcatheters were used to access and embolize BAVMs [41]. In the 1990s, the use of microcatheters and microguidewires advanced substantially. A 2.4F guidewire-directed Tracker catheter-18 (Target Therapeutic, Fremont, CA) and a 1.8F flow-directed Magic catheter (Balt Extrusion, Montmorency, France) were developed and used to embolize BAVMs [38, 42]. Tracker catheter-18 can be used to match taper [0.013″] guidewires (Target Therapeutics, Fremont, CA) and seeker (0.014″) guidewires (Target Therapeutics, Fremont, CA) [41]. A Terumo 0.010 guidewire (Terumo, Japan) can be used to help the Magic catheter through a tortuous feeding artery [34, 43]. In addition, Pursil catheters (Balt Extrusion, Montmorency, France), MiniTorquer catheters (Ingenor, Paris, France) and transit microcatheters (Cordis Endovascular Systems, Miami Lakes, Fla) have been reported to deliver NBCA [44, 45]. In the late 1990s, microcatheters and catheters had hydrophilic coatings, such as hydrophilic Fastracker-18 and Fasguide guiding coatings (Target Therapeutics, Fremont, CA), which are less thrombogenic and therefore increase the safety of EVT for treating BAVMs [45].

After the 2000s

After the 2000s, BAVM embolization became convenient because of the development and improvement of microcatheters to deliver embolic agents, coaxial distal access catheters to support microcatheters, and liquid embolic agents.

Currently, a vast array of guidewire-directed and flow-directed microcatheters are standard tools used to embolize BAVMs. Classic guidewire-directed microcatheters include Echelon-10 (Medtronic, Irvine, CA, USA) and SL-10 (Stryker Neurovascular, Fremont, CA, USA) microcatheters. The classic flow-directed microcatheters included the 1.5F tip of the Marathon (Medtronic, Minneapolis, Minnesota, USA) and the 1.2F tip of the Magic (Balt Extrusion, Montmorency, France) microcatheters. Two new microcatheters with a detachable tip, the Sonic microcatheter (Balt Extrusion, Montmorency, France) and the 1.5F tip of the Apollo (Medtronic, Minneapolis, MI, USA) microcatheter, increased the safety and convenience of BAVM embolization [46-48]. In addition, the 1.6F tip of the headway Duo microcatheter (Microvention, Aliso Viejo, California, USA) has flow-directed properties and can be used to embolize BAVMs [49]. As another example, a dual-lumen Scepter mini balloon catheter (Microvention, Tustin, CA, USA) can be used to embolize BAVMs [50]. These microcatheters have hydrophilic coatings.

Guidewire-directed microcatheters can match 0.014″ microguidewires, including 0.014″ Synchro (Stryker, Kalamazoo, MI, USA), 0.014″ Transend (Boston Scientific), 0.014″ Traxcess (MicroVention, Tustin, CA, USA) and Hybrid 1214D (Balt Extrusion, Montmorency,

France) microguidewires. The flow-directed microcatheters can match 0.010″ Synchro (Stryker Neurovascular, Fremont, CA, USA), 0.014’ Traxcess (Microvention, Tustin, CA, USA) and Hybrid 1214D (Balt Extrusion, Montmorency, France) microguidewires. These microguidewires are hydrophilic and can pass through microcatheters easily.

After 2000, the main liquid embolic agents used to embolize BAVMs included EVOH and NBCA [51, 52]. NBCA products included Glubran 2 (GEM SRL, Viareggio, Italy), Magic glue (Balt, Montmorency, France) and TruFill (Cerenovus, Irvine, CA, USA). A representative EVOH is the Onyx liquid embolic system [Medtronic, Irvine, CA, USA], which includes Onyx 18, 20, and 34 [53]. Onyxes 18 and 20 are used to embolize plexiform BAVMs, and Onyx 34 is used to embolize arteriovenous fistulas in BAVMs [54]. The nonadhesive property of Onyx eliminates the risk of microcatheter adhesion. Each injection lasted for several minutes to more than one hour. When Onyx reflux in the feeding pedicle or early filling of draining veins is noted, the injection can be paused for 1–2 minutes, allowing the Onyx to solidify and change direction. Similar to Onyx, other EVOH products, including Squid (Emboflu, Switzerland) and precipitating hydrophobic injectable liquid (PHIL) (Microvention, Tustin, CA, USA), are useful for embolizing BAVMs [55-58]. The squid product has 6 different formulations, namely, Squid-12, 12LD, 18, 18LD, 34 and 34LD, which provides convenience for EVT for BAVM [56]. In 2024, the CLARIDAD clinical trial showed that $_{iht}$Obtura [Iberhospitex, Lliçà de Vall, Spain) was safe and effective in treating BAVMs. It is a novel EVOH-based liquid embolic with proprietary technology, allowing the conjugation of iodine to the embolic material with postprocedural gradual and progressive elimination of radiopacity from the deposited liquid embolic agent [59].

Recently, the use of various long sheaths and intracranial support catheters (distal access catheters, intermediate catheters) via the transfemoral or transradial approach has increased the convenience of EVT for BAVM [60-64].

Understanding the EVT Status for BAVM Management

In general, the role of EVT in BAVMs remains uncertain; however, it is important for the management of BAVMs. The risks of EVT for BAVMs must be weighed against the natural history of risk [65].

EVT for Ruptured BAVMs

EVT for ruptured BAVM can play two roles. First, preoperative embolization can facilitate surgical resection of the BAVM (Figure 2). In addition, for acutely ruptured BAVMs, EVT can be used to embolize intranidal or flow-related aneurysms and fistulous structures to prevent rebleeding in the acute period; this allows time for subsequent treatment when these weak structures are likely sources of bleeding, especially when they are correlated with the hemorrhage pattern (Figures 3-4). However, for ruptured BAVMs without definite ruptured weak structures, the long-term outcome of EVT is uncertain (Figures 5-6). In 2023, the registry of Multimodality Treatment for Brain Arteriovenous Malformation in Mainland China (MATCH) compared long-term outcomes in ruptured diffuse BAVMs between interventional therapy and conservative management. The study suggested that interventional therapy may be more favorable than conservative management [66]. To confirm the conclusions of the MATCH study, further evidence is needed.

EVT for Unruptured BAVMs

To date, no level I or II data are available in the literature to guide the use of EVT for unruptured BAVMs. There are three important recommendations and a study on EVT for BAVMs that affect the decision to perform EVT. Two recommendations from the American Heart Association (AHA) and American Stroke Association (ASA) were published in 2001 and 2017 [4, 67]. Another recommendation was from the ARISE (Aneurysm/BAVM/cSDH Roundtable Discussion with Industry and Stroke Experts) I consensus on the management of BAVM in 2024 [65]. One study was the ARUBA (A Randomized Trial of Unruptured Brain Arteriovenous Malformations (AVMs)) on unruptured BAVMs published in 2014 [68].

In the AHA and ASA recommendations, for Spetzler–Martin (SM) grade II-III BAVMs, EVT can be used before surgery or radiosurgery; for SM grade IV-V lesions, EVT should not be used unless it is performed in conjunction with other treatments to achieve complete care (Figure 7). The exceptions are SM grade IV-V BAVMs with venous outflow obstruction, and palliative EVT can be used to reduce blood inflow to control edema; another exception is in BAVMs with true "stealing" from high-flow fistulas, in which EVT is used to relieve the amount of shunting through the BAVM. For these lesions, the goal of EVT is flow reduction to minimize or halt symptom progression (Figure 8) [4, 67]. Finally, EVT for flow-related aneurysms, fistulous structures and pseudoaneurysms in the nidus may be possible (Figure 9).

In 2014, the ARUBA study represented a turning point in the history of BAVM management, as it showed that conservative management was superior to interventions in the prevention of death or stroke in unruptured BAVMs, which challenged the existing practices supporting intervention for unruptured BAVMs [68]. In the results of the ARUBA study published in 2020, after extended follow-up, medical management alone remained superior to interventional therapy for the prevention of death or symptomatic stroke in patients with an unruptured BAVM [69]. Therefore, many surgeons have been hesitant to treat patients with unruptured BAVMs since the publication of the ARUBA results [70]. However, this study has been criticized. In 2017, Magro et al. questioned ARUBA's drawbacks in the primary design of designating the intervention group as the control group and the conservative treatment test group as the experimental group. Magro et al. also further questioned ARUBA's choice of analysis methods by grouping all interventional methods into one arm but not individually to validate individual risks and benefits [71]. In 2024, Chen reported that the ARUBA study did not prevent EVT for unruptured BAVMs in the U.S. cases, suggesting that trends moved counter to the conclusions of the ARUBA study and that clinicians rejected the findings of the ARUBA study in managing unruptured BAVMs [72]. In 2024, after performing a retrospective analysis of prospectively collected data from ARUBA-eligible patients who underwent intervention at 18 participating centers, Alrohimi et al. reported that intervention for unruptured BAVMs at comprehensive stroke centers across the United States was safe [73].

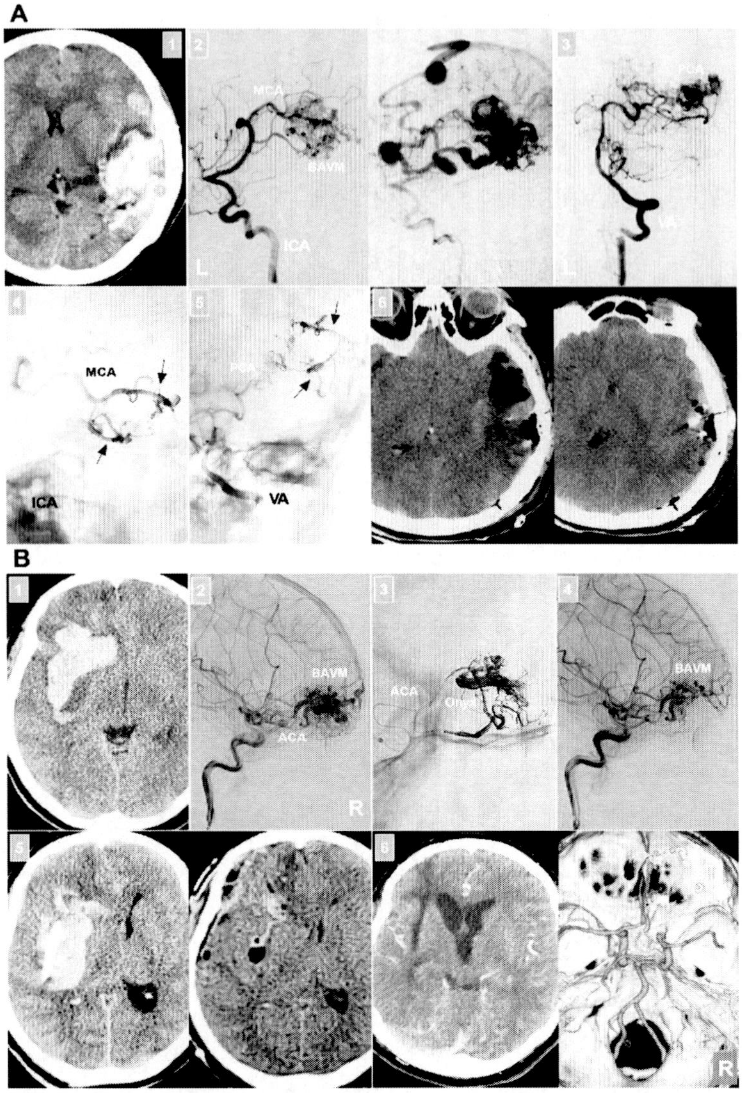

Abbreviations: ACA: anterior cerebral artery; BAVM: brain arteriovenous malformation; CT: computed tomography; CTA: CT angiography; DSA: digital subtraction angiography; ICA: internal carotid artery; L: left; MCA: middle cerebral artery; PCA: posterior cerebral artery; R: right; VA: vertebral artery.

Figure 2. Surgical resection of BAVMs after embolization. A: Number 1 panel: CT image showing left temporal lobe hemorrhage; Number 2 panel: Arterial phase (left) and venous phase (right) DSA of the left ICA showing that the BAVM was supplied by the MCA and had extensive venous drainage; Number 3 panel: DSA of the left VA showing that the PCA was supplied to the BAVM; Numbers 4-5 panels: Unsubtracted DSA images of the ICA and VA showing that the feeding arteries of the BAVM were occluded by the Onyx (arrows); Number 6 panel: CT showing that both the hematoma and the BAVM were removed. B: Number 1 panel: CT image showing right frontal lobe hemorrhage. Number 2 panel: DSA image of the right ICA showing that the BAVM was supplied by the ACA. Number 3 panel: X-ray image showing Onyx casting in the nidus. Number 4 panel: DSA image of the right ICA showing that the BAVM was partially embolized. Number 5 panel: CT image showing that the hematoma was drained by a bur hole; however, the occupying effect was not solved (left). Then, craniectomy was performed to evacuate the hematoma (right). Number 6 panel: Six-month follow-up CT and CTA images showing that the BAVM was removed.

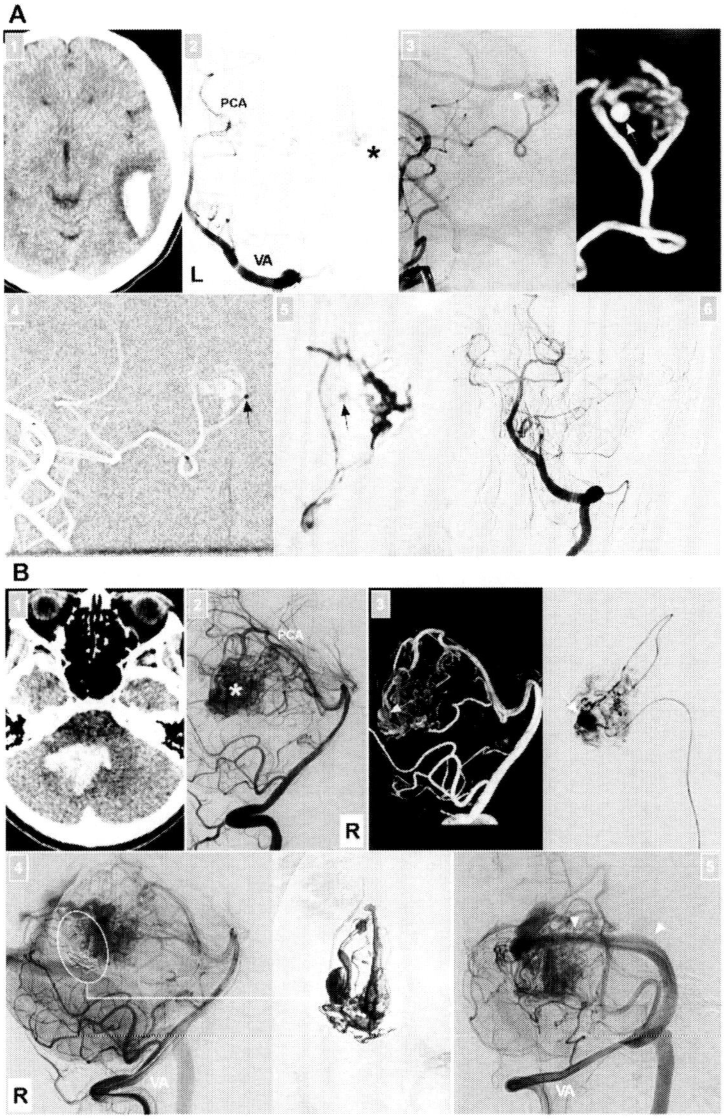

Abbreviations: BAVM: brain arteriovenous malformation; CT: computed tomography; DSA: digital subtraction angiography; EVT: endovascular treatment; L: left; PCA: posterior cerebral artery; R: right; VA: vertebral artery.

Figure 3. EVT for BAVMs with intranidal aneurysms. A: Number 1 panel: CT image showing left temporal lobe hemorrhage; Number 2 panel: DSA of the left VA showing a small BAVM (asterisk) supplied by the branch of the PCA; Number 3 panel: DSA (left) and three-dimensional DSA (right) showing an intranidal aneurysm (arrows); Number 4 panel: Roadmap image showing the Apollo microcatheter (arrow) accessing the nidus; Number 5 panel: Roadmap image showing Onyx casting in the nidus, where the intranidal aneurysm (arrow) was obliterated; Number 6 panel: Six-month follow-up DSA showing that the BAVM was completely embolized and had no residual. B: Number 1 panel: CT image showing cerebellar hemorrhage; Number 2 panel: DSA of the right VA showing that the BAVM (asterisk) was supplied by the PCA; Number 3 panel: Three-dimensional DSA (left) and microcatheter DSA (right) showing an intranidal aneurysm (arrow); Number 4 panel: DSA of the right VA showing that the BAVM region containing an intranidal aneurysm (ellipse) was embolized, and the arrow indicating Onyx casting; Number 5 panel: DSA showing that the venous drainage (arrowheads) of the BAVM was patent.

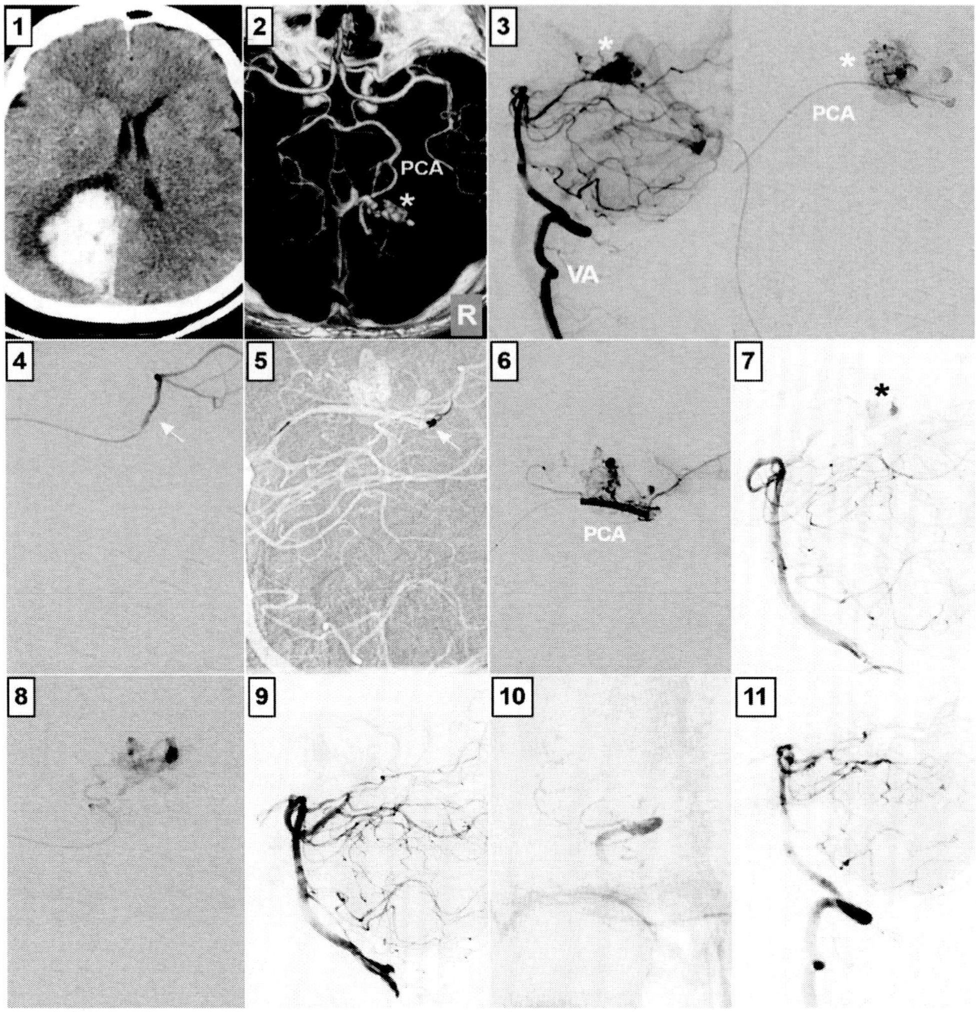

Abbreviations: BAVM: brain arteriovenous malformation; CT: computed tomography; DSA: digital subtraction angiography; EVT: endovascular treatment; PCA: posterior cerebral artery; R: right; VA: vertebral artery.

Figure 4. EVT for BAVMs with intranidal aneurysms. A: Number 1 panel: CT image showing right occipital lobe hemorrhage; Number 2 panel: CT angiography image showing that a BAVM (asterisk) was supplied by a branch of the PCA; Number 3 panel: DSA (left) and microcatheter DSA (right) showing the BAVM (asterisk); Number 4 panel: Microcatheter DSA image showing that the microcatheter was navigated into the distal PCA (arrow) beyond the BAVM; Number 5 panel: Roadmap image showing that the distal PCA beyond the BAVM was coiled (arrow). Panel Number 6: Microcatheter DSA image showing the angioarchitecture of the nidus; Panel Number 7: DSA image after BAVM embolization showing the residual nidus (asterisk); Panel 8: Microcatheter DSA image showing the angioarchitecture of the residual BAVM; Panel 9: DSA image showing the curative embolization of the BAVM; Panel 10: X-ray image showing the Onyx casting in the nidus; Panel 11: Six-month follow-up DSA image showing that the BAVM was cured and had no recurrence.

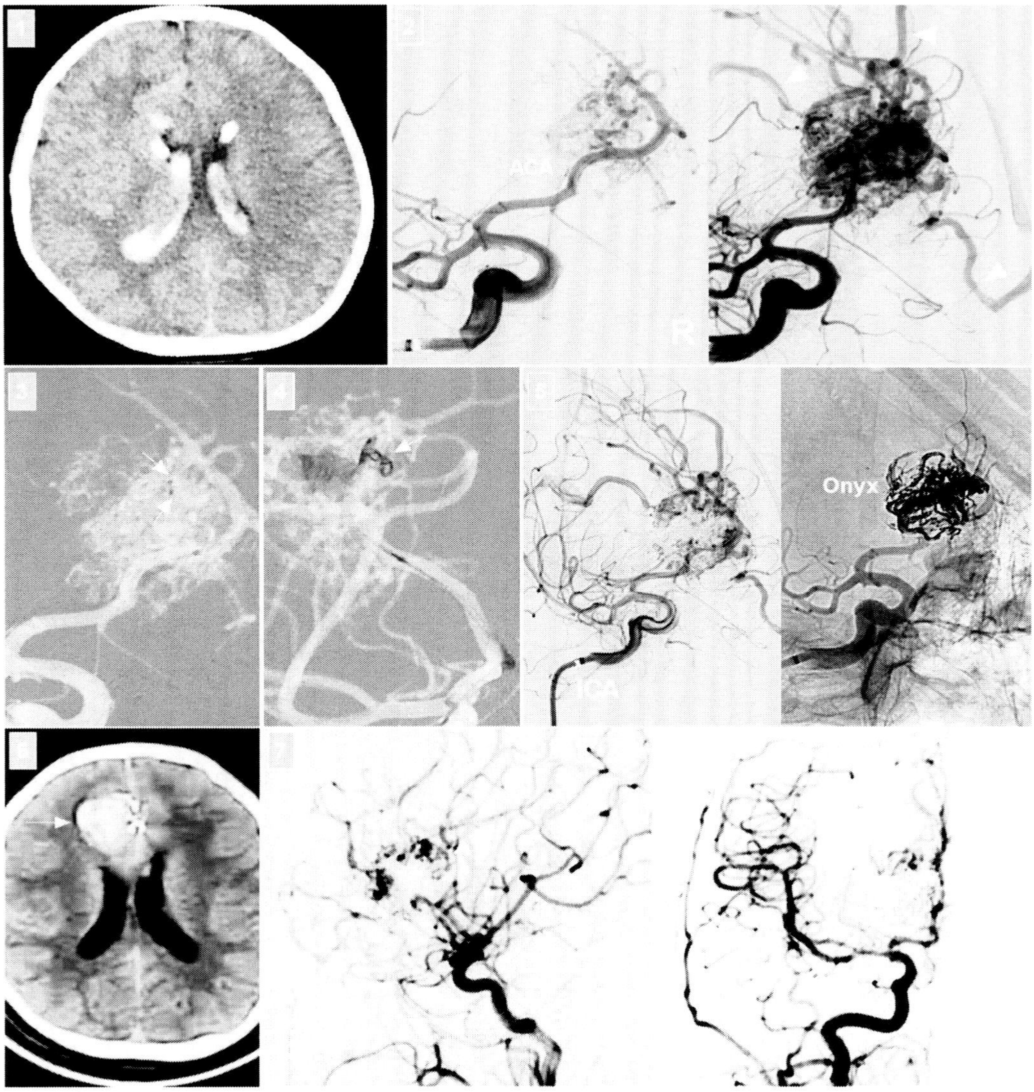

Abbreviations: ACA: anterior cerebral artery, BAVM: brain arteriovenous malformation, CT: computed tomography, DSA: digital subtraction angiography, EVT: endovascular treatment, ICA: internal carotid artery, R: right.

Figure 5. Rebleeding after EVT for a BAVM. A: Number 1 panel: CT image showing intraventricular hemorrhage; Number 2 panel: Arterial phase (left) and venous phase (right) DSA of the right ICA showing that the BAVM was supplied by the ACA and drained by multiple veins (arrowheads); Number 3 panel: Roadmap image showing that a feeding artery was catheterized by two microcatheters (arrows); Number 4 panel: Roadmap image showing that the feeding artery was coiled (arrow) via a microcatheter to establish a "pressure-cooker" effect; Number 5 panel: DSA of the right ICA showing that most of the nidus was embolized (left panel), unsubtracted DSA showing that the Onyx casting in the nidus (right panel); Number 6 panel: Postoperative four-month CT showing rebleeding (arrow) from the BAVM; and Number 7 panel: Lateral view (left) and anterior posterior view (right) DSA of the right ICA showing that most of the nidus was embolized and that no weak risky structures could be detected.

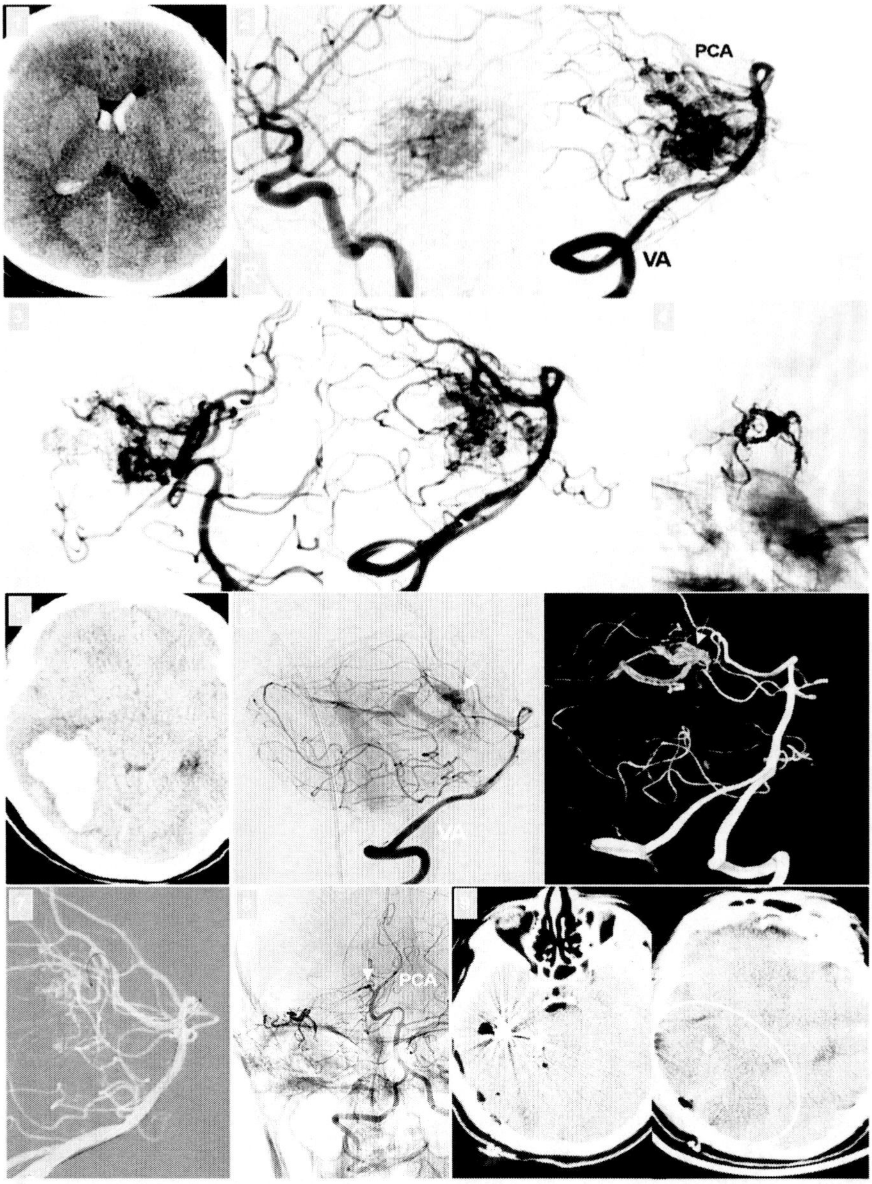

Abbreviations: BAVM: brain arteriovenous malformation; CT: computed tomography; DSA: digital subtraction angiography; EVT: endovascular treatment; ICA: internal carotid artery; PCA: posterior cerebral artery; R: right.

Figure 6. Rebleeding after EVT and radiotherapy for a BAVM. A: Number 1 panel: CT image showing intraventricular hemorrhage; Number 2 panel: DSA of the right ICA (left panel) and left VA (right panel) showing that the BAVM was supplied by the PCA; Number 3 panel: Anterior posterior (left panel) and lateral (right panel) DSA images of the left VA showing that the BAVM was partially embolized and that the BAVM volume was reduced; Number 4 panel: X-ray image showing the Onyx casting in the nidus; Number 5 panel: CT image showing right temporal hemorrhage; Number 6 panel: DSA (left panel) and three-dimensional DSA (right panel) of the VA showing only a small residual of the nidus (arrow); Number 7 panel: Roadmap image showing that the feeding artery was catheterized to plan the reembolization (arrow); Number 8 panel: Unsubtracted DSA showing that the main feeding artery was occluded (arrow); Number 9 panel: Postoperative CT image showing that the BAVM and hematoma were removed and that the edema (ellipse).

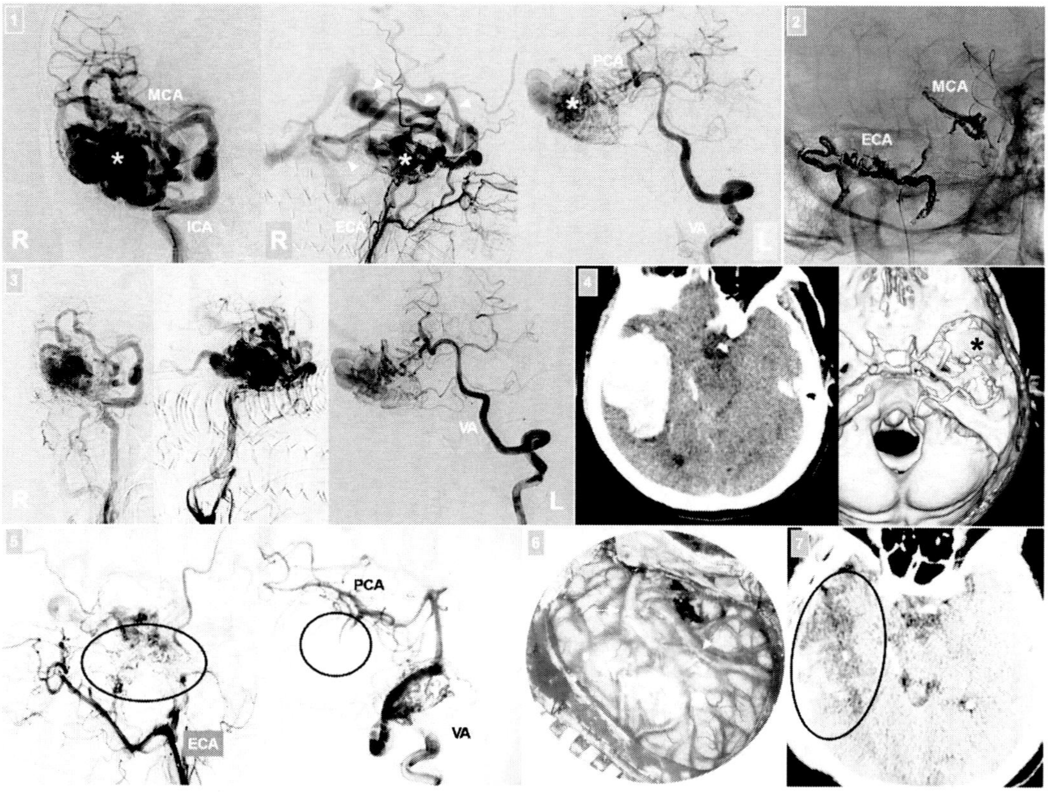

Abbreviations: BAVM: brain arteriovenous malformation; CT: computed tomography; DSA: digital subtraction angiography; ECA: external carotid artery; EVT: endovascular treatment; ICA: internal carotid artery; L: left; MCA: middle cerebral artery; PCA: posterior cerebral artery; R: right.

Figure 7. Rebleeding after EVT for a BAVM. A: Number 1 panel: DSA images of the right ICA (left panel), right ECA (middle panel) and left VA (right VA) showing a BAVM (asterisk) supplied by the MCA, ECA and PCA; Number 2 panel: X-ray image showing Onyx casting in the MCA and ECA; Number 3 panel: Six-month follow-up DSA images of the right ICA (left panel), right ECA (middle panel) and left VA (right VA) showing no volume reduction of the BAVM; Number 4 panel: Post-EVT eighteen-month CT showing hemorrhage of the right temporal lobe (left panel), and CT bone reconstruction showing the location of Onyx casting (asterisk) (right panel); Number 5 panel: DSA images of the right ECA (left panel) and VA (right panel) showing that the main feeding arteries were occluded and that the blood flow into the nidus was reduced (ellipse); Number 5 panel: Intraoperative image showing swollen brain and arterialized veins (arrows); Number 6 panel: CT showing that the BAVM and hematoma were removed (ellipse).

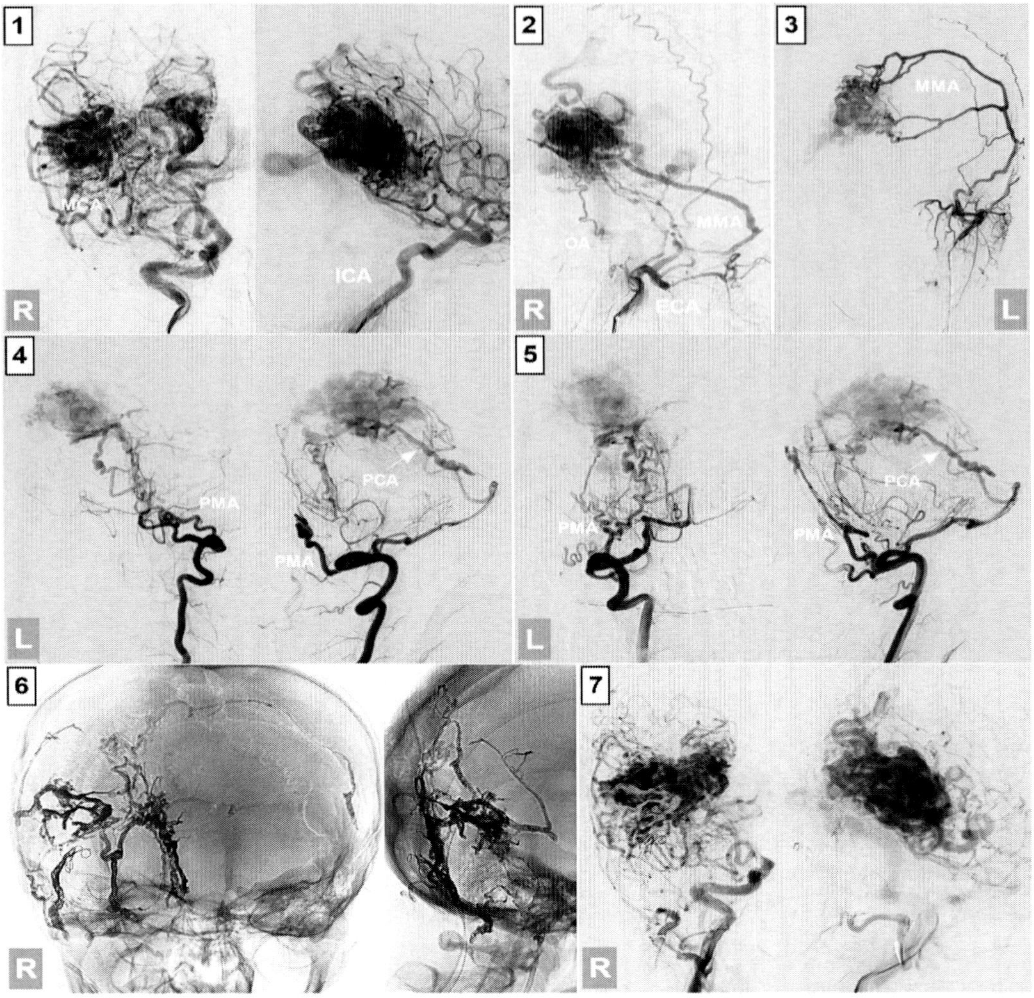

Abbreviations: BAVM: brain arteriovenous malformation; CT: computed tomography; DSA: digital subtraction angiography; ECA: external carotid artery; EVT: endovascular treatment; ICA: internal carotid artery; L: left; MCA: middle cerebral artery; MMA: middle meningeal artery; OA: occipital artery; PCA: posterior cerebral artery; PMA: posterior meningeal artery; R: right.

Note: This patient was a middle-aged male who had been experiencing dizziness and hypophrenia for two years. After EVT, she improved.

Figure 8. Palliative EVT for a BAVM with transdural circulation. A: Number 1 panel: Anterior posterior view (left panel) and lateral view (view) DSA images of the right ICA showing a BAVM (asterisk) supplied by the MCA; B: Number 1 panel: DSA of the right ECA showing a BAVM supplied by the right MMA and OA; C: Number 3 panel: DSA of the left ECA showing a BAVM supplied by the left MMA; D: Number 4-5 panels: DSA images of the right VA (Number 4 panel) and left VA (Number 5 panel) showing a BAVM supplied by bilateral PMAs and the right artery of Davidoff and Schechter (arrows); Number 6 panels: X-ray image showing Onyx casting via the bilateral MMA, right OA, and right PMA. Number 7 Panel: Anterior posterior view (left panel) and lateral view (view) DSA images of the right ICA showing blood flow reduction in the BAVM.

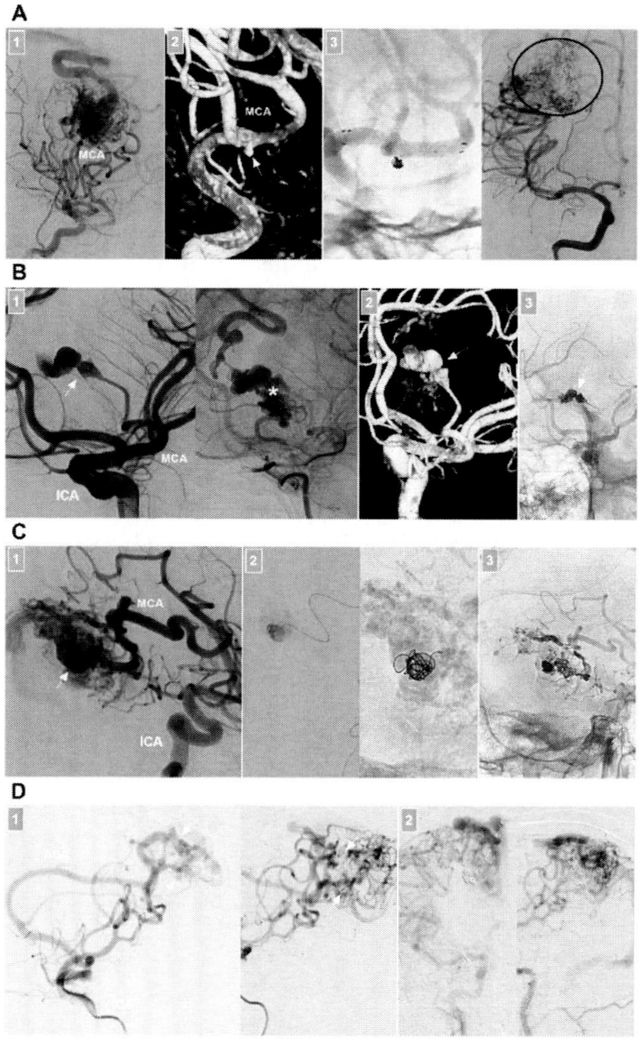

Abbreviations: BAVM: brain arteriovenous malformation; DSA: digital subtraction angiography; EVT: endovascular treatment; ICA: internal carotid artery; MCA: middle cerebral artery.

Figure 9. EVT for weak structures associated with BAVMs. A: Coiling of a saccular flow-related aneurysm on the feeding artery: Number 1 panel: DSA of the ICA showing a BAVM supplied by the MCA; Number 2 panel: Three-dimensional DSA showing an aneurysm of MCA bifurcation (arrow); Number 3 panel: Unsubtracted DSA showing that the aneurysm was coiled with the assistance of stenting (left panel), where the BAVM was partially embolized (right panel); B: Embolizing a flow-related dissecting aneurysm on the feeding artery: Number 1 panel: Arterial phase (left panel) and venous phase (right panel) DSA images of the ICA showing a BAVM (asterisk), where the feeding artery from the MCA was dissected (arrow) near the nidus; Number 2 panel: Three-dimensional DSA showing that the dissecting feeding artery; Number 3 panel: Unsubtracted DSA showing that the aneurysm was embolized by Onyx casting (arrow). C: Coiling of an intranidal aneurysm: Number 1 panel: DSA image showing an aneurysm (arrow) in the nidus; Number 2 panel: Microcatheter DSA image showing the aneurysm (left panel), the aneurysm was coiled (right panel); Number 3 panel: Unsubtracted DSA image showing that the BAVM was partially embolized; D: Coiling of fistulous structures in the nidus: Number 1 panel: DSA image showing a BAVM with fistulous structures (arrows) in the nidus (left panel), which were coiled (arrows) (right panel); Number 2 panel: Anterior posterior view (left panel) and lateral view (view) DSA images of six-month follow-up DSA image showing the complete embolization of fistulous structures.

Clinical Trials

To overcome the drawbacks of ARUBA, several clinical trials have been designed to explore the role of EVT in BAVMs. The international, multicenter Treatment of Brain Arteriovenous Malformations Study (TOBAS) was launched in 2014 [74]. By May 2021, over 1000 patients had been recruited. The clinical outcomes of patients included in the surgical and endovascular registries have been published. In a report in 2022, TOBAS revealed that embolization as a curative treatment for BAVMs was often incomplete, and hemorrhagic complications were frequent [75]. In a report in 2023, TOBAS reported that surgical treatment of BAVMs was curative in 88% of patients [76]. The results of EVT registries have been disappointing [77]. Although TOBAS provided some suggestions for EVT to treat BAVMs, patients included in this randomized trial differ significantly from registry patients, mainly in terms of presentation, size, SM grade, and eloquence. Whether the study provides meaningful results depends on the participation of many more centers, clinicians, and patients in randomized trials [77].

Other trials may provide more results in the future, such as the safety and efficacy of EVT and gamma knife surgery for BAVMs in China [78], the transvenous approach for the treatment of cerebral arteriovenous malformations (TVIAMs) [79] and the multicenter arteriovenous malformation Research Study (MARS) [80].

Curative EVT for BAVMs

Curative EVT for BAVMs has highly variable outcomes and can be associated with poor radiographic outcomes and an increased risk of complications, depending on the patient selection and technique used [81, 82]. According to the recommendations of the AHA and ASA, curative EVT can be performed only for BAVMs with simple angioarchitectures [83-86].

Curative TAE for BAVMs

TAE is the most effective method when the BAVM has only a few feeding arteries and when EVT is performed with a minimal number of sessions (Figure 10) [65].

In terms of overall TAEs for BAVMs with various SM grades, the rate of curative EVT was not high. In a report by Frizzel et al. in 1995, in the embolization of 1246 BAVMs, the curative rates of embolization were 4% in reports of 708 patients published before 1990 and 5% in reports of 538 patients published since 1990. Temporary morbidity from embolization was 10%, and permanent morbidity was 8%. Permanent morbidity was 9% before 1990 and 8% after 1990. Death after embolization occurred in 1% of patients. The incidence of mortality associated with embolization was 2% before 1990 and 1% after 1990 [23].

In recent years, high rates of total or near-total occlusion of BAVMs have been achieved with multiple sessions of Onyx embolization, with acceptable morbidity and mortality [87]. In a report by Katsaridis et al. in 2008, during the 4-year study period, 219 BAVM embolization procedures for TAE were performed in 101 patients; total and near-total occlusions were obtained in 45.5% of patients, and permanent neurological deficits resulted in a morbidity rate of 8% and a mortality rate of 3% [87]. In a report by van Rooij et al. in 2012, in selected patients with small- and medium-sized superficial BAVMs, complete angiographic obliteration of the BAVM with Onyx via TAE was achieved in all 24 patients; there were no hemorrhagic or ischemic complications and no new neurologic deficits [88]. In a 2019 report by Iosif et al. curative EVT was performed in 73 low-grade SM BAVMs, including 64% [47/73] of the lesions treated by TAE; the prognosis was good, the procedure-related morbidity rate was 2.7%, and the mortality rate was 0% [86].

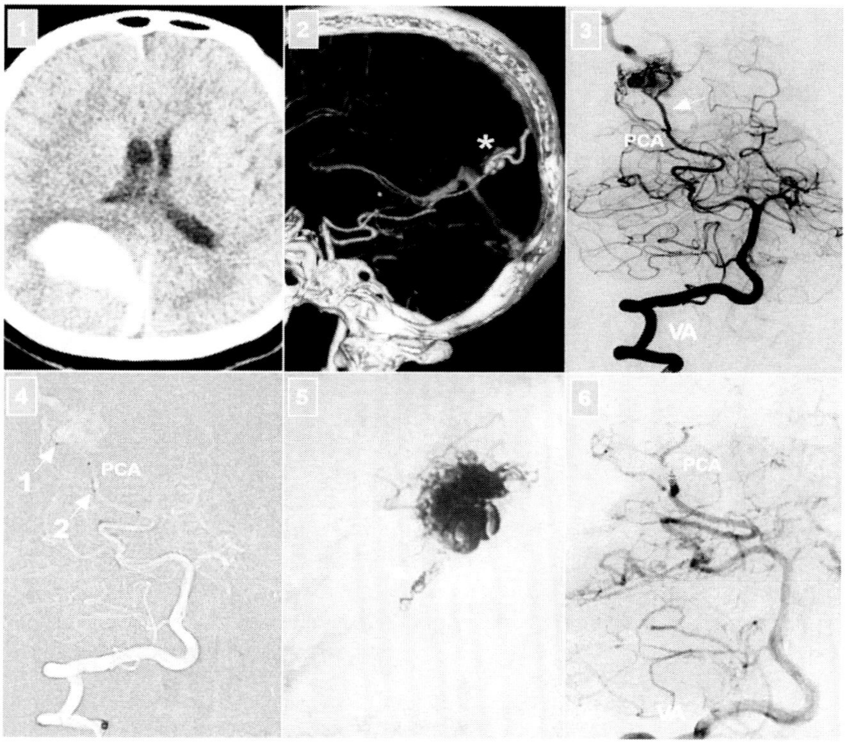

Abbreviations: TAE: transarterial embolization, BAVM: brain arteriovenous malformation, CT: computed tomography, DSA: digital subtraction angiography, EVT: endovascular treatment, PCA: posterior cerebral artery.

Figure 10. Curative TAE for BAVMs. Number 1 panel: CT image showing a left occipital lobe hematoma; Number 2 panel: CT angiography image showing a BAVM (asterisk); Number 3 panel: DSA of the VA showing a BAVM supplied by the PCA; Number 4 panel: Roadmap image showing two microcatheters (arrows with numbers 1 and 2) accessing the nidus; Number 1 microcatheter was planned to cast Onyx; Number 2 microcatheter was planned to coil the feeding artery to establish the "pressure cooker" effect; Number 5 panel: X-ray image showing Onyx casting in the nidus and coiling feeding artery (arrow); Number 6 panel: Six-month follow-up DSA showing that the BAVM was cured and had no residual.

However, curative TAE is not recommended. In 2022, 106 patients with curative embolization were treated with TOBAS. Embolization was confirmed to occlude the BAVM in 30% of the curative attempts, and new symptomatic hemorrhages occurred in 20% of the curative embolizations. The primary outcome of death or disability (mRS >2) occurred in 14% of patients who underwent curative embolization. Research has shown that EVT as a curative treatment for BAVMs is often incomplete, and hemorrhagic complications are frequent (Figure 11) [75].

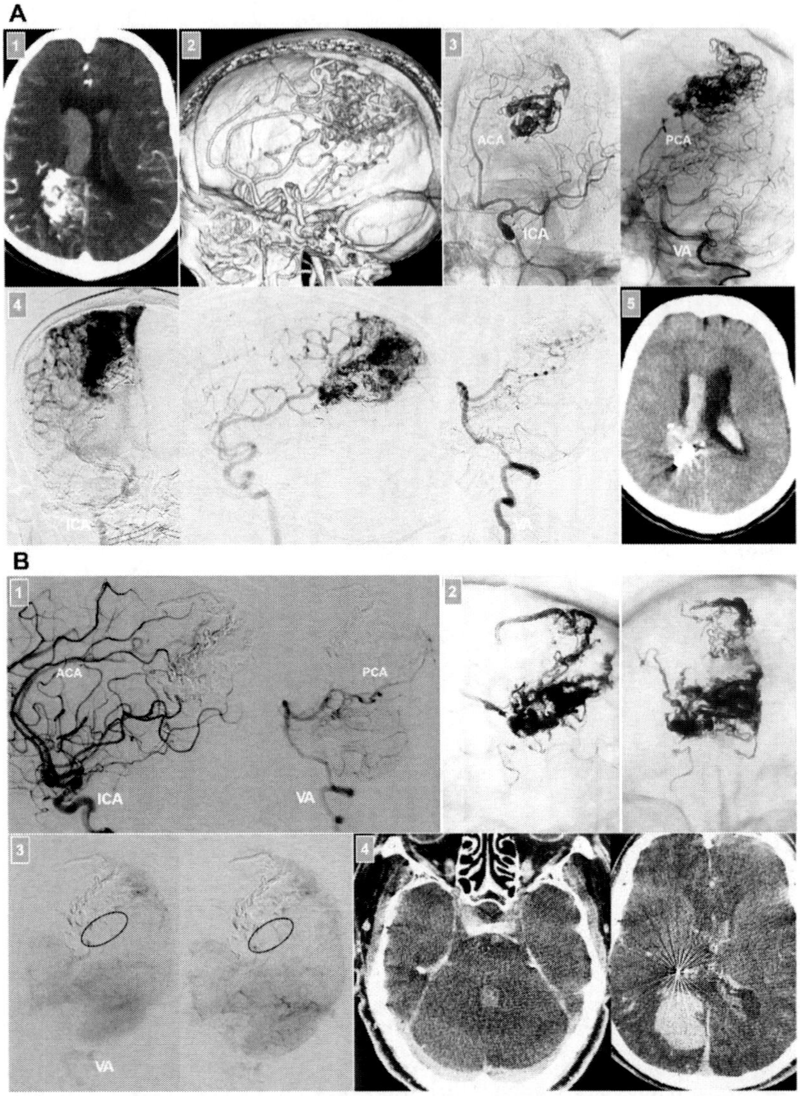

Abbreviations: ACA: anterior cerebral artery, BAVM: brain arteriovenous malformation, CT: computed tomography, DSA: digital subtraction angiography, EVT: endovascular treatment, PCA: posterior cerebral artery, TAE: transarterial embolization.

Figure 11. Hemorrhagic complications in a BAVM with curative TAE. A: First EVT: Number 1 panel: CT image showing that the BAVM ruptured into the lateral ventricle; Number 2 panel: CT angiography image showing a large BAVM; Number 3 panel: Unsubtracted DSA image of the ICA (left panel) and VA (right panel) showing that the BAVM had been embolized via the ACA and PCA; Number 4 panel: Six-month follow-up DSA image of the ICA (left and middle panels) and VA (right panel) showing residual BAVM; Number 5 panel: Eight-month follow-up CT image showing rerupture of the BAVM. B: Second EVT: Number 1 panel: DSA of the ICA (left panel) and VA (right panel) showing that the BAVM had been completely embolized via the ACA and PCA; Number 2 panel: X-ray image showing Onyx casting in the nidus; Number 3 panel: DSA of the VA showing active bleeding (ellipse); Number 4 panel: Xper-CT showing rebleeding.

Curative TVE for BAVMs

Concept and Proposal of TVE for BAVMs

Pioneering works on TVE for dural arteriovenous fistula (DAVF) continued in the 1980s [89, 90]. However, this success did not translate into a similar management paradigm for BAVMs [91]. In 1991, Houdart et al. considered the theory of TVE for BAVMs [92]. In 1992, it was proposed that in TVE, specifically designed balloon catheters should be used to temporarily occlude the feeding arteries [93]. In 1993, Houdart et al. suggested that TVE is contraindicated in plexiform and nonfistulous BAVMs [94]. In 1994, Mullan et al. proposed that TVE can be used as a curative standalone modality to treat BAVM [95]. In 1999, Massoud et al. proposed the famous principle of TRENSH (transvenous retrograde nidus sclerotherapy under controlled hypotensive anesthesia) in a swine model to guide TVE for BAVMs [96].

The first study with TVE for a ruptured BAVM supplied by an enpassant arterial feeder was reported by Nguyen et al. in 2010 [97], followed by Kessler et al. with a larger series of patients in 2011 [98]. Since then, TVE for BAVMs has gradually increased, and experience has accumulated. Most influential studies were reported from 2010 approximately 2018; French and German authors served as pioneers, and other authors in the US, China, Brazil, Spain, Switzerland, Canada, Iran and Italy also contributed [46]. The top 10 authors with the most published research on the TVE of BAVMs were from France, and the most cited study was published by Iosif C in 2015, followed by Consoli A in 2013 and Chen CJ in 2018 [46].

Case Selection and Expansion of TVE for BAVMs

In general, the venous drainage system of BAVMs is simpler, and the draining veins are considerably fewer and larger in caliber than their counterpart arterial feeders are, which enables the possibility of TVE [94]. However, TVE can be performed only in highly selected BAVMs, but it should not be considered a first-line treatment [99]. For BAVMs with larger niduses and an increased number of venous collectors, the risk of hemorrhagic complications when TVE is implemented may increase, as reported by De Sousa et al. in 2020 [100]. In addition, TVE may not be a favored approach for loose and diffuse plexiform BAVMs, as early venous occlusion without securing multiple arterial feeders results in a high risk for venous hypertension, resulting in cerebral edema and hemorrhage [90]. BAVM compactness refers to the score proposed by Beslow et al. in 2024, in which a score of 1 represents an ill-defined BAVM with a diffuse nidus, a score of 2 represents a better-defined BAVM with a few areas of diffuse nidus, and a score of 3 represents a compact BAVM [101].

The current consensus is that TVE can be used only in selected cases (Figures 12-13), such as those with small niduses (<3 cm), deep-seated lesions, supplication by very thin or perforating arterial branches and the absence of potential feeders, and the presence of a single draining vein, which was described in the reports of Kessler et al. in 2015 [98], Choudhri et al. in 2015 [91], Iosif et al. in 2015 [7], Mendes et al. in 2016 [102], Viana et al. in 2017 [103], Mendes et al. in 2018 [104], De Sousa et al. in 2020 [100], Koyanagi et al. (2021) [105], and Saal-Zapata et al. (2023) et al. [46]. A small nidus size and a single draining vein were associated with a good prognosis after TVE for BAVMs. In 2019, in the study protocol of a randomized controlled trial of the transvenous approach for the treatment of cerebral arteriovenous malformations (TATAMs), TVE indications included a small nidus (<3 cm) and a single draining vein [79].

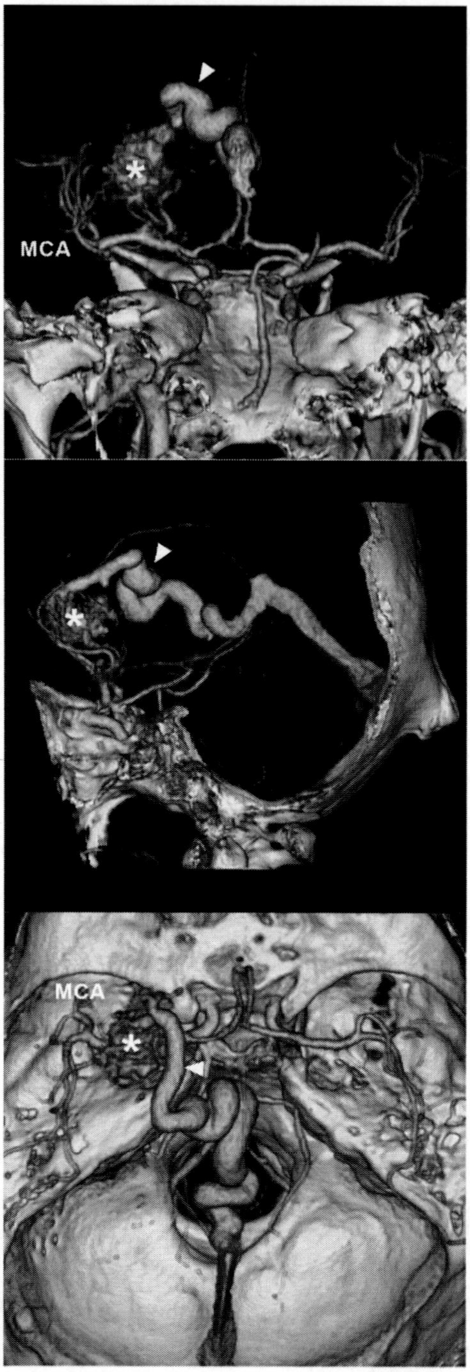

Abbreviations: BAVM: brain arteriovenous malformation, CT: computed tomography, TVE: transvenous embolization.

Figure 12. A BAVM appropriate for TVE. Upper, middle and lower panels: CT angiography of different views showing a BAVM supplied by lenticulostriate arteries from the MCA and draining into the deep vein.

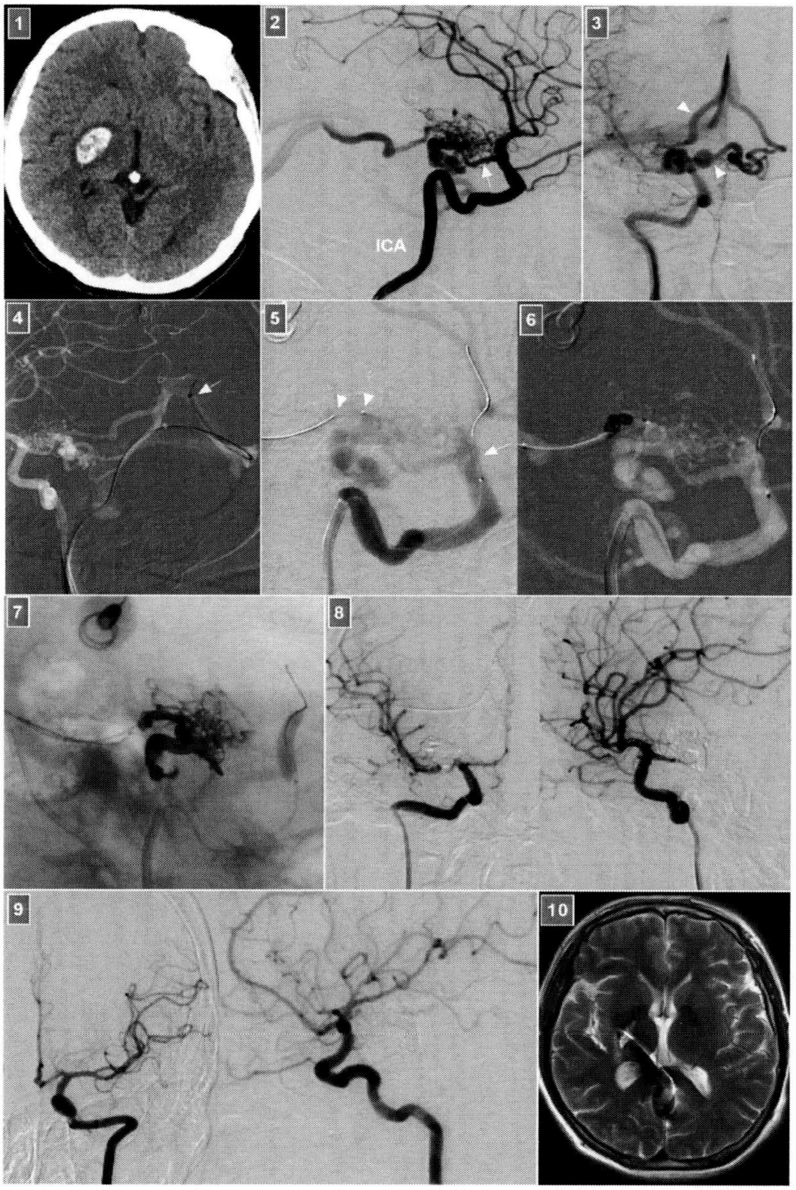

Abbreviations: BAVM: brain arteriovenous malformation, CT: computed tomography, DSA: digital subtraction angiography, EVT: endovascular treatment, ICA: internal carotid artery, TVE: transvenous embolization.

Figure 13. Curative TVE for BAVMs. Panel 1: CT image showing a right internal capsule hematoma; Panel 2: DSA of the ICA showing a BAVM supplied by the anterior choroidal artery (arrow); Panel 3: DSA image showing that the BAVM has two deep veins as the draining route (arrowheads); Panel 4: Roadmap image showing a distal access catheter in the straight sinus (arrow); Panel 5: DSA image showing two microcatheters (arrowheads) in the distal draining vein and a balloon catheter (arrow) placed in the ICA to cover the anterior choroidal artery; Panel 6: Roadmap image showing that the draining vein was coiled to establish the "pressure cooker" effect; Panel 7: X-ray image showing the casting of the Onyx in the nidus with the assistance of the feeding artery being occluded by the balloon. Number 8 panel: Postoperative immediate DSA image showing that the BAVM was obliterated. Number 9 panel: Six-month follow-up DSA image showing that the BAVM was cured. Number 10 panel: Six-month follow-up magnetic resonance image showing that the hemorrhage was absorbed.

Currently, the scope of case selection for TVE for BAVMs is expanding. TVE for BAVMs may be used for complex high Spetzler–Martin grade lesions. In 2015, Iosif et al. reported that single-session TVE seems to be a safe and effective curative treatment for complex BAVMs with high Spetzler–Martin (SM) III-V grades [7]. In 2020, Koyanagi et al. reported that curative TVE for BAVMs can be used for high-SM-grade lesions [105]. However, more clinical experience and data are required.

TVE Technique Development

Arterial Control

To increase the ability of the liquid embolic agent to penetrate the nidus retrogradely from the venous side, the arterial inflow into the nidus should be reduced or stopped, which can be realized by temporary systemic hypotension. In 1999, the TRENSH model proposed by Massoud et al. suggested reducing the mean systemic pressure to 40–50 mmHg or targeting 20% of the mean arterial pressure below baseline [96]. In 2000, Massoud et al. reported that induced systemic hypotension may reduce the risk of iatrogenic hemorrhage [106]. In addition to reducing the mean systemic pressure, selective systemic flow arrest by asystole can be attempted to facilitate the TVE procedure for BAVMs, such as in a report by Lim et al. in 2020 [107] and by Ghorbani et al. in 2021 [108]. Intraoperative and postoperative hypotension remains an important cornerstone of BAVM care for preventing hemorrhage and edema after TVE.

In addition, balloon inflation in major feeders or occlusion of the ostium of the feeders can reduce the pressure gradient and blood flow to the nidus to allow the injection of the liquid embolisates to overcome feeding arterial pressure. The currently available balloons include the Scepter or mini-Scepter microcatheter balloon, Eclipse or Eclipse 2 L (Balt Extrusion, Montmorency, France), Ascent (DePuy Synthes, Raynham, Massachusetts, USA), and Hyperglide or Hyperform (Medtronic, Minneapolis, Minnesota, USA) [9, 109, 110]. The balloon was inflated before each embolis was injected; every 5 min, the balloon was deflated, and every 2 min, the balloon was inflated [9]. To reduce arterial inflow into the BAVM nidus, for BAVMs with large feeding arteries, TVE may be accompanied by TAE in the same session to reduce arterial inflow into the BAVM nidus.

Venous Access and Embolization

When the primary draining vein is thick and ≥5 mm in diameter, reflux of a liquid embolic agent on the order of 3 cm cannot be tolerated. The reverse "pressure cooker" technique using coils or NBCA glue as a venous plug can be used [9]. The earliest description of a precipitating embolic agent with the transvenous "pressure cooker" technique dates back to 2003 during the ABC WIN seminar in Val d'Isère (France) by Houdak, followed in 2005 by Houdart and Chapot at the same meeting [105]. After TVE, it may be difficult to remove the working microcatheter of the casting liquid embolates; if TVE is performed via transjugular access, the microcatheter can be cut at the neck [98].

Two new flow-directed detachable-is microcatheters, the Sonic microcatheter and the Apollo microcatheter, which led to the development and modification of the "pressure cooker" technique after TVE [47]. In 2014, René Chapot et al. described in detail the "pressure cooker" technique, which consists of the navigation of 2 microcatheters (1 detachable tip and the other nondetachable tip) as close as possible to the nidus via an enlarged and arterialized primary vein [111].

With the development and advancement of microcatheters, when routine microcatheters for delivering coils have difficulty reaching the ideal position to establish a venous plug, a 1.5F Apollo or Marathon microcatheter can be used to deliver certain detachable coils, such as ED coils (Kaneka Medix Corporation, Osaka, Japan), barricade coils (Blockade Medical, Irvine, CA), Visee coils (Visee Medical Devices Co., Ltd., Shandong, China) and Jasper®SS-10 coils (Achieva Medical Co., Ltd., Shanghai, China) [105, 112-114].

With respect to liquid embolic agents, before 2005, the most commonly used embolic agent for BAVM treatment was adhesive NBCA [98]. Owing to the rapidity of polymerization, NBCA is not suitable for TVE for BAVMs, as immediate occlusion of the draining vein can be disastrous [90, 98]. Since its initial use in 2005, Onyx has been approved for BAVM treatment, and it is most suited for TVE because it is more cohesive and has milder adhesive properties. Onyx can be injected over a period of several minutes to over an hour for more controlled embolization [90, 98]. During TVE for BAVM, the Onyx begins to adhere along the wall of the vein before occlusion of the lumen, and retrograde filling of the nidus occurs when there is restriction of anterograde flow before total occlusion of the vein occurs [96].

Proposal and Development of BAVM Endovascular Grading Scales

Several grading systems for the treatment of BAVMs have been proposed to predict the prognosis and complications of interventions (Table 1). In 1986, the SM BAVM grading system was proposed, which is based on size, location (eloquence or not) and venous drainage of the BAVM [115]. In 2010, the Lawton–Young BAVM grading system supplemented the SM system by incorporating additional factors important for surgical selection and outcome, including patient age, hemorrhagic presentation, and compactness of the nidus [116]. In 2011, the SM BAVM grading system was revised to the Spetzler-Ponce system [117]. Although these grading systems can predict deficits in EVT, they do not reflect major anatomical issues in EVT.

In 2010, Feliciano et al. proposed a new BAVM grading scale for EVT, which is based on the number of arterial pedicles, the eloquence of adjacent areas, and the presence of arteriovenous fistulas [118]. In 2015, the Buffalo scoring system was proposed for EVT of BAVMs on the basis of the number of arterial pedicles, diameter of the arterial pedicles, and eloquent location of the BAVM [119]. In 2016, the BAVM embocure score was proposed to assess the curative risk of EVT on the basis of the number of arterial pedicles and draining veins, size of the BAVM nidus, and degree of vascular eloquence [120]. In 2024, the Tsinghua grading system was proposed by Lv et al. This grading system is a simple radio-clinical grading scale that includes a ruptured or unruptured status, a superficial or deep location [arterial feeders are amenable to selective catheterization], a small or large nidus size, a coexisting arterial aneurysm and a fistula compartment or not [121]. The above grading systems were designed for TAE, and they can predict the complication risk of TAE.

However, a grading system designed for TVE for BAVMs has not been proposed, and the patterns of the arterial feeder, nidus and venous drainage should be considered. This grading system, which is designed for TVE for BAVMs, is desirable.

Table 1. Grading systems for the TAE of BAVMs

Classification	Graded feature	Points
Puerto Rico scale	Number of arterial pedicles	
	<3	1
	3-6	2
	>6	3
	Eloquence of adjacent areas	
	Noneloquent	0
	Eloquent	1
	Presence of arteriovenous fistula	
	No	0
	Yes	1
Buffalo grading system	Number of arterial pedicles	
	1 or 2	1
	3 or 4	2
	5 or more	3
	Diameter of arterial pedicles	
	Most >1 mm	0
	Most ≤1 mm	1
	Nidus location	
	Noneloquent	0
	Eloquent	1
AVM embocure score	Nidus size	
	<3 cm	1
	3-6 cm	2
	>6 cm	3
	Arterial pedicles	
	1-3	1
	4-6	2
	>6	3
	Draining veins	
	1-3	1
	4-6	2
	>6	3
	Vascular eloquence	
	Noneloquent	0
	Eloquent	1
Tsinghua grading system	Presentation	
	Ruptured	1
	Unruptured	0
	Location	
	Superficial	1
	Deep	0
	Size	
	Small ≤3 cm	1
	Large >3 cm	0
	Arterial aneurysm	
	Yes	1
	No	0
	Fistula compartment	
	Yes	1
	No	0

Abbreviations: BAVM: brain arteriovenous malformation; TAE: transarterial embolization.

Future of EVT for BAVMs

The future of TVE for BAVMs is not known but is worthy of investigation. The popularity of TVE for treating BAVMs depends on the development of basic studies of BAVM models, improvements in engineering and imaging technologies, the development and evolution of microcatheter or balloon microcatheter technology, the evolution of nanoparticles and bioactive embolic agents and the accumulation of clinical experience [122]. Currently, imaging techniques, such as three-dimensional rotational angiography and three-dimensional roadmapping techniques, have improved, making EVT for BAVMs more convenient [123-125]. In the future, artificial intelligence can be applied in EVT for BAVMs, including analyzing angioarchitectures, helping EVT designation and predicting prognosis [126, 127].

Conclusion

Currently, EVT plays an important role in the treatment of BAVMs. Further developments in EVT technologies, the evolution of microcatheters, embolic agents and the accumulation of clinical experience will improve the safety and efficacy of EVT.

References

[1] Hou K, Song Y, Guo Y, Yu J. Brain arteriovenous malformations and dural arteriovenous fistulas with extensive venous congestive encephalopathy. *Acta Neurol Belg*. 2022;122 (1):1-9.

[2] Doppman JL. The nidus concept of spinal cord arteriovenous malformations. A surgical recommendation based upon angiographic observations. *Br J Radiol*. 1971;44 (526):758-63.

[3] Lawton MT, Rutledge WC, Kim H, Stapf C, Whitehead KJ, Li DY, et al. Brain arteriovenous malformations. *Nat Rev Dis Primers*. 2015;1:15008.

[4] Ogilvy CS, Stieg PE, Awad I, Brown RD, Jr., Kondziolka D, Rosenwasser R, et al. AHA Scientific Statement: Recommendations for the management of intracranial arteriovenous malformations: a statement for healthcare professionals from a special writing group of the Stroke Council, American Stroke Association. *Stroke*. 2001;32 (6):1458-71.

[5] Luessenhop AJ, Spence WT. Artificial Embolization Of Cerebral Arteries: Report Of Use In A Case Of Arteriovenous Malformation. *JAMA*. 1960;172 (11):1153-5.

[6] Yang R, Ren Y, Maingard J, Thijs V, Le DVA, Kok HK, et al. The 100 most cited articles in the endovascular treatment of brain arteriovenous malformations. *Brain Circulation*. 2021;7 (2):49-64.

[7] Iosif C, Mendes GA, Saleme S, Ponomarjova S, Silveira EP, Caire F, et al. Endovascular transvenous cure for ruptured brain arteriovenous malformations in complex cases with high Spetzler-Martin grades. *J Neurosurg*. 2015;122 (5):1229-38.

[8] Batista S, Almeida Filho JA, Oliveira LB, Koester S, Pinheiro AC, Dinato RA, et al. Evaluating the safety and efficacy of transvenous embolization for brain arteriovenous malformation: A systematic review and meta-analysis. *Interv Neuroradiol*. 2023:15910199231204922.

[9] Iosif C, Almeida Filho JA, Gilbert CE, Nazemi Rafie A, Saleme S, Rouchaud A, et al. Selective arterial temporary flow arrest with balloons during transvenous embolization for the treatment of brain arteriovenous malformations: a feasibility study with MRI-monitored adverse events. *J Neurointerv* Surg. 2022;14 (12):1234-8.

[10] Luessenhop AJ, Velasquez AC. Observations On The Tolerance Of The Intracranial Arteries To Catheterization. *J Neurosurg*. 1964;21:85-91.

[11] Doppman JL, Zapol W, Pierce J. Transcatheter embolization with a silicone rubber preparation. Experimental observations. *Invest Radiol*. 1971;6 (5):304-9.

[12] Serbinenko FA. Balloon catheterization and occlusion of major cerebral vessels. J Neurosurg. 1974;41 (2):125-45.

[13] Kricheff II, Madayag M, Braunstein P. Transfemoral catheter embolization of cerebral and posterior fossa arteriovenous malformations. *Radiology*. 1972;103 (1):107-11.

[14] Kerber C. Balloon catheter with a calibrated leak. A new system for superselective angiography and occlusive catheter therapy. *Radiology*. 1976;120 (3):547-50.

[15] Fleischer AS, Kricheff I, Ransohoff J. Postmortem findings following the embolization of an arteriovenous malformation. Case report. J Neurosurg. 1972;37 (5):606-9.

[16] Djindjian R, Cophignon J, Rey Théron J, Merland JJ, Houdart R. Superselective arteriographic embolization by the femoral route in neuroradiology. Study of 50 cases. 3. Embolization in craniocerebral pathology. *Neuroradiology*. 1973;6 (3):143-52.

[17] Djindjian R, Cophignon J, Théron J, Merland JJ, Houdart R. Embolization by superselective arteriography from the femoral route in neuroradiology. Review of 60 cases. 1. Technique, indications, complications. *Neuroradiology*. 1973;6 (1):20-6.

[18] Wolpert SM, Stein BM. Catheter embolization of intracranial arteriovenous malformations as an aid to surgical excision. *Neuroradiology*. 1975;10 (2):73-85.

[19] Djindjian R. Superselective internal carotid arteriography and embolization. *Neuroradiology*. 1975;9 (3):145-56.

[20] Debrun G, Lacour P, Caron JP, Hurth M, Comoy J, Keravel Y. Detachable balloon and calibrated-leak balloon techniques in the treatment of cerebral vascular lesions. *J Neurosurg*. 1978;49 (5):635-49.

[21] Romodanov AP, Zozulia YA, Shcheglov VI. Balloon catheter occlusion of the feeding vessels of arteriovenous malformations of the brain. *Zentralbl Neurochir*. 1979;40 (1):21-8.

[22] Berenstein A, Kricheff II. Catheter and material selection for transarterial embolization: technical considerations. I. Catheters. *Radiology*. 1979;132 (3):619-30.

[23] Frizzel RT, Fisher WS, 3rd. Cure, morbidity, and mortality associated with embolization of brain arteriovenous malformations: a review of 1246 patients in 32 series over a 35-year period. *Neurosurgery*. 1995;37 (6):1031-9; discussion 39-40.

[24] Podlas H, Lipschitz R, Allen ML. Selective arterial embolization of the brain in an inoperable arteriovenous malformation in the thalamus. A case report. S Afr Med J. 1979;55 (24):1000-2.

[25] Cromwell LD, Harris AB. Treatment of cerebral arteriovenous malformations: a combined neurosurgical and neuroradiological approach. J Neurosurg. 1980;52 (5):705-8.

[26] Viñuela FV, Debrun GM, Fox AJ, Girvin JP, Peerless SJ. Dominant-hemisphere arteriovenous malformations: therapeutic embolization with isobutyl-2-cyanoacrylate. *AJNR Am J Neuroradiol*. 1983;4 (4):959-66.

[27] Debrun G, Vinuela F, Fox A, Drake CG. Embolization of cerebral arteriovenous malformations with bucrylate. *J Neurosurg*. 1982;56 (5):615-27.

[28] ApSimon HT, Khangure MS. Improved technique of bucrylate embolisation in brain arteriovenous malformation. The use of additional temporary balloon occlusion. *Acta Radiol Suppl*. 1986;369:618-20.

[29] Brothers MF, Kaufmann JC, Fox AJ, Deveikis JP. n-Butyl 2-cyanoacrylate--substitute for IBCA in interventional neuroradiology: histopathologic and polymerization time studies. *AJNR Am J Neuroradiol*. 1989;10 (4):777-86.

[30] van Rooij WJ, Sluzewski M, Beute GN. Brain AVM embolization with Onyx. *AJNR Am J Neuroradiol*. 2007;28 (1):172-7; discussion 78.

[31] Taki W, Yonekawa Y, Iwata H, Uno A, Yamashita K, Amemiya H. A new liquid material for embolization of arteriovenous malformations. *AJNR Am J Neuroradiol*. 1990;11 (1):163-8.

[32] Terada T, Nakamura Y, Nakai K, Tsuura M, Nishiguchi T, Hayashi S, et al. Embolization of arteriovenous malformations with peripheral aneurysms using ethylene vinyl alcohol copolymer. Report of three cases. *J Neurosurg*. 1991;75 (4):655-60.

[33] Germano IM, Davis RL, Wilson CB, Hieshima GB. Histopathological follow-up study of 66 cerebral arteriovenous malformations after therapeutic embolization with polyvinyl alcohol. *J Neurosurg.* 1992;76 (4):607-14.

[34] Debrun GM, Aletich V, Ausman JI, Charbel F, Dujovny M. Embolization of the nidus of brain arteriovenous malformations with n-butyl cyanoacrylate. *Neurosurgery.* 1997;40 (1):112-20; discussion 20-1.

[35] Wallace RC, Flom RA, Khayata MH, Dean BL, McKenzie J, Rand JC, et al. The safety and effectiveness of brain arteriovenous malformation embolization using acrylic and particles: the experiences of a single institution. *Neurosurgery.* 1995;37 (4):606-15; discussion 15-8.

[36] Jafar JJ, Davis AJ, Berenstein A, Choi IS, Kupersmith MJ. The effect of embolization with N-butyl cyanoacrylate prior to surgical resection of cerebral arteriovenous malformations. *J Neurosurg.* 1993;78 (1):60-9.

[37] Mizoi K, Takahashi A, Yoshimoto T, Sugawara T, Saito K. Surgical excision of giant cerebellar hemispheric arteriovenous malformations following preoperative embolization. Report of two cases. *J Neurosurg.* 1992;76 (6):1008-11.

[38] Sorimachi T, Koike T, Takeuchi S, Minakawa T, Abe H, Nishimaki K, et al. Embolization of cerebral arteriovenous malformations achieved with polyvinyl alcohol particles: angiographic reappearance and complications. *AJNR Am J Neuroradiol.* 1999;20 (7):1323-8.

[39] Guglielmi G, Viñuela F, Sepetka I, Macellari V. Electrothrombosis of saccular aneurysms via endovascular approach. Part 1: Electrochemical basis, technique, and experimental results. *J Neurosurg.* 1991;75 (1):1-7.

[40] Guglielmi G, Viñuela F, Duckwiler G, Dion J, Lylyk P, Berenstein A, et al. Endovascular treatment of posterior circulation aneurysms by electrothrombosis using electrically detachable coils. *J Neurosurg.* 1992;77 (4):515-24.

[41] Willinsky R, TerBrugge K, Montanera W, Wallace C, Aggarwal S. Micro-arteriovenous malformations of the brain: superselective angiography in diagnosis and treatment. *AJNR Am J Neuroradiol.* 1992;13 (1):325-30.

[42] Fox AJ, Pelz DM, Lee DH. Arteriovenous malformations of the brain: recent results of endovascular therapy. *Radiology.* 1990;177 (1):51-7.

[43] Aletich VA, Debrun GM, Koenigsberg R, Ausman JI, Charbel F, Dujovny M. Arteriovenous malformation nidus catheterization with hydrophilic wire and flow-directed catheter. *AJNR Am J Neuroradiol.* 1997;18 (5):929-35.

[44] Hodes JE, Aymard A, Casasco A, Rüfenacht D, Reizine D, Merland JJ. Embolization of arteriovenous malformations of the temporal lobe via the anterior choroidal artery. *AJNR Am J Neuroradiol.* 1991;12 (4):775-80.

[45] Kallmes DF, McGraw JK, Evans AJ, Mathis JM, Hergenrother RW, Jensen ME, et al. Thrombogenicity of hydrophilic and nonhydrophilic microcatheters and guiding catheters. *AJNR Am J Neuroradiol.* 1997;18 (7):1243-51.

[46] Saal-Zapata G, Visconti-Lopez FJ. Worldwide Research Trends on Transvenous Embolization of Brain Arteriovenous Malformations: A Bibliometric and Visualized Study. *World Neurosurg.* 2023;178:20-7.

[47] Flores BC, See AP, Weiner GM, Jankowitz BT, Ducruet AF, Albuquerque FC. Use of the Apollo detachable-tip microcatheter for endovascular embolization of arteriovenous malformations and arteriovenous fistulas. *J Neurosurg.* 2018;130 (3):963-71.

[48] Maimon S, Strauss I, Frolov V, Margalit N, Ram Z. Brain arteriovenous malformation treatment using a combination of Onyx and a new detachable tip microcatheter, SONIC: short-term results. AJNR Am *J Neuroradiol.* 2010;31 (5):947-54.

[49] Heit JJ, Faisal AG, Telischak NA, Choudhri O, Do HM. Headway Duo microcatheter for cerebral arteriovenous malformation embolization with n-BCA. *J Neurointerv* Surg. 2016;8 (11):1181-5.

[50] Clarençon F, Papagiannaki C, Saleme S, Rouchaud A, Shotar E, Rius E, et al. Balloon Pressure Technique with the Scepter Mini Balloon as Part of the Endovascular Strategy for Brain Arteriovenous Malformations Embolization: Preliminary Multicenter Experience. *Clin Neuroradiol.* 2023;33 (4):1055-65.

[51] Weber W, Kis B, Siekmann R, Kuehne D. Endovascular treatment of intracranial arteriovenous malformations with onyx: technical aspects. *AJNR Am J Neuroradiol*. 2007;28 (2):371-7.
[52] Lv X, Liang S. Update Onyx embolization for plexiform arteriovenous malformation: Ante-grade drifting technique. *Neuroradiol J*. 2020;33 (5):386-92.
[53] Jahan R, Murayama Y, Gobin YP, Duckwiler GR, Vinters HV, Viñuela F. Embolization of arteriovenous malformations with Onyx: clinicopathological experience in 23 patients. *Neurosurgery*. 2001;48 (5):984-95; discussion 95-7.
[54] Saatci I, Geyik S, Yavuz K, Cekirge HS. Endovascular treatment of brain arteriovenous malformations with prolonged intranidal Onyx injection technique: long-term results in 350 consecutive patients with completed endovascular treatment course. J Neurosurg. 2011;115 (1):78-88.
[55] Leyon JJ, Chavda S, Thomas A, Lamin S. Preliminary experience with the liquid embolic material agent PHIL [Precipitating Hydrophobic Injectable Liquid] in treating cranial and spinal dural arteriovenous fistulas: technical note. *J Neurointerv* Surg. 2016;8 (6):596-602.
[56] Ch'ng LS, Zaki Z, Sobri Muda A. Embolization of brain arteriovenous malformations with squid co-polymer embolic material: Initial experience. *J Interv Med*. 2023;6 (4):176-9.
[57] Akmangit I, Daglioglu E, Kaya T, Alagoz F, Sahinoglu M, Peker A, et al. Preliminary experience with squid: a new liquid embolizing agent for AVM, AV fistulas and tumors. *Turk Neurosurg*. 2014;24 (4):565-70.
[58] Sirakov SS, Sirakov A, Minkin K, Hristov H, Ninov K, Penkov M, et al. Initial experience with precipitating hydrophobic injectable liquid in cerebral arteriovenous malformations. *Interv Neuroradiol*. 2019;25 (1):58-65.
[59] Llibre-Guerra JC, Guimaraens L, Kadziolka KB, Siddiqui AH, Chapot R, Gil A. *Obtura: A novel liquid embolic agent with post-embolization radiopacity loss, in endovascular treatment of brain arteriovenous malformations, dural arteriovenous fistulas, and tumors: CLARIDAD trial. *J Neurointerv* Surg. 2024.
[60] Wong JHY, Do HM, Telischak NA, Moraff AM, Dodd RL, Marks MP, et al. Initial experience with SOFIA as an intermediate catheter in mechanical thrombectomy for acute ischemic stroke. *J Neurointerv Surg*. 2017;9 (11):1103-6.
[61] Puri AS, Kühn AL, Hou SY, Wakhloo AK. Use of intermediate guide catheters as an adjunct in extracranial embolization to avoid onyx reflux into the anastomotic vasculature. A technical note. *Interv Neuroradiol*. 2014;20 (4):424-7.
[62] Liu P, Zhang H, Qiu T, Zhu W. Trans-radial artery microcatheter angiography-assisted juvenile ruptured brainstem arteriovenous malformation resection. *Acta Neurochir* (Wien). 2024;166 (1):53.
[63] Liu X, Luo W, Wang M, Huang C, Bao K. Feasibility and Safety of Flow Diversion in the Treatment of Intracranial Aneurysms via Transradial Approach: A Single-Arm Meta-Analysis. *Front Neurol*. 2022;13:892938.
[64] Campos JK, Zarrin DA, Meyer BM, Khan MW, Laghari FJ, Collard de Beaufort JC, et al. Use of a large-bore 088 intracranial access support catheter for delivery of large intracranial devices: case series with the TracStar LDP in 125 cases. *J Neurointerv Surg*. 2024.
[65] Samaniego EA, Dabus G, Meyers PM, Kan PT, Frösen J, Lanzino G, et al. Most Promising Approaches to Improve Brain AVM Management: ARISE I Consensus Recommendations. *Stroke*. 2024;55 (5):1449-63.
[66] Lu C, Han H, Ma L, Li R, Li Z, Zhang H, et al. Comparison of Long-Term Outcomes in Ruptured Diffuse Brain Arteriovenous Malformations Between Interventional Therapy and Conservative Management. *Transl Stroke Res*. 2023.
[67] Derdeyn CP, Zipfel GJ, Albuquerque FC, Cooke DL, Feldmann E, Sheehan JP, et al. Management of Brain Arteriovenous Malformations: A Scientific Statement for Healthcare Professionals From the American Heart Association/American Stroke Association. *Stroke*. 2017;48 (8):e200-e24.
[68] Mohr JP, Parides MK, Stapf C, Moquete E, Moy CS, Overbey JR, et al. Medical management with or without interventional therapy for unruptured brain arteriovenous malformations [ARUBA]: a multicentre, non-blinded, randomised trial. *Lancet*. 2014;383 (9917):614-21.
[69] Mohr JP, Overbey JR, Hartmann A, Kummer RV, Al-Shahi Salman R, Kim H, et al. Medical management with interventional therapy versus medical management alone for unruptured brain

arteriovenous malformations [ARUBA]: final follow-up of a multicentre, non-blinded, randomised controlled trial. *Lancet Neurol*. 2020;19 (7):573-81.

[70] Wahood W, Alexander AY, Doherty RJ, Bhandarkar A, Lanzino G, Bydon M, et al. Elective intervention for unruptured cranial arteriovenous malformations in relation to ARUBA trial: a National Inpatient Sample study. *Acta Neurochir* (Wien). 2021;163 (9):2489-95.

[71] Magro E, Gentric JC, Darsaut TE, Ziegler D, Msi, Bojanowski MW, et al. Responses to ARUBA: a systematic review and critical analysis for the design of future arteriovenous malformation trials. *J Neurosurg*. 2017;126 (2):486-94.

[72] Chen KS, Khawaja A, Xu E, Mekary RA, Vaitkevicius H, Aziz-Sultan A, et al. Changes in inpatient brain arteriovenous malformation management in the United States following the ARUBA trial: analysis of an interrupted time series design. *Clin Neurol Neurosurg*. 2024;242:108293.

[73] Alrohimi A, Achey RL, Thompson N, Abdalla RN, Patterson T, Moazeni Y, et al. Treatment outcomes for ARUBA-eligible brain arteriovenous malformations: a comparison of real-world data from the NVQI-QOD AVM registry with the ARUBA trial. *J Neurointerv Surg*. 2024.

[74] Darsaut TE, Magro E, Gentric JC, Batista AL, Chaalala C, Roberge D, et al. Treatment of Brain AVMs [TOBAS]: study protocol for a pragmatic randomized controlled trial. *Trials*. 2015;16:497.

[75] Raymond J, Gentric JC, Magro E, Nico L, Bacchus E, Klink R, et al. Endovascular treatment of brain arteriovenous malformations: clinical outcomes of patients included in the registry of a pragmatic randomized trial. *J Neurosurg*. 2023;138 (5):1393-402.

[76] Darsaut TE, Magro E, Bojanowski MW, Chaalala C, Nico L, Bacchus E, et al. Surgical treatment of brain arteriovenous malformations: clinical outcomes of patients included in the registry of a pragmatic randomized trial. *J Neurosurg*. 2023;138 (4):891-9.

[77] Raymond J, Benomar A, Gentric JC, Magro E, Nico L, Bacchus E, et al. Patient Selection in a Pragmatic Study on the Management of Patients with Brain Arteriovenous Malformations. *World Neurosurg*. 2023;172:e611-e24.

[78] Jin H, Huo X, Jiang Y, Li X, Li Y. Safety and efficacy of endovascular therapy and gamma knife surgery for brain arteriovenous malformations in China: Study protocol for an observational clinical trial. *Contemp Clin Trials Commun*. 2017;7:103-8.

[79] Fahed R, Darsaut TE, Mounayer C, Chapot R, Piotin M, Blanc R, et al. Transvenous Approach for the Treatment of cerebral Arteriovenous Malformations [TATAM]: Study protocol of a randomised controlled trial. *Interv Neuroradiol*. 2019;25 (3):305-9.

[80] Kim H, Al-Shahi Salman R, Flemming KD, Flint AC, Hess CP, Hetts S, et al. Abstract TP585: Long-Term Outcomes in Unruptured Brain Arteriovenous Malformation Patients: The Multicenter Arteriovenous Malformation Research Study [MARS]. *Stroke*. 2019;50 (Suppl_1):ATP585-ATP.

[81] Dabhi N, Sokolowski J, Zanaty M, Kellogg RT, Park MS, Mastorakos P. Primary Embolization of Cerebral Arteriovenous Malformations With Intention to Cure: A Systematic Review of Literature and Meta-Analysis. *Neurosurgery*. 2024.

[82] De Leacy R, Ansari SA, Schirmer CM, Cooke DL, Prestigiacomo CJ, Bulsara KR, et al. Endovascular treatment in the multimodality management of brain arteriovenous malformations: report of the Society of NeuroInterventional Surgery Standards and Guidelines Committee. *J Neurointerv Surg*. 2022;14 (11):1118-24.

[83] Gobin YP, Laurent A, Merienne L, Schlienger M, Aymard A, Houdart E, et al. Treatment of brain arteriovenous malformations by embolization and radiosurgery. *J Neurosurg*. 1996;85 (1):19-28.

[84] van Beijnum J, van der Worp HB, Buis DR, Al-Shahi Salman R, Kappelle LJ, Rinkel GJ, et al. Treatment of brain arteriovenous malformations: a systematic review and meta-analysis. *JAMA*. 2011;306 (18):2011-9.

[85] Viñuela F, Dion JE, Duckwiler G, Martin NA, Lylyk P, Fox A, et al. Combined endovascular embolization and surgery in the management of cerebral arteriovenous malformations: experience with 101 cases. *J Neurosurg*. 1991;75 (6):856-64.

[86] Iosif C, de Lucena AF, Abreu-Mattos LG, Ala VHE, El-Ghanam A, Saleme S, et al. Curative endovascular treatment for low-grade Spetzler-Martin brain arteriovenous malformations: a single-center prospective study. *J Neurointerv Surg*. 2019;11 (7):699-705.

[87] Katsaridis V, Papagiannaki C, Aimar E. Curative embolization of cerebral arteriovenous malformations [AVMs] with Onyx in 101 patients. *Neuroradiology*. 2008;50 (7):589-97.

[88] van Rooij WJ, Jacobs S, Sluzewski M, van der Pol B, Beute GN, Sprengers ME. Curative embolization of brain arteriovenous malformations with onyx: patient selection, embolization technique, and results. *AJNR Am J Neuroradiol*. 2012;33 (7):1299-304.

[89] Halbach VV, Higashida RT, Hieshima GB, Hardin CW, Pribram H. Transvenous embolization of dural fistulas involving the cavernous sinus. *AJNR Am J Neuroradiol*. 1989;10 (2):377-83.

[90] Zaki Ghali G, Zaki Ghali MG, Zaki Ghali E. Transvenous embolization of arteriovenous malformations. *Clin Neurol Neurosurg*. 2019;178:70-6.

[91] Choudhri O, Ivan ME, Lawton MT. Transvenous Approach to Intracranial Arteriovenous Malformations: Challenging the Axioms of Arteriovenous Malformation Therapy? *Neurosurgery*. 2015;77 (4):644-51; discussion 52.

[92] Houdart E. *Angioarchitecture des malformations arterio-veneuses cerebrales de l'adulte: Correlations radio-cliniques*. Paris, Universite de Paris VII, 1991 [dissertation].

[93] University of California at Los Angeles. New catheter for alternative embolization of brain arteriovenous malformations: Nonconfidential synopsis number LA92-023-01, in Technologies Available for Licensing. Los Angeles, UCLA, 1994, p 25.

[94] Houdart E, Gobin YP, Casasco A, Aymard A, Herbreteau D, Merland JJ. A proposed angiographic classification of intracranial arteriovenous fistulae and malformations. *Neuroradiology*. 1993;35 (5):381-5.

[95] Mullan S. Reflections upon the nature and management of intracranial and intraspinal vascular malformations and fistulae. J Neurosurg. 1994;80 (4):606-16.

[96] Massoud TF, Hademenos GJ. Transvenous retrograde nidus sclerotherapy under controlled hypotension [TRENSH]: a newly proposed treatment for brain arteriovenous malformations--concepts and rationale. *Neurosurgery*. 1999;45 (2):351-63; discussion 63-5.

[97] Nguyen TN, Chin LS, Souza R, Norbash AM. Transvenous embolization of a ruptured cerebral arteriovenous malformation with en-passage arterial supply: initial case report. *J Neurointerv Surg*. 2010;2 (2):150-2.

[98] Kessler I, Riva R, Ruggiero M, Manisor M, Al-Khawaldeh M, Mounayer C. Successful transvenous embolization of brain arteriovenous malformations using Onyx in five consecutive patients. *Neurosurgery*. 2011;69 (1):184-93; discussion 93.

[99] He Y, Ding Y, Bai W, Li T, Hui FK, Jiang WJ, et al. Safety and Efficacy of Transvenous Embolization of Ruptured Brain Arteriovenous Malformations as a Last Resort: A Prospective Single-Arm Study. *AJNR Am J Neuroradiol*. 2019;40 (10):1744-51.

[100] De Sousa JMB, Iosif C, Sganzerla LZ, Rafie AN, Borodetsky V, Rouchaud A, et al. Selection of Patients for Treatment of Brain Arteriovenous Malformations by the Transvenous Approach: Relationship with Venous Anatomy and Risk of Hemorrhagic Complications. *AJNR Am J Neuroradiol*. 2020;41 (12):2311-6.

[101] Beslow LA, Vossough A, Kim H, Nelson J, Lawton MT, Pollak J, et al. Brain AVM compactness score in children with hereditary hemorrhagic telangiectasia. *Childs Nerv Syst*. 2024;40 (7):2101-8.

[102] Mendes GA, Silveira EP, Caire F, Boncoeur Martel MP, Saleme S, Iosif C, et al. Endovascular Management of Deep Arteriovenous Malformations: Single Institution Experience in 22 Consecutive Patients. *Neurosurgery*. 2016;78 (1):34-41.

[103] Viana DC, de Castro-Afonso LH, Nakiri GS, Monsignore LM, Trivelato FP, Colli BO, et al. Extending the indications for transvenous approach embolization for superficial brain arteriovenous malformations. J Neurointerv Surg. 2017;9 (11):1053-9.

[104] Mendes GAC, Kalani MYS, Iosif C, Lucena AF, Carvalho R, Saleme S, et al. Transvenous Curative Embolization of Cerebral Arteriovenous Malformations: A Prospective Cohort Study. *Neurosurgery*. 2018;83 (5):957-64.

[105] Koyanagi M, Mosimann PJ, Nordmeyer H, Heddier M, Krause J, Narata AP, et al. The transvenous retrograde pressure cooker technique for the curative embolization of high-grade brain arteriovenous malformations. *J Neurointerv Surg*. 2021;13 (7):637-41.

[106] Massoud TF, Hademenos GJ, Young WL, Gao E, Pile-Spellman J. Can induction of systemic hypotension help prevent nidus rupture complicating arteriovenous malformation embolization?: analysis of underlying mechanism achieved using a theoretical model. *AJNR Am J Neuroradiol.* 2000;21 (7):1255-67.

[107] Lim J, Shallwani H, Vakharia K, Siddiqui AH. Adenosine-Induced Cardiac Arrest for Transvenous Embolization of Midbrain Arteriovenous Malformation. *Oper Neurosurg* (Hagerstown). 2020;18 (6):E184-e90.

[108] Ghorbani M, Griessenauer CJ, Wipplinger C, Jabbour P, Asl MK, Rahbarian F, et al. Adenosine-induced transient circulatory arrest in transvenous embolization of cerebral arteriovenous malformations. *Neuroradiol J.* 2021;34 (5):509-16.

[109] He Y, Bai W, Li T, Hui FK, He Y, Xu B. Curative Transvenous Embolization for Ruptured Brain Arteriovenous Malformations: A Single-Center Experience from China. *World Neurosurg.* 2018;116:e421-e8.

[110] Pop R, Harsan O, Martin I, Mihoc D, Richter JS, Manisor M, et al. Balloon-assisted coiling of intracranial aneurysms using the Eclipse 2L double lumen balloon. *Interv Neuroradiol.* 2020;26 (3):291-9.

[111] Chapot R, Stracke P, Velasco A, Nordmeyer H, Heddier M, Stauder M, et al. The pressure cooker technique for the treatment of brain AVMs. *J Neuroradiol.* 2014;41 (1):87-91.

[112] Wang X, Yu J. Coiling of an iatrogenic aneurysm of the distal posterior inferior cerebellar artery via a Marathon microcatheter. Interdisciplinary *Neurosurgery.* 2024;36:101950.

[113] Zhou Z, Yu J. Coiling an aneurysm in the twig-like MCA via a Marathon microcatheter: A case report. *Int J Surg Case Rep.* 2024;119:109661.

[114] Li B, Yu J. Embolization of an arteriovenous malformation using the "pressure cooker" technique in the AICA via a marathon microcatheter: A case report. *Int J Surg Case Rep.* 2024;120:109905.

[115] Spetzler RF, Martin NA. A proposed grading system for arteriovenous malformations. J Neurosurg. 1986;65 (4):476-83.

[116] Lawton MT, Kim H, McCulloch CE, Mikhak B, Young WL. A supplementary grading scale for selecting patients with brain arteriovenous malformations for surgery. *Neurosurgery.* 2010;66 (4):702-13; discussion 13.

[117] Spetzler RF, Ponce FA. A 3-tier classification of cerebral arteriovenous malformations. Clinical article. *J Neurosurg.* 2011;114 (3):842-9.

[118] Feliciano CE, de León-Berra R, Hernández-Gaitán MS, Rodríguez-Mercado R. A proposal for a new arteriovenous malformation grading scale for neuroendovascular procedures and literature review. *P R Health Sci J.* 2010;29 (2):117-20.

[119] Dumont TM, Kan P, Snyder KV, Hopkins LN, Siddiqui AH, Levy EI. A proposed grading system for endovascular treatment of cerebral arteriovenous malformations: Buffalo score. *Surg Neurol Int.* 2015;6:3.

[120] Lopes DK, Moftakhar R, Straus D, Munich SA, Chaus F, Kaszuba MC. Arteriovenous malformation embocure score: AVMES. *J Neurointerv Surg.* 2016;8 (7):685-91.

[121] Zhang H, Su Y, Liang S, Lv X. Transarterial AVM embolization using Tsinghua grading system: Patient selection and complete obliteration. *Neuroscience Informatics.* 2024;4 (2):100160.

[122] Rivera R, Cespedes A, Cruz JP, Rouchaud A, Mounayer C. Brain Arteriovenous Malformation In Vitro Model for Transvenous Embolization Using 3D Printing and Real Patient Data. *AJNR Am J Neuroradiol.* 2024;45 (5):612-7.

[123] R BS, Korkmazer B, Süleyman K, Hikmat E, Kocer N, Islak C, et al. Dynamic [live] 3D roadmap as navigational tool in multiplug brain arteriovenous malformation embolization: technical note. *Neuroradiology.* 2024;66 (1):129-33.

[124] Xiang W, Yan L, Zhao Y, Yang M, Bai S, Ma L, et al. Four-dimensional digital subtraction angiography to assess cerebral arteriovenous malformations. *J Neuroimaging.* 2023;33 (1):67-72.

[125] Falk KL, Schafer S, Speidel MA, Strother CM. 4D-DSA: Development and Current Neurovascular Applications. *AJNR Am J Neuroradiol.* 2021;42 (2):214-20.

[126] Li X, Xiang S, Li G. Application of artificial intelligence in brain arteriovenous malformations: Angioarchitectures, clinical symptoms and prognosis prediction. *Interv Neuroradiol*. 2024:15910199241238798.

[127] Hao Q, Zhang H, Han H, Jin H, Ma L, Li R, et al. Recurrence of Cerebral Arteriovenous Malformation Following Complete Obliteration Through Endovascular Embolization. *Transl Stroke Res*. 2023.

Chapter 18

The History and Development of DAVFs Embolization and Classifications

Chao Ma*, PhD
Department of Neurosurgery, Beijing Chaoyang Hospital, Capital Medical University, Beijing, China

Abstract

This article reviewed the history and development of embolization for dural arteriovenous fistulas (DAVFs) and discusses the evolution of classification systems. It highlighted the limitations of early surgical treatments and describes the shift towards embolization as imaging technology and minimally invasive endovascular techniques advanced. The introduction of liquid embolic agents, such as N-butyl cyanoacrylate (NBCA) and Onyx, significantly improved treatment outcomes by providing better occlusion and reducing complications. The article also presented two case studies, illustrating the successful application of modern liquid embolic agents and endovascular techniques in treating complex DAVFs. Future directions in DAVF treatment are expected to focus on further improvements in embolic materials and the integration of advanced imaging techniques to enhance the safety and efficacy of embolization procedures.

Keywords: dural arteriovenous fistula, embolization, endovascular techniques

Introduction

Intracranial DAVFs account for 10%–15% of all intracranial vascular malformations [1]. These lesions derive their arterial supply primarily from meningeal vessels, and the venous drainage is either via dural venous sinuses, through the cortical veins or via perimedullary veins. While the etiology of DAVFs is not fully understood, many cases are believed to be acquired, potentially due to factors like dural sinus thrombosis, trauma, or previous surgery. These lesions are typically found near major dural venous sinuses, such as the transverse-sigmoid, cavernous, and superior sagittal sinuses (SSS). The pattern of venous drainage observed on dynamic

* Corresponding Author's Email: machao3270@163.com

In: World History of Neurointerventional Surgery
Editors: Xianli Lv and Zhongxue Wu
ISBN: 979-8-89530-792-2

vascular imaging determines the type of DAVF and correlates with the severity of symptoms and the risk of hemorrhage [2].

The clinical manifestations of DAVFs can range from asymptomatic to severe, depending on the angioarchitecture, particularly the venous drainage pattern. Aggressive DAVFs, characterized by leptomeningeal venous reflux, are associated with a high risk of intracranial hemorrhage and other neurological complications, necessitating prompt and effective treatment.

With an understanding of the pathophysiology and clinical manifestations of dural arteriovenous fistulas, it becomes imperative to explore the advances in treatment modalities and the nuanced classification systems that have been developed. These classifications not only aid in the understanding of DAVFs but also guide the selection of appropriate therapeutic strategies, including the increasingly refined techniques in endovascular embolization. By delving into both the classifications and treatment options, we can appreciate the evolution of DAVF management from a rudimentary understanding to the sophisticated approaches utilized in modern neurosurgery.

Conservative Management and Challenges

The initial management of intracranial DAVFs was predominantly surgical. During the mid-20th century, the standard treatment for DAVFs involved direct surgical resection of the fistula, often necessitating craniotomy. These early surgeries aimed to directly obliterate the abnormal arteriovenous connections by either resecting the involved dura or interrupting the feeding arteries and draining veins [3]. However, surgical approaches were often limited by the complexity of the fistula's angioarchitecture, particularly in cases with deep-seated or extensive fistulas.

One of the main challenges of surgical treatment was the high morbidity and mortality associated with craniotomy, particularly for fistulas located in critical areas, such as the cavernous sinus or near the brainstem. These surgeries required extensive brain exposure, which increased the risk of complications such as infection, hemorrhage, and neurological deficits. As a result, surgical treatment was often reserved for life-threatening cases or those refractory to other treatments [4].

In the 1960s and 1970s, as the understanding of DAVFs improved, there was a gradual shift towards more conservative management strategies for non-aggressive, asymptomatic fistulas. Observation with serial imaging became a viable option for patients with DAVFs that did not pose an immediate risk of hemorrhage or neurological decline. This conservative approach was particularly recommended for older patients or those with significant comorbidities, where the risks of surgery outweighed the benefits [5].

The development of stereotactic radiosurgery in the 1980s provided an alternative, non-invasive treatment for DAVFs. Radiosurgery, particularly gamma knife and linear accelerator-based treatments, became popular for their ability to target and obliterate the fistula with high precision, reducing the need for craniotomy. Radiosurgery was particularly advantageous for small, deep-seated fistulas that were difficult to access surgically. However, the main limitation of radiosurgery was the delayed effect, as complete obliteration of the fistula often took months to years, during which the risk of hemorrhage persisted [4].

History and Development of Intracranial DAVFs Embolization

Advent of Endovascular Techniques

The real paradigm shifts in DAVF treatment occurred with the advent of endovascular techniques in the 1980s. This minimally invasive approach revolutionized the management of DAVFs, offering a safer and more effective alternative to surgery and radiosurgery. Early endovascular treatments primarily involved the use of embolic materials such as polyvinyl alcohol (PVA) particles and detachable balloons to occlude the feeding arteries or the fistula itself [6].

Initially, these procedures were performed via a transarterial approach, where the embolic agent was delivered directly into the arterial feeders of the DAVF. While these early techniques showed promise, they were associated with significant limitations, including incomplete occlusion, recanalization, and difficulty in navigating tortuous arteries. Despite these challenges, the success of early endovascular treatments paved the way for further innovations in embolization [5, 6].

Development and Refinement of Embolic Materials

In the late 1980s and 1990s, the development of liquid embolic agents marked a major advancement in the endovascular treatment of DAVFs. One of the first widely used liquid agents was N-butyl cyanoacrylate (NBCA), a fast-acting glue that polymerized upon contact with blood. NBCA allowed for deeper penetration into the fistula and better occlusion compared to particulate embolic agents. However, NBCA's rapid polymerization and adhesive properties made it challenging to control, leading to complications such as non-target embolization and catheter entrapment [7, 8].

Embolizing external carotid branches with particles is a relatively simple procedure that can effectively reduce shunt flow. However, achieving total obliteration through transarterial particulate embolization is typically difficult because some feeding arteries are inaccessible, and collateral arteries may continue to supply blood to the lesion [9]. Consequently, this method is primarily used to alleviate symptoms or in conjunction with other treatments such as irradiation, surgery, or transvenous embolization (TVE).

Using glue to occlude the collecting vein or fistula via the transarterial route can potentially cure the condition, but it poses a higher risk due to its less controllable nature compared to coil embolization. N-butyl-2-cyanoacrylate (NBCA) is often used in transarterial embolization (TAE) for complex DAVFs when percutaneous transvenous catheterization is not feasible [10]. The early 2000s saw the introduction of Onyx (ethylene-vinyl alcohol copolymer), which addressed many of the limitations of NBCA. Onyx, a newer non-adhesive liquid embolic agent composed of EVOH, DMSO, and tantalum, precipitates upon contact with blood to occlude vessels without adhering to the vessel walls. This unique property prevents the microcatheter from becoming glued to the vessels, allowing for a slow, prolonged injection with real-time angiographic monitoring. Proper positioning of the microcatheter and a controlled injection can achieve a complete fill of the fistula, leading to a potential cure. Onyx is currently available in two FDA-approved concentrations in the United States for presurgical cerebral AVM embolization [11]. Depending on the specific requirements, Onyx or glue in concentrations of 20%, 25%, or 33% may be used. Onyx is a non-adhesive liquid embolic agent that allows for slow, controlled injections, enabling more precise delivery to the target site. The non-adhesive nature of Onyx also reduced the risk of catheter entrapment, making it a safer and more effective option for DAVF embolization. Onyx quickly became the standard of care for endovascular treatment of DAVFs, especially for those with complex angioarchitecture or extensive cortical venous reflux [4].

More recently, other liquid embolic agents like SQUID have been developed, offering different viscosity formulations for greater flexibility in treatment. These advancements have further improved the safety and efficacy of endovascular embolization, allowing for the treatment of increasingly complex and high-risk DAVFs [6, 12].

The following two case presentations illustrate the successful use of these materials in the embolization of intricate DAVF structures, demonstrating how modern advancements in liquid embolic agents and endovascular techniques have revolutionized treatment outcomes (Figures 1 to 4).

Evolution of Endovascular Techniques

Alongside the development of new embolic materials, endovascular techniques have also evolved. Initially, transarterial embolization (TAE) was the primary approach for most DAVFs. However, as understanding of DAVF angioarchitecture improved, transvenous embolization (TVE) became more widely adopted, particularly for DAVFs involving the transverse-sigmoid sinus or the superior sagittal sinus. TVE involves navigating a catheter through the venous system to reach the fistula, where coils or liquid embolic agents are deployed to occlude the fistula.

In some cases, a combined transarterial and transvenous approach is used to achieve complete occlusion, particularly in complex or recurrent DAVFs. Direct puncture of the affected sinus has also been employed in challenging cases where traditional arterial or venous access is not feasible.

Coils are frequently employed for curative purposes, with studies indicating their effectiveness, achieving complete occlusion in 80-100% of cases [13]. An angiographically non-visualized inferior petrosal sinus (IPS) can be successfully catheterized in 30-50% of patients [14]. If the IPS is thrombosed, alternative transvenous access routes, such as the superior petrosal sinus (SPS), facial vein, angular vein, pterygoid sinus, and superior ophthalmic vein (SOV), may be attempted [15]. Inadequate embolization can lead to worsening symptoms. Using detachable coils before injecting Onyx or glue helps slow and reduce flow in the fistula, providing a stable foundation for the Onyx or glue cast.

Stents have been explored as a method to close shunts in dural arteriovenous fistulas. According to Kieran et al. it is possible to recanalize a chronically occluded dural venous sinus and achieve complete closure of multiple DAVF feeders through stent deployment. [16] However, the long-term outcomes of stent use in treating DAVFs are still unknown. Stents can restore antegrade sinus flow by exerting radial force to close the shunts within the sinus wall [17].

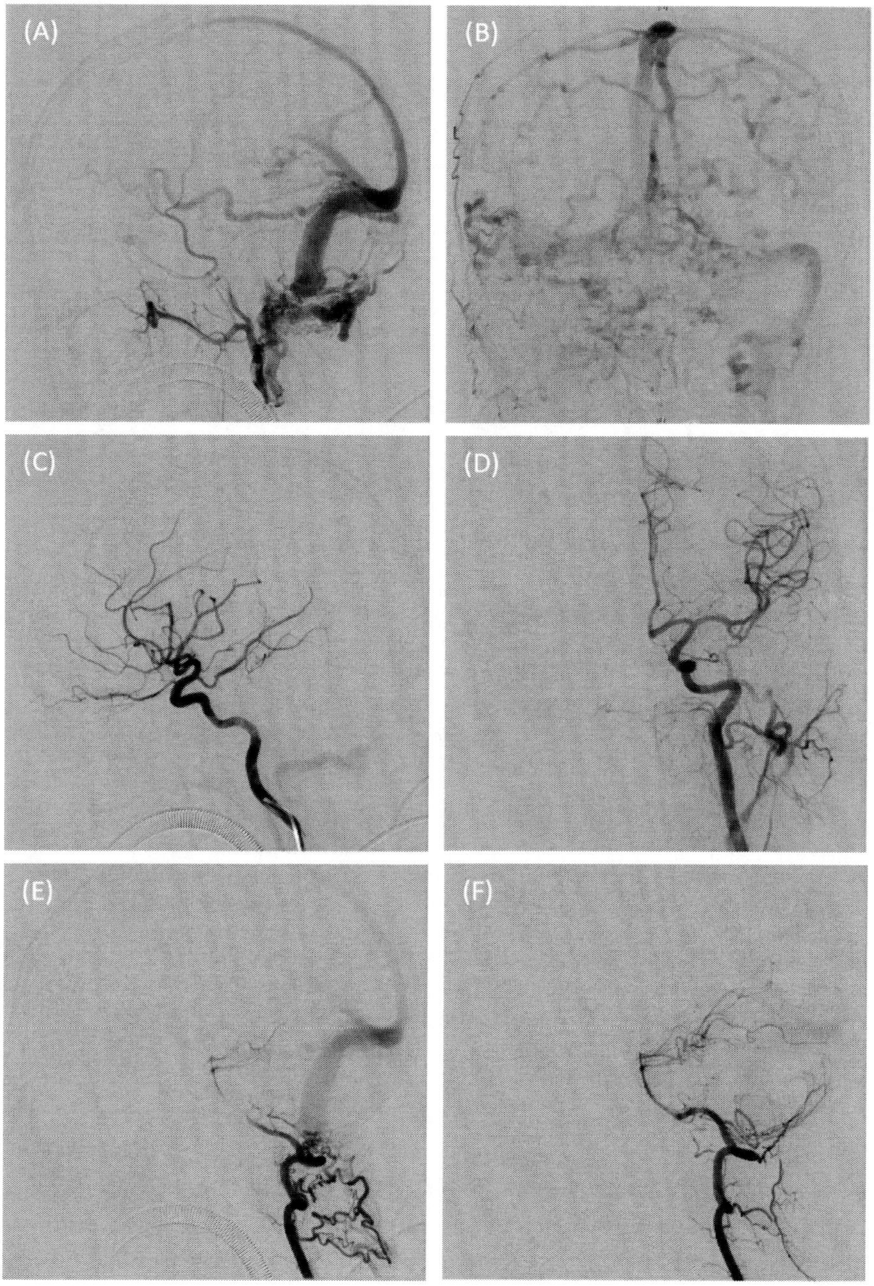

Figure 1. A 37-year-old male patient presented with intermittent headaches, nausea, and vomiting for 20 days with no apparent cause. Cranial DSA revealed a dural arteriovenous fistula (DAVF) in the right transverse-sigmoid sinus region. (A) Angiography of the right external carotid artery shows retrograde blood flow within the venous sinus with pressure transmission in the reverse direction. (B) Retrograde venous sinus flow caused cortical venous dilation and late-stage dynamic occlusion. (C) Angiography of the right internal carotid artery shows no blood supply to the DAVF. (D) Angiography of the left common carotid artery shows no blood supply to the DAVF. (E) Angiography of the right vertebral artery. (F) Angiography of the left vertebral artery.

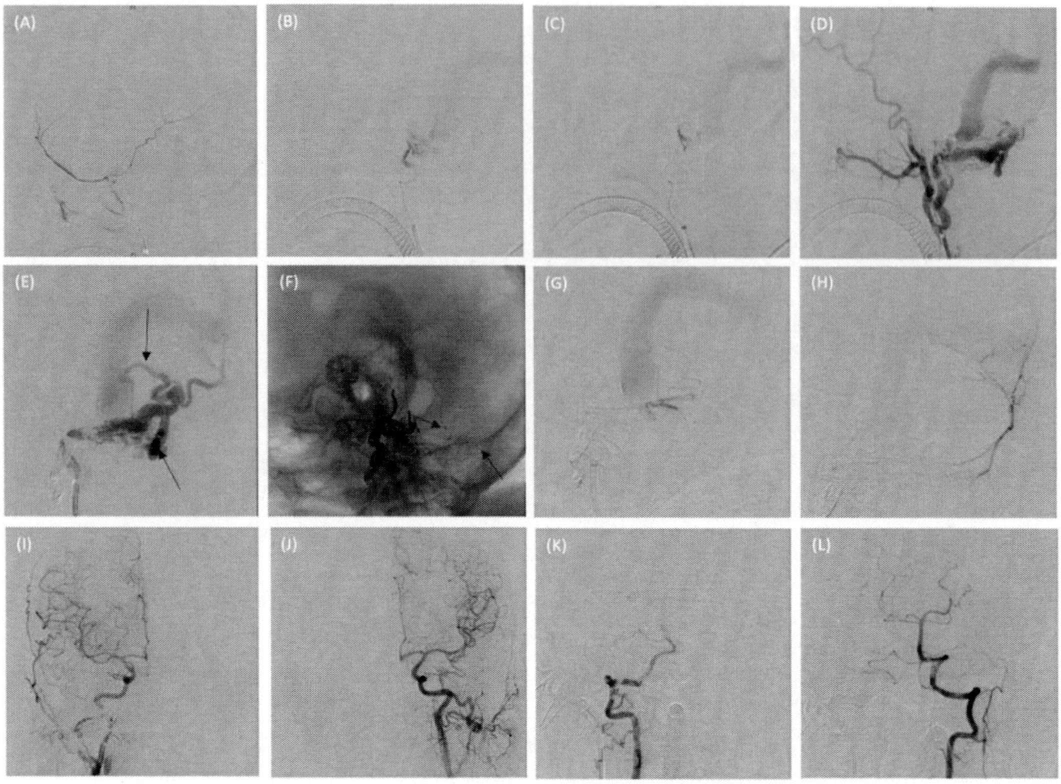

Figure 2. (A) Minimal contrast injection shows no blood supply from the right middle meningeal artery. (B-C) An Echelon10 microcatheter was super-selectively advanced into the ascending pharyngeal artery, and partial embolization of the fistula was performed using Onyx. (D-E) Post-embolization angiography of the ascending pharyngeal artery shows residual blood supply from branches of the occipital artery (indicated by red arrows). (F-G-H) Two additional Echelon10 microcatheters were super-selectively advanced into branches of the occipital artery (indicated by red arrows) with minimal contrast injection, and the fistula was completely embolized using Onyx. (I-J-K-L) Post-procedural angiography demonstrates complete embolization of the fistula.

Current Approaches and Future Directions

Today, the treatment of DAVFs is highly individualized for the specific angioarchitecture of the fistula, the presence of cortical venous reflux, and the patient's overall health status. The continued evolution of embolic materials and techniques has made it possible to treat even the most complex DAVFs with high success rates and low morbidity. However, challenges remain, particularly in achieving complete occlusion in high-grade DAVFs with extensive arterial supply or in cases where the fistula located in a critical area.

Future advancements in DAVF treatment are likely to focus on the development of new embolic agents with improved control and safety profiles, as well as the integration of advanced imaging techniques to better visualize and assess the fistula before and during treatment. The goal is to continue reducing the risks associated with DAVF embolization while improving long-term outcomes for patients.

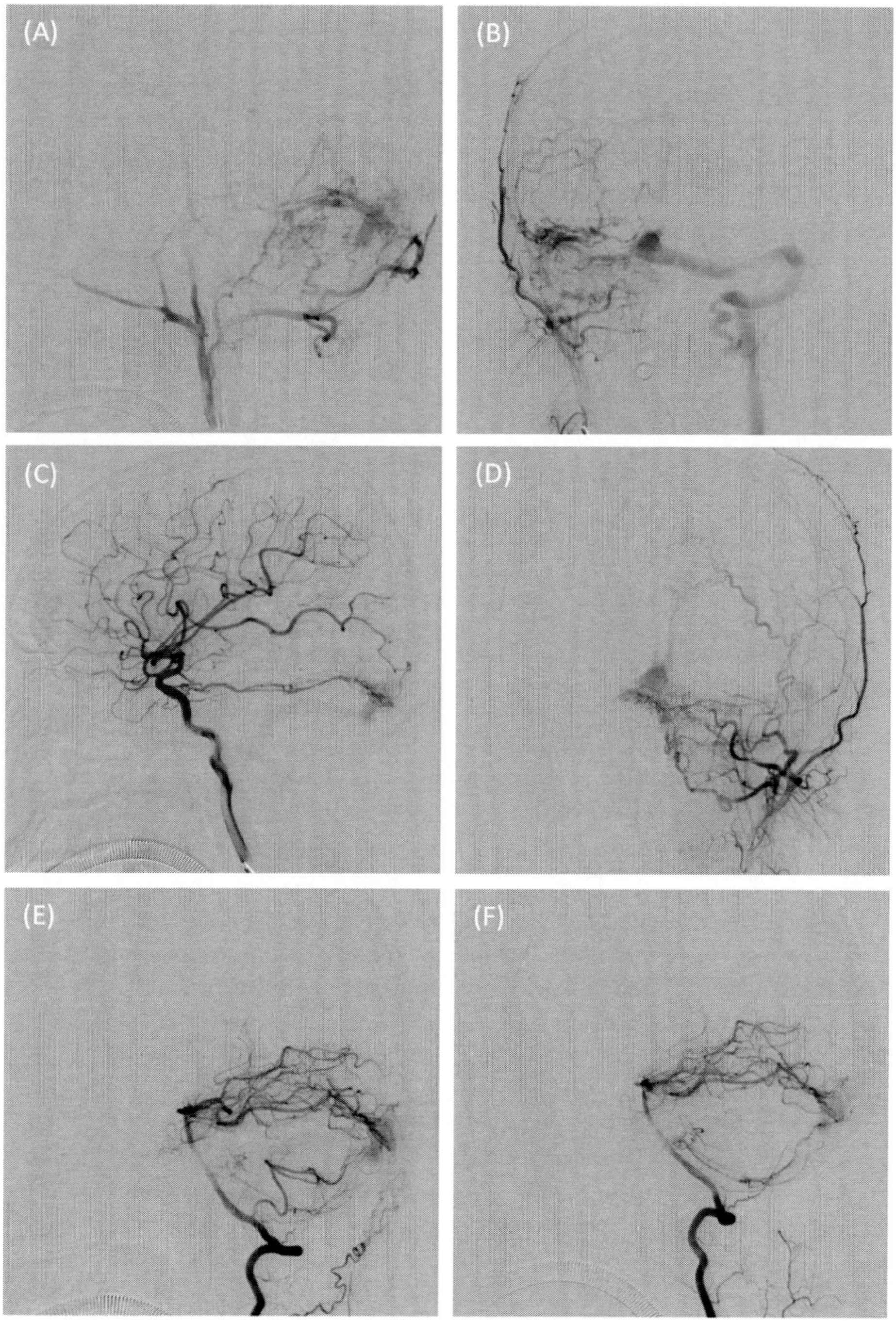

Figure 3. A 45-year-old male patient presented with pulsatile tinnitus for six months, blurred vision for three months, and a diagnosis of dural arteriovenous fistula (DAVF) one month ago. The DAVF located in the right transverse-sigmoid sinus region. (A-B) Angiography of the right external carotid artery shows blood supply to the fistula without retrograde flow in the venous sinus. (B) Retrograde venous sinus flow caused cortical venous dilation and late-stage dynamic occlusion. (C) Angiography of the right internal carotid artery shows no blood supply to the DAVF. (D) Angiography of the left external carotid artery shows blood supply to the DAVF. (E) Angiography of the right vertebral artery shows no arterial supply. (F) Angiography of the left vertebral artery shows no arterial supply.

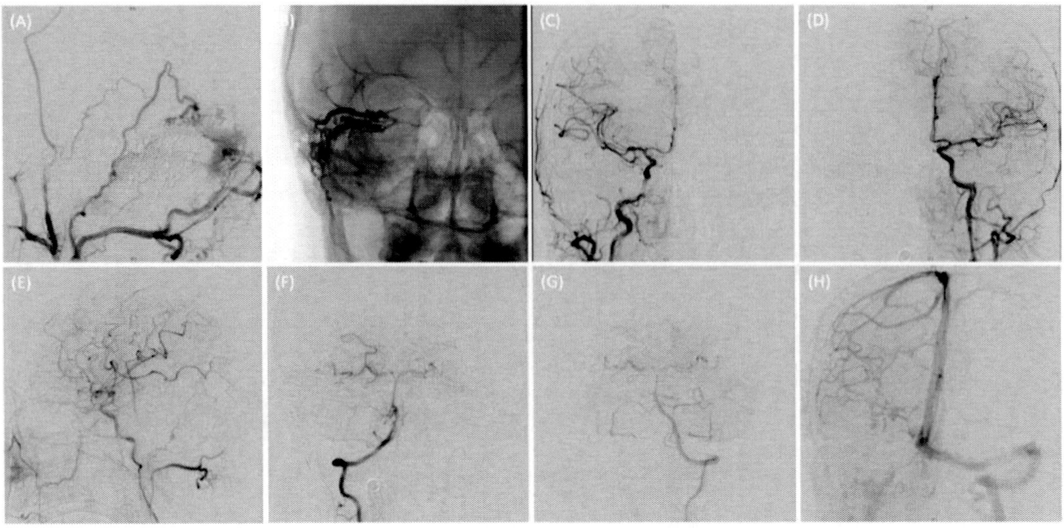

Figure 4. (A-B) The Echelon10 microcatheter was advanced into the petrosquamous branch of the middle meningeal artery, and Onyx was intermittently injected to achieve complete embolization of the fistula. (C-D) Post-procedural bilateral common carotid artery angiography demonstrates complete embolization of the fistula. (E) Lateral view of right common carotid artery angiography shows complete fistula embolization. (F-G) Bilateral vertebral artery angiography. (H) Venous phase of right common carotid artery angiography shows no retrograde flow in the venous sinus.

History and Development of Spinal Dural Arteriovenous Fistula Embolization

In 1968, Doppman et al. conducted the first embolization of a spinal dural arteriovenous fistula, marking a significant advancement in the treatment of this condition [18]. Currently, endovascular treatment is often the first-line therapy for dural arteriovenous fistulas of the spine due to its low morbidity rate and high potential for cure [19]. If initial endovascular treatment is unsuccessful, surgery or repeat angiography/embolization may be considered [19].

Endovascular intervention has evolved significantly over the years, transitioning from an adjunct to a viable alternative to surgery [20]. The success rate of endovascular management ranges between 70% and 89.5% [21]. In a study involving 61 patients treated with N-Butyl-2-cyanoacrylate, the success rate was 77% [21]. Despite advancements, the endovascular treatment group still experiences a significant failure rate of 23%, although this has been steadily decreasing over the past decade due to improvements in interventional neuroradiology techniques and experience [21].

Embolization, which is less invasive than surgery, can be performed in the same session as spinal angiography [22]. The penetration of adhesive material to the proximal vein during angiography indicates successful endovascular treatment [21]. However, inadequate glue distribution between the arterial and venous segments can lead to fistula recurrence [22]. Particle embolization is not recommended due to high recanalization rates; instead, liquid embolization materials are essential to prevent recanalization [22, 23].

Performing the treatment under general anesthesia allows for better imaging, particularly in the thoracic spine where respiration can cause artifacts [22]. Diagnostic angiography is performed prior to embolization to fully delineate the vascular anatomy and select the best feeder vessel for approaching and embolizing the fistula [21, 23]. Post-embolization, these vessels should be rechecked to ensure no fistula remnants remain [21, 23]. Most patients undergo a transfemoral approach [21]. The choice of catheter for the guide catheter is crucial for stability within the involved segmental artery during the procedure, considering the aorta's diameter and the segmental arteries' angle of origin [21]. The microcatheter tip is positioned as close as possible to the fistula [21]. Two main causes of treatment failure are the inability to position the microcatheter in the wedge position and placing it too far from the lesion due to navigation difficulties [21, 23].

Embolization is considered safe for lumbar lesions, provided the artery of Adamkiewicz does not originate from the same segmental artery as the radiculomeningeal artery feeding the fistula [22]. A relative contraindication exists if the same segmental artery supplying the fistula also contributes to the posterior spinal artery [22]. Suitable candidates for endovascular therapy are those without a common origin for the arteries supplying the spinal cord and the dural fistula, and those without stenosis or occlusion of the relevant segmental artery [21].

When performed by an experienced team, endovascular management has a very low morbidity rate [23]. Additionally, as endovascular treatment is less invasive than open surgery, patients experience less postoperative pain and shorter hospital stays [23]. Microsurgical treatment is recommended if the arteriovenous shunt persists after one or more endovascular procedures [21]. The effectiveness and overall durability of endovascular intervention have improved with the development of better embolic agents, though it remains somewhat inferior to surgical occlusion [20].

Classification Systems of DAVF

1. Traditional Classifications

The first classification of DAVFs that correlated their patterns of venous drainage with symptoms was published in 1977 by Djindjian, Merland and Theron [24]. The authors assumed that those DAVFs that drained freely into a sinus cause only benign symptoms, whereas those with cortical venous drainage might cause aggressive neurologic symptoms and hemorrhage. DAVFs were first classified into four types: type I, with immediate drainage into a sinus or a meningeal vein; type II, with drainage into a sinus with reflux into other sinuses or cortical veins; type III, with drainage into a cortical vein; and type IV, with drainage into a cortical vein with a giant venous pouch [24]. The Borden classification has three subtypes and is more user-friendly [25]. This classification was modified by Cognard, Merland et al. in 1995 after reviewing a series of 205 consecutive patients with DAVFs over 18 years [26]. They statistically correlated the new classification and various clinical and angiographic features with the aggressive neurologic behaviour of DAVFs. The revised classification was more complex and inclusive because of the high variability of type II DAVFs and the addition of type V DAVFs, with spinal venous drainage responsible for myelopathy.

Borden classification [25]	
1	Venous drainage directly into dural venous sinus or meningeal vein
2	Venous drainage into dural venous sinus with cortical venous reflux
3	Venous drainage directly into subarachnoid veins (cortical venous reflux only)

Cognard classification [26]	
I	Venous drainage into dural venous sinus with antegrade flow
II a	Venous drainage into dural venous sinus with retrograde flow
II b	Venous drainage into dural venous sinus with antegrade flow and CVR
II a + b	Venous drainage into dural venous sinus with retrograde flow and CVR
III	Venous drainage directly into subarachnoid veins (CVR only)
IV	Type III with venous ectasias of the draining subarachnoid veins
V	Direct drainage into spinal perimedullary veins (CVR indicates cortical venous reflux)

2. New Classification Methods

Casasco et al. [27] noted a potential subtype of venous pattern in type 4 fistulas: intracranial dural AV fistulas with drainage into pial veins, venous ectasia, and reflux into spinal perimedullary veins. This DAVF variant integrates two aggressive drainage patterns, not included in the initial classification. Further extensive research is required to understand this condition. They hypothesize these patients face higher risks of intracranial or spinal hemorrhage and aggressive neurological progression with myelopathy. If verified, its diagnosis may necessitate urgent treatment.

A new subtype of intracranial dural AVF according to the patterns of venous drainage [27]	
"Benign"	
I	Dural sinus with antegrade flow
IIa	Dural sinus with reflux only into the sinus
"Aggresive"	
IIb	Dural sinus with reflux into cortical veins
IIa + b	Dural sinus with reflux into sinus and cortical veins
III	Directly into cortical veins
IV	Directly into cortical veins with venous ectasia
V	Spinal perimedullary veins
Iv + v	Into cortical veins with venous ectasia and spinal perimedullary veins

Becerril-Gaitan et al. [28] introduce the VEBAS scoring system, a practical tool designed to predict the success rate of treatments for intracranial dural arteriovenous fistulas (dAVFs). Developed using data from over 1000 dAVF cases in a multicenter database, the VEBAS scoring system is based on five key components:

the VEBAS scoring system [28]
Venous stenosis: Presence vs. absence
Elderly age: <75 years vs. ≥75 years
Borden classification: I vs. II-III
Arterial feeders: Single vs. multiple
Surgery: Presence vs. absence of past cranial surgery

The name "VEBAS" is derived from the first letters of these five components. Each component is assigned a different weight based on its odds ratio for predicting complete obliteration, with the total score ranging from 0 to 12. Higher VEBAS scores indicate a greater likelihood of complete dAVF obliteration. The system has been validated using ROC curves and AUC values, demonstrating high predictive accuracy in clinical practice.

The current classification systems for cavernous sinus dural arteriovenous fistula (CS-DAVF), primarily the Barrow classification system and the Cognard classification system, are inadequate for modern clinical practice: Barrow Classification System primarily categorizes based on arterial supply and venous drainage anatomy, but it fails to adequately address the morphological and hemodynamic characteristics of the lesions. This system is not effective in describing the draining anatomy and hemodynamics of CS-DAVF, which are crucial for understanding the natural history, prognosis, and treatment of the condition. Cognard Classification System considers some morphological and hemodynamic features but is limited in its application to CS-DAVF. For instance, it struggles to accurately classify lesions with significant orbital drainage but no retrograde leptomeningeal venous drainage [29].

To address the shortcomings of existing systems, Wenderoth et al. [29] proposes a new classification system. The new system categorizes CS-DAVF based on the presence of unilateral or bilateral arteriovenous shunting, ipsilateral, contralateral, or bilateral venous drainage, the patency or occlusion of the relevant inferior petrosal sinus (IPS), and the presence or absence of retrograde leptomeningeal venous drainage.

Wenderoth classification [29]
Type 1: Lesions with unilateral or bilateral cavernous sinus involvement and patent IPS.
Type 2: Lesions with unilateral or bilateral cavernous sinus involvement with one IPS patent and the other occluded.
Type 3: Lesions with unilateral or bilateral cavernous sinus involvement with both IPS occluded.

The new classification system allows for a more accurate and reproducible description of the primary arterial feeding and venous drainage patterns of CS-DAVF. Hemorrhage Risk Marker: It incorporates a marker for the risk of intracranial hemorrhage, based on the presence of retrograde leptomeningeal venous drainage. The classification provides insights into the preferred treatment route and urgency for a given lesion type based on its characteristics. Wenderoth's proposed classification system offers significant improvements over the existing Barrow and Cognard systems by more accurately reflecting the morphological and hemodynamic features of CS-DAVF. This enhanced classification allows for better description of the lesions, assessment of hemorrhage risk, and guidance on treatment decisions.

3. Comparative Analysis of Classification Systems for Carotid Cavernous Fistula (CCF)

Carotid cavernous fistula (CCF) is a complex vascular condition characterized by abnormal communication between the carotid artery and the cavernous sinus. Various classification systems have been proposed to describe its diverse manifestations.

The Barrow classification is widely used and focuses primarily on the arterial characteristics of the fistula:

Barrow Classification [30]
Type A: Direct shunt between the internal carotid artery (ICA) and the cavernous sinus.
Type B: Shunt between branches of the ICA and the cavernous sinus.
Type C: Shunt between branches of the external carotid artery (ECA) and the cavernous sinus.
Type D: Shunt involving both ICA and ECA branches.

The Thomas classification provides a more detailed description of the venous drainage patterns:

Thomas Classification [31]
Type 1: Drainage posteriorly (inferior and/or superior petrosal sinuses) and/or inferiorly (pterygoid and parapharyngeal plexus).
Type 2: Drainage posterior/inferior and anterior (superior and inferior ophthalmic veins).
Type 3: Anterior drainage only.
Type 4: Retrograde drainage into cortical veins.
Type 5: High-flow direct shunt between cavernous ICA and cavernous sinus (Barrow type A) with multiple venous drainage routes.

Each classification system for CCF has its own strengths and limitations. The Barrow classification is straightforward and easy to use but lacks detail on venous drainage. The Thomas classification adds valuable information about venous patterns, enhancing its clinical utility.

A newly proposed API-ACE classification integrates both arterial and venous characteristics:

API-ACE Classification [32]
A±I: Anterior drainage (superior and inferior ophthalmic veins) ± inferior (pterygoid and parapharyngeal plexus).
P±I: Posterior drainage (inferior and/or superior petrosal sinuses) ± inferior (pterygoid and parapharyngeal plexus).
A1: Direct fistula (Barrow type A).
A0: Indirect fistula.
C1: Presence of cortical efflux.
C0: Absence of cortical efflux.
E1: Presence of external carotid supply.
E0: Absence of external carotid supply.

The API-ACE classification offers a comprehensive view that integrates both arterial and venous characteristics, making it a powerful tool for understanding CCF's complex anatomy and guiding treatment. However, its complexity may limit its practical application.

4. Historical Classification of Spinal Arteriovenous Lesions:

Since Foix and Alajouanine first described spinal dural arteriovenous fistulas (DAVFs) in 1926, advancements in diagnostic tools have greatly enhanced our understanding of the angioarchitecture of these spinal vascular lesions. Despite these advancements, there remains a lack of consensus in the classification and terminology of spinal arteriovenous lesions. [33] These lesions have been described by various names and classified according to clinical features, anatomical location, and angioarchitecture. [34]

Generally, spinal vascular lesions are categorized into two main groups: arteriovenous shunting lesions, which include spinal arteriovenous malformations (AVMs) and arteriovenous fistulas (AVFs), and non-shunting lesions, such as capillary telangiectasia and cavernous malformations. This chapter will focus on spinal arteriovenous shunting lesions.

In 1971, Di Chiro et al. introduced the first classification of spinal AV shunts, categorizing them as type I (single coiled vessel), type II (glomus), and type III (juvenile). The majority of type I fistulas align with the current concept of spinal DAVFs, while the other types correspond to intramedullary AVMs. In 1986, a direct spinal AVF, now termed a perimedullary fistula, was added as type IV, described as a direct arteriovenous shunt between the anterior spinal artery and vein located ventral to the spinal cord.

Rosenblum's 1987 classification [35], which is the most widely accepted, includes:

Rosenblum's 1987 classification [35]
Type I: Dural AVF
Type II: Intradural intramedullary glomus AVM
Type III: Intradural intramedullary juvenile AVM
Type IV: Intradural direct AVF.

Since 1993, type IV intradural direct AVFs have been referred to as perimedullary AVFs. These were further classified based on the number of feeding arteries and the size of the AVF [36]: Type I: Single feeder and single small AVF; Type II: Multiple feeders and multiple medium AVFs; Type III: Multiple feeders and a single giant AVF. More recently, extradural AVFs have been incorporated into this classification system and are subdivided into three types according to the presence of intradural venous drainage and associated neurological deficits [37]. Takai proposed a revised version of these classifications, offering further refinements to the existing framework [38].

Revised classification of spinal AV shunt by Takai (2017) [38]			
Type	Academic name	Subtype	Feeder, AVF, and venous drainage
I	Dural AVF		
II	Intramedullary glomus AVM		
III	Intramedullary juvenile AVM		
IV	Perimedullary AVF	IVa	A single feeder and small AVF
		IVb	Multiple feeders and medium AVF
		IVc	Multiple feeders and a giant AVF
V	Extradural AVF	Va	With intradural venous drainage
		Vb	Without intradural venous drainage
AVF, arteriovenous fistulas; AVM, arteriovenous malformation			

In 2008, Geibprasert and Lasjaunias proposed a classification encompassing both intracranial and spinal AVFs, dividing arteriovenous shunts into three groups based on the embryologic development of venous drainage: the ventral, lateral, and dorsal epidural groups [39]. According to this system, spinal DAVFs are categorized as lateral epidural AVFs.

Conclusion

This chapter reviews the history and development of embolization for the treatment of dural arteriovenous fistula (DAVF) and discusses the evolution of the classification system. The chapter emphasizes the limitations of early surgical treatment and describes the shift toward embolization with the development of imaging and minimally invasive endovascular techniques. The introduction of liquid embolic agents, such as n-butyl cyanoacrylate (NBCA) and Onyx, has significantly improved outcomes by providing better occlusion and reducing complications.

References

[1] Newton TH, Weidner W, Greitz T. Dural arteriovenous malformation in the posterior fossa. *Radiology*. 1968;90 (1):27-35.

[2] Gandhi D, et al. Intracranial dural arteriovenous fistulas: classification, imaging findings, and treatment. *AJNR Am J Neuroradiol*. 2012;33 (6):1007-13.

[3] Kurabe S, Kumagai T, Abe H. A Comprehensive Analysis of Dural Arteriovenous Fistula Involving the Superior Sagittal Sinus: A Systematic Review. *J Neuroendovasc Ther*. 2021;15 (1):1-7.

[4] Tsai LK, Liu HM, Jeng JS. Diagnosis and management of intracranial dural arteriovenous fistulas. *Expert Rev Neurother*. 2016;16 (3):307-18.

[5] Luo CB, Chang FC, Teng MM. Update of embolization of intracranial dural arteriovenous fistula. *J Chin Med Assoc*. 2014;77 (12):610-7.

[6] Gioppo A, et al. Medial Tentorial Dural Arteriovenous Fistula Embolization: Single Experience with Embolic Liquid Polymer SQUID and Review of the Literature. *World Neurosurg*. 2017;107:1050.e1-1050.e7.

[7] Halbach VV, et al. Dural fistulas involving the transverse and sigmoid sinuses: results of treatment in 28 patients. *Radiology*. 1987;163 (2):443-7.

[8] Rabinov JD, et al. ONYX versus n-BCA for embolization of cranial dural arteriovenous fistulas. *J Neurointerv Surg*. 2013;5 (4):306-10.

[9] Kawaguchi S, et al. Surgery for dural arteriovenous fistula in superior sagittal sinus and transverse sigmoid sinus. *J Clin Neurosci*. 2000;7 Suppl 1:47-9.

[10] Tomak PR, et al. Evolution of the management of tentorial dural arteriovenous malformations. *Neurosurgery*. 2003;52 (4):750-60; discussion 760-2.

[11] Troffkin NA, et al. Combined transvenous and transarterial embolization of a tentorial-incisural dural arteriovenous malformation followed by primary stent placement in the associated stenotic straight sinus. *J Neurosurg*. 2003;99 (3):579-83.

[12] Vollherbst DF, et al. LIQUID—Treatment of high-grade dural arteriovenous fistulas with Squid liquid embolic agent: a prospective, observational multicenter study. *J Neurointerv Surg*. 2023;15 (11):1111-6.

[13] Quinones D, et al. Embolization of dural cavernous fistulas via superior ophthalmic vein approach. *AJNR Am J Neuroradiol*. 1997;18 (5):921-8.

[14] Viñuela F, et al. Unusual clinical manifestations of dural arteriovenous malformations. *J Neurosurg*. 1986;64 (4):554-8.

[15] Suzuki S, et al. Transvenous treatment of spontaneous dural carotid-cavernous fistulas using a combination of detachable coils and Onyx. *AJNR Am J Neuroradiol*. 2006;27 (6):1346-9.

[16] O'Leary S, et al. Intracranial dural arteriovenous malformations: results of stereotactic radiosurgery in 17 patients. *Clin Oncol* (R Coll Radiol). 2002;14 (2):97-102.

[17] Murphy KJ, et al. Endovascular treatment of a grade IV transverse sinus dural arteriovenous fistula by sinus recanalization, angioplasty, and stent placement: technical case report. *Neurosurgery*. 2000;46 (2):497-500; discussion 500-1.

[18] Doppman JL, Di Chiro G, Ommaya A. Obliteration of spinal-cord arteriovenous malformation by percutaneous embolisation. *Lancet*. 1968;1 (7540):477.

[19] Steinmetz MP, et al. Outcome after the treatment of spinal dural arteriovenous fistulae: a contemporary single-institution series and meta-analysis. *Neurosurgery*. 2004;55 (1):77-87; discussion 87-8.

[20] *J Neurosurg Spine.* Open and endovascular treatment of spinal dural arteriovenous fistulas: a 10-year experience. 2017;26 (4):519-523.

[21] Kirsch M, et al. Endovascular management of spinal dural arteriovenous fistulas in 78 patients. *Neuroradiology*. 2013;55 (3):337-43.

[22] Oh Y, et al. Microsurgery Versus Endovascular Treatment—Which Is Adequate for Initial Treatment of Spinal Dural Arteriovenous Fistula: A Case Series. *Neurospine*. 2021;18 (2):344-354.

[23] Maimon S, Luckman Y, Strauss I. Spinal Dural Arteriovenous Fistula: A Review. *Adv Tech Stand Neurosurg*. 2016;43:111-37.

[24] Djindjian R. Super-selective arteriography of branches of the external carotid artery. *Surg Neurol.* 1976;5 (3):133-42.

[25] Borden JA, Wu JK, Shucart WA. A proposed classification for spinal and cranial dural arteriovenous fistulous malformations and implications for treatment. *J Neurosurg.* 1995;82 (2):166-79.

[26] Cognard C, et al. Cerebral dural arteriovenous fistulas: clinical and angiographic correlation with a revised classification of venous drainage. *Radiology.* 1995;194 (3):671-80.

[27] Casasco A, et al. A new subtype of intracranial dural AVF according to the patterns of venous drainage. *Interv Neuroradiol.* 2021;27 (1):121-128.

[28] Becerril-Gaitan A, et al. The VEBAS score: a practical scoring system for intracranial dural arteriovenous fistula obliteration. J Neurointerv Surg. 2024;16 (3):272-279.

[29] Wenderoth J. Proposal for an improved classification system for cavernous sinus dural arteriovenous fistula (CS-DAVF). *J Neurointerv Surg.* 2017;9 (3):220-224.

[30] Barrow DL, et al. Classification and treatment of spontaneous carotid-cavernous sinus fistulas. *J Neurosurg.* 1985;62 (2):248-56.

[31] Thomas AJ, et al. Proposal of venous drainage-based classification system for carotid cavernous fistulae with validity assessment in a multicenter cohort. *Neurosurgery.* 2015;77 (3):380-5; discussion 385.

[32] Mishra K, et al. Carotid cavernous fistula: redefining the angioarchitecture. J Cerebrovasc Endovasc *Neurosurg.* 2022;24 (4):356-365.

[33] Chaudhary MY, et al. Dural arteriovenous malformation of the major venous sinuses: an acquired lesion. *AJNR Am J Neuroradiol.* 1982;3 (1):13-9.

[34] Sivakumar W, et al. Endovascular management of spinal dural arteriovenous fistulas: a review. *Neurosurg Focus.* 2009;26 (5):E15.

[35] Rosenblum B, et al. Spinal arteriovenous malformations: a comparison of dural arteriovenous fistulas and intradural AVM's in 81 patients. *J Neurosurg.* 1987;67 (6):795-802.

[36] Mourier KL, et al. Intradural perimedullary arteriovenous fistulae: results of surgical and endovascular treatment in a series of 35 cases. *Neurosurgery.* 1993;32 (6):885-91; discussion 891-2.

[37] Rangel-Castilla L, et al. Spinal extradural arteriovenous fistulas: a clinical and radiological description of different types and their novel treatment with Onyx. J Neurosurg Spine. 2011;15 (5):541-9.

[38] Takai K. Spinal Arteriovenous Shunts: angioarchitecture and historical changes in classification. *Neurol Med Chir* (Tokyo). 2017;57 (7):356-365.

[39] Geibprasert S, et al. Dural arteriovenous shunts: a new classification of craniospinal epidural venous anatomical bases and clinical correlations. *Stroke.* 2008;39 (10):2783-94.

Chapter 19

The History and Development of Stroke-Related Scores

Leen Rikan Azzam[1,*]
Abdulrahman Alomar[1,†]
Ahmed Muthana[2,‡], MD
and Samer S. Hoz[3,§], MD
[1]School of Medicine, Royal College of Surgeons in Ireland, Bahrain
[2]Department of Neurosurgery, University of Baghdad, Baghdad, Iraq
[3]Department of Neurosurgery, University of Cincinnati Medical Center, Cincinnati, OH, USA

Abstract

The development of stroke-related scores has evolved significantly over the past years, reflecting advancements in diagnostic techniques, treatment modalities, and understanding of stroke pathophysiology. Stroke-related scores are fundamental tools in neurointerventional surgery, aiding in the assessment of stroke severity, guiding treatment decisions, and predicting patient outcomes. The chapter discusses different score systems, with their advantages and disadvantages, and provides a comparative analysis of each other. The chapter underscores the pivotal role of stroke-related scores in shaping the landscape of neurointerventional surgery by highlighting key milestones and advancements in this field.

Keywords: stroke-related score, ASPECTS, TICI, ASTRAL, THRIVE, SPAN-100, AISS

Introduction

Over the years, the development of stroke-related scores has evolved significantly, reflecting advancements in diagnostic techniques, treatment modalities, and understanding of stroke pathophysiology. Stroke-related scores are fundamental tools in neurointerventional surgery,

* Corresponding Author's Email: leenrakan28@gmail.com
† Corresponding Author's Email: aalomar836@gmail.com
‡ Corresponding Author's Email: ahmed.m.najm@gmail.com
§ Corresponding Author's Email: hozsamer2055@gmail.com

In: World History of Neurointerventional Surgery
Editors: Xianli Lv and Zhongxue Wu
ISBN: 979-8-89530-792-2

aiding in the assessment of stroke severity, guiding treatment decisions, and predicting patient outcomes. The evolution of stroke-related scores can be traced back to seminal works such as the National Institutes of Health Stroke Scale (NIHSS) and the Glasgow Coma Scale (GCS), which laid the groundwork for standardized neurological assessment in stroke patients. Subsequent refinements led to the development of specialized scoring systems tailored to specific stroke subtypes and treatment modalities. Among these, the Alberta Stroke Program Early CT Score (ASPECTS) emerged as a pioneering tool for the assessment of early ischemic changes on imaging, providing valuable insights on patients with middle cerebral artery strokes. The Thrombolysis in Cerebral Infarction (TICI) scale revolutionized the evaluation of revascularization outcomes, guiding endovascular therapy decisions. Advancements in predictive modeling gave rise to scores such as the ASTRAL and THRIVE scores, offering valuable prognostic information for stroke patients undergoing neurointerventional procedures. More recently, the integration of artificial intelligence and machine learning techniques has led to the development of innovative scoring systems, such as the Stroke Prognostication using Age and NIH Stroke Scale (SPAN-100) score and the Artificial Intelligence Stroke Scale (AISS), further enhancing risk stratification and treatment optimization.

Initial Challenges and Milestones

Several obstacles arose during the early developmental stages of stroke-related scoring. Clinicians recognized the need for standardized evaluation techniques to accurately determine stroke severity, but early attempts were frequently unsuccessful and without validation. The National Institutes of Health Stroke Scale (NIHSS), one of the first comprehensive tools, had major challenges during its adoption. The NIHSS was developed in 1989, however, it required substantial modification to ensure consistent administration. The main challenges encountered were associated with inter-rater reliability [1]. However, despite these challenges, it became a stroke assessment staple due to its capacity to give a systematic examination of neurological impairments.

The National Institutes of Health Stroke Scale (NIHSS) was introduced at a critical point, as validation studies established its efficacy in predicting outcomes and guiding thrombolytic therapy decisions, establishing it as a standard tool in clinical practice [2]. Another significant milestone was the Modified Rankin Scale (mRS), which was first developed in 1957 and received renewed attention in the 1990s as a measure of functional outcomes following a stroke. The mRS was a simple yet successful approach for assessing the degree of disability or dependency in daily tasks, and its extensive use in therapeutic trials demonstrated its significance [3].

In 2000, the Alberta Stroke Program Early CT Score (ASPECTS) was introduced where it represented a significant advance in stroke imaging by providing a rapid and reliable method to identify patients who are likely to benefit from thrombolytic therapy, by assessing early ischemic changes on CT scans [4]. Additionally, the Thrombolysis in Cerebral Infarction (TICI) Score was developed in the early 2000s to assess the efficacy of revascularization operations in acute ischemic stroke. The score offered a systematic technique for grading the level of reperfusion achieved following endovascular therapy, which was critical for directing post-intervention care and predicting long-term results [5].

Scoring Systems

Stroke-Related Score

The National Institutes of Health Stroke Scale (NIHSS) is arguably the most utilized rating scale in the discipline of neurology [6]. It has proven to be a critical tool used in the evaluation of stroke severity and has significantly impacted stroke patient's care ever since its development.

The NIH stroke scale was developed in the early 1980s in a collaborative effort between researchers from the Stroke Branch of the National Institute of Health (NIH) and the National Institute of Neurological Disorders and Stroke (NINDS). During the early days of development, stroke deficit rating scales were already in use [7-9]. An NIH-sponsored trial of naloxone for acute stroke combined several scales in an attempt to come up with a scale that represented the size of the infarction. During the naloxone study, investigators combined the scales of the University of Cincinnati, the Canadian neurological scale, the Edniburgh-2 coma scale, and the Oxbury initial severity scale [1, 10]. At the end of this study, a new fully formed revolutionary scale was approved and is now widely accepted as the NIH stroke scale [6].

The NIH stroke scale is a rigorous assessment composed of 11 different elements, each developed to assess a specific function of stroke-related symptoms: the level of consciousness, best gaze, vision, facial palsy, motor arm, motor leg, limb ataxia, sensory, best language, dysarthria, and extinction and attention [6].

Advantages

The NIHSS possesses several advantages, one being that it provides a rapid yet comprehensive evaluation of neurological function, supporting the early assessment of stroke severity [10]. The rapid assessment subsequently enables rapid intervention, which is critical in the management of stroke. It assists in administering thrombolytic therapy, such as tissue plasminogen activator (tPA), as soon as possible, given that it is best administered within 4.5 hours of a stroke onset. Furthermore, studies have shown a correlation between the effectiveness of medical intervention and the stroke score. It was revealed that patients who presented with an NIH stroke scale score of 0-2 had favorable functional outcomes at discharge when compared to those with a higher score [11]. Moreover, regardless of the treatment, the NIHSS allows medical professionals to predict patient outcomes. A higher score predicts a poorer functional outcome regardless of treatment [12].

Another important advantage of the NIH stroke scale is its wide use in research. It has been routinely used in clinical trials and demographic and epidemiological studies. NIHS scores can accurately be reproduced from adequately documented neurological examinations. This provides researchers the ability to thoroughly carry out studies pertaining to strokes, without the need to be clinically experienced [13].

Disadvantages

One of the main limitations faced with the NIH stroke scale is its subjectivity. Each item in the stroke scale is graded on a scale, some items are graded on a scale of 0 to 2, some 0 to 3, and others 0 to 4. Regardless of the item scale, such an entity may be evaluated differently by different providers, thus affecting reproducibility and accuracy.

The NIH stroke scale has been shown to be anatomically biased, producing scores that vary in accuracy according to the location of the lesion. Several trials have shown that the NIHSS system favors strokes that affect anterior circulation, which presents with motor function and cortical signs, in contrast to posterior strokes which are associated more with cranial nerve abnormalities and ataxia. Furthermore, a bias towards left-sided strokes is observed.

Redundancy is another aspect of the NIHSS system. Firstly, in cases where a patient has an altered mental status, evaluating some of the elements of NIH stroke becomes challenging, especially items that require patient cooperation.

ASPECTS

The Alberta Stroke Program Early CT Score (ASPECTS) was created to give a consistent and accurate tool for detecting early ischemia alterations on non-contrast CT scans in individuals suffering from acute ischemic stroke. It was first introduced in 2000 and due to its capacity to guide treatment decisions and predict outcomes, immediately became a helpful tool in neurointerventional surgery [4, 14].

Advantages

ASPECTS has a wide range of important benefits, which have contributed to its broad use in clinical practice. One of the key advantages is its ease of use and speedy application. ASPECTS scores 10 areas of the middle cerebral artery territory, which allows doctors to swiftly identify the amount of ischemia damage. This is crucial in the time-sensitive setting of acute stroke therapy.

The score has demonstrated good inter-rater reliability. Studies have shown that due to ASPECTS' strong correlation with clinical outcomes, it has been proven to be a valid prognostic predictor. This is necessary for consistent and repeatable assessments among various doctors and institutions. Higher ASPECTS scores are linked with better results following reperfusion therapies, such as endovascular thrombectomy and intravenous thrombolysis [15]. Furthermore, the broad availability and ease of use of non-contrast CT improves the use of ASPECTS in a variety of healthcare contexts, including those with restricted access to cutting-edge imaging modalities. According to Demchuk, accessibility guarantees that a larger number of patients may be evaluated immediately and precisely, enabling timely and relevant therapies [16].

Disadvantages

While ASPECTS has shown to have several benefits, it also has its setbacks. One significant drawback is its reliance on non-contrast CT might lead to undetectable early ischemic changes in such areas as the posterior circulation. Those undetectable changes could have an impact on the treatment modalities and results, due to the underestimated ischemic damage [4].

Another disadvantage is the variations in the ischemic changes that are not taken into account. Due to the binary nature of the ASPECTS system, ischemic changes in each region can go undetected. For instance, subtle ischemia that will not alter the ASPECTS might be clinically significant and will go undetected. The lack of this crucial detail can have an impact on clinical decision-making and treatment modalities [17].

Furthermore, non-clinical factors can also have an impact on the accuracy of ASPECTS. Variables such as patient movement, radiologists' skills and experience, and the CT scanner technology could all lead to variability in image quality, which may have an effect on the interpretation, the therapeutic decisions, and the results [15].

TICI

Developed in the early 2000s, the scoring system known as Thrombolysis in Cerebral Infarction (TICI) has since been an essential tool in assessing the effectiveness of revascularization procedures in acute ischemic stroke. The TICI score originated from the Thrombolysis in Myocardial Infarction (TIMI) score, which was first utilized in cardiology for assessing reperfusion following coronary artery procedures. In the early 2000s, there was a recognized need for a specific and dependable grading system to evaluate cerebral perfusion, leading to the development of the TICI score [18].

The purpose of TICI was to offer a more precise evaluation of reperfusion in the intricate vascular structure of the brain in comparison to the TIMI scale, which had various operational versions in stroke trials. This scoring system offers a standardized approach for assessing the level of reperfusion attained following endovascular treatment, which is essential for determining the appropriate management after the intervention and predicting the long-term results [5].

Advantages

TICI has proven to be an essential tool since its adoption in clinical practice. Its capability to offer standardized and consistent duplicatable measures of reperfusion has made it one of the key benefits in comparing outcomes across various studies and clinical trials. In addition, it has contributed to enhancing the assessment of treatment efficacy and refining therapeutic modalities [19].

The TICI grading scale spans from 0, indicating no perfusion, to 3, indicating complete perfusion. This scale enables a thorough evaluation of revascularization success, providing clinicians with detailed information for making well-informed decisions about additional interventions and post-procedural care. Research indicates that higher TICI scores correlate with improved clinical outcomes, establishing it as a dependable predictor of patient prognosis [5].

Disadvantages

With all the benefits that the scoring systems provide there are limitations, and this applies to the TICI score. The inter-variability in grading perfusion of this score is one of its significant drawbacks. This could lead to inconsistencies between different operators resulting in an impact on the results being compared from various studies and clinical settings [5].

Furthermore, while achieving a high degree of reperfusion is associated with better patient outcomes, the TICI score does not take into account factors such as the size and location of the infarct, the time to reperfusion, and the patient's comorbidities, which could significantly impact the clinical outcomes. This is due to the fact that the TICI score focuses primarily on angiographic outcomes rather than clinical ones. In addition, this limitation may also influence the poor measures of TICI in detecting small, distal vessels [20, 21].

ASTRAL

The ASTRAL score is a newly developed prognostic tool that can be used to predict long-term outcomes in stroke patients. Researchers developed this scoring system to be used in the emergency room, providing a prognostic assessment at 3 months of stroke patients within 24 hours of arrival. The scoring system uses 6 readily accessible parameters to perform the assessment rapidly at the bedside.

The development of the ASTRAL score started due to the widespread need for a practical and accurate tool to predict outcomes following an acute ischemic stroke. Prior to its development, several scales and scoring systems were available, however, they mostly faced issues of being either too complex or insufficient validity. Therefore, researchers initiated the ASTRAL project with the objective of producing an easy-to-use and reliable scoring system.

The ASTRAL scoring system was developed using a linear regression analysis of cohorts of patients from the Acute Stroke Registry and Analysis of Lausanne, identifying factors predicting unfavorable outcomes. A wide variety of such factors were analyzed to determine which factors most significantly influenced outcome, subsequently, of those factors, 6 were selected based on ease of measurement, and predictive value.

The 6 parameters of the ASTRAL score are age, severity of stroke on admission as measured by the NIH Stroke Scale score, stroke onset to admission time, range of visual fields, acute glucose, and level of consciousness. Table 1 illustrates the parameters and associated scores.

The study revealed that there was a strong correlation between the ASTRAL score and the possibility of an unfavorable outcome within 3 months. A score of 31 is deemed the midway, wherein, it predicts a 50% chance of an unfavorable outcome within 3 months.

Table 1. The parameters of ASTRAL score

Parameter	Score Points
Age: For every 5 years	1
Severity: for every NIHSS point	1
Time delay from onset to admission >3 h	2
Range of visual field defect	2
Acute glucose >7.3 or <3.7 mmol/L	1
Level of consciousness decreased	3

Advantages

The ASTRAL scoring system has several significant advantages. One of the major advantages associated with this system is its predictive accuracy. Contrary to several other systems, the ASTRAL system has been validated by multiple studies and proven to be accurate in providing prognostic predictions. This makes the ASTRAL score a reliable tool for clinicians [22]. Furthermore, the ASTRAL scoring system does not require information from brain imaging, further simplifying its use [23].

Additionally, the ASTRAL score was designed to be a simple, rapid, and easy-to-use assessment tool. Composed of only 6 rapidly accessible items, the scoring system is relatively easy to use and does not require any additional training, nor is it time-consuming.

The prognostic prediction provided by the ASTRAL score plays a role in resource allocation. Patients who present with higher scores can be deemed a higher priority with treatment allocation.

Disadvantages

One notable disadvantage of the ASTRAL scoring system is its reliance on the NIH stroke scale. The NIH stroke scale is a complex and operator-dependent stroke scale that can be time-consuming if there are too many NIHSS-trained physicians. This may impede the ability to perform an ASTRAL assessment, as it is dependent on the NIH stroke score.

Another issue arises as the parameters may not always be readily available. One main parameter that is commonly misrepresented or unrepresented is the onset to admission time. It is not always possible to provide an accurate estimate of the time of stroke onset, which is one of the 6 parameters of the ASTRAL scoring system [24].

THRIVE

The development of the Totaled Health Risks in Vascular Events (THRIVE) score was primarily to provide a comprehensive assessment of patient risk factors and to predict outcomes following an acute ischemic stroke. The score was designed to combine key non-modifiable risk factors, such as age, stroke severity as measured by the National Institutes of Health Stroke Scale (NIHSS), and the presence of chronic health conditions such as hypertension, diabetes, and atrial fibrillation, into a single predictive metric tool [21].

The score was validated using data from the Virtual International Stroke Trials Archive and the TREVO-2 trials, among others. This modality deemed the score reliable for predicting clinical outcomes, including the mortality and risk of hemorrhage following thrombolytic therapy. Such development helped achieve the aim of offering a more holistic view of the patient risk factors and guiding physicians in therapeutic modalities in acute stroke management [21, 25].

Advantages

The primary and one key advantage of THRIVE lies in its design to incorporate multiple risk factors. Compared to single-factor models, this score can provide an accurate prediction of patient outcomes which aids clinicians to rank their patients based on their overall risk profile. In addition, studies have shown that this holistic approach, which helps in designing personalized treatment plans for the patient is deemed reliable as a valuable tool and a strong predictor for both short-term and long-term outcomes [25].

Another key feature is the simplicity and the ease of use of THRIVE score. The score can be used at the bedside of the patient and can be calculated in a span of minutes. As a result, it has been integrated into routine clinical practice as it can be consistently applied across different healthcare settings, enhancing its utility and reliability [25].

Disadvantages

Despite its strength, like any score, the THRIVE score has its own limitations. One key disadvantage is that it doesn't take into account imaging findings, which is essential in providing critical information regarding stroke etiology and the extent of brain damage or injury. This potentially limits the accuracy of THRIVE in predicting outcomes, as it might not fully capture the complexity of certain cases [25].

Additionally, while the score includes several high-yield risk factors, it doesn't take into account factors that influence patient prognosis, such as pre-stroke patient status, socio-economic status, and access to rehabilitation services. These factors can significantly impact the recovery of patients. This drawback highlights the need for additional scores and tools to aid THRIVE in providing more detailed evaluation of patient outcomes [21].

SPAN-100

A common treatment modality of acute ischemic stroke is thrombolysis, particularly the use of tissue plasminogen activator (tPA). While age and stroke severity are the most important factors affecting stroke outcomes, evidence has shown that they also impact thrombolysis treatment outcomes [25-27]. Randomized trials and observational studies have shown worse outcomes and higher bleeding risks in the elderly undergoing thrombolysis [28, 29].

With a lack of a system predicting outcomes of thrombolysis in ischemic stroke patients, researchers began developing the SPAN-100 index, which aimed at providing clinicians and patients with quantifiable information about the likelihood of a negative outcome or intracranial hemorrhage associated with thrombolysis [29].

The SPAN-100 index was developed on the basis of 3 rationales. Firstly, age and stroke severity are the two most important prognostic factors. Secondly, patients aged 80 and above with a high NIH stroke score have poorer outcomes. Lastly, a simple index is needed to help clinicians estimate outcomes. Therefore, the researchers proposed a system that only relies on 2 parameters: Age and NIH stroke score. A SPAN index of 100 or greater indicates that the patient is SPAN-100-positive and therefore at a higher risk of a worse outcome.

The study developing the SPAN-100 index utilized available information from the NINDS tPA trial. Data from the trial was used to compare SPAN-100-positive and SPAN-100-negative patients where clinical outcomes risk of intracranial hemorrhages were evaluated. The results of the study revealed that out of the 624 patients, 62 of them were SPAN-100-positive, and 42% of them had intracranial hemorrhages post-tPA, compared to 12% in the SPAN-100-negative cohort. Furthermore, secondary outcomes involved include fatal ICH, catastrophic outcome defined as a mRS of 4 to 6 at 3 months, death at 3 months, and a lack of neurologic improvement. Results revealed that the 3-month mortality of SPAN-100-positive patients post-tPA was 50% compared to 13% in SPAN-100-negative patients. These results solidify the ability of the SPAN-100 index to provide outcome estimates for patients and therefore optimize patient care [30].

Advantages

One key advantage of the SPAN-100 index is that is a simple system, applicable in almost all clinical settings. It entails only 2 parameters, that are easy to add up without the need for any special equipment or training. Clinicians are able to rapidly assess a patient and form an evaluation that helps in guiding treatment using this easy-to-remember formula. Furthermore, the ability of the SPAN-100 to provide healthcare workers as well as patients and their families with a quantifiable risk associated with outcomes and treatment. This helps in providing guidance with treatment and counseling. Identifying patients with a worse predicted outcome may help in better preparing for said outcomes, for both healthcare workers and family members.

Disadvantages and Limitations

Just as with any scoring system, the SPAN-100 index has its limitations. One limitation underlined by the researchers was that the use of only 2 variables could be too simplistic. Many different factors affect the outcome of a stroke, and it is not enough to merely rely on the age and stroke severity. Furthermore, it is argued that the weight of age and stroke severity are not equal in predetermining outcomes, wherein, patients aged > 80 years with a low NIHS score may still have good outcomes. Another limitation of the SPAN-100 index is the study design. The results of the study should be cautiously interpreted, given that the system was developed using a relatively small cohort of 624 patients. The small number of patients and more specifically SPAN-100-positive patients could potentially affect the accuracy of the results.

Future Directions

The development of stroke-related scores such as ASPECTS, TICI, THRIVE, and SPAN-100 has greatly contributed to neurointerventional surgery in such a way that it enhanced the assessment and management of stroke patients. However, future advancements and contributions are required to address the limitations and improve patient outcomes.

One key advancement is the possibility of integrating artificial intelligence and machine learning into stroke-related scoring systems. This model would aid in analyzing large datasets and patient information that would predict outcomes more accurately than current modalities. One such solution would be the integration of AI or MI into existing scores or the developing of new ones, offering personalized treatment plans based on the patient's individual profile [31].

Furthermore, the integration of imagining findings such as MRI, CT, and perfusion imaging, into the stroke-related scores. Incorporating such data would provide comprehensive insight into stroke pathology, therefore, allowing for a more holistic assessment of stroke severity and predicting potential outcomes [31].

Conclusion

Overall, the history and development of stroke-related scores have been marked by key advancements that have improved the accuracy of stroke assessment, guided physicians in treatment decision-making, and successfully determined patient outcomes. Each score has its own benefits and limitations, reflecting the need for diverse assessment tools. Future advancements are likely to build on the existing foundations of the stroke-related scores, to create more personalized patient-related scores.

References

[1] Brott T, et al. Measurements of acute cerebral infarction: a clinical examination scale. *Stroke*. 1989;20 (7):864-870.

[2] Goldstein LB, Bertels C, Davis JN. Interrater reliability of the NIH stroke scale. *Arch Neurol*. 1989;46 (6):660-662.

[3] Rankin J. Cerebral vascular accidents in patients over the age of 60: II. Prognosis. *Scott Med J*. 1957;2 (5):200-215.

[4] Barber PA, et al. Validity and reliability of a quantitative computed tomography score in predicting outcome of hyperacute stroke before thrombolytic therapy. *Lancet*. 2000;355 (9216):1670-1674.

[5] Zaidat OO, et al. Recommendations on angiographic revascularization grading standards for acute ischemic stroke: a consensus statement. *Stroke*. 2013;44 (9):2650-2663.

[6] Lyden P. Using the national institutes of health stroke scale: a cautionary tale. *Stroke*. 2017;48 (2):513-519.

[7] Lyden PD, Lau GT. A critical appraisal of stroke evaluation and rating scales. *Stroke*. 1991;22 (11):1345-1352.

[8] Gilroy J, Barnhart MI, Meyer JS. Treatment of acute stroke with dextran 40. *JAMA*. 1969;210 (2):293-298.

[9] Muir KW, et al. Comparison of neurological scales and scoring systems for acute stroke prognosis. *Stroke*. 1996;27 (10):1817-1820.

[10] Marsh EB, et al. The NIH Stroke Scale has limited utility in accurate daily monitoring of neurologic status. *Neurohospitalist*. 2016;6 (3):97-101.

[11] Wang L, et al. Intravenous thrombolysis for mild stroke: NIHSS 3–5 versus NIHSS 0–2. *J Stroke Cerebrovasc Dis*. 2023;32 (5):107070.

[12] Wouters A, et al. Prediction of outcome in patients with acute ischemic stroke based on initial severity and improvement in the first 24 h. *Front Neurol*. 2018;9:308.

[13] Kasner SE, et al. Reliability and validity of estimating the NIH stroke scale score from medical records. *Stroke*. 1999;30 (8):1534-1537.

[14] Ryu CW, et al. Alberta Stroke Program Early CT Score in the prognostication after endovascular treatment for ischemic stroke: a meta-analysis. *Neurointervention*. 2017;12 (1):20-30.

[15] Puetz V, et al. CT angiography source images predict final infarct extent in patients with basilar artery occlusion. *AJNR Am J Neuroradiol*. 2009;30 (10):1877-1883.

[16] Demchuk AM, et al. Importance of early ischemic computed tomography changes using ASPECTS in NINDS rtPA Stroke Study. *Stroke*. 2005;36 (10):2110-2115.

[17] Mair G, et al. Sensitivity and specificity of the hyperdense artery sign for arterial obstruction in acute ischemic stroke. *Stroke*. 2015;46 (1):102-107.

[18] Fugate J, Klunder A, Kallmes DF. What is meant by "TICI"? AJNR *Am J Neuroradiol*. 2013;34 (9):1792-1797.

[19] Higashida RT, Furlan AJ. Trial design and reporting standards for intra-arterial cerebral thrombolysis for acute ischemic stroke. *Stroke*. 2003;34 (8):e109-e137.

[20] Goyal M, et al. Endovascular thrombectomy after large-vessel ischaemic stroke: a meta-analysis of individual patient data from five randomised trials. *Lancet*. 2016;387 (10029):1723-1731.

[21] Lansberg MG, et al. MRI profile and response to endovascular reperfusion after stroke (DEFUSE 2): a prospective cohort study. *Lancet Neurol*. 2012;11 (10):860-867.

[22] Papavasileiou V, et al. ASTRAL score predicts 5-year dependence and mortality in acute ischemic stroke. *Stroke*. 2013;44 (6):1616-1620.

[23] Ntaios G, et al. An integer-based score to predict functional outcome in acute ischemic stroke: the ASTRAL score. *Neurology*. 2012;78 (24):1916-1922.

[24] Drozdowska BA, Singh S, Quinn TJ. Thinking about the future: a review of prognostic scales used in acute stroke. *Front Neurol*. 2019;10:274.

[25] Weimar C, et al. Age and National Institutes of Health Stroke Scale Score within 6 hours after onset are accurate predictors of outcome after cerebral ischemia: development and external validation of prognostic models. *Stroke*. 2004;35 (1):158-162.

[26] Collaboration GSS. Predicting outcome after acute ischemic stroke: an external validation of prognostic models. *Neurology*. 2004;62 (4):581-585.
[27] König IR, et al. Predicting long-term outcome after acute ischemic stroke: a simple index works in patients from controlled clinical trials. *Stroke*. 2008;39 (6):1821-1826.
[28] Mishra NK, et al. Thrombolysis in very elderly people: controlled comparison of SITS international stroke thrombolysis registry and virtual international stroke trials archive. *BMJ*. 2010;341:c6046.
[29] Sylaja P, et al. Thrombolysis in patients older than 80 years with acute ischaemic stroke: Canadian Alteplase for Stroke Effectiveness Study. *J Neurol Neurosurg Psychiatry*. 2006;77 (7):826-829.
[30] Saposnik G, et al. Stroke prognostication using age and NIH stroke scale: SPAN-100. *Neurology*. 2013;80 (1):21-28.
[31] Ospel JM, Goyal M. A review of endovascular treatment for medium vessel occlusion stroke. *J Neurointerv Surg*. 2021;13 (7):623-630.

Chapter 20

The History and Development of Stroke Trials

Abdullah M. Al-Qudah[1,*]
Aseel K. Fakhri[2,†]
Ahmed Aljuboori[3,‡], MD
Ahmed Muthana[4,§], MD
and Samer S. Hoz[5,‖], MD
[1]UPMC Stroke Institute, University of Pittsburgh Medical Center, PA, USA
[2]University of Baghdad, College of Medicine, Baghdad, Iraq
[3]Department of Neurosurgery, Geisinger Clinic, PA, USA
[4]Department of Neurosurgery, University of Baghdad, Baghdad, Iraq
[5]Department of Neurosurgery, University of Cincinnati Medical Center, Cincinnati, OH, USA

Abstract

Stroke is the major cause of disability and the second leading cause of death worldwide. The chapter explores the history of stroke trials, provides insight into the current and ongoing trials, and delineates how they have led to advancements in neurointerventional surgery for managing acute strokes. The chapter also demonstrates the technique's evolution over the past decade, resulting in significant improvements in reperfusion safety, speed, and completeness. Moreover, the chapter discusses the initial efforts to develop endovascular treatment 50 years ago, and critical gaps in device technology and treatment selection through successful and failed randomized clinical trials. By the end of this chapter, the reader will have a clear vision of how this field started and how it came after all the advancements and evolution.

Keywords: stroke, trials, endovascular thrombectomy, large vessel occlusion

---

[*] Corresponding Author's Email: qudah.m.a@gmail.com
[†] Corresponding Author's Email: asilk6195@gmail.com
[‡] Corresponding Author's Email: ahmedaljuboori9494@gmail.com
[§] Corresponding Author's Email: ahmed.m.najm@gmail.com
[‖] Corresponding Author's Email: hozsamer2055@gmail.com

In: World History of Neurointerventional Surgery
Editors: Xianli Lv and Zhongxue Wu
ISBN: 979-8-89530-792-2

Introduction

Stroke remains a leading cause of death and disability worldwide, with a significant global burden [1, 2]. In 2016, there were 13.7 million new stroke cases globally, with approximately 87% being ischemic strokes [3]. Large vessel occlusion (LVO) accounts for 10-20% of acute ischemic strokes (AIS) [3]. Despite declining age-standardized rates, the absolute number of people affected by stroke has increased due to population growth and aging [4]. Low- and middle-income countries bear the highest burden, comprising 75.2% of stroke deaths and 81.0% of stroke-related disability-adjusted life years (DALYs) [5]. The global economic impact of stroke is substantial, necessitating improved prevention and management strategies [6]. Primary prevention remains crucial, as demonstrated by Japan's success in reducing stroke mortality through decreased salt intake [7].

Importance of Endovascular Thrombectomy (EVT)

Endovascular thrombectomy (EVT) has revolutionized acute ischemic stroke treatment, becoming the standard of care for large vessel occlusions [8, 9]. This breakthrough evolved from early intra-arterial thrombolysis to modern stent retrievers and aspiration techniques [10]. EVT's efficacy has been validated through numerous randomized controlled trials, demonstrating significant improvements in patient outcomes with a number needed to treat as low as 2.6 [8, 11]. The treatment window has expanded from 6 to 24 hours for selected patients based on perfusion imaging [9, 12]. Ongoing research focuses on optimizing first-pass complete reperfusion, developing new devices and techniques, and expanding indications to include large core infarctions, medium vessel occlusions, and tandem lesions [8, 11, 12]. Despite its success, challenges remain in prehospital detection, rapid diagnosis, and post-EVT care [9].

Early Efforts in Stroke Treatment (50 Years Ago)

Historical Background of Endovascular Treatment

The history of endovascular treatments for intracranial aneurysms spans nearly two centuries, with early attempts dating back to the 1800s [13]. Pioneers like Phillips and Velpeau experimented with needle insertion and electrical current to induce clot formation [13]. The field progressed through various eras, including pre-balloons, balloons, and coils [14]. Significant milestones include Luessenhop and Velasquez's first intracranial vessel catheterization in 1964 [14] and Forssmann's self-catheterization in 1929 [15]. Technological advancements, such as microcatheters and detachable coils, revolutionized the field [16, 17]. Despite initial skepticism, endovascular techniques gained acceptance as their efficacy improved, offering minimally invasive alternatives to traditional surgery [17, 18]. Today, endovascular neurosurgery continues to evolve, providing vascular neurosurgeons with an expanding array of treatment options [15].

Early Devices and Techniques

Endovascular thrombectomy for acute ischemic stroke has evolved significantly over the past decades. Early techniques included intra-arterial thrombolysis in the late 1990s, followed by first-generation mechanical devices like the Merci Retriever and Penumbra System [10, 19]. Despite initial setbacks, the introduction of stent retrievers in 2008 revolutionized stroke treatment, enabling recanalization rates exceeding 90% [20]. The superiority of mechanical thrombectomy over intravenous thrombolysis was established through landmark trials in 2015 [21, 22]. Current mainstreams in thrombectomy techniques include stent retriever thrombectomy and direct clot aspiration, with the Solitaire and Trevo retrievers being prominent devices [21]. Combination techniques like ADAPT, FAST, and Solumbra have also emerged [23-25]. These advancements have significantly improved clinical outcomes for acute ischemic stroke patients.

Failed Stroke Trials and Lessons Learned

Early trials like PROACT II demonstrated the potential of intra-arterial thrombolysis for acute ischemic stroke, showing improved outcomes within 6 hours of onset [26]. Subsequent mechanical thrombectomy devices, such as the Merci Retriever, achieved recanalization rates of 48-57% [27, 28]. However, early randomized trials (SYNTHESIS, IMS-III, MR-RESCUE) failed to show clear benefits of endovascular treatment, likely due to suboptimal patient selection and outdated devices [29]. The introduction of stent retrievers marked a significant advancement, leading to higher recanalization rates compared to older devices [30]. Despite initial setbacks, lessons learned from failed trials informed subsequent studies, emphasizing the importance of proper patient selection, faster treatment times, and improved imaging techniques [31, 32]. These insights paved the way for successful trials in 2015 that established endovascular therapy as the standard of care for large vessel occlusion strokes [10].

Successes and Breakthroughs

Recent landmark trials have demonstrated the effectiveness of endovascular thrombectomy (EVT) for acute ischemic stroke caused by large vessel occlusion. MR CLEAN, ESCAPE, EXTEND-IA, SWIFT PRIME, and REVASCAT trials showed significant improvements in functional outcomes and established EVT as a new standard of care [33-35]. These trials selected patients based on occlusion location, time from stroke onset, and infarct burden [35]. The DAWN and DEFUSE-3 trials extended the treatment window to 24 hours in selected patients [35]. Meta-analyses confirmed the safety and efficacy of stent retrievers for acute stroke management [36]. Despite these breakthroughs, complete recovery is not achieved in all patients, highlighting the need for adjunct neuroprotective therapies [37]. The success of these trials has significant implications for healthcare systems, necessitating the establishment of well-equipped stroke centers and trained personnel [38].

Milestones in Stroke Trials

Endovascular Stroke Trials for Anterior Circulation

The evolution of endovascular thrombectomy for acute ischemic stroke has seen significant advancements over the past two decades. These advancements have transformed acute stroke treatment, offering hope for better outcomes in patients who do not meet the criteria for intravenous thrombolysis [19]. Anterior circulation stroke trials can be divided into three main categories: early window trials, extended window trials, and large core trials. These trials helped guide the current guidelines for treating patients who presented with acute stroke within 24 hours which improves the medical care for stroke patients.

Early Window Trials

In 2015, five randomized trials (MR CLEAN, ESCAPE, SWIFT PRIME, REVASCAT, and EXTEND-IA) showed the efficacy of EVT over standard medical care in patients with acute ischemic stroke caused by occlusion of arteries of the proximal anterior circulation within 6 hours after stroke onset [39-43], summaries below:

1. MR CLEAN [39]: The first trial to demonstrate a clear benefit of EVT in patients with ischemic stroke due to large vessel occlusion (LVO) in the anterior circulation.
2. ESCAPE [41]: This trial highlighted the importance of faster time to treatment significantly improved outcomes in stroke patients treated with EVT.
3. SWIFT PRIME [43]: Focused on the early treatment of stroke patients with EVT and showed better functional outcomes at 90 days compared to standard care alone.
4. REVASCAT [42]: Reinforced the importance of EVT in reducing disability among patients with ischemic stroke due to large vessel occlusion.
5. EXTEND-IA [40]: Demonstrated that EVT was associated with improved reperfusion rates and better clinical outcomes in stroke patients.

These trials together transformed the management of acute ischemic stroke by establishing EVT as the standard of care for patients presenting with large vessel occlusion within the specified time window.

A meta-analysis at the patient level was conducted using the combined data set from the MR CLEAN, ESCAPE, SWIFT Prime, REVASCAT, and EXTEND-IA trials. A total of 1287 individuals (634 endovascular thrombectomy patients and 653 control patients) were enrolled in the Highly Effective Reperfusion Evaluated in Multiple Endovascular Stroke Trials (HERMES) collaboration [44], resulting in a substantial impact on clinical guidelines for the management of acute ischemic stroke. Therefore, supporting the increased use of EVT as a standard treatment method, which enhances patient care for stroke.

There were 2 additional studies that were conducted around the same time that were not included in the HERMES collaboration.

1. The THRACE (Thrombectomie des Artères Cérébrales) trial [45]: has shown that individuals with acute cerebral ischemia can achieve considerable improvements in functional independence when EVT is paired with routine intravenous thrombolysis (IVT). The trial found no evidence of increased mortality among patients who received this combined treatment. This suggests that bridging therapy (IVT + EVT) should be considered.
2. The Pragmatic Ischemic Thrombectomy Evaluation (PISTE) trial [46]: was a multicenter, randomized clinical trial to evaluate the effectiveness of combining intravenous thrombolysis (IVT) with adjunctive mechanical thrombectomy (MT) in patients with acute ischemic stroke due to large vessel occlusion. The trial, which was conducted at several sites, sought to ascertain whether thrombectomy, in addition to routine thrombolysis, could result in better functional outcomes after 90 days. Overall, while the PISTE trial did not conclusively demonstrate improved outcomes from the addition of MT to IVT in all cases, it emphasized the need for further exploration and the potential for tailored approaches in managing acute ischemic stroke.

Table 1 lists the summary of each early window trial that was included in HERMES collaboration including Baseline characteristics and inclusion criteria in addition to outcomes [47].

Extended Window Trials

Recent trials have demonstrated the efficacy of endovascular thrombectomy (EVT) for anterior circulation large vessel occlusion strokes beyond the traditional 6-hour window. The DAWN [48] and DEFUSE-3 [49] trials showed benefits up to 24 hours in carefully selected patients [50]. Those two were the main Trials for extended window patients, there were also POSITIVE [51] and RESILIENT [52] trials including patients in the extended window period.

1. DAWN [48]: Investigated endovascular therapy (EVT) for stroke patients 6 to 24 hours from the last known well time, showing significantly improved functional outcomes compared to standard care, particularly in patients with favorable imaging profiles.
2. DEFUSE 3 [49]: Evaluated endovascular therapy (EVT) for patients with ischemic stroke between 6 to 16 hours from the time last known well, demonstrating significantly better functional outcomes in patients selected based on perfusion imaging.
3. POSITIVE [51]: A collaborative trial focused on using perfusion imaging to select ischemic stroke patients for endovascular therapy, but it was terminated early due to the overwhelming success of previous trials, including those in the HERMES collaboration.
4. RESILIENT [52]: Conducted in Brazil, this trial confirmed the effectiveness of mechanical thrombectomy in treating acute ischemic stroke caused by large vessel occlusion, showing significantly improved functional outcomes in a public healthcare setting.

Table 1. Summary of each early window trial included in HERMES collaboration

Variable	MR CLEAN	ESCAPE	SWIFT PRIME	REVASCAT	EXTEND-IA
Baseline characteristics and inclusion criteria					
Geographical location	16 Medical centers in the Netherlands	22 Centers worldwide	39 Centers in the United States and Europe	4 Centers in Catalonia, Spain	14 Centers in Australia and New Zealand
Age, y Median (IQR) Mean ± SD	≥18 65.8 (54.5–76)	≥18 71 (60–81)	18–80 66.3 ± 11.3	18–80 65.7 ± 11.3	No age limits 70.2 ± 11.8
NIHSS score Median (IQR)	≥2 17 (14–2)	≥6 16 (13–20)	≥8 and <30 17 (13–19)	≥6 17 (14–20)	Any 13 (9–19)
Time window, h	6	12	6	8	6
Ischemic core volume/ASPECTS	Any	>5	≥6 or ischemic core <50 mL on CTP	>6 on NCCT >5 (DWI-MRI)	Ischemic core <70 mL, mismatch of >1.2 CTP
Site of occlusion	Intracranial ICA, MCA M1 or M2, or ACA A1 or A2	ICA or MCA M1 or M2	ICA or MCA M1	ICA or MCA M1	ICA or MCA M1 or M2
Premorbid mRS score	Any	Barthel index ≥90	0–1	0–1	0–1
IV-tPA	87.1% vs 90.6%	72.7% vs 79.7%	100% in both	68% vs 77.7%	100% in both
Outcome					
Reperfusion rates	75.4% vs 32.9%*	72.4% vs 31.2%*	83% vs 40%*	66% with core laboratory, 80% self-assessment; not reported in control group	89% vs 34%*
sICH	7.7% vs 6.4%	3.6% vs 2.7%	0% vs 3%,	1.9% in both groups	0% vs 6%
90-d mRS score 0–2	33% vs 19%*	53% vs 29.3%*	60% vs 35%*	43.7% vs 28.2%*	71% vs 40%*
Shift of 90-d mRS scores	cOR, 1.67 (95% CI, 1.21–2.30)	cOR, 2.6 (95% CI, 1.7–3.8)	*P*<0.001 by the Cochran-Mantel-Haenszel test	Adjusted OR, 1.7 (95% CI, 1.05–2.8)	Generalized OR, 2.0 (95% CI, 1.2–3.8)
90-d Mortality	21% vs 22%	10.4% vs 19%*	9% vs 12%	18.4% vs 15.5%	9% vs 20%

*Indicates significance.

ACA anterior cerebral artery; ASPECTS, Alberta Stroke Program Early CT Score; cOR, common OR; CTP, computed tomography perfusion; DAWN, DWI or CTP Assessment With Clinical Mismatch in the Triage of Wake-Up and Late Presenting Strokes Undergoing Neurointervention With Trevo; DEFUSE 3, Endovascular Therapy Following Imaging Evaluation for Ischemic Stroke 3; DWI, diffusion-weighted imaging; ESCAPE, Endovascular Treatment for Small Core and Anterior Circulation Proximal Occlusion With Emphasis on Minimizing CT to Recanalization Times; EXTEND-IA, Extending the Time for Thrombolysis in Emergency Neurological Deficits With Intra-Arterial Therapy; ICA, internal carotid artery; IST-3, Third International Stroke Trial Computed Tomography Angiography (IST-3 CTA) score; IQR, interquartile range; IV-tPA, intravenous tissue-type plasminogen activator; MCA, middle cerebral artery; MR CLEAN, Multicenter Randomized Clinical Trial of Endovascular Treatment for Acute Ischemic Stroke in the Netherlands; MRI, magnetic resonance imaging; mRS, modified Rankin Scale; NCCT, noncontrast computed tomography; NIHSS, National Institutes of Health Stroke Scale; OR, odds ratio; PISTE, Pragmatic Ischemic Thrombectomy Evaluation; RESILIENT, Randomization of Endovascular Treatment With Stent-Retriever and/or Thromboaspiration Versus Best Medical Therapy in Acute Ischemic Stroke Due to Large Vessel Occlusion Trial; REVASCAT, Revascularization With Solitaire FR Device Versus Best Medical Therapy in the Treatment of Acute Stroke Due to Anterior Circulation Large Vessel Occlusion Presenting Within 8 Hours of Symptom Onset; sICH, symptomatic intracranial hemorrhage; SWIFT PRIME, Solitaire With the Intention for Thrombectomy as Primary Endovascular Treatment for Acute Ischemic Stroke; and THRACE, Thrombectomie des Artères Cerebrales [47].

Table 2. Summary of each extended window trial included in the AURORA collaboration and was not a part of HERMES collaboration

Variable	DEFUSE 3	DAWN	RESILIENT
Inclusion criteria and baseline characteristics			
Geographical location	38 US centers	32 Centers worldwide	12 Public hospitals in Brazil
Age, y Median (IQR) Mean±SD	18–90 70 (59–79)	≥18 69.4±14.1	>18 65 (54–77)
NIHSS score Median (IQR)	≥6 16 (10–20)	≥10 17 (13–21)	≥8 18 (14–21)
Time window, h	6–16	6–24	8
Ischemic core volume/ASPECTS	Infarct size <70 mL, mismatch ratio ≥1.8	A. Aged ≥80 y: infarct volume of <21 mL B. Aged <80 y: infarct volume of <31 mL C. Age <80 y and NIHSS score ≥20: infarct volume of 31 to <51 mL	≥6 Infarct size <70 mL, mismatch ratio ≥1.8 Penumbra ≥15 mL
Site of occlusion	ICA or MCA M1	ICA or MCA M1	ICA or MCA M1
Premorbid mRS score	0–2	0–1	0–1
IV-tPA	11% vs 9%	5% vs 13%	68.5% vs 71.8%
Outcome			
Reperfusion rates	79% vs 18%*	77% vs 36%*	80.2% vs 46.3*
sICH	7% vs 4%	6% vs 3%	4.5% in both groups
90-d mRS score 0–2	45% vs 17%*	49% vs 13%*	35.1% vs 20%*
Shift of 90-d mRS scores	OR, 2.77 (95% CI, 1.63–4.70)	Not reported	OR, 2.28 (95% CI, 1.41–3.69)
90-d Mortality	14% vs 26%	19% vs 1	24.3% vs 30.0%

*Indicates significance.

ACA indicates anterior cerebral artery; ASPECTS, Alberta Stroke Program Early CT Score; cOR, common OR; CTP, computed tomography perfusion; DAWN, DWI or CTP Assessment With Clinical Mismatch in the Triage of Wake-Up and Late Presenting Strokes Undergoing Neurointervention With Trevo; DEFUSE 3, Endovascular Therapy Following Imaging Evaluation for Ischemic Stroke 3; DWI, diffusion-weighted imaging; ESCAPE, Endovascular Treatment for Small Core and Anterior Circulation Proximal Occlusion With Emphasis on Minimizing CT to Recanalization Times; EXTEND-IA, Extending the Time for Thrombolysis in Emergency Neurological Deficits With Intra-Arterial Therapy; ICA, internal carotid artery; IST-3, Third International Stroke Trial Computed Tomography Angiography (IST-3 CTA) score; IQR, interquartile range; IV-tPA, intravenous tissue-type plasminogen activator; MCA, middle cerebral artery; MR CLEAN, Multicenter Randomized Clinical Trial of Endovascular Treatment for Acute Ischemic Stroke in the Netherlands; MRI, magnetic resonance imaging; mRS, modified Rankin Scale; NCCT, noncontrast computed tomography; NIHSS, National Institutes of Health Stroke Scale; OR, odds ratio; PISTE, Pragmatic Ischemic Thrombectomy Evaluation; RESILIENT, Randomization of Endovascular Treatment With Stent-Retriever and/or Thromboaspiration Versus Best Medical Therapy in Acute Ischemic Stroke Due to Large Vessel Occlusion Trial; REVASCAT, Revascularization With Solitaire FR Device Versus Best Medical Therapy in the Treatment of Acute Stroke Due to Anterior Circulation Large Vessel Occlusion Presenting Within 8 Hours of Symptom Onset; sICH, symptomatic intracranial hemorrhage; SWIFT PRIME, Solitaire With the Intention for Thrombectomy as Primary Endovascular Treatment for Acute Ischemic Stroke; and THRACE, Thrombectomie des Artères Cerebrales [47].

The AURORA (Analysis of Pooled Data From Randomized Studies of Thrombectomy More Than 6 Hours After Last Known Well) [42] Collaboration in order to provide a more comprehensive assessment of the safety and effectiveness of thrombectomy in the 6–24 hour window, pooled individual patient data from the DAWN (6–24 hours; n = 206) and DEFUSE 3 (6–16 hours; n = 182) as well as from the subset of patients from the ESCAPE (6–12 hours; n = 49), POSITIVE (6–12 hours; n = 21) [51], REVASCAT (6–8 hours; n=21), and RESILIENT (6–8 hours; n = 26) [52] trials who were treated after 6 hours from the time last seen well. Patient-level data from 505 subjects (266 intervention, 239 control) were included.

There was a strong benefit of thrombectomy in the primary analysis. Real-world data from registries and retrospective studies also support the safety and effectiveness of EVT beyond 6 hours, with outcomes comparable to earlier treatment [53, 54]. Some studies even report successful outcomes for EVT performed beyond 24 hours [55, 56]. Patient selection typically involves the assessment of the infarct core, penumbra, and collateral circulation using advanced imaging techniques [57]. While strict trial criteria exclude many patients, off-label treatment of trial-ineligible patients has shown promising results [55]. These findings suggest that a larger population of stroke patients may benefit from extended time window EVT with more permissive selection criteria.

Table 2 listed the summary of each extended window trial that was included in the AURORA collaboration and was not a part of HERMES collaboration, including Baseline characteristics and inclusion criteria in addition to outcomes [47].

Large Core Trials

Six randomized controlled trials (RCT) were conducted to evaluate the outcomes of patients who presented with acute ischemic stroke who presented with large core infarctions; defined as infarct sizes determined by an ASPECTS less or equal to 5 and/or an estimated ischemic-core volume greater than 50 ml.

These patients were managed either with endovascular thrombectomy (EVT) in addition to medical management or with medical management alone. Those trials are summarized below:

1. The SELECT2 trial [58]: was a multicentral international, randomized controlled trial. Patients treated with EVT had much better functional outcomes than those treated solely with medical treatment. This was especially noticeable when looking at functional independence using the modified Rankin Scale (mRS). The trial did, however, also highlight how important it is to act quickly and implement effective transfer procedures in order to maximize the advantages of EVT. For patients with large core strokes, healthcare professionals can increase overall survival rates and maximize patient outcomes by reducing delays and guaranteeing prompt transport to EVT-capable hospitals.
2. The ANGEL-ASPECT trial [59]: was a multicentral, randomized controlled trial conducted in 46 sites in China. Patients treated with EVT had much better functional outcomes than those treated solely with medical treatment. This was especially noticeable when looking at functional independence using the modified Rankin Scale (mRS). Additionally, the study demonstrated the potential of EVT even in patients with significant infarction, even though there was no significant interaction between baseline imaging characteristics and treatment benefits. Still, the EVT group experienced a higher frequency of complications, such as symptomatic intracerebral hemorrhage. These results underline the need for more research into how to optimize patient selection and post-treatment outcomes, and they support the use of EVT as a therapy option for patients with large infarct cores.
3. The RESCUE-Japan LIMIT trial [60]: was a multicentral, randomized controlled trial conducted in 45 sites in Japan. The percentage of patients who achieved functional

independence varied noticeably between the EVT and medical care groups (20% in the former and 7% in the latter). The results showed that EVT considerably improved functional outcomes. Concerns about safety were also raised by the study; notable among these was the slightly elevated frequency of symptomatic intracerebral hemorrhage in the EVT group. The trial demonstrates that EVT can be beneficial even in more severe cases of stroke and supports it as a therapy option for patients with large infarct cores.

4. TESLA [61]: was a multicentral international, randomized controlled trial conducted in up to 65 centers in the US and 15 centers in Europe. The aim of the trial was to demonstrate the treatment benefits of EVT in improving disability outcomes at 90 days and one-year post-stroke, using the utility-weighted mRS as a primary measure of efficacy, alongside safety outcomes such as mortality rates at 90 days. The primary endpoint which is functional independence at 90 days was not met. However, it did indicate a potential benefit of EVT treatment in a large core infract population. This was shown on one-year follow-up for the patients favoring thrombectomy in patients with large core stroke.
5. TENSION [62]: was a multicentral international randomized controlled trial conducted in 40 sites across Canada and Europe. The primary outcome was assessed using the modified Rankin Scale at 90 days. It was stopped early due to significant efficacy findings following the first interim analysis. Which demonstrated that EVT was associated with improvement in functional outcomes compared to medical treatment alone. In addition, the EVT group showed reduced mortality rates and controllable rates of symptomatic intracerebral hemorrhage, which occurred in 6% of EVT patients as opposed to 5% in the control group.
6. LASTE [63]: was a multicentral international randomized controlled trial conducted in 24 sites in France and 6 sites in Spain. It aimed to determine whether endovascular thrombectomy within 24 hours after stroke onset could lead to better functional outcomes compared to standard medical care alone in patients with unrestricted large infarcts. It concluded that EVT plus medical care resulted in better functional outcomes and decreased mortality. However, it was associated with higher rates of symptomatic intracerebral hemorrhage. Owing to ethical concerns raised after the publication of other large core trials, the LASTE trial was terminated early.

Endovascular Stroke Trials for Basilar Artery Occlusion

Acute basilar artery occlusion (BAO) is a devastating condition with high mortality and disability rates. Recent randomized trials and meta-analyses have demonstrated that EVT significantly improves functional outcomes and reduces mortality compared to standard medical treatment alone [64-66]. Successful recanalization rates with EVT are high, ranging from 72% to 94.4% [67, 68]. Time to treatment is crucial, with shorter onset-to-treatment times associated with better outcomes [69]. However, EVT is associated with a higher risk of symptomatic intracerebral hemorrhage [70]. Patient selection using imaging criteria and consideration of collateral status may improve outcomes [67]. Overall, evidence supports the use of EVT for BAO within 24 hours of symptom onset in patients with moderate to severe stroke.

Recently, 4 randomized controlled trials were conducted for EVT management of basilar artery occlusion, 3 of them were conducted in China. Their summaries are listed below 2 were neutral trials (BEST and BASICS) and 2 were positive (ATTENTION and BAOCHE):

1. The BEST (Basilar Artery Occlusion Endovascular Intervention Versus Standard Medical Treatment) [71]: was a multicentral randomized controlled trial conducted at 28 centers in China. It aimed to evaluate the efficacy of EVT compared to standard medical management alone in patients with acute vertebrobasilar artery occlusion (VBAO) to assess if successful reperfusion could be associated with improved functional outcomes including functional independence and mortality at 90 days. When comparing patients undergoing endovascular therapy to those receiving standard medical care alone, there was no evidence that the former group had better outcomes. Loss of equipoise during the trial may have confounded the results, leading to low adherence to the prescribed study treatment and a smaller sample size as a result of the study's early termination. However, the trend towards better functional outcomes and lower mortality in the patients who received EVT.
2. BASICS (Basilar Artery International Cooperation Study) [72]: was a multicentral international randomized controlled trial conducted at 27 centers in seven countries. It aimed to evaluate the efficacy of EVT compared to standard medical management alone in patients with acute vertebrobasilar artery occlusion (VBAO) to assess if successful reperfusion could be associated with improved functional outcomes including functional independence at 90 days. The primary safety outcomes were symptomatic intracranial hemorrhage within 3 days after the initiation of treatment and mortality at 90 days. This trial found no difference in favorable outcomes between the two groups.
3. ATTENTION (Endovascular Treatment for Acute Basilar Artery Occlusion) [73]: was a multicentral randomized controlled trial conducted at 36 centers in China. It aimed to evaluate the efficacy of EVT compared to standard medical management alone in patients with acute vertebrobasilar artery occlusion (VBAO) to assess if successful reperfusion could be associated with improved functional outcomes including functional independence mRS (0-3) at 90 days. Secondary outcomes included mRS (0-2). While the safety outcomes were symptomatic intracranial hemorrhage at 24-72 hours, 90-days mortality, and procedural complications. In this trial, EVT was superior to medical care alone regarding functional outcomes at 90-days. However, it was associated with more safety concerns in terms of higher rates of intracerebral hemorrhages and procedural complications.
4. BAOCHE (Basilar Artery Occlusion Chinese Endovascular Trial) [74]: was a multicentral randomized controlled trial conducted over 5-year period in China. It aimed to evaluate the efficacy of EVT plus medical therapy compared to medical therapy alone in the extended window period (6 to 24 hours). The primary outcome was an mRS score of 0-4 at 90 days, which was changed later to an mRS of 0-3. The primary safety outcomes were symptomatic intracranial hemorrhage at 24 hr and 90-day mortality. In this trial, EVT plus medical therapy achieved a higher percentage of good functional outcomes at 90 days. However, it was associated with procedural complications and more cerebral hemorrhages.

Despite the safety concerns that were associated with the EVT group. Available evidence indicates that EVT is effective in treating BAO patients within 24 hours of the start of symptoms in moderate-to-severe neurological deficits. Those trials (ATTENTION and BAOCHE) showed similar efficacy compared to patients with anterior circulation ischemic strokes (AURORA [75] and HERMES collaborations [44], which highlight the importance of using EVT in BAO strokes. Currently, there is a collaboration (VERITAS) to pool patient-level data from the BEST and BASICS trials, which found that EVT has favorable functional outcomes and lower mortality rates compared to medical management alone. While rates of symptomatic intracerebral hemorrhage were higher in the EVT group [64].

Conclusion

Since its implementation as part of stroke management practice, EVT has changed the way acute ischemic stroke (AIS) is managed, turning a disease that was formerly fatal into one that has a significant chance of recovery. Initially, the sole option for treating AIS was intravenous thrombolysis (IVT) using tissue plasminogen activator (tPA). While this was helpful, it only worked for a small percentage of patients and had a narrow therapeutic window. By enabling the removal of significant large vessels occlusions, EVT revolutionized therapy options and enhanced patient outcomes.

This evolution of EVT has been fueled by improvements in imaging methods and medical devices technology in addition to an increasing amount of clinical evidence that support its effectiveness. Important clinical trials including ESCAPE, EXTEND-IA, and MR CLEAN played a pivotal role in proving the effectiveness and safety of EVT in lowering disability in stroke patients. These trials have increased the scope of EVT to cover more patients who would not have been eligible in the past, along with improvements to patient selection criteria and longer time windows for intervention.

Future developments in device technology, the use of artificial intelligence (AI) in imaging to enhance precisely patients' selection, and efforts to shorten treatment times will all likely have an impact on EVT. Given the substantial discrepancies in stroke care across the globe, one significant challenge will be ensuring fair access to EVT across various demographics and geographical areas. Optimizing pre-hospital stroke evaluation and transfer protocols is also essential in reducing delays and improving outcomes of EVT. As research in this field grows, advances in neuroprotection techniques, maybe in conjunction with EVT, could further minimize brain damage during ischemic events.

As EVT becomes increasingly essential for treating stroke patients, logistical and infrastructural barriers to provide timely care will remain one of the challenges. Additionally, ensuring the necessary training requirements for healthcare providers will be crucial.

References

[1] Feigin VL, Norrving B, Mensah GA. Global burden of stroke. *Circ Res*. 2017;120 (3):439–448.

[2] Katan M, Luft A. Global burden of stroke. In: *Semin Neurol*. 2018;Thieme Medical Publishers.

[3] Saini V, Guada L, Yavagal DR. Global epidemiology of stroke and access to acute ischemic stroke interventions. *Neurology*. 2021;97 (20_Supplement_2):S6–S16.

[4] Feigin VL, et al. Update on the global burden of ischemic and hemorrhagic stroke in 1990–2013: the GBD 2013 study. *Neuroepidemiology*. 2015;45 (3):161–176.
[5] Feigin VL, et al. Atlas of the global burden of stroke (1990–2013): the GBD 2013 study. *Neuroepidemiology*. 2015;45 (3):230–236.
[6] Mukherjee D, Patil CG. Epidemiology and the global burden of stroke. *World Neurosurg*. 2011;76 (6):S85–S90.
[7] Kalache A, Aboderin I. Stroke: the global burden. *Health Policy Plan*. 1995;10 (1):1–21.
[8] Ospel JM, et al. Evolution of stroke thrombectomy techniques to optimize first-pass complete reperfusion. In: *Semin Intervent Radiol*. 2020;Thieme Medical Publishers.
[9] Wassélius J, et al. Endovascular thrombectomy for acute ischemic stroke. *J Intern Med*. 2022;291 (3):303–316.
[10] Bageac DV, Gershon BS, De Leacy RA. The evolution of devices and techniques in endovascular stroke therapy. In: *Exon Publications*. 2021:149–170.
[11] Starikova N, et al. Endovascular thrombectomy for anterior circulation large vessel occlusion stroke: an evolution of trials. In: *Semin Ne*urol. 2023;Thieme Medical Publishers, Inc.
[12] Yeo LL, et al. Evidence-based updates to thrombectomy: targets, new techniques, and devices. *Front Neurol*. 2021;12:712527.
[13] Siddique K, et al. Treatment of aneurysms with wires and electricity: a historical overview. *J Neurosurg*. 2003;99 (6):1102–1107.
[14] Guglielmi G. The beginning and the evolution of the endovascular treatment of intracranial aneurysms: from the first catheterization of brain arteries to the new stents. *BMJ Publishing Group*. 2009:53–55.
[15] Costello JS, et al. Endovascular approach to cerebral revascularization: historical vignette. *World Neurosurg*. 2020;136:258–262.
[16] Kanaan Y, et al. Evolution of endovascular therapy for aneurysm treatment: historical overview. *Neurosurg Focus*. 2005;18 (2):1–4.
[17] Richling B. History of endovascular surgery: personal accounts of the evolution. *Neurosurgery*. 2006;59 (5):S3–30.
[18] Prestigiacomo CJ. Historical perspectives: the microsurgical and endovascular treatment of aneurysms. *Neurosurgery*. 2006;59 (5):S3–39.
[19] Spiotta AM, et al. Evolution of thrombectomy approaches and devices for acute stroke: a technical review. *J Neurointerv Surg*. 2015;7 (1):2–7.
[20] Buecke P, et al. The history of endovascular stroke treatment: from local intraarterial fibrinolysis to stent retriever thrombectomy. *RöFo*. 2023;Georg Thieme Verlag KG.
[21] Kang DH, Park J. Endovascular stroke therapy focused on stent retriever thrombectomy and direct clot aspiration: historical review and modern application. *J Korean Neurosurg Soc*. 2017;60 (3):335–347.
[22] Pierot L, et al. Techniques for endovascular treatment of acute ischemic stroke: from intra-arterial fibrinolytics to stent-retrievers. *Stroke*. 2015;46 (3):909–914.
[23] Leung V, et al. Mechanical thrombectomy in acute ischaemic stroke: a review of the different techniques. *Clin Radiol*. 2018;73 (5):428–438.
[24] Munich SA, Vakharia K, Levy EI. Overview of mechanical thrombectomy techniques. *Neurosurgery*. 2019;85 (Suppl_1):S60–S67.
[25] Przybylowski CJ, et al. Evolution of endovascular mechanical thrombectomy for acute ischemic stroke. *World J Clin Cases*. 2014;2 (11):614.
[26] Furlan A, et al. Intra-arterial prourokinase for acute ischemic stroke: the PROACT II study—a randomized controlled trial. *JAMA*. 1999;282 (21):2003–2011.
[27] Smith WS, et al. Mechanical thrombectomy for acute ischemic stroke: final results of the Multi MERCI trial. *Stroke*. 2008;39 (4):1205–1212.
[28] Smith WS, et al. Safety and efficacy of mechanical embolectomy in acute ischemic stroke: results of the MERCI trial. *Stroke*. 2005;36 (7):1432–1438.
[29] Gomis M, Dávalos A. Recanalization and reperfusion therapies of acute ischemic stroke: what have we learned? *Front Neurol*. 2014;5:226.
[30] Broderick JP, Schroth G. What the SWIFT and TREVO II trials tell us about the role of endovascular therapy for acute stroke. *Stroke*. 2013;44 (6):1761–1764.

[31] Goyal M, et al. Challenges of acute endovascular stroke trials. *Stroke*. 2014;45 (10):3116–3122.

[32] Gupta R. Reflections on the lessons of the recent endovascular stroke trials. *BMJ*. 2015;350:h575.

[33] Alberts MJ, Shang T, Magadan A. Endovascular therapy for acute ischemic stroke: dawn of a new era. *JAMA Neurol*. 2015;72 (10):1101–1103.

[34] Ding D. Endovascular mechanical thrombectomy for acute ischemic stroke: a new standard of care. *J Stroke*. 2015;17 (2):123.

[35] Jadhav AP, Desai SM, Jovin TG. Indications for mechanical thrombectomy for acute ischemic stroke: current guidelines and beyond. *Neurology*. 2021;97 (20_Supplement_2):S126–S136.

[36] Marmagkiolis K, et al. Safety and efficacy of stent retrievers for the management of acute ischemic stroke: comprehensive review and meta-analysis. *JACC Cardiovasc Interv*. 2015;8 (13):1758–1765.

[37] Lapchak PA. Critical early thrombolytic and endovascular reperfusion therapy for acute ischemic stroke victims: a call for adjunct neuroprotection. *Transl Stroke Res*. 2015;6:345–354.

[38] Pereira VM, Krings T. Comeback victory. *AJNR Am J Neuroradiol*. 2015;36:821–824.

[39] Berkhemer OA, et al. A randomized trial of intraarterial treatment for acute ischemic stroke. *N Engl J Med*. 2015;372 (1):11–20.

[40] Campbell BCV, et al. Endovascular therapy for ischemic stroke with perfusion-imaging selection. *N Engl J Med*. 2015;372 (11):1009–1018.

[41] Goyal M, et al. Randomized assessment of rapid endovascular treatment of ischemic stroke. *N Engl J Med*. 2015;372 (11):1019–1030.

[42] Jovin TG, et al. Thrombectomy within 8 hours after symptom onset in ischemic stroke. *N Engl J Med*. 2015;372 (24):2296–2306.

[43] Saver JL, et al. Stent-retriever thrombectomy after intravenous t-PA vs. t-PA alone in stroke. *N Engl J Med*. 2015;372 (24):2285–2295.

[44] Goyal M, et al. Endovascular thrombectomy after large-vessel ischaemic stroke: a meta-analysis of individual patient data from five randomised trials. *Lancet*. 2016;387 (10029):1723–1731.

[45] Bracard S, et al. Mechanical thrombectomy after intravenous alteplase versus alteplase alone after stroke (THRACE): a randomised controlled trial. *Lancet Neurol*. 2016;15 (11):1138–1147.

[46] Muir KW, et al. Endovascular therapy for acute ischaemic stroke: the PISTE randomised controlled trial. *J Neurol Neurosurg Psychiatry*. 2017;88 (1):38–44.

[47] Mohammaden MH, Haussen DC, Nogueira RG. Therapeutic advancements in the endovascular management of acute ischemic stroke. *Stroke Vasc Interv Neurol*. 2021;1 (1):e000168.

[48] Nogueira RG, et al. Thrombectomy 6 to 24 hours after stroke with a mismatch between deficit and infarct. *N Engl J Med*. 2018;378 (1):11–21.

[49] Albers GW, et al. Thrombectomy for stroke at 6 to 16 hours with selection by perfusion imaging. *N Engl J Med*. 2018;378 (8):708–718.

[50] Vidale S, et al. Mechanical thrombectomy in strokes with large-vessel occlusion beyond 6 hours: a pooled analysis of randomized trials. *J Clin Neurol*. 2018;14 (3):407–412.

[51] Mocco J, et al. POSITIVE: perfusion imaging selection of ischemic stroke patients for endovascular therapy. *J Neurointerv Surg*. 2022;14 (2):126–132.

[52] Martins SO, et al. Thrombectomy for stroke in the public health care system of Brazil. *N Engl J Med*. 2020;382 (24):2316–2326.

[53] Casetta I, et al. Endovascular thrombectomy for acute ischemic stroke beyond 6 hours from onset: a real-world experience. *Stroke*. 2020;51 (7):2051–2057.

[54] Mokin M, et al. Real-world stent retriever thrombectomy for acute ischemic stroke beyond 6 hours of onset: analysis of the NASA and TRACK registries. *J Neurointerv Surg*. 2019;11 (4):334–337.

[55] Desai SM, et al. Thrombectomy 24 hours after stroke: beyond DAWN. *J Neurointerv Surg*. 2018;10 (11):1039–1042.

[56] Manning NW, et al. Endovascular thrombectomy >24-hr from stroke symptom onset. *Front Neurol*. 2018;9:501.

[57] Motyer R, et al. Endovascular thrombectomy beyond 12 hours of stroke onset: a stroke network's experience of late intervention. *J Neurointerv Surg*. 2018;10 (11):1043–1046.

[58] Sarraj A, et al. Trial of endovascular thrombectomy for large ischemic strokes. *N Engl J Med*. 2023;388 (14):1259–1271.

[59] Huo X, et al. Trial of endovascular therapy for acute ischemic stroke with large infarct. *N Engl J Med.* 2023;388 (14):1272–1283.

[60] Yoshimura S, et al. Endovascular therapy for acute stroke with a large ischemic region. *N Engl J Med.* 2022;386 (14):1303–1313.

[61] Zaidat OO, et al. TESLA trial: rationale, protocol, and design. *Stroke Vasc Interv Neurol.* 2023;3 (4):e000787.

[62] Bendszus M, et al. Endovascular thrombectomy for acute ischaemic stroke with established large infarct: multicentre, open-label, randomised trial. *Lancet.* 2023;402 (10414):1753–1763.

[63] Costalat V, et al. Trial of thrombectomy for stroke with a large infarct of unrestricted size. *N Engl J Med.* 2024;390 (18):1677–1689.

[64] Alemseged F, et al. Endovascular therapy for basilar artery occlusion. *Stroke.* 2023;54 (4):1127–1137.

[65] Asif KS, et al. Endovascular treatment in acute basilar artery occlusion stroke: a brief practice update from the Society of Vascular and Interventional Neurology. *Stroke Vasc Interv Neurol.* 2023;3 (6):e000885.

[66] Ghozy S, et al. Endovascular treatment for basilar artery occlusion: revisiting evidence from randomized clinical trials. *Stroke Vasc Interv Neurol.* 2023:e000655.

[67] Pasarikovski CR, et al. Outcomes of endovascular thrombectomy for basilar artery occlusion. *Can J Neurol Sci.* 2020;47 (4):479–485.

[68] Sun X, et al. Endovascular treatment for acute basilar artery occlusion: a single center retrospective observational study. *BMC Neurol.* 2019;19:1–8.

[69] Dorňák T, et al. Endovascular treatment of acute basilar artery occlusion: time to treatment is crucial. *Clin Radiol.* 2015;70 (5):e20–e27.

[70] Zi W, et al. Assessment of endovascular treatment for acute basilar artery occlusion via a nationwide prospective registry. *JAMA Neurol.* 2020;77 (5):561–573.

[71] Liu X, et al. Endovascular treatment versus standard medical treatment for vertebrobasilar artery occlusion (BEST): an open-label, randomised controlled trial. *Lancet Neuro*l. 2020;19 (2):115–122.

[72] Langezaal LC, et al. Endovascular therapy for stroke due to basilar-artery occlusion. *N Engl J Med.* 2021;384 (20):1910–1920.

[73] Tao C, et al. Trial of endovascular treatment of acute basilar-artery occlusion. *N Engl J Med.* 2022;387 (15):1361–1372.

[74] Jovin TG, et al. Trial of thrombectomy 6 to 24 hours after stroke due to basilar-artery occlusion. *N Engl J Med.* 2022;387 (15):1373–1384.

[75] Jovin TG, et al. Thrombectomy for anterior circulation stroke beyond 6 h from time last known well (AURORA): a systematic review and individual patient data meta-analysis. *Lancet.* 2022;399 (10321):249–258.

Chapter 21

The History of the Neurointerventional Industry and Interventional Neuroradiology in Europe

Weiming Kong
and Xianli Lv*
Department of Neurosurgery, Beijing Tsinghua Changgung Hospital, School of Clinical Medicine, Tsinghua Medicine, Tsinghua University, Beijing, China

Abstract

There are numerous products utilized in interventional neuroradiology, including catheter sheaths, catheters, guidewires, connectors, neurostents, and embolic materials. All of these devices must possess the ability to resist breakage, as it is critical that catheters do not fracture within the blood vessels of the brain. Simultaneously, they should be designed to be exceptionally fine and flexible to minimize complications such as vascular damage, vascular spasm, and perforation of small cerebral arteries. This chapter focuses on the development and design of interventional neuroradiology devices tailored for complex and challenging neurovascular conditions. To fully comprehend the performance of these interventional neuroradiology products, it is essential to first understand their manufacturing processes.

Keywords: interventional neuroradiology, neurointervention, device, production

Introduction

To become an interventional neuroradiologist, one must engage in extensive study and cultivate a flexible mindset. The accuracy of three-dimensional imaging is continually improving. The X-rays produced by advanced digital imaging equipment necessitate the use of heavy lead protective clothing, which is becoming increasingly standard. The anatomical structure of the brain is highly intricate, and only with a calm and meticulous approach can physicians accurately identify the location of aneurysms—sometimes as small as a grain of wheat—and employ minimally invasive techniques for treatment. Interventional neuroradiologists do not

* Corresponding Author's Email: lvxianli000@163.com

In: World History of Neurointerventional Surgery
Editors: Xianli Lv and Zhongxue Wu
ISBN: 979-8-89530-792-2

perform craniotomy surgeries; instead, they utilize vascular access devices such as microwires and microcatheters to guide their procedures. These tools enable them to navigate to the aneurysm and either occlude it with a platinum coil or implant a microvascular device known as an "intracranial stent" for treatment. These precise surgical interventions require the surgeon to control movements and gestures via a screen while the patient remains under general anesthesia. The entire surgical process can last from one to three hours. There are numerous types of interventional neuroradiology products, and it is essential to understand their manufacturing and development processes to comprehend their characteristics. This knowledge is crucial for selecting the appropriate product during treatment to achieve optimal therapeutic outcomes.

From Extruded Catheters to Braided Catheters

The production of interventional neuroradiological catheters, including arterial angiography catheters for brain and spinal cord examinations, has evolved from extruded/non-braided to braided types.

In 2008, the B. Burdenko Neurosurgery Institute in Moscow unveiled a bronze bust of Professor Fiodor Serbinenko (1928-2002) to honor his invention of detachable balloons in 1974 (Figure 1). Professors Debrun and Ingenor in Paris have also developed similar balloons [1].

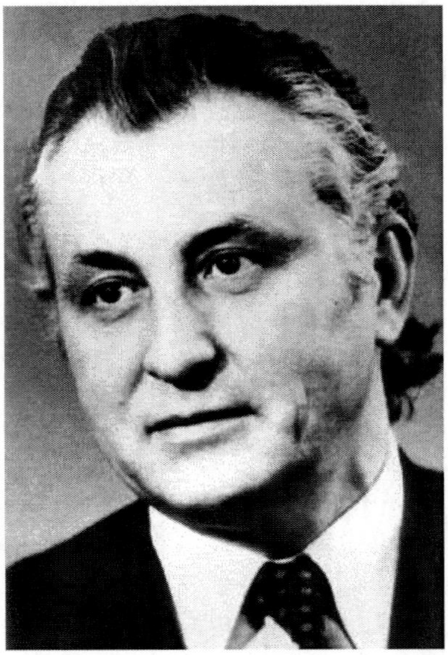

Figure 1. Professor Fedor Serbinenko (1928-2002), Founder of Endovascular Neurosurgery. Burdenko Neurosurgical Institute, Moscow, Russia.

To insert a detachable balloon into intracranial blood vessels, a very thin and flexible tube is essential. However, at that time, no one had successfully created a tube thin enough for use in intracranial blood vessels. Léopold Plowiecki began researching and developing micro-tools, such as extruders, punches, and molds, and subsequently founded BALT Extrusion. In 1977, BALT Extrusion successfully manufactured a very thin tube, the PE ROSE 1F tube, which has an inner diameter of 0.2 mm and an outer diameter of 0.33 mm. This tube was utilized for detachable balloons (Figure 2) [1].

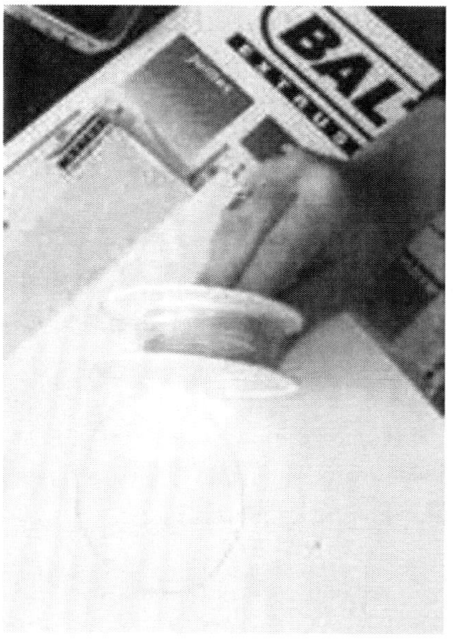

Figure 2. Roll of PE ROSE 1F tube with inner diameter of 0.2 mm and outer diameter of 0.33 mm. Illustration extracted from Leopold Plowiecki's book "The art and savoir faire of interventional neuroradiology – Memoirs of a manufacturer."

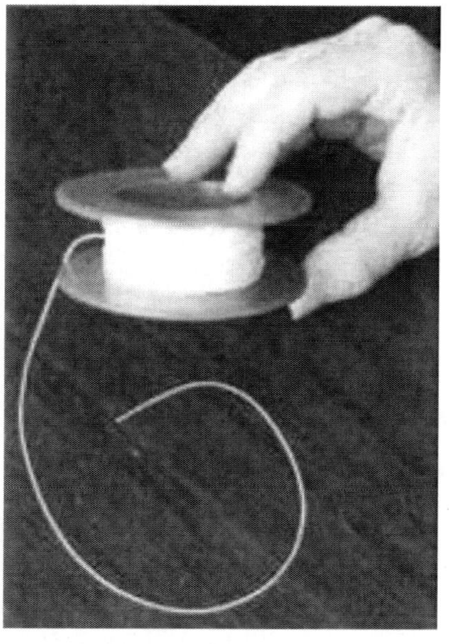

Figure 3. The PURSIL 1.8 F with an inner diameter of 0.4mm and an outer diameter of 0.6mm. Illustration extracted from Leopold Plowiecki's book "The art and savoir faire of interventional neuroradiology – Memoirs of a manufacturer."

In 1980, the plastic conversion industry struggled to produce high-quality, ultra-soft catheters. BALT Extrusion developed a synthetic material that combines the mechanical resistance of polyurethane with the flexibility of silicone. This synthetic material catheter is named "PURSIL," which is the commercial name given by Léopold Plowiecki and is invented for Pr. Jean-Jacques Merland. As it is made of PolyURethane (PUR) and SILicone (SIL), he simply named it "PURSIL." It is very soft, has strong tensile strength, is compatible with blood, and is easy to observe under X-rays. The product is white in color, feels very smooth to the touch, and has a good hand feel. PURSIL 1.8F with an inner diameter of 0.4mm and an outer diameter of 0.6mm is very soft and needs to be used in conjunction with a guiding catheter (Figure3). During the same period, several doctors were using various types of injection glass chambers made by glass blowing factories. Some doctors also assemble two large syringes for injecting contrast agents. These tools had been used for several years [1].

At the suggestion of Professor Luc Picard of Nancy, BALT extrusion made the proximal end of the microcatheter as hard as a contrast catheter and the distal end as soft as a PURSIL. Professor Jacques Moret tested the new prototype catheter in 1987 and found that it could quickly pass through increasingly thin and curved arterial vessels. The world's first floating microcatheter was called the Magic Catheter because it really is magic. There were a few imitations, including the "Zephir" from Target in San Francisco and the "Minitorquer" from Ingenor in Paris. But these imitations disappeared because they did not outperform the Magic catheter [1].

In 1980, several major cardiac catheter manufacturers in the United States, including Cardiovascular, Cordis and William Cook, did not recognise the potential of interventional neuroradiology. At the time, there were only three small manufacturers interested in interventional neuroradiology: ITC (Interventional Therapy Company) in the United States, Ingenor and BALT Extrusion in Europe. But the development of interventional neuroradiology later attracted Cordis, William Cook and Target, a San Francisco-based manufacturer founded in 1985 [1]. Target had the largest market in the world (at the time, the US market was estimated to be 10 times larger than the European market), so it developed rapidly. Target pioneered the interventional neuroradiology medical market with its Tracker microcatheter and a range of microwire products.

In 1985, BALT Extrusion's main business was extruded tube catheters. However, it became the first manufacturer in Europe to produce metal braided catheters. At that time, the American manufacturers Cordis and Cook had already mastered selective arterial angiography and braided catheter technology for many years (Figure 4). The stainless steel braided catheters could effectively transmit torque and pressure (Figure 5). Therefore, in 1985, the detachable balloon had not only a release system but also a delivery system via the femoral or carotid artery. The carotid route was quickly abandoned because it was dangerous for both physicians and patients (physicians had a high risk of X-rays being too close and thrombotic complications). The new type of braided microcatheters have a perfectly calibrated inner cavity, good flexibility and sufficient lubrication of the inner coating compared to extruded microcatheters. The commonly used sizes of braided microcatheters are 17 (the diameter of the inner cavity is 0.017 inch), 21 (the diameter of the inner cavity is 0.021 inch) and 27 (the diameter of the inner cavity is 0.027 inch). For these metal braided catheters, the gradual softness gradient effect is achieved by welding several sections of tubing together, sometimes requiring 4 to 5 tubes to be welded together. Without these metal braided microcatheters, it would be impossible to deliver platinum coils or self-expanding nickel-titanium alloy stents into the brain to embolize aneurysms. To improve the delivery of detachable coils, calibrated lumen of braided catheters and lubricating coatings are required. The delivery performance of non-braided catheters is not ideal.

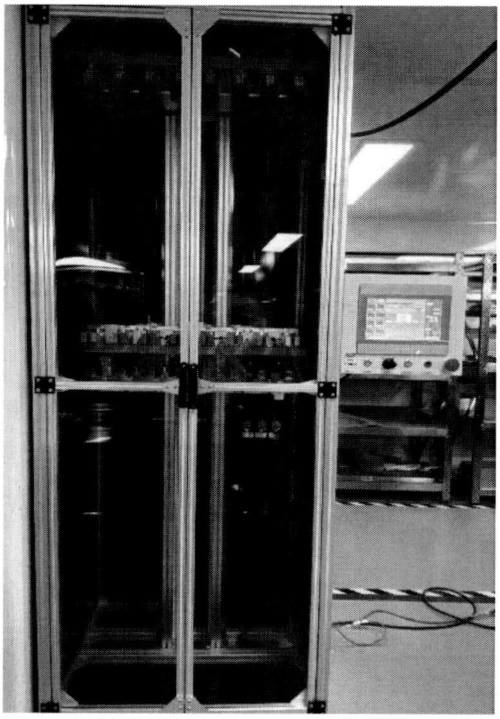

Figure 4. A tube laminating machine is used to laminate braided tube and polymer tube together to produce stainless steel braided catheters.

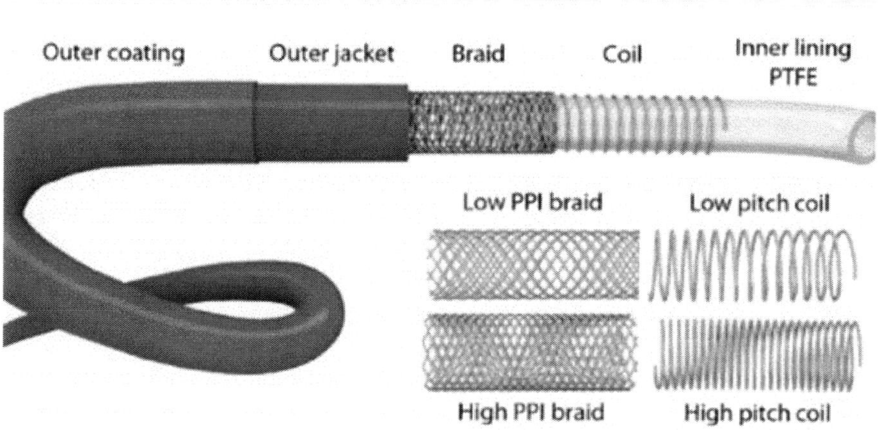

Figure 5. The production of stainless steel braided catheter involves placing these layers on a core shaft and then using equipment to laminate them together.

From Free Coils to Retrievable Coils

In the 1980s, there was an increasing use of very small, tightly coiled coils for embolization of arterial aneurysms and arteriovenous fistulas. The initial utilized coil is designated as the "Hillal Coil." Fabricated from stainless steel, this coil boasts a diameter of less than 1 millimeter and a length of less than 1 centimeter. The substance under consideration is characterized by its linear configuration and substantial rigidity. To administer the substance, it is necessary to inject it through a syringe and a microcatheter. This is a matter of significant concern, as the object in question possesses a degree of sharpness that is comparable to that of a nail. The technology of coils has undergone rapid development, resulting in a progressive shift towards greater softness and slenderness. In order to eliminate artifacts (distortions of magnetic resonance images) caused by coils, stainless steel was substituted with platinum or tungsten (non-ferromagnetic metals). Notwithstanding, the implantation of the coils into the aneurysm proved to be a challenging procedure. For instance, if the coil is excessively long and not completely inserted into the aneurysm, its removal becomes unfeasible. In 1991, Target Corporation introduced a controllable detachable coil system known as the GDC (Guglielmi Detachable Coil). This innovation was named after Italian neurosurgeon Dr. Guglielmi, who holds the patent for the technology [2].

The development of detachable coil systems represents a major step forward in using coil technology for aneurysm embolization. This product uses the process of electrolysis. This coil is welded onto a stainless steel pusher wire. To achieve detachment, the solder joint must be pushed to the end of the microcatheter. The positive pole of a 4V battery is connected to the coil's pusher wire, and the negative pole is connected to a needle that pierces the skin. Then, the solder joint will be dissolved by electrolysis. This method may seem simple, but the initial design release was not as easy as imagined. Sometimes it took half an hour for the coil to come off, and sometimes it just wouldn't come off. In 1993, Balt invented the Mechanical Detachable Coil System (MDS) and applied for a technology patent to protect the intellectual property of the quick mechanical detachable system. It's inspired by bicycle wire rope: the handle at one end of the coil is held in place by the hook of the pusher. If the hook is still in the catheter, the coil cannot be released. As soon as the hook leaves the catheter, the ball on the coil is released because it is no longer held in place by the inner wall of the catheter.

When you're moving the coil, it's important to keep the microcatheter stable. The push rod of the coil should be softer than the microcatheter. The push rod is made of a special alloy with a very small diameter, similar to a hair line (8% of 1 mm). It has a hook at the end that catches the 0.15 mm handle at the end of the coil. The catheter's tip reaches the neck of the aneurysm. The doctor pushes the coil (a tightly coiled microcoil) forward with a push rod. The doctor needs to insert a 2-meter push rod from the patient's groin puncture site, pass it through the femoral artery, and insert the coil into the aneurysm. The pushing and releasing of the coil are both controlled by angiography and displayed on the screen of the DSA machine (DSA is digital subtraction angiography). DSA shows a black and white 2D image. Although the mechanical design of MDS was very good, the calibration of the inner cavity size of the extruded microcatheter used as a pathway was too poor. This usually caused the hook on the MDS push rod to get stuck or the coil to detach inside the catheter. It is especially important to use metal braided microcatheters, whose inner lumen is much better calibrated.

The MDS coil, made of tungsten, is colorful. These coils have a special design that uses a "shape memory" effect. After they are heated, the coils will change color. They can look light golden yellow, green, purple, or blue. The coils have different colors because they were cooled at different rates, but they all work well.

The Guglielmi detachable coil (GDC; Boston Scientific, Massachusetts, USA) was approved by the US Food and Drug Administration in 1995 [2]. These platinum coils are soft and can be used to make aneurysms of different sizes, lengths, and shapes. The two-marker coil delivery microcatheter is made with the two markers at the end separated by 3 centimeters. A similar marker also exists on GDC pusher wire. This is located 3 centimeters from the fusion point of the platinum coil and pusher wire. The position of the proximal catheter marker and the coil marker shows that the detachment zone of the GDC system is at the tip of the catheter, where it can be detached. There are two types of GDC coils: 0.010-inch diameter (GDC-10) and 0.018-inch diameter (GDC-18). GDC-10 and GDC-18 coils are available in different lengths and diameters. There is also a more flexible version that allows for tighter and less traumatic packing of the aneurysmal cavity. Stretch-resistant coils have been developed to help prevent damage or unraveling when they are retrieved from an aneurysm.

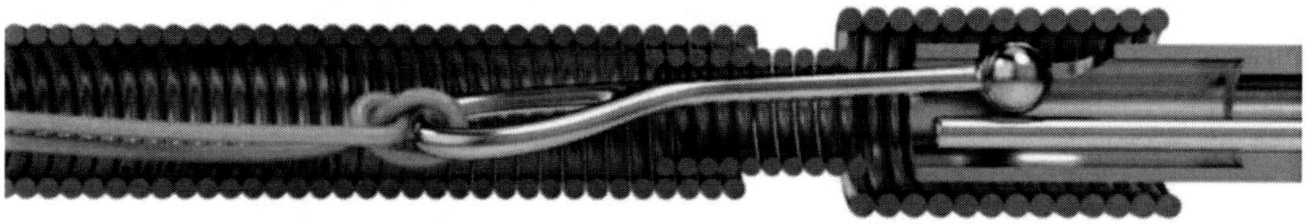

Figure 6. A new mechanical detachment design.

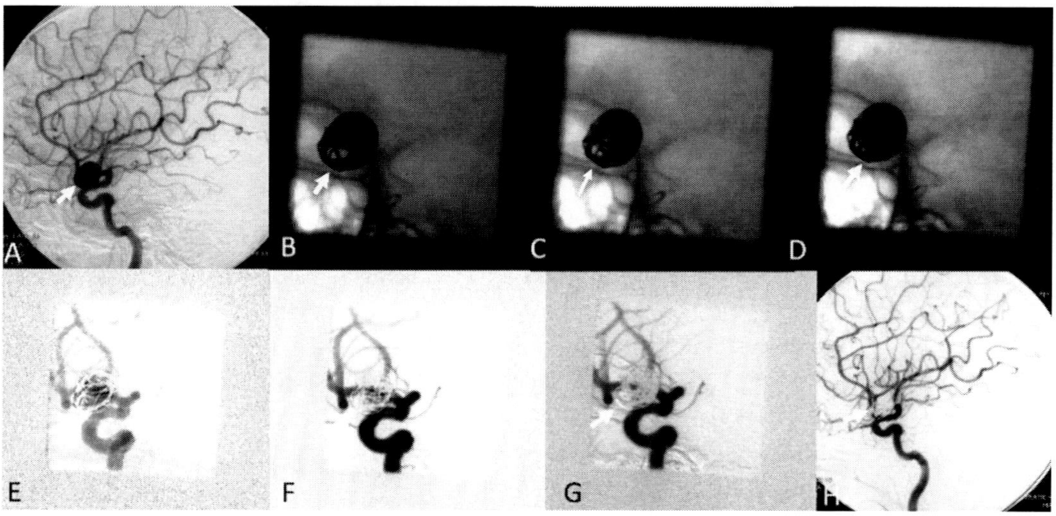

Figure 7. A 54-year-old woman with an unruptured large supraclinoid aneurysm of the right internal carotid artery was coiled. A, lateral view of the right internal carotid artery injection showing the large aneurysm of the supraclinoid segment (arrow). B-D, unsubtracted images, lateral projection, showing the coils (Microplex 20mm×50cm, 10mm×30cm; Orbit 10mm×30cm, 8mm×15cm; Hydrocoil 6mm×15cm, 5mm×10cm, 5mm×8cm, 6mm×10cm; Microplex 5mm×20cm) were inserted through an Echelon-14 microcatheter (ev3, Medtronic, USA) (arrows). E-G, subtracted angiography during coil embolization, lateral projection, showing the aneurysm was embolized step by step (arrows). H, lateral view of the right internal carotid artery injection after 5 months of aneurysm coil embolization showing the aneurysm was completely occluded (arrow).

The technologies of electrolytic and mechanical detachment are constantly being improved (Figure 6). In addition, hydraulic detachment technology has been developed [3]. Hydraulic and mechanical detachment technologies are better than electrolytic detachment technology because there is no metal where the coil and the pusher wire connect. This may not make the coil system stiffer. It's important to note that electrolytic detachment can be improved by having more consistent second separation times and success rates.

The development of new platinum coils that are more flexible and shaped, as well as platinum coils covered with biomaterials, has led to better results for patients receiving endovascular coiling treatment. Some examples of detachable coils that are available for commercial use include the Guglielmi detachable coil (GDC) (Stryker), Orbit (Codman Neurovascular), Micrus Presidio (Codman Neurovascular), Target 360 (Stryker) coils, Cosmos (MicroVention/Terumo, Inc.; Aliso Viejo, Calif.), Axium (Covidien/ev3), and Target Nano 360 (Stryker) coils (Figure 7). At the same time, scientists have created many different modified coils. These coils can improve outcomes for embolism by promoting blood clotting or by allowing for higher packing densities. Some examples of these coils include polyglycolic acid (PGA)-core coils, polylactic-co-glycolic acid (PLGA)-coated coils, PLGA-coated coils, and nylon fibers attached or expandable hydrogel coils. The last type is also called "bioactive coils" [3].

Three-Way Valve

In 1978, there was only one company that made injection molded valves (single-way and three-way). That company was American "Pharmacile." There are also new valve manufacturers in Europe. They provided all the valve introduction sheaths needed for embolization systems [1].

Hydrophilic Layer

The development of medical hydrophilic coating materials began in 1956, when DuPont first published the first patent for a double-layer hydrophilic coating. This coating was initially used on primary products such as urinary catheters. Then in 1995, Surmodics (Inc., Eden Prairie, MN, US) published a patent related to photopolymerization. In the 1990s, new methods for treating heart and blood vessel problems led to the use of high-performance materials like polyvinylpyrrolidone (PVP) and polyvinyl alcohol (PVA). Right now, PVP material is the most important medical hydrophilic coating material. Its safety and effectiveness are well-known. It is most often used with catheters, guide wires, and stents.

In the early 1990s, the first catheters and guide wires with hydrophilic coating technology were introduced. A patent in the United States has improved the lubrication of micro-guidewires. Micro wire is another field that focuses on very small mechanical parts, such as grinding and making very small coils and welding tiny parts together. This process greatly improves how easily the catheter and guide wire slide, creating new possibilities for intracranial positioning. So, we go deeper into the brain, reaching smaller and more distant blood vessels.

Hydrophilic treatment is a type of surface treatment that changes the surface of an object so that it can absorb water and form a thin layer that helps it slide in liquid without much friction. Hydrophilic treatment has been used in industry for a long time. For example, rowing and sailing boats have a hydrophilic coating on their surfaces. This reduces friction, which increases speed. To develop a hydrophilic coating process based on water-absorbing molecules, such as acrylamide, requires the joint efforts of physical, chemical, and surface treatment experts.

Laser-Cut or Braided Stent

In the late 1990s, some doctors started using stents to treat aneurysms inside the head. Some doctors who specialize in interventions to treat neurological problems tried to put special tubes into the arteries in the brain. These stents, which are used to treat coronary artery stenosis, have been in use for over a decade. However, their design is not suitable for intracranial arteries [4]. These stents are not soft enough to go deep enough into the cavernous segment and distal siphon of the internal carotid artery. So, scientists are making stents that are specially designed for intracranial arteries.

Stent is the name of a British doctor who invented a stainless steel tube used to widen narrow blood vessels. This type of bracket is made by a machine that cuts steel pipes (which have a diameter of about 1.5 mm) into a grid shape using laser cutting. The width of the cut steel struts is less than 0.1 mm, and the length of the bracket is about 10 mm. The stent was pressed onto a balloon that was 1 mm wide. The stent is inflated to a diameter of 2 to 4 mm. This is done to withstand a pressure of approximately 20 bar. The best bracket laser cutting machine is made in Germany. Stainless steel can sometimes make MRI images less clear, but it can be used with electrolytic polishing technology. This technology is important for making the implant so that it doesn't cause any damage to the artery it is put into. Some manufacturers have also tried using platinum to make stents, but platinum cannot be damaged by any acid. We can only use mechanical techniques for polishing, but it's hard to do because of the device's small size. Platinum stents haven't been very successful, and they cost a lot of money. Stainless steel brackets are popular and in high demand, so their prices have dropped significantly.

The introduction of the Neuroform stent (Boston Scientific/Target, California, USA) in 2002 changed this. It was the first stent specifically designed for cerebral blood vessels. Neuroform is a nickel-titanium stent that expands on its own. It has a special design with open cells. This design allows coils to pass through the stent's support struts. In 2007, after the development of the Neuroform stent, the Solitaire AB (formerly Solo stent; ev3 MTI, Irvine, CA, USA) and Enterprise stent (Cordis Neurovascular, Lake Miami, Florida, USA) were also launched. Neuroform, Solitaire AB, and Enterprise stents are different because they have a closed-cell design. This design allows the stents to be partially deployed, recaptured, and redeployed. This helps to achieve the best possible positioning and coil retention (Figure 8) [4].

In 2001, stents were hard to make using laser cutting and forming methods. Research is now focusing on woven stents. The first braided stent was the WalStent carotid stent from Scientific Boston in the USA, which has been around for about 20 years. It is made from stainless steel wire or covered with polyester or PTFE fibers, and it can be used to treat the iliac artery and aorta. Now, we need to figure out how to make it smaller. The first weaving machine used was a modified machine used for textiles in the early 1980s. It can weave 16 stainless steel wires and can be used to manufacture braided catheters. However, this machine is not suitable for producing woven stents because once the small sleeve on the machine is cut, the 16 metal wires at both ends of the bracket will scatter. This type of stent is hard to manipulate and can easily damage blood vessels. So, they started looking for workers who had been tailors in the workshop and who were good with their hands. They weave the stents by hand using a nickel titanium wire, which makes the ends of the stents very smooth. This kind of bracket is still a miracle. You can pull it in any direction, and it will always return to its original shape, with a soft touch. The intracranial stent delivery system has three parts: the stent microcatheter, the guiding catheter, and the pusher wire.

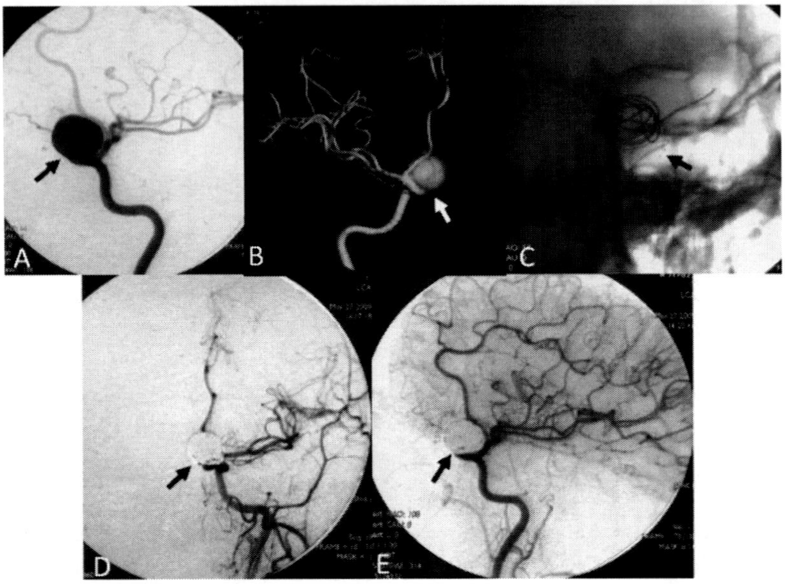

Figure 8. A 67-year-old woman presented with blurred vision of the left eye caused by a large paraclinoid aneurysm of the internal carotid artery. A, oblique view of the left internal carotid artery injection showing a large aneurysm of the paraclinoid segment of the internal carotid artery (arrow). B, 3-D reconstruction of the left internal carotid artery injection showing the 16mm×17mm paraclinoid aneurysm of the internal carotid artery (arrow), which was treated with 4mm×30mm Neuroform stent and coils. C, the unsubtracted image showing the Neuroform stent and the first 3-D coil (arrow). Frontal view (D) and lateral view (E) of the left internal carotid artery injection after coiling (17 coils and 533cm in total length) showing the aneurysm was occluded completely (arrows).

The first set of woven, self-expanding intracranial stents, known as the LEO system, was introduced in 2002 (Figure 9) [4]. After the Leo system, the Low-Profile Visualized Intraluminal Support (LVIS) stent and LVIS Jr. stent (Microvention, Aliso Viejo, CA, USA) were approved by the FDA in 2018. These braided stents are closed cell stents with a braided design, allowing the stent to more easily adapt to irregular blood vessel walls. The newest generation of woven scaffolds has higher visibility and smaller cells. Shortly after the LVIS stent was approved, the Neuroform Atlas (Stryker Neurovascular, Fremont, California, USA) was approved in 2019. Like the first generation Neuroform stent, it is self-expanding and does not shorten, making it easier for operators to measure the length of the stent. Neuroform Atlas is different from other stents because it is laser cut. It can be delivered through a 0.0165 inch microcatheter. This makes it easy to navigate in small blood vessels [5].

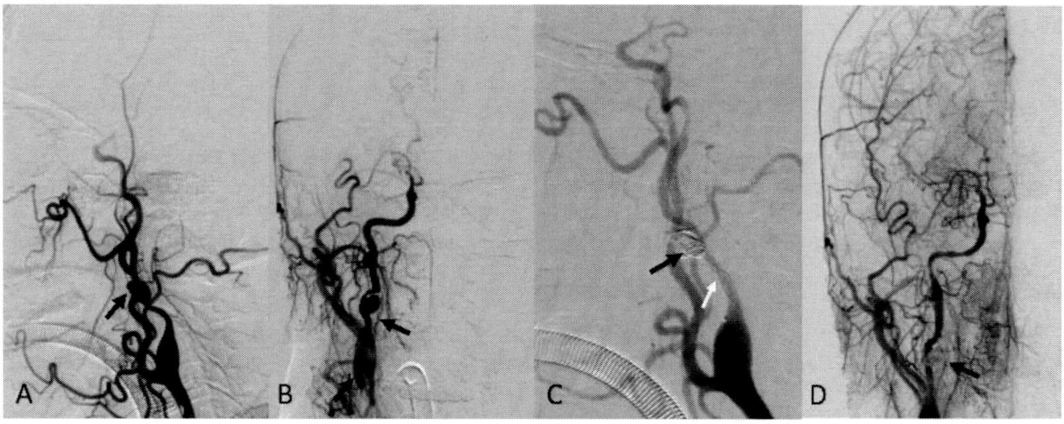

Figure 9. A 55-year-old woman presented with an extracranial dissecting aneurysm of the internal carotid artery coexisting Moyamoya disease. Lateral view (A) and frontal view (B) of the right carotid artery injection showing an extracranial dissecting aneurysm of the right internal carotid artery (arrows). Lateral view (C) and frontal view (D) of the right carotid artery injection showing the aneurysm was treated with 5.0mm×50mm Leo stent (Balt, France) (white arrow) and coils (black arrow).

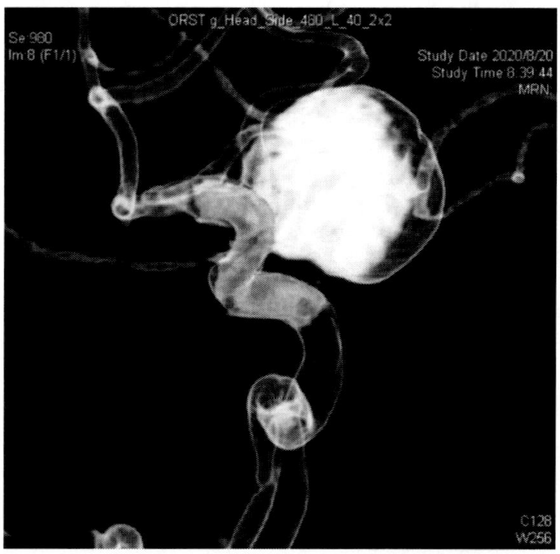

Figure 10. Image reconstruction showing a giant carotid aneurysm and a flow diversion device deployment without coil embolization.

Researchers are learning that they can make stents that are lighter and denser than woven stents. This research has created a denser stent. This stent is so dense that it can contain aneurysms outside the circulatory system without the need to fill them with coils (Figure 10). The stent is called a blood flow diversion device. Implanting a flow diversion device can quickly change blood flow in and around the aneurysm. After testing the device on animals and using it in many clinical trials, the results show that the flow diversion device is dense enough, and vascular endothelial cells can quickly grow on its surface and form a covering for aneurysms (Figure 11). Blood flow diversion devices are now more than just stents. It has become a vascular endothelial prosthesis. The weaving machine that is currently being used can weave 48 wires and 96 metal wires. These wires can be used to manufacture blood flow diversion devices (Figure 12) [6].

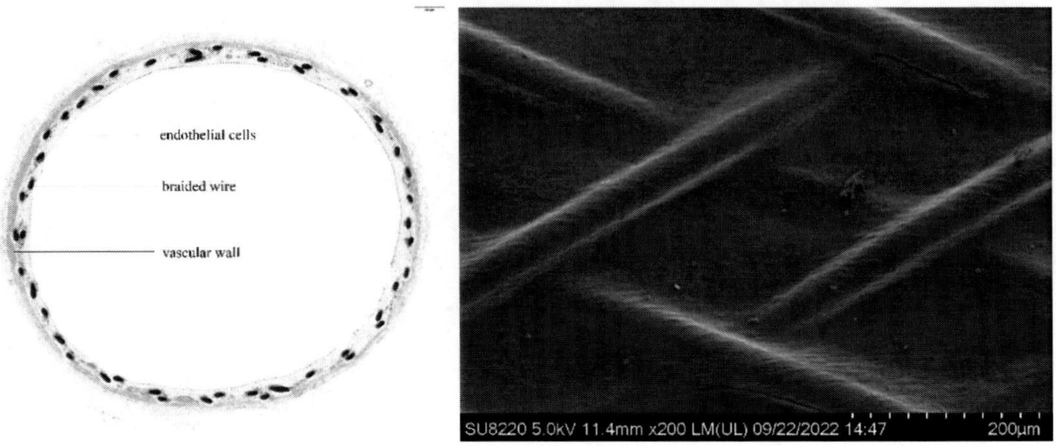

Figure 11. Histological specimen demonstrating subintimal incorporation of a flow diversion device within a rabbit carotid artery (from top to bottom: endothelial cells, vascular wall, braided wire of the flow diversion device) (left) and the electron microscopy scan of the arterial intima (right) at one month after the implantation of the flow diversion device.

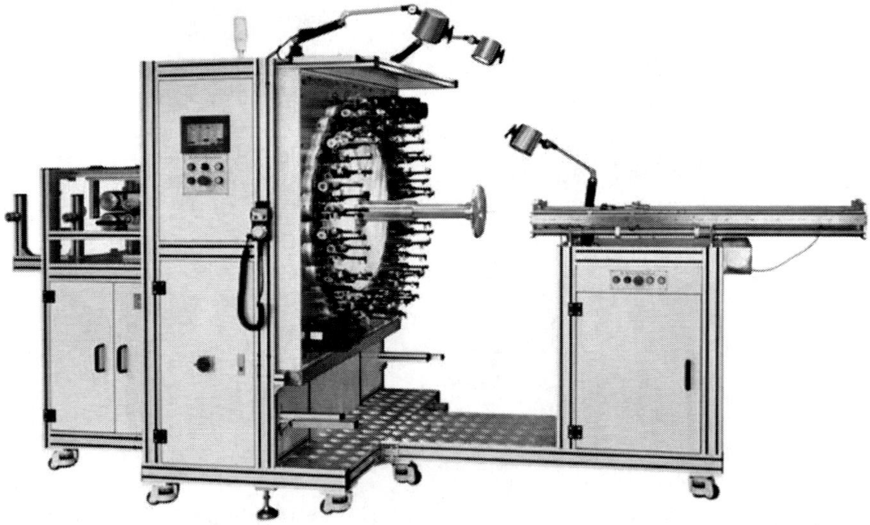

Figure 12. A metal weaving machine used for manufacturing flow diversion devices.

Development of Interventional Neuroradiology of Europe

Dr. René Djindjian died in 1977 at the age of 56. Jean Jacques Merland then became the head of the Department of Neuroradiology at Lariboisière Hospital (Figure 13). Professor Jean Jacques Merland spoke softly, but he was a big deal in the industry. Under his leadership, the department gained a great reputation in the medical field. Professor Merlan loved teaching. Many young doctors from different countries who were interested in this new area of medicine came to his department. This department has three operating rooms that can fit about ten doctors at the same time. It was the largest training center in Europe and has trained numerous outstanding practitioners, including Ms. Ling Feng from Beijing, Alfredo Casasco from Buenos Aires, Léopoldo Guimarens from Barcelona, Eduardo Servigo from La Corunia, Paulo Passos from Porto Alegre, Paulo de Sousa from Curitiba, Daniel Rüfenacht from Geneva, Wilhelm Brassel from Hamburg, and Siegfried Bien from Marburg, René Chapot from Essen.

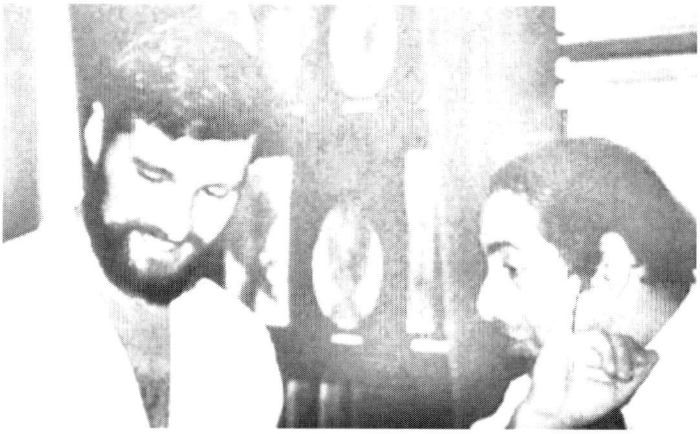

Figure 13. Dr. Jean-Jacques Merland (9.2.1942 – 17.5.2023) and Dr. René Djindjian in 1976. Picture extracted from Leopold Plowiecki's book "The art and savoir faire of interventional neuroradiology – Memoirs of a manufacturer."

Lariboisière Hospital is more than just a teaching center for interventional neuroradiology. Also, students from different countries come here to talk about professional topics with each other. This makes it a place where different ideas meet and clash. These discussions have led to new research and new treatments.

In 1980, a meeting was held in Santa Barbara. Several American doctors attended, including Berenstein, Kerber, Vinuela, Bank. Several French professors also attended, including Debrun, Picard, Merland, Lasjaunias, and Moret. This conference is important because it led to the creation of the International Interventional Neuroradiology Organization. In the 1980s, Lariboisière Hospital, Adolphe de Rothschild Hospital (Professor Jacques Moret), and Nancy University Teaching Hospital (Professor Luc Picard) were the three most important places for training and practicing interventional neuroradiology in France and even Europe (Figure14).

Since 1982, Professor Luc Picard had held an annual meeting of interventional neuroradiologists from around the world at the ski resort Val d'Isère in the French Alps. This meeting is called WIN, which stands for Working Group of Interventional Neuroradiology. This meeting often attracted many stars, including Luc Picard from France, Pierre Lajaunias, Jacques Moret, as well as Michel Mawad from Houston, Alex Berenstein from New York, Karel TerBrugge from Toronto, and several other outstanding professors. Professor Luc Picard was the most experienced and spirited of all the pioneers in the field of interventional neuroradiology. Marco Leonardi had admitted that he had learned a lot from Professor Picard.

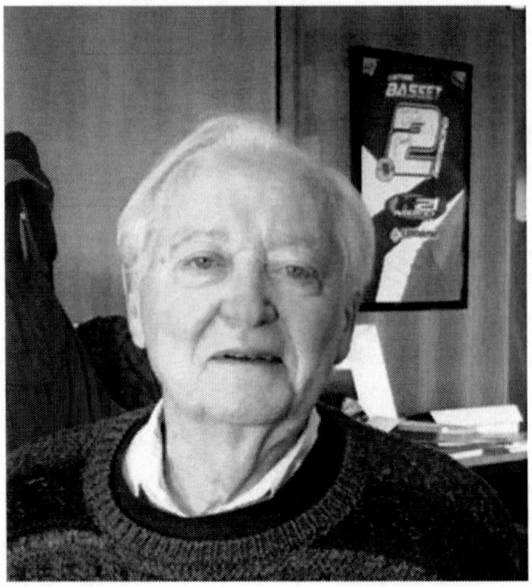

Figure 14. Professor Luc Picard (1937-2021) in 2019, Professor of Neuroradiology of the Faculty of Medicine in Nancy, France. He is one of the pioneers of Interventional Neuroradiology.

Professor Marco Leonardi is the head of the teaching hospital at the University of Bologna (Figure 15). He is not only a great doctor and a hard worker, but he's also really good at running meetings. He organized the WFITN conference (World Federation of Interventional and Therapeutic Neuroradiology) in Venice in 2005, and he was the chairman of the 19th Neuroradiology Symposium held in Venice in 2010. These symposiums are held every four years.

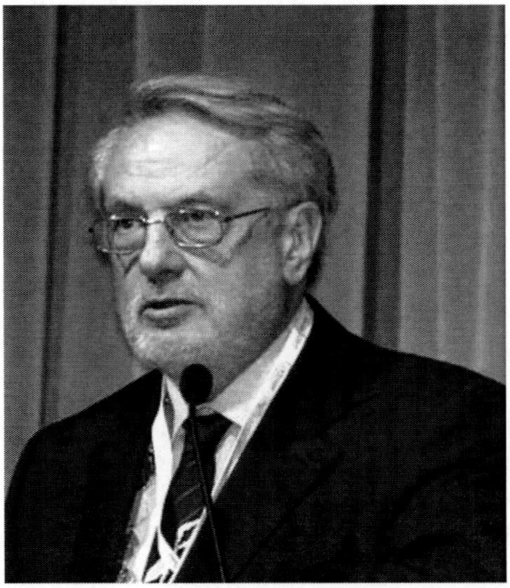

Figure 15. Professor Marco Leonardi (1944-2017), Head of Neuroradiology, University of Bologna, Italy.

Another professor who was very close to Professor Luc Picard was Pierre Lasjaunias (Figure16), who unfortunately passed away on Tuesday, July 1, 2008, at the European Congress of Neuroradiology in Zurich due to a myocardial infarction at the age of 56 years. Professor

Pierre Lasjaunias had a passion for teaching, and his teachings were not only expressed orally, but also in his papers and books. He had written the most books: a total of six, each with over 1000 pages (coauthored with Alex Berenstein), and had also contributed many papers to professional journals. He cofounded the journal of Interventional Neuroradiology with Marco Leonardi. In addition to attending Professor Luc Picard's annual conference in Val d'Isère, Professor Pierre Lasjaunias had also participated in almost all major international conferences and seminars, or hosted related conferences. He may suffer from overwork and illness as a result.

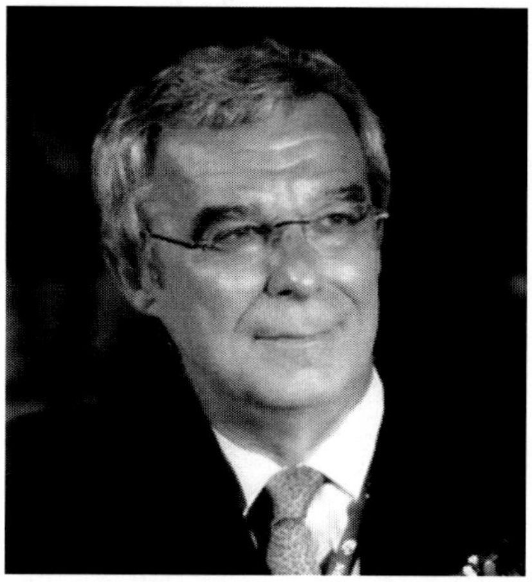

Figure 16. Professor Pierre Lasjaunias (1948–2008), Head of Neurosciences at Bicêtre Hospital in Paris, France.

Over the past decade, Professor Jacques Moret has regularly organized LINNC (Interventional Neuroradiology and Neurosurgery Live Courses) in Paris (Figure17). The audience came from France, Germany, Belgium, the United Kingdom, Spain, the Netherlands, Italy, Poland, South America, the Baltic States, Russia and Türkiye. Although Michel Mawad from Houston also organizes LINNC courses in North America, Professor Jacques Moret's courses also have a large audience from North America.

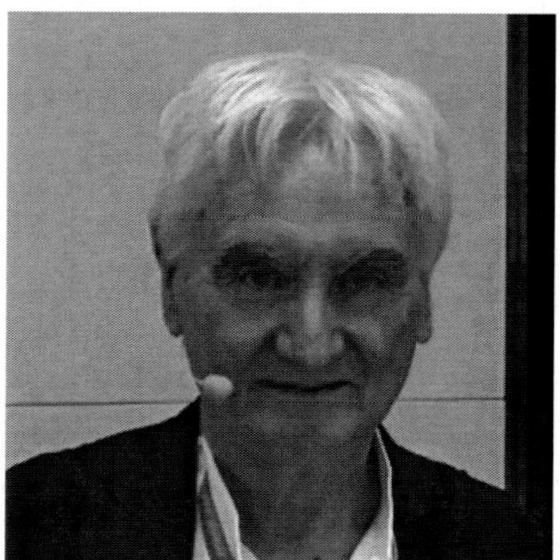

Figure 17. Dr. Jacques Moret, Adolphe de Rothschild Hospital.

In Eastern Europe, interventional neuroradiology is a small discipline. In Poland, which is not wealthy, neurosurgeons are applying interventional neuroradiology in practice, and this practice is gradually becoming popular. There are currently about 10 interventional neuroradiologists in Poland. There are also practices of interventional neuroradiology in the Czech Republic, Hungary and Bulgaria. Although Professor Fiodor Serbinenko, the inventor of the detachable balloons, is Russian, the development of interventional neuroradiology in Russia is still very slow.

It's interesting that the development of interventional neuroradiology in Latin American countries was faster than in Northern Europe during its early stages. In Argentina, in the early 1980s, Dr. Claudio Schünholtz studied interventional neuroradiology under the talented Dr. Tonnelier at the CCN (Northern Heart Center) in Saint Denis. Dr. Pedro Lylyk is a very skilled doctor who treats vascular diseases of the brain and spine. He is the most dynamic interventional neuroradiologist in Latin America. In addition to Dr. Pedro Lylyk, there are about ten interventional neuroradiologists in Argentina.

Professor Shimon Maimon is a leading figure in Israel's field of neuroradiology, which is the branch of medicine concerned with the diagnosis and treatment of diseases of the nervous system. He trains doctors from other countries (including the UK, Spain, Italy, and Russia) in his department in Tel Aviv, and travels around the world to share his knowledge and skills with other doctors. In Turkey, there are two interventional neuroradiologists who are particularly active: Dr. Cekirge is in Ankara and Dr. Islak is in Istanbul. They are the doctors who use the American embolization product Onyx the most in their practice. Finally, Dr. Paulo Passos from Porto Alegre, Brazil was trained at Lariboisière Hospital.

In 2006, medical imaging made significant progress. This was due to the increasing number of 3D DSA (digital subtraction angiography) and 3D CTA (computed tomography angiography) machines (Figure18).

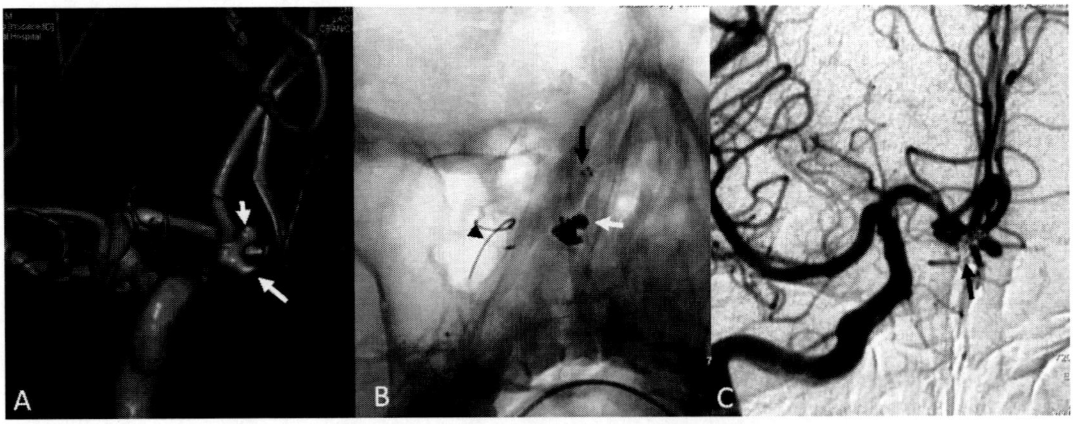

Figure 18. A 49-year-old man presented with subarachnoid hemorrhage. A, the 3D color image of the carotid artery reconstructed by DSA can clearly showing 2 aneurysms arising from the anterior communicating artery (arrows), which was treated with 4.0mm×15mm Solitaire AB stent and coils. B, the unsubtracted image showing the head (black arrow) and the end (arrowhead) of the Solitaire AB stent and the coil mass (white arrow). C, frontal view of the right internal carotid artery injection after coiling showing the 2 aneurysms were occluded completely (arrow).

Conclusion

A good interventional neuroradiology manufacturer needs to have two types of technology: plastic and latex conversion technology, as well as micromechanics technology. In the field of making medical devices used to treat neurological conditions, the United States is much more advanced than Europe. Of the seven top manufacturers (Balt Extrusion, Scientific Boston/Stryker, Coock, Cordman, Medtronic/EV3, Microvention, and Micrus), Balt Extrusion is the only one based in Europe. It is rare for researchers to invent new products or techniques. Research on products or techniques should focus on what doctors need, what they're already using, and what they've tried before. The goal is to make these products and techniques better. Technological progress takes time. New ideas must find the right techniques, and new products need to be tested in both lab and real-world settings. To be successful, you need to know what to do and how to do it. Learning can help you gain knowledge, but it's not enough on its own to make you a good researcher, someone who can find answers to problems. The ability to solve problems is a natural talent that cannot be taught. We love devices that are soft, small, and beautiful, and that last a long time. It is very important for a therapy to make progress if highly skilled and enthusiastic doctors and medical product manufacturers work together.

References

[1] Plowiecki L. The art and savoir faire of interventional neuroradiology – memoirs of a manufacturer. *Self-published memoir*. 2023.

[2] Tong FC, Cloft HJ, Dion JE. Endovascular treatment of intracranial aneurysms with Guglielmi detachable coils: emphasis on new techniques. *J Clin Neurosci*. 2000;7 (3):244-253.

[3] Zhu Y, Zhang H, Zhang Y, et al. Endovascular metal devices for the treatment of cerebrovascular diseases. *Adv Mater*. 2019;31 (8):e1805452.

[4] Lv X, Wu Z, eds. *Neurointerventional Surgery: Current Status and Future Prospects*. Nova Science; 2022.

[5] Lauzier DC, Huguenard AL, Srienc AI, et al. A review of technological innovations leading to modern endovascular brain aneurysm treatment. *Front Neurol*. 2023;14:1156887.

[6] Deshmukh AS, Priola SM, Katsanos AH, et al. The management of intracranial aneurysms: current trends and future directions. *Neurol Int*. 2024;16 (1):74-94.

Chapter 22

The History of Endovascular Neurosurgery: Europe, Russia and Americas

Kirill Orlov*
Federal Center of Brain Research and Neurotechnologies of Federal Medical Biological Agency of Russia, Moscow, Russian Federation

Abstract

The history of endovascular neurosurgery reflects a transformative journey, marked by technological advancements, pioneering techniques, and influential figures. The following is an overview of the key developments and personalities that have shaped this field.
The origins of endovascular procedures can be traced back to the early 20th-century. In 1904, Dawbarn described the direct embolization of head and neck tumors using wax. Later, in 1933, Hamby and Gardner employed muscle beads to embolize carotid-cavernous fistulae (CCF). A practical method of selective cerebral angiography via direct puncture of the carotid and vertebral arteries was developed by Portuguese neurosurgeons, Antonio Agas Moniz and Pedro Almeida Lima, between 1927 and 1933. In 1953, the Swedish radiologist Sven Ivar Seldinger introduced the Seldinger technique, a method for safe percutaneous access to major blood vessels. In the 1960s, Dotter and Judkins developed tools and techniques for navigating the major arteries using coaxial plastic catheters and steerable guidewires. They also popularized femoral and radial arterial access.
In the early 1960s, Alfred Luessenhop (USA), Boris Samotokin, and Vitaly Khilko (USSR) began using calibrated plastic balls for non-selective embolization in treating cerebral arteriovenous malformations (AVMs) and dural arteriovenous fistulae (dAVFs). In 1962, Alfred Luessenhop was the first to perform selective catheterization of cerebral arteries using a flow-guided microcatheter. In 1964, he performed the first temporary occlusion of an intracranial artery with a non-detachable flow-guided balloon. However, these procedures were experimental and not intended for widespread clinical application. Several minimally invasive techniques for treating intracranial aneurysms (IAs) have been explored, with varying degrees of success. These early methods included direct injection of aneurysms with animal hair (Gallagher, 1962), stereotactic electrothrombosis (Mullan, 1964), stereotactic embolization using magnetically guided iron particles (Alksne, 1966), and techniques involving local blood flow reduction and artificial clotting (Samotokin and Khilko, 1966).

* Corresponding Author's Email: kirill.orlov@rens-russia.org

In: World History of Neurointerventional Surgery
Editors: Xianli Lv and Zhongxue Wu
ISBN: 979-8-89530-792-2

At the turn of the 1960s and the 1970s, Soviet neurosurgeon Fedor Serbinenko developed the first practical technique for selective catheterization and therapeutic occlusion of cerebral vessels using flow-guided detachable balloons and began performing such interventions in a systematic fashion. Serbinenko's method was adopted worldwide and became the backbone of endovascular procedures in neurosurgery until the 1990s. He is generally acknowledged as "the father of endovascular neurosurgery." Significant contributions to the flow-guided balloon technique and the advent of new neuroendovascular field were made by Gerard Debrun (France - USA), Yury Zubkov (USSR), Viktor Shcheglov (USSR), Charles Kerber (USA), Alejandro Berenstein (USA), Michael DiTullio (USA), Jean-Jacques Merland (France), Luc Picard (France), Jacques Moret (France), Fernando Vinuela (USA) and others. In the mid-1970s, Kerber introduced a calibrated leak balloon and performed the first intranidal embolization of cerebral AVM using liquid cyanoacrylate.

During the same period, French neurologist Rene Djindjian pioneered spinal angiography and embolization techniques while introducing several new embolic agents. In the 1980s, Soviet neurosurgeon Theodor Tissen advanced spinal angiography and embolization techniques. In the latter half of the 1980s, the development of new variable-stiffness microcatheters and microguidewires marked a significant shift from flow-guided to over-the-wire techniques for cerebral vascular navigation. In the turn of the 1980s and 1990s, the Italian-American neuroradiologist Guido Guglielmi invented electrically detachable coils and developed a novel technique for intracranial aneurysm treatment: endosaccular coiling (EC). By the 1990s, Guglielmi Detachable Coils (GDC), together with advanced microcatheters, had replaced balloons in most neuroendovascular applications.

Between 1992 and 1997, Moret introduced a technique called balloon-assisted coiling (BAC), which utilizes non-detachable balloons. He employed his own flow-guided balloons ("Moret catheters") and over-the-wire coronary balloons. Later, in the 2000s, dedicated neurovascular balloons emerged. These were made of new super-compliant polymers and guided over the microwires. In the mid-1990s, Randall Higashida and Pedro Lylyk pioneered the use of stent-assisted coiling (SAC) for treating intracranial aneurysms (IAs). Balloon-expanded coronary stents were initially used. Subsequently, in the 2000s, the first dedicated neurovascular stent was developed. The stents were self-expanding and delivered via microcatheters.

In the late 2000s, flow diverters (FDs) were introduced based on earlier studies conducted by Ajay Wakhloo, Barukh Lieber, M. Aenis, and others. These stent-like endoluminal devices, made of fine metallic mesh, divert blood flow away from the aneurysm sac, inducing thrombosis within the aneurysm. This represents a novel concept in IA treatment that focuses on parent-vessel reconstruction without direct manipulation of the aneurysm. Since the 1990s, non-adhesive liquid embolic agents have been used to treat cerebral arteriovenous malformations (AVMs) and dural arteriovenous fistulas (dAVFs). By the 2000s, these compounds had gained widespread acceptance. Together with new microcatheters featuring detachable tipsintroduced in the late 2000s and the early 2010s, they significantly transformed cerebral AVM and dAVF embolization from an auxiliary or palliative measure into a first-line treatment method with curative intent. Altogether, these techniques and personalities have shaped the modern practice of endovascular neurosurgery.

Keywords: history, endovascular, neurosurgery, Europe, Russia, Americas

Introduction

The history of endovascular neurosurgery is similar to that of spatial exploration. From theorists and dreamers to scientific practitioners. From the first homemade rockets that barely got off the ground to the launch of the first satellites and then to the first manned space flight. From unique risky missions to the current routine work of launching the most complex high-tech devices into orbit, enabling communication, navigation, and research without which our everyday life is impossible.

Endovascular neurosurgery is a special area of vascular neurosurgery that addresses the treatment of cerebral artery aneurysms, cerebral and spinal arteriovenous malformations (AVM), dural arteriovenous fistulas (dAVF), carotid-cavernous fistulas (CCF) and other pathological arteriovenous shunts of the nervous system, as well as vascular tumors of cranial and spinal localization. Endovascular neurosurgery has evolved through attempts to solve the problems posed by these diseases to neurosurgeons, neuroradiologists, and neurologists.

Pre-Angiographic Era

At the end of the 19th century, the outstanding pioneer of neurosurgery, Victor Horsley, prophetically asserted that the most rational access to the cerebral vessels is the lumen of these particular vessels [1].

The first attempt in history that we may classify as "endovascular neurosurgery" was made by the American neurosurgeon James Dawbarn. In 1904, he proposed a method for embolizing face and head tumors: cutting off the branches of the external carotid artery that fed the tumor and injecting liquid beeswax, petrolatum, paraffin, and other similar organic substances. Dawbarn mentioned that he had performed several similar interventions, but their exact number and results are unknown [2].

Next, to use embolization in neurosurgery, Hamby and Gardner. In 1933, they undertook several relatively successful interventions to embolize traumatic carotid-cavernous fistulas (CCF) with small pieces of muscle labelled with a silver wire. Muscle emboli were placed into the lumen of the temporarily clamped internal carotid artery (ICA) through an incision, and the clamps were removed from the artery. The emboli were supposed to move with blood flow towards the fistula [3].

The authors referred to the fact that their method was proposed in 1930 by the American surgeon Barney Brooks; however, none of the Brooks' publications described this technique. Brooks mentioned his only attempt to occlude the ICA using a thin muscle band inserted into the ICA lumen. The anastomosis was occluded, as was the artery along its entire length. Brooks did not continue with such procedures and warned his colleagues against them [4].

The Soviet neurosurgeons Alexander Arutyunov and Alexander Burlutsky supplemented the Hamby and Gardner method by clipping ICA in the intracranial region and ligating the artery in the neck. Until the early 1960s, this technique was the only "endovascular" intervention in neurosurgery [5].

An insurmountable obstacle to the development of endovascular techniques in the first decades of the 20th century was the lack of methods for the indirect visualization of cerebral blood vessels.

In 1927, Portuguese neurosurgeons Antonio Egaz Moniz and Pedro Almeida Lima performed the first selective cerebral angiography. The successful procedure was preceded by multiple experiments on animals and cadavers as well as eight unsuccessful attempts in humans, with one patient dying from complications following the intervention. Moniz obtained high-quality images of the cerebral arteries only in the ninth patient [6].

In the early stages, Moniz and Lima surgically exposed the carotid and subclavian arteries and injected them with bromine-, lithium-, and strontium-based contrast agents (Figure 1). Subsequently, they switched to percutaneous arterial puncture and less aggressive and toxic iodine- and thorium-based contrast agents. By 1931, Moniz performed the first cerebral panangiography and improved the technique such that it could be used widely [7].

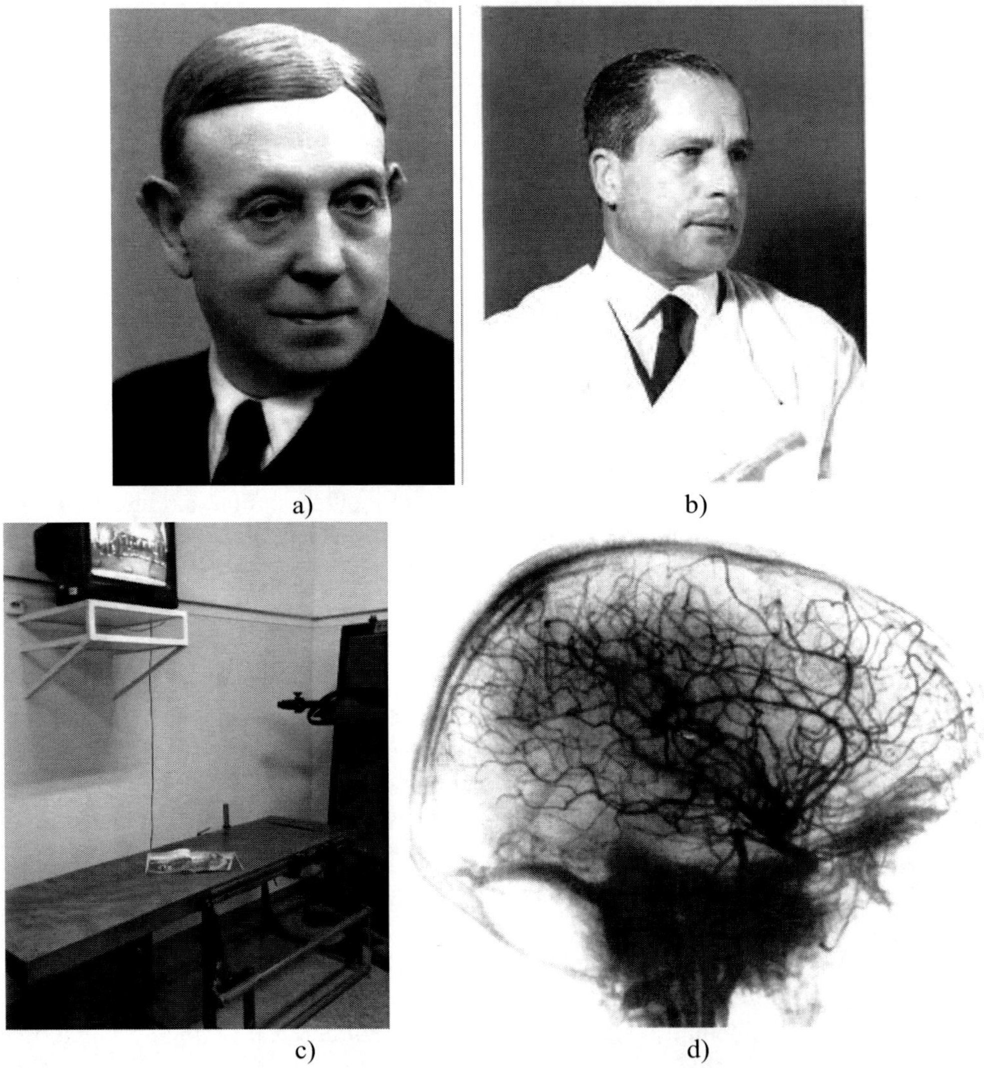

Figure 1. a) Antonio Egaz Moniz (1874-1955). b) Pedro Almeida Lima (1903-1985). c) Original Moniz angiosuite. d) One of the first cerebral angiograms obtained by Moniz et al.

Moniz did more than 300 cerebral angiography procedures during his career and authored over 200 publications on the anatomy of the cerebral circulatory system and the use of angiography. Until the advent of computed tomography in the late 1970s, cerebral angiography remained the most informative neuroimaging method.

In 1930, The Lancet prophetically wrote: "... in the future, cerebral angiography will probably have not only diagnostic but also therapeutic applications..." At that time, there were no instruments enabling the remote manipulation of the lumen of the blood vessels. It took three more decades to develop such instruments and endovascular catheters, and to start the first experiments using the angiographic method for therapeutic purposes.

The word "catheter" is of Greek origin. In the past, people have attempted to insert various objects into body openings since ages ago. Hollow tubes made of various materials and designed specifically for this purpose are referred to as catheters. The Latin word "cannula" and the German "sonde" (probe) mean the same thing; the first version, however, is firmly established in endovascular medicine.

Emergence of Endovascular Medicine

The German urologist Werner Frossmann pioneered vascular catheterization in humans. In 1929, he inserted a rubber urinary catheter through the brachial vein into the right atrium, and radiography was X-ray (Figure 2). At that time, a popular belief was that entering foreign bodies into heart chambers would inevitably lead to tragic consequences. Frossmann proved the opposite with a bold experiment on himself, thus, laying the foundation for endovascular (or interventional) medicine [8].

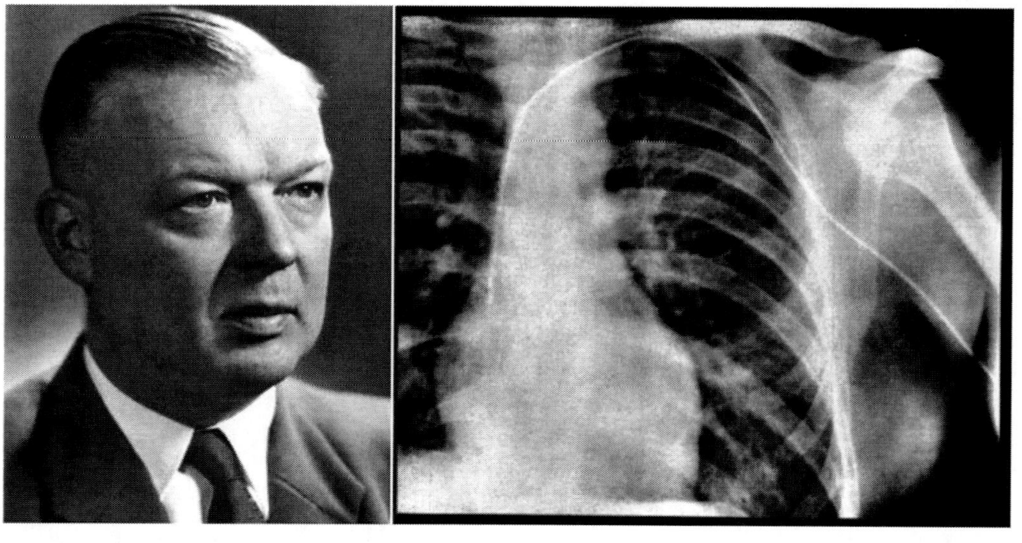

Figure 2. Werner Frossmann (1904-1979). The X-ray image depicting a catheter within the heart.

Another outstanding invention was achieved by Swedish radiologist Sven Ivar Seldinger. In 1953, he developed relatively safe and atraumatic catheterization of blood vessels (and later on, of virtually any hollow structures of the body). Seldinger proposed puncturing vessels with a thick needle and inserting a thread-like guide. The needle was then removed, and a blunt atraumatic cannula was inserted into the vessel lumen with a guide. No damaging objects were left inside the vessel, and various devices with smaller diameters could be inserted through the cannula [9].

Before the introduction of specialized endovascular catheters, the Seldinger cannula was the main instrument for intravascular access, particularly in neurosurgery, and currently Seldinger's vascular catheterization technique is still applies (Figure 3).

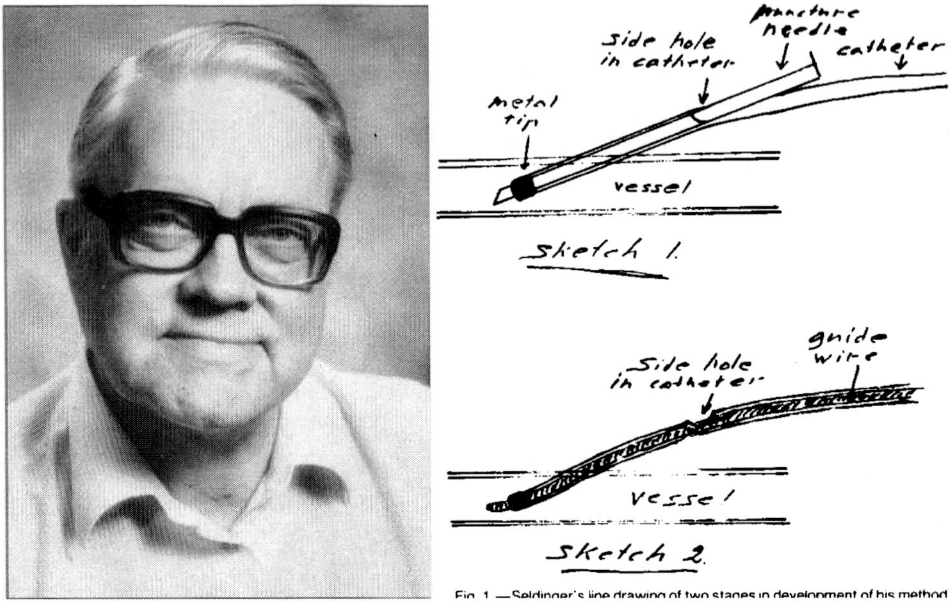

a) b)

Figure 3. a) Sven Ivar Seldinger (1921 – 1998) b) Seldinger's original drawings, depicting his method.

At the time of Frossmann and Moniz, medical catheters were made of metal or rubber; unfortunately, these materials are not suitable for safe remote manipulations within the vascular bed. The emergence of specialized endovascular catheters became possible no earlier than the middle of the 20th century, when synthetic polymers such as polyethylene, fluoroplastics (Teflon), nylon, silicone, and polyurethane entered widespread medical use.

In the 1940s, American entrepreneurs David Sheridan and Norman Jeckel founded the world's first company to manufacture disposable medical catheters using synthetic polymers. Catheter and Instrument Corp.

At the turn of the 1950s and 1960s, the American radiologist Charles Dotter performed systematic endovascular interventions on large arteries for the first time using homemade Teflon and polyethylene catheters (Figure 4). He was also the first to employ a coaxial system for such interventions, consisting of a short and rigid cannula (introducer), into which a long and flexible guiding catheter was inserted. Moreover, Dotter improved the Seldinger intravascular guidewire by adding a flexible "J"-shaped tip to it. The Dotter guidewire allows purposeful navigation through arterial bifurcations and selective catheterization of the arterial branches [10].

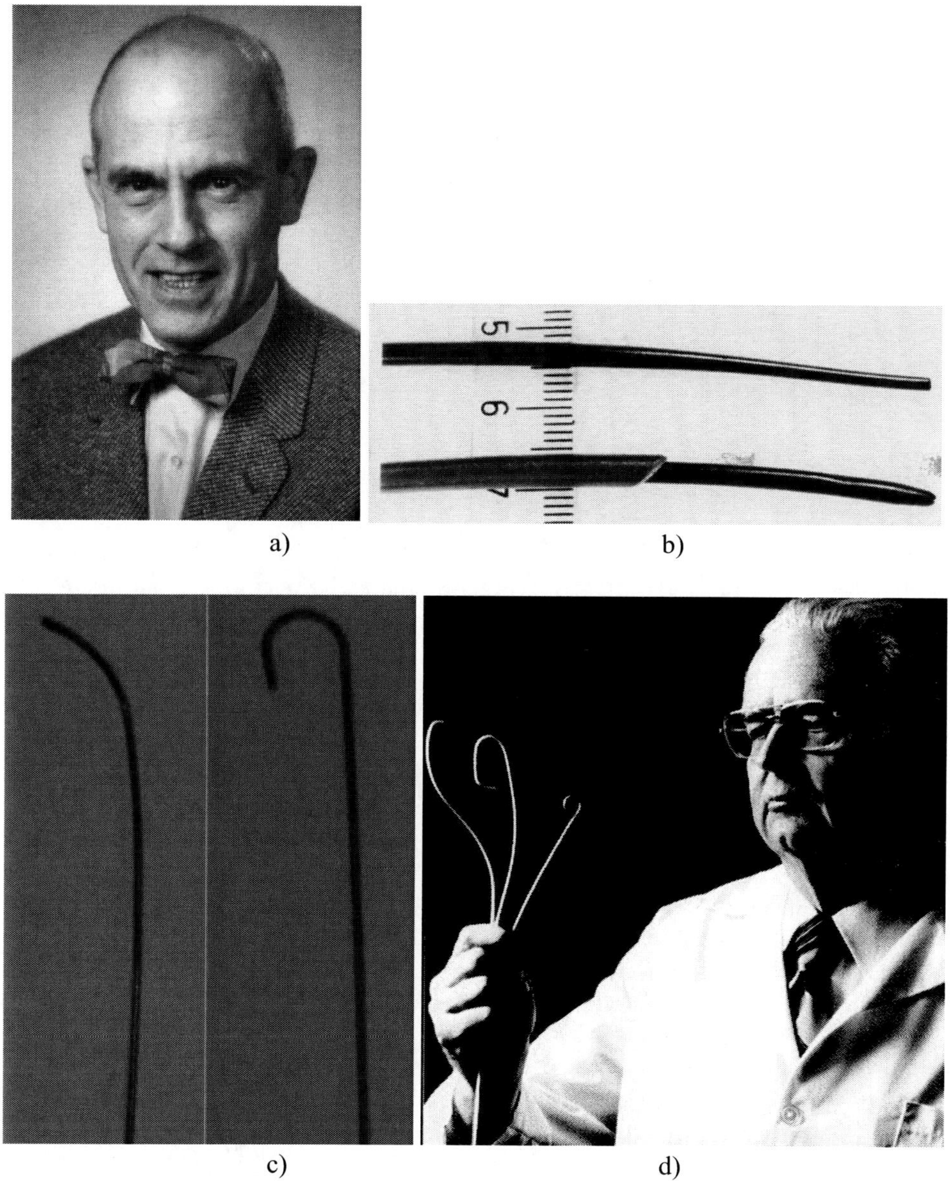

Figure 4. a) Charles Dotter (1920 - 1985). b) Dotter's early coaxial catheters. c) Dotter's J-wires. d) Melvin Judkins (1922 - 1985) with his pre-shaped catheters.

In 1963, Dotter began collaborating with the American entrepreneur and inventor Bill Cook. Together, they founded the first company to industrially manufacture catheters and other instruments for endovascular interventions (Cook Medical) and later became one of the largest manufacturers of endovascular devices.

In the second half of the 1960s, Dotter's student Melvin Judkins introduced endovascular catheters with preformed tips into practice. Judkins obtained tips of various shapes by heating catheter blanks on a curved metal rod.

He devised several configurations of endovascular catheters that are currently being used and are considered standard both in interventional cardiology and endovascular neurosurgery:

Judkins Right, Cobra, Headhunter, Pigtail, and others. In addition, Judkins was the first to propose a hydrophilic polymer coating for intravascular guidewires and catheters, which reduces friction and is less traumatic to the vascular wall; it is a mandatory component of most modern endovascular instruments [11].

It would be quite correct to say that the technique of endovascular interventions on large arteries in its current form was mostly established in the early 1970s. Dotter and Judkins popularized transfemoral and transradial intravascular approaches and developed most instruments necessary for such manipulations. Until the 1990s, however, direct carotid and vertebral punctures were preferred in neurosurgery. The reasons for this include both the anatomical features of the cerebral vascular anatomy and some objective technical problems, as described further in this paper.

Pre-Endovascular Era in Vascular Neurosurgery

In the 1960s, open neurosurgical procedures for cerebral aneurysms, AVMs, CCFs, dAVFs, and cranial vascular tumors were already being systematically performed, but the results were not uniformly encouraging. As a result, physicians were already looking for minimally invasive methods to treat these diseases.

In 1938, American neurosurgeons Sidney Werner and Arthur Blakemore performed percutaneous electrothrombosis of a giant aneurysm of the ophthalmic artery. They inserted a needle through the orbit into the aneurysm cavity, placed a silver thread-like electrode there, and then passed an electric current that caused the aneurysm to occlude. The case described was anecdotal. Such an intervention became possible because the giant aneurysm destroyed the bone wall of the orbit [12].

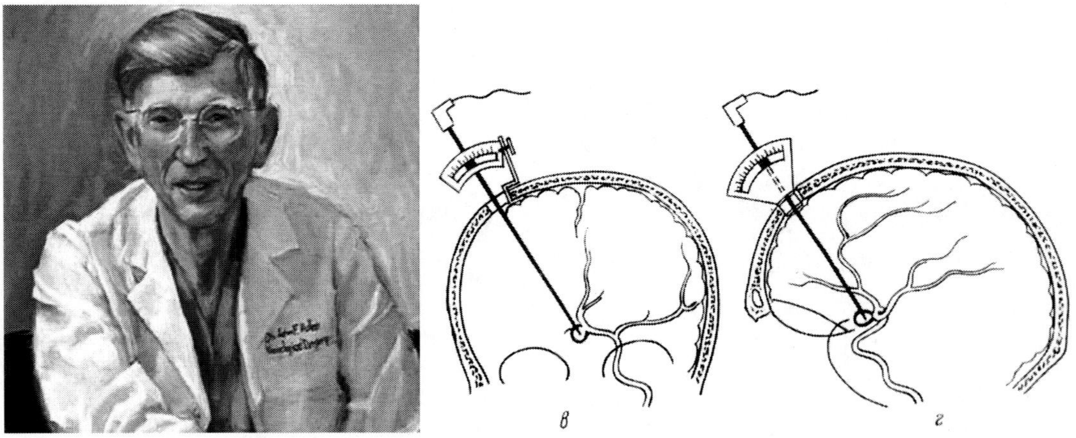

a) b)

Figure 5. a) Sean Mullan (1925 - 2015) b) Mullan's method of stereotactic electrothrombosis (from Khilko and Samotokin, 1973 [15]).

In 1964, the American neurosurgeon Sean Mullan described a method of stereotactic electrothrombosis of cerebral aneurysms (Figure 5). A set of needle electrodes (approximately 0.2 mm in diameter) was inserted into the aneurysm wall through a trephine opening using a stereotactic frame. A low current was then applied to the needles for an extended period of time, and control angiograms were taken every 15-30 minutes to assess the degree of aneurysm thrombosis. Over the course of two years, Mullan performed 12 such procedures. Adequate aneurysm occlusion was achieved in 6 cases with no operative mortality [13].

In 1963, another American neurosurgeon, John Gallagher, proposed pilojection - the introduction of horse and pig hair into aneurysms - to thrombose cerebral aneurysms. A small craniotomy was performed, which was sufficient to bring a pilojector (a specially designed pneumatic pistol, similar in size and shape to a pencil) to the aneurysm wall (Figure 6). This device was used to shoot sterilized animal hair into the aneurysm wall at high velocity. From 3-4 to 10-12 hairs were needed to occlude the aneurysm. Gallagher performed 15 such procedures. Acceptable occlusion was achieved in half of the observations, while the mortality rate due to surgical complications was 2 patients [14].

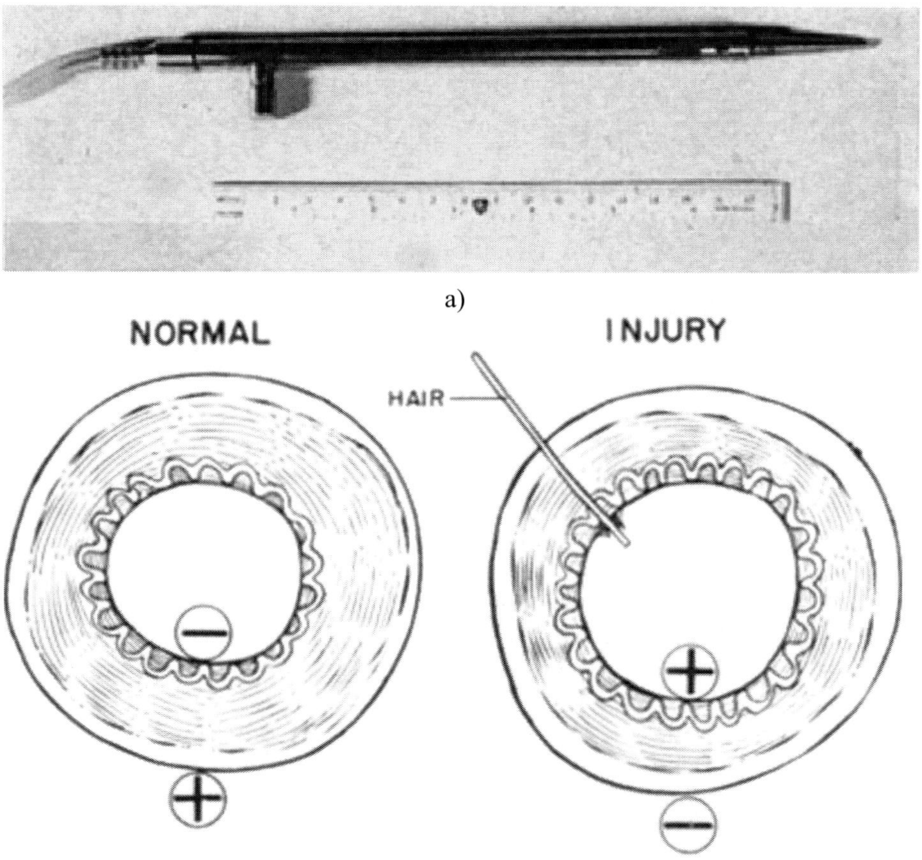

Figure 6. a) The pilojector device. b) A drawing from Gallagher's original publication showing the effect of animal hair on the aneurysm wall [14].

In 1966-1968, Soviet neurosurgeons Boris Samotokin, Vitaly Khilko, and Raymond Kikut performed artificial thrombosis of cerebral aneurysms by introducing coagulants (aminocaproic acid, vitamin K, calcium chloride) and temporarily narrowing the ICA in the cervical region with a muscle cuff. 35 operations were performed, but acceptable results were achieved only in carotid aneurysms, where complete occlusion was observed in 7 out of 10 cases. There were no surgical deaths [15].

The disadvantage of all of the above methods was that the thrombus obtained often dissolved later, resulting in only a temporary effect of the operation [15].

In an attempt to create a stable thrombus within the aneurysm, the American neurosurgeon John Alksne developed a method that is still admired today (Figure 7). In the mid-1960s, he proposed to thrombose aneurysms with iron particles held in the aneurysm cavity by a magnet. A magnetic probe in the form of an approximately 6 mm thick rod was stereotactically inserted into the aneurysm wall through a trephine opening. In the central part of the probe, there was a continuous channel through which a thin needle was inserted into the aneurysm cavity and a suspension of iron particles 3-5 microns in size was injected. The magnetic probe was attached to the skin and left for 3-5 days until a stable thrombus formed in the aneurysm, after which the probe was removed [16].

Alksne performed 39 procedures between 1966 and 1971. The mortality rate was 12 patients (33%), but it should be emphasized that all procedures were performed on acutely ruptured aneurysms. Of the 27 patients who survived, 22 (81%) had complete aneurysm occlusion, an excellent result even by today's standards. Technically, the Alksne method was well ahead of its time. The rather modest capabilities of the angiographic equipment of those years did not allow reliable control of the process of introducing iron particles, and they were washed out of the aneurysm in significant quantities. In about a quarter of the cases, neurological complications were caused by distal embolization of the cerebral arteries.

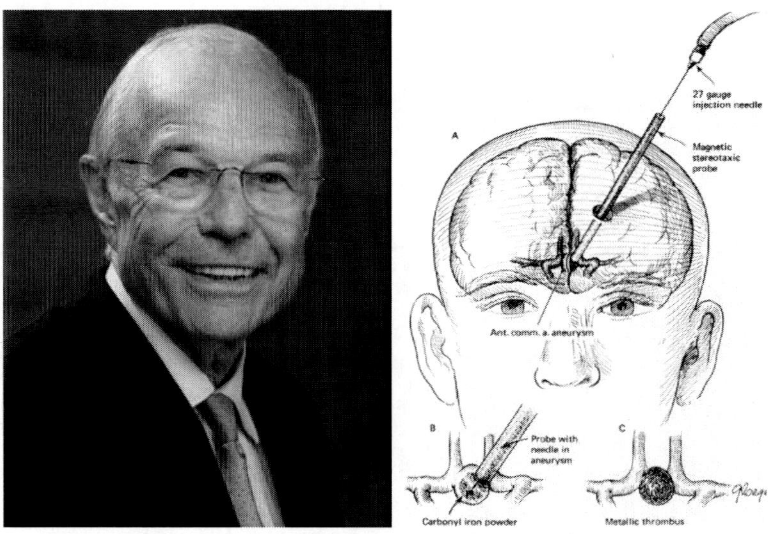

a) b)

Figure 7. a) John Alksne (1933 - 2024). b) A stereotactic magnet-assisted aneurysm thrombosis using metallic particles (from Alksne's original publication, 1971 [16]).

Prerequisites for Endovascular Neurosurgery

In 1959 at the latest, the American neurosurgeon Alfred Luessenhop began non-selective embolization of cerebral AVMs with plastic beads. Initially, methacrylate (protacryl) and later silicone were used as embolic material. To deliver the emboli into the blood stream, Luessenhop designed an original device, a propulsion chamber: a glass flask with several branches. The chamber was attached to the common carotid artery (CCA) bifurcation with a cuff from the external carotid artery (ECA), which was cut at the mouth. The ECA was ligated at the end of the procedure.

Emboli 1 to 5 mm in size were placed in the chamber, pushed into the arterial lumen by a fluid jet, and carried away by the blood flow in the direction of the malformation. The diameter of the emboli was chosen so that they could freely pass through the dilated AVM afferents but could not enter the intact arterial branches, which have a smaller diameter. In practice, however, emboli often got stuck before reaching the malformation or entered the wrong arteries.

To solve this problem, Luessenhop attached silk threads to the emboli (Figure 8). If the embolus was in a non-target artery, the thread traction allowed the embolus to be repositioned or even removed. If the embolus was in a satisfactory position, the thread was cut and pushed into the arterial lumen.

During one such procedure in 1963, a silicone microcatheter was attached to the embolus and successfully passed through the carotid siphon and into the middle cerebral artery. Luessenhop injected a contrast agent and performed the first selective angiography of a cerebral artery [17, 18].

Luessenhop and colleagues performed 94 embolizations in 55 patients with AVMs between 1960 and 1975. The rate of neurological complications from non-target embolization was approximately 15% [19].

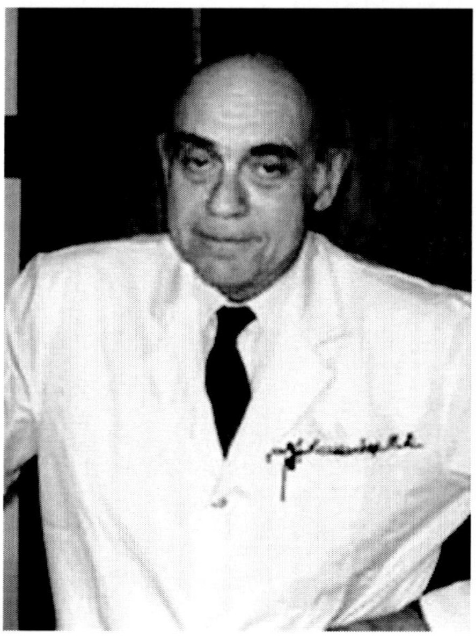

a)

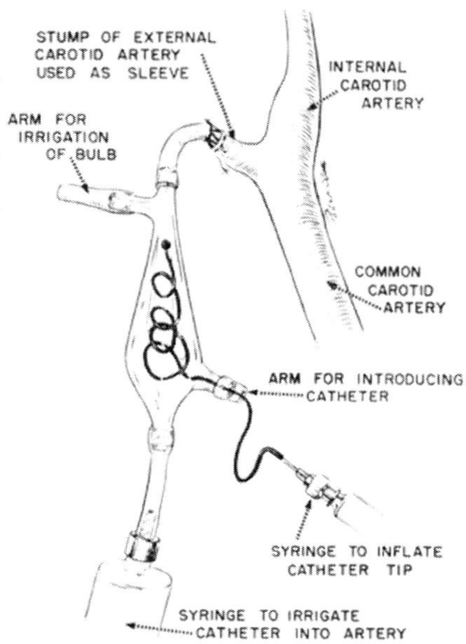

b)

Figure 8. a) Alfred Luessenhop (1925 - 2009). b) Luessenhop's embolization technique and propulsion chamber (from Luessenhop's original publication, 1964 [17]).

Around the same time, Soviet neurosurgeons Vitaly Khilko, Boris Samotokin, and Yury Zubkov used non-selective embolization of AVMs with expanded polystyrene beads (Figure 9). They exposed the common carotid artery in the neck, made an incision in its wall, and inserted a flexible plastic tube that was attached to the artery with a purse-string suture. Emboli were placed in the tube, either individually or in a series, and propelled into the lumen of the artery with a stream of fluid. At the end of the procedure, the artery wall was sutured. Unlike the Lussenhop method, this technique allowed for multistage embolization and the introduction of larger diameter emboli.

From 1965 to 1975, more than 250 embolizations were performed in 130 patients. The incidence of neurological complications from non-target embolization did not exceed 10-15% with later versions of the technique. Neurosurgeons also embolized with ferromagnetic alloy beads, which they attempted to direct with an external magnet. Apparently, this technique fell short of expectations, as few such procedures were performed [15, 20].

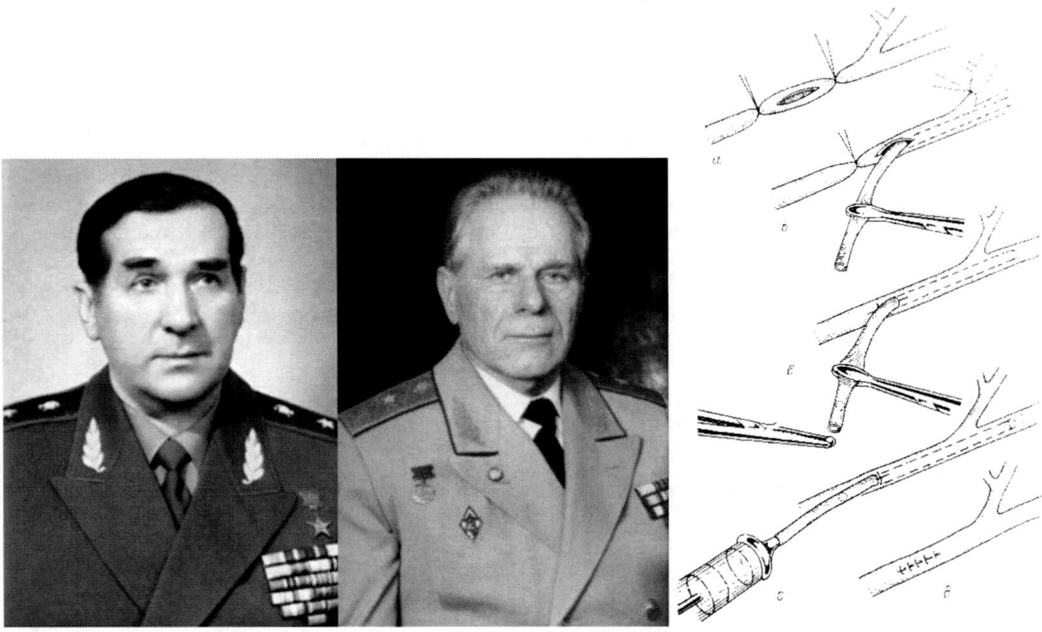

a) b)

Figure 9. a) Boris Samotokin (1915 - 1994) b) Vitaly Khilko c) Samotokin and Khilko's embolization technique (from the original monograph, 1973 [15]).

Until the late 1960s, one of the major obstacles to the development of endovascular neurosurgery was the carotid siphon and the tortuosity of the vertebral artery at the craniovertebral junction. The crude endovascular catheters of those years rested on one of the turns of the artery, and any attempt to pass them more distally typically resulted in vessel dissection or even rupture. In 1963, Lussehnop was the first to overcome this "neurosurgical Karman line," but his attempts at selective catheterization of cerebral arteries were anecdotal and had no practical application.

In the second half of the 1960s, a group of American and Israeli neuroradiologists and neurosurgeons - Ephroim Frei, Jack Dirller, Sadek Hilal and colleagues - tackled the "carotid siphon problem" with a solution that was technically ahead of its time and remains an outstanding example of research thinking even by today's standards (Figure 10). In several publications between 1966 and 1974, they described their work with the so-called POD (para-operational device) - a microcatheter controlled by an external magnetic field.

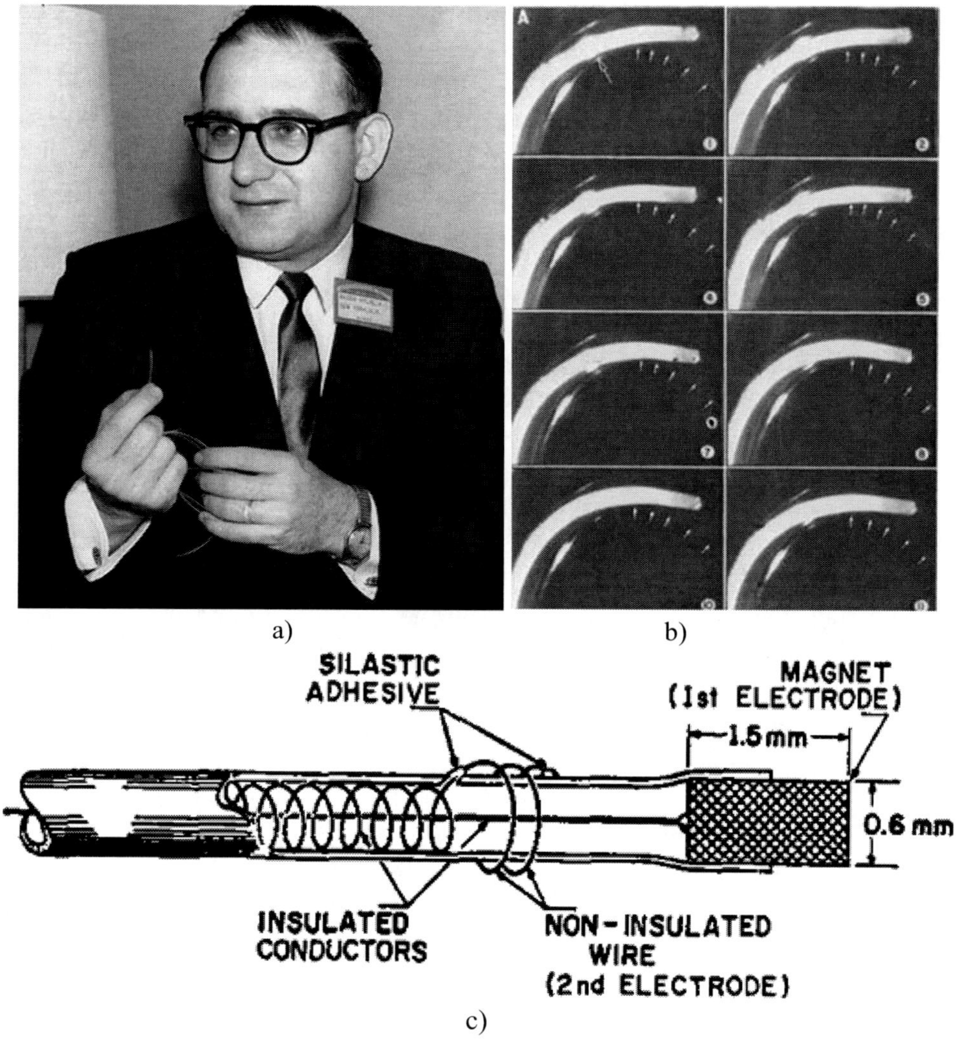

Figure 10. a) Sadek Hilal (1930 - 2000). b) A vibrating tip of the POD device. c) A magnetic rigging of the POD tip (from the original publication by Hilal et al. 1974 [24]).

A thin copper-beryllium alloy coil was placed inside a 1 mm diameter silicone microcatheter, and an approximately 1.5 mm samarium-cobalt magnet was attached to the tip of the device like a bung. The microcatheter was inserted via a transcarotid approach using a Seldinger needle. Strong direct and alternating electromagnets mounted on movable stands were applied to the patient from the outside.

An alternating magnetic field caused the microcatheter to vibrate at tens of Hz. The hydrodynamic waves generated by this vibration moved the microcatheter forward along the artery without mechanical resistance, while the tip of the microcatheter was deflected in the desired direction by a permanent magnet. As a result, the microcatheter easily overcame the carotid siphon and penetrated the cerebral arteries. In 1969, one of the first superselective angiograms of cerebral arteries in history was performed with such manipulations.

The metal coil inside the microcatheter could be used as an electrode for electrothrombosis and for recording electrical potentials of the brain. The magnetic tip of the microcatheter could be separated by introducing liquid into the microcatheter and used as a free embolus. In addition, it was proposed to introduce liquid embolizing materials through the microcatheter.

POD has been used in numerous successful experimental procedures in animals; however, the actual clinical application of this technique is limited to a few observations. For example, two cases of successful electrothrombosis of cerebral saccular aneurysms, one case of tumor (hemangioma) embolization with cyanoacrylate, and several cases of intravascular electroencephalography in patients with epilepsy have been described [21-24].

The complex, technology-intensive, and essentially experimental magnetic equipment required for this method was hardly suitable for widespread use and poorly compatible with the angiographic and anesthetic technology of the time. Presumably, the problems would have been solved over time, but by the mid-1970s, more accessible and understandable to neurosurgeons, detachable balloons guided by blood flow had become widely used.

The Rise of Endovascular Neurosurgery: The Era of Flow-Guided Balloons

The first endovascular balloon catheter was invented in 1961 by American cardiac surgeon Thomas Fogarthy. The device was a Teflon catheter that blindly ended in a latex balloon (Figure 11a). The Fogarthy catheter was designed for open thrombectomy of the pulmonary and peripheral arteries and is still used for these purposes today. In the 1960s, attempts were made to use this device in combination with other techniques to occlude carotid-cavernous fistulas [25].

No later than 1962, Charles Dotter, of whom we are already aware, began to use Teflon “dilatation catheters” of his own invention, which were nothing more than some of the first endovascular balloons (Figure 11b). Dotter authored many variations of balloon catheters, both single and double lumen, guided by a guidewire. Dotter also invented the first flow-guided balloon catheter designed for pulmonary artery catheterization [10, 26].

The first balloon catheter designed specifically for the needs of neurosurgery was developed in 1962 by the American neurosurgeon Sanford Rothenberg. His device consisted of a neoprene bladder placed between two halves of a metal ball. A specially folded polyester cuff was placed over the bladder. The device was placed on the tip of a Cournand-type cardiac catheter. As the neoprene balloon was inflated, the cuff straightened and pressed against the vessel wall, where it remained. Thus, the Rothenberg device was also the first stent graft in history, having been “officially” invented more than two decades earlier by Puhl and Zigwart (1986) [27].

Rothenberg planned to use his invention to occlude cerebral aneurysms and CCF (Figure 11c). He performed several successful embolizations in experimental models of aneurysms and fistulas in dogs. However, the device was never used on real patients. Most likely, Rothenberg was never able to solve the “carotid siphon” problem.

In 1964, Luessenhop, mentioned earlier in this paper, performed the first flow-directed balloon catheterization of cerebral arteries and the first temporary balloon occlusion of the ICA in a patient with a cerebral AVM and a flow-directed aneurysm of the posterior communicating artery (PCA) [17, 18].

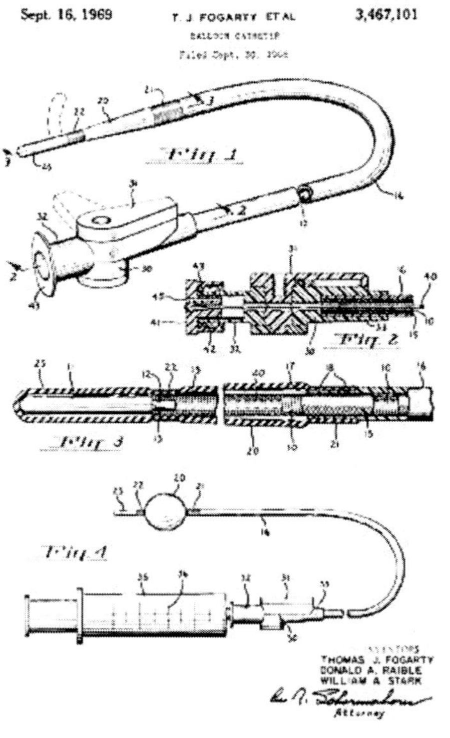

a)

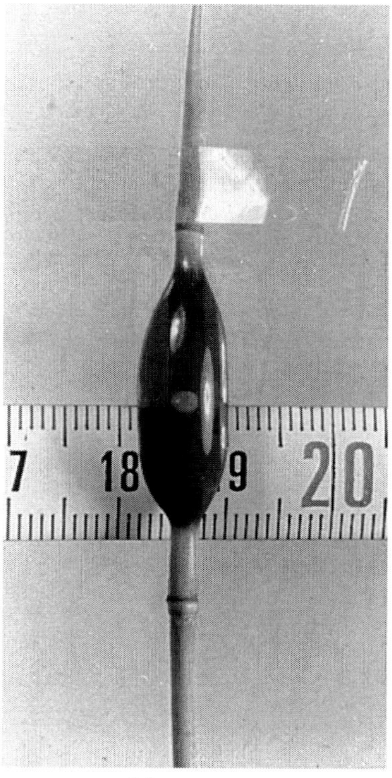

b)

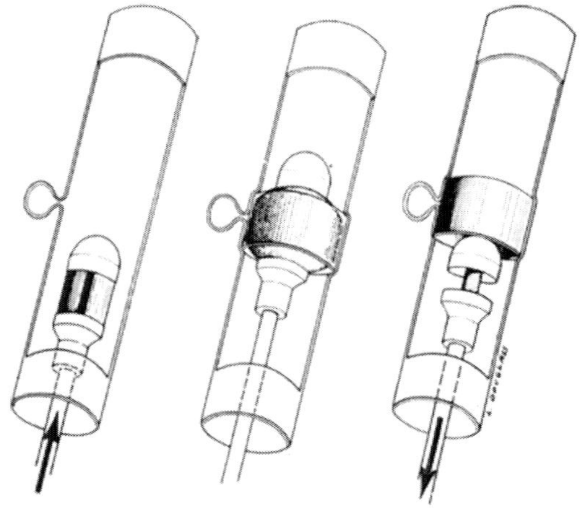

c)

Figure 11. a) Fogarty's balloon (from original patent, 1969). b) Dotter's early balloon. c) Rothenberg's device (from his original publication, 1962 [27]).

During one of the embolization sessions, Luessenhop inserted a 1-mm diameter silicone microcatheter into the patient with a blind distal end that was mechanically stretched. When contrast was introduced into the microcatheter, its tip spontaneously inflated. This improvised balloon was placed at the ICA bifurcation, in the protrusion of the neck of the flow aneurysm, and then inflated to a diameter of approximately 5 mm, completely blocking the blood flow in the artery. A few minutes later, the balloon was removed and the temporary occlusion of the

ICA led to thrombosis of the aneurysm. Based on this experience, Luessenhop concluded that "...cerebral arteries are tolerant of catheterization and temporary occlusion...." This procedure was experimental, and Luessenhop's balloon was not intended for stable, long-term occlusion of cerebral arteries.

In the second half of the 1960s, Soviet neurosurgeon Fedor Serbinenko invented the first detachable balloon catheter suitable for long-term occlusion of cerebral arteries. He developed the world's first applied method of selective catheterization, temporary (diagnostic) and permanent (therapeutic) occlusion of cerebral arteries with detachable and non-detachable balloons guided by blood flow. He is also the author of the first ever reconstructive endovascular interventions on cerebral vessels, namely balloon occlusion of cerebral saccular aneurysms and CCF with preservation of the patency of the affected artery.

In the 1970s, the Serbinenko balloon technique became popular abroad, and until the 1990s it was the main method of endovascular treatment of cerebrovascular diseases in the world. Fedor Serbinenko is the founder of endovascular neurosurgery as a separate field of medicine.

According to his contemporaries, Serbinenko came up with the idea of flow-driven balloons after observing the behavior of helium-filled balloons at a May Day celebration in 1959. Serbinenko began working on the balloon technology in 1960 at the latest. Over the course of several years, he experimented with various materials and designs of endovascular balloons and microcatheters, and tested various X-ray contrast agents and fillers. Finally, in 1964, he performed the first selective angiography of the external carotid artery (ECA) by temporarily occluding the ICA with a non-detachable balloon [28].

From 1964 to 1969, Serbinenko was mainly involved in diagnostic procedures. He refined the technique of selective catheterization of cerebral arteries, studied the peculiarities of cerebral hemodynamics in various vascular diseases, the possibilities and limits of cerebral collateral circulation, and evaluated the tolerance of various cerebral vessels to temporary and permanent occlusion. It should be noted that at that time all these aspects were understudied, and Serbinenko carried out a huge amount of preparatory work to anatomically and physiologically substantiate the applicability of his method.

The first balloon deconstruction of the ICA was performed in 1969 in a patient with CCF and the following year in a patient with a giant aneurysm of the ophthalmic artery. In 1971, Serbinenko performed the first balloon occlusion of CCF while maintaining patency of the affected artery. Subsequently, he systematically performed balloon occlusions of feeding arteries in patients with cerebral AVMs and dAVFs, as well as superselective injections of chemotherapeutic agents for brain tumors. Finally, in 1973, Serbinenko performed the first balloon occlusion of a cerebral saccular aneurysm (CSA), maintaining patency of the affected artery. By the mid-1970s, he had performed more than 300 diagnostic and more than 160 therapeutic endovascular interventions for various cerebrovascular diseases (Figure 12) [29].

In 1974, Serbinenko published his extensive experience in neurosurgery. In 1975, the N. Burdenko Neurosurgical Institute, where Serbinenko worked, was visited by the French (later Canadian) neuroradiologist Gerard Debrun, who at that time was working on his own endovascular balloon. He studied Serbinenko's method, improved it, and then popularized it in the West [30].

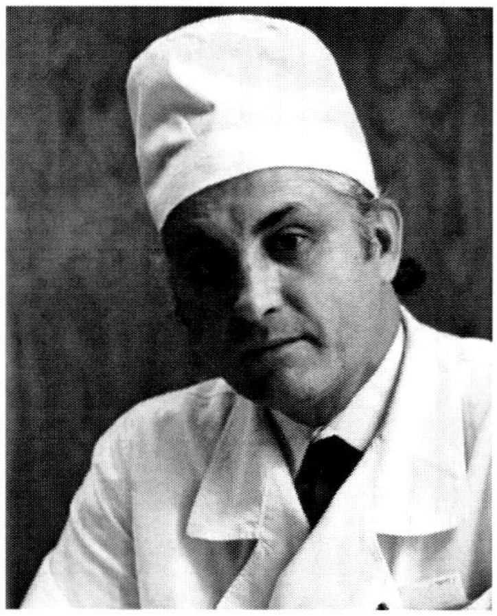

a)

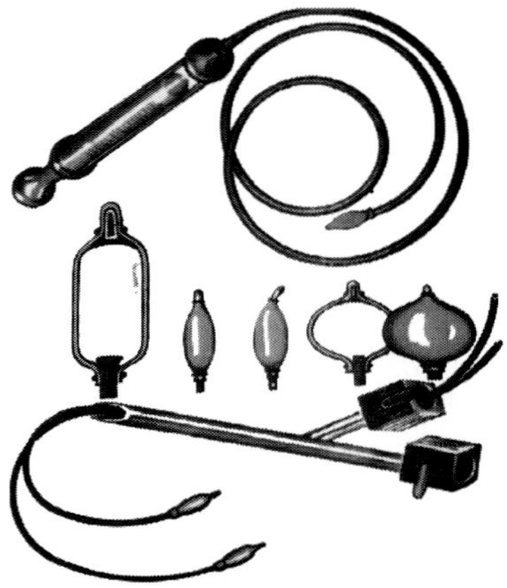

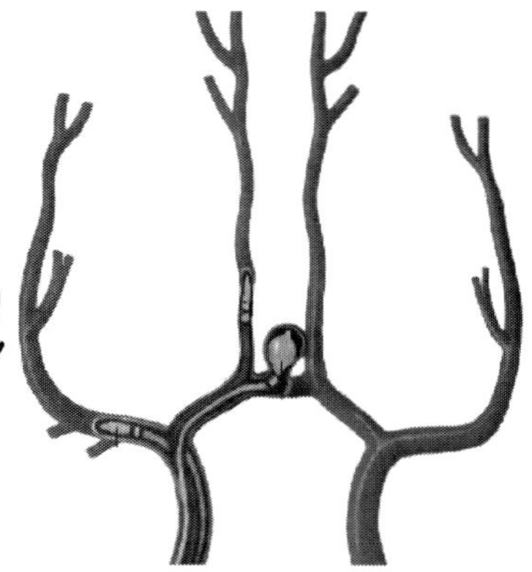

b) c)

Figure 12. a) Fedor Serbinenko (1928 - 2002). b) Serbinenko's balloons, microcatheters, and delivery cannula. c) Aneurysm treatment using multiple balloons. To guide a detachable balloon into the aneurysm, alternative vessels are temporarily occluded with non-detachable auxiliary balloons. (from the monograph of A. Romodanov, 1986 [36]).

The "classic" version of the Serbinenko method relied on two types of microcatheters: more flexible, made of polyethylene, and more rigid, made of fluoroplastic (Teflon). Microcatheters consisted of polymer tubes 1-1.5 mm in diameter with an internal lumen of 0.3 to 0.6 mm. The distal end of a tube was heated and mechanically stretched 1.5-2 times. A rim was fused to the distal end to which a balloon was then attached. The length of the microcatheter varied from 30 to 100 cm or more, depending on the location of the pathological focus and the particular intravascular access (transcarotid, transvertebral, or transfemoral).

The balloons were dipped from high quality natural latex. The balloon blank was a paper clip or a syringe needle with the tip cut off. The blank was dipped in liquid latex 3-5 times, air dried, and placed in an oven and then in a water bath for vulcanization. A radiopaque marker made of a piece of silver or tantalum wire was attached to the distal (blind) end of the microcatheter. The proximal (open) end of the balloon was placed on the rim of the microcatheter (Figure 13).

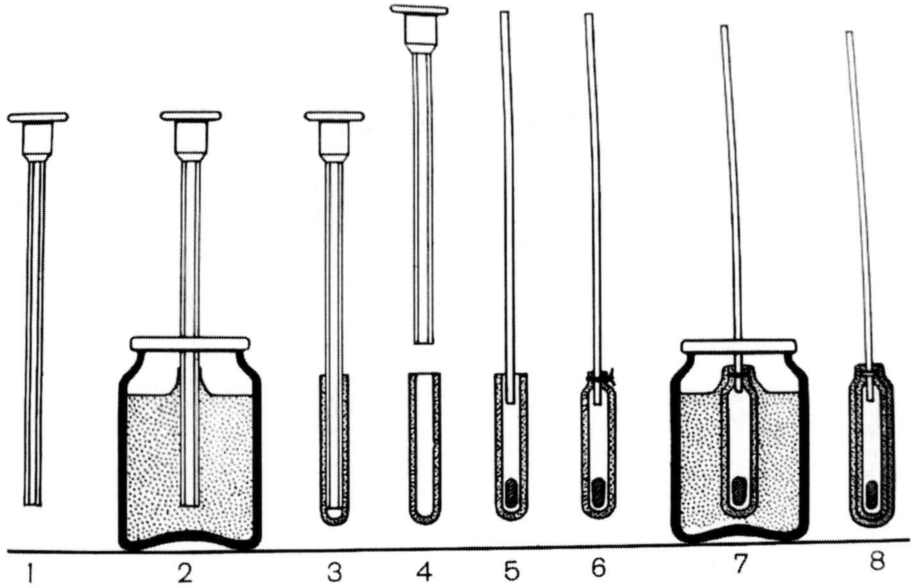

Figure 13. A technique for making a latex detachable balloon (from the original monograph by Khilko and Zubkov, 1982 [20]. 1-3 Dipping and drying of the mold, vulcanization not shown 4 - Cutting to usable length, 5 - Introducing a radiopaque marker and mounting on the microcatheter, 6 - Tying to the microcatheter with elastic ligature, 7-8 - Making a final layer of latex.

If a balloon was not intended to be detachable, its proximal end was tied to the microcatheter with a monofilament thread. If a balloon was intended to be detachable, its proximal end was folded inward to form a simple elastic sphincter. When the balloon was placed on a microcatheter, it was covered with a layer of latex. In addition to solid balloons, perforated balloons were also used, which were punctured in the distal part. When inflated to a certain degree, these balloons released part of their contents. This option was designed for superselective angiography and introduction of various drugs (e.g., during pharmacological tests).

To introduce a balloon into the cerebral arteries, it was partially inflated (to 1/2 - 2/3 of the artery diameter) and allowed to move with the blood flow. In some cases, the balloon was given positive buoyancy by introducing a small amount of air, and the patient's head was positioned so that the target vessel was at the highest point. Balloon navigation at arterial bifurcations was accomplished by temporarily blocking blood flow in the alternative branch with a second (auxiliary) balloon. The inflated balloon was detached by gentle traction on the microcatheter [20, 29, 31].

The early version of a detachable balloon had many technical shortcomings. One was the tendency of the balloon to detach prematurely because a simple sphincter did not provide a reliable connection to the microcatheter. At the same time, the balloon was often dislodged. Delayed deflation of the balloon was also a significant problem, as the sphincter did not provide adequate sealing. To prevent this, Serbinenko suggested that the final inflation of the balloon be performed with fast-curing silicone. However, the silicone did not harden immediately or completely and could leak from the balloon, causing distal thromboembolism. In addition, a certain amount of radiopaque material always remained in the lumen of the microcatheter, making it impossible to fill the entire volume of the balloon with silicone. When the volume of the balloon was comparable to the dead space of the microcatheter, silicone inflation became virtually impossible. These two phenomena were referred to as the "dead space problem. [32-34] Balloon technology continued to evolve. In 1976, Zubkov and Debrun independently modified the Serbinenko balloon in a similar fashion (Figure 14). They suggested attaching the proximal end of the balloon to the microcatheter with an elastic ligature or latex rings. To separate such a balloon, an auxiliary microcatheter of larger diameter was used. It was placed on the outside of the main microcatheter, pushed distally, and "pushed" the balloon. Such a design significantly increased the resistance of the balloon to delayed deflation and prevented its migration during detachment [34, 35].

One year later, in 1977, Zubkov developed a technique for balloon angioplasty for subarachnoid hemorrhage, which was also widely used abroad [36].

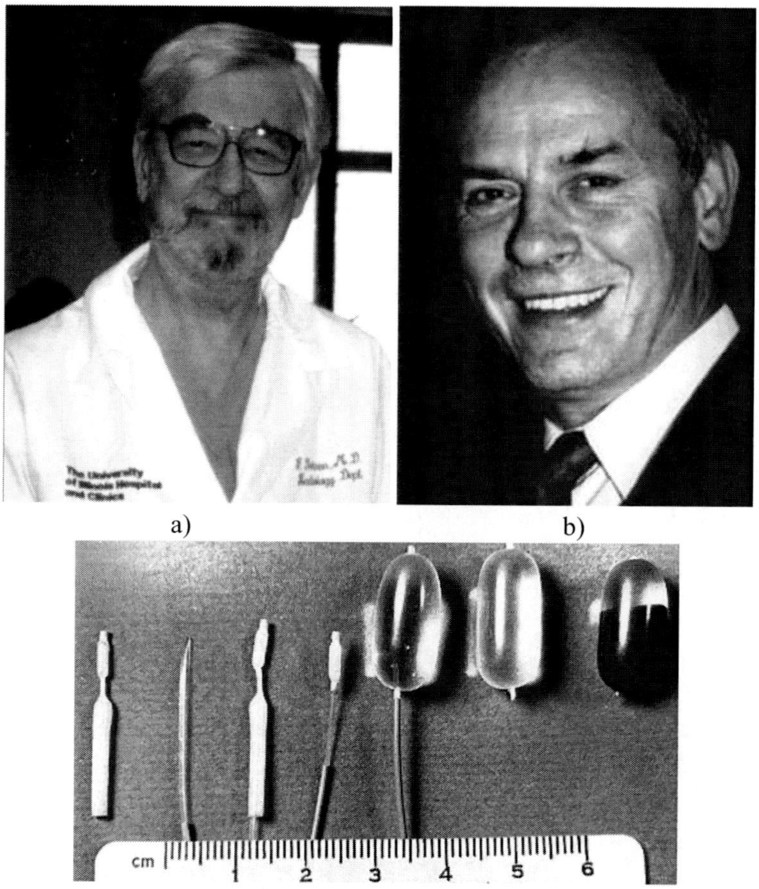

a) b) c)

Figure 14. a) Gerard Debrun. b) Yury Zubkov (1940-1997) c) Later modifications of Serbinenko's balloons, introduced independently by Debrun and Zubkov (from the original publication by Debrun, 1978 [34]).

In 1976-1977, Michael DiTullio and Paul Pevsner independently developed detachable silicone balloons (Figure 15a). Compared to latex balloons, silicone balloons had both advantages and disadvantages. Silicone was less thrombogenic and caused less inflammation, reducing the likelihood of ascending thrombosis and distal thromboembolism of cerebral arteries. Silicone balloons were less prone to delayed deflation and biodegradation. At the same time, they were less elastic (more traumatic), had worse endothelialization, and were more prone to delayed migration due to less adhesion to the vessel wall (compared to latex). Both types of balloons were used in parallel, depending on the specific task and surgeon preference [37, 38].

In 1978, Alejandro Berenstein and John Aberle developed a dual lumen detachable balloon (Figure 15b). A microcatheter had two channels - round (larger diameter) and crescent-shaped (smaller diameter). The first was used to temporarily inflate the balloon with a contrast agent, and the second was used for final inflation with a hardening filler. This innovation eliminated the "dead space" problem; however, dual-lumen balloons were never able to completely replace single-lumen balloons [39].

In 1979, the French company Balt extrusion, founded by the Polish-French engineer Leopold Plowiecki, introduced the first factory-made detachable balloon. This device was designed with the direct participation of Fyodor Serbinenko and the French neuroradiologist Jean-Jacques Merland [40].

In 1980, Waro Taki developed an electrically detachable balloon. The balloon had a fusible junction of polyvinyl alcohol and a radiofrequency electrode [41].

During the 1980s, homemade detachable balloons created by enthusiasts gave way to factory-made models such as Gold Valve and DeBrun Tie-On (Nycomed, Switzerland), Gold Balloon (Balt extrusion, France), DSB (Target therapeutics, USA), and others. Such balloons usually had higher manufacturing quality and standardized parameters (dimensions, volume and inflation pressure, etc.), which made their use safer and more predictable [42, 43].

Detachable balloons showed very good results in occlusion of direct arteriovenous fistulas (mainly CCF) and in deconstructive interventions of cerebral aneurysms. The radicality of such operations exceeded 90%, and the frequency of neurological complications was low, subject to careful functional testing of patients and observance of the principles of physiological acceptability.

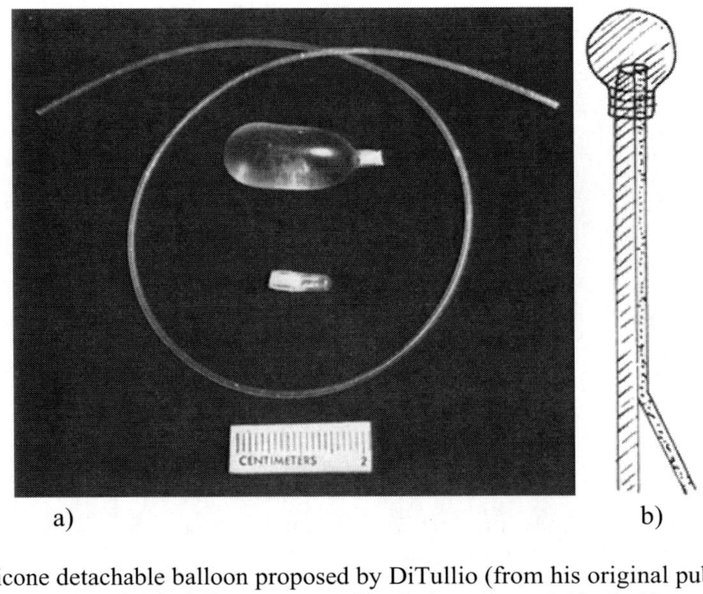

a) b)

Figure 15. a) Silicone detachable balloon proposed by DiTullio (from his original publication, 1978 [38]). b) Double lumen detachable balloon proposed by Berenstein and Aberle (from the publication by Debrun, 1978 [34]).

In a series of observations by Debrun (1989) of 143 patients with direct arteriovenous fistulas, complete occlusion was achieved in 133 (93%) with no neurological morbidity or mortality [44].

Fox (1987) described 68 deconstructive balloon interventions for inoperable proximal cerebral aneurysms. Complete aneurysm occlusion was achieved in 65 cases (96%), the incidence of neurological complications was 8 cases (12%), and permanent morbidity was observed in only 1 case (1.5%). There were no deaths [45].

At the same time, deconstructive surgery is often impossible, and balloon occlusion of saccular aneurysms while maintaining patency of the affected artery has been associated with significant technical difficulties and high surgical risk.

Typically, the balloons refused to spontaneously enter the aneurysms. Various maneuvers had to be performed, such as inflating the balloons with air, temporarily occluding the distal part of the artery with an auxiliary balloon, and others. In more favorable cases, the neck of the aneurysm was aligned with the track of the balloon catheter [20, 31].

Another problem was that the shape of the balloon often did not match the shape of the aneurysm. When the balloon was inflated, an "angioplasty" of the aneurysm cavity actually occurred, which was a very risky manipulation. Intraoperative rupture of the aneurysm by the balloon was a frequent and usually fatal complication [32].

According to a series of observations published by Randall Higashida in 1989, out of 84 patients who underwent balloon occlusion of saccular aneurysms with preserved patency of the affected artery, complete aneurysm occlusion was achieved in 65 cases (77%), while intraoperative aneurysm rupture occurred in 8 patients (9%), surgical morbidity was observed in 9 cases (11%), and mortality - in 15 cases (18%) [46].

The largest series of observations using this method (617 patients) was reported by Viktor Shcheglov in 1990. According to his data, the frequency of complete occlusion of aneurysms was 80%, the patency of the affected artery was preserved in 90% of cases, while the operative mortality in non-acutely ruptured aneurysms was 5.5%. These results were comparable to the results of microsurgical clipping of aneurysms at that time [47].

Reconstructive balloon occlusion of saccular aneurysms performed by Shcheglov, Serbinenko and Zubkov showed good results. At the same time, according to most foreign authors, such interventions were accompanied by an unacceptably high rate of surgical complications, disability and mortality. For this reason, reconstructive balloon occlusion was most often considered a "last resort" treatment for aneurysms unsuitable for other methods. In those years, no more than 10% of all cerebral aneurysms underwent intravascular occlusion, which was a significant limitation for endovascular neurosurgery. The situation began to change in the 1990s with the introduction of detachable coils into neurosurgical practice. However, before moving on to this stage of endovascular neurosurgery, several other issues need to be addressed.

In the 1970s, neurosurgeons began using selective occlusion of feeding arteries with detachable balloons to treat cerebral AVMs, dAVFs, and vascular tumors. However, these procedures were almost never radical. Once the main afferent arteries are occluded, the arterial collaterals typically begin to function and blood flow within the pathological formation is restored.

In the second half of the 1960s, the French neuroradiologist Rene Djindjian provided anatomical and physiological explanations for the fact that radical occlusion of the above-mentioned diseases can only be achieved by direct embolization of the AVM nidus or tumor stroma. At the same time, American neurosurgeons Paul Zanetti and Frank Sherman proposed direct embolization of the malformation node with cyanoacrylate glue ("Bucrylate") during microsurgical removal of cerebral AVMs [48, 49].

In 1973, the American neuroradiologist Charles Kerber developed a calibrated leak balloon (Figure 16). The device was based on the same principles as Serbinenko's perforated balloons and was intended for superselective catheterization and angiography of cerebral arteries, as well as the delivery of liquid embolic materials. Due to its compliance and small size, this device allowed catheterization of 4th-5th order cerebral arteries, including intranidal catheterization of AVMs, whereas the capabilities of the Serbinenko balloons were limited to 2nd-3rd order arteries. Interestingly, the Kerber balloon was invented independently of Serbinenko, even before his technique became known in the West, and conceptually became a "descendant" of the Luessenhop balloons [50, 51].

The early Kerber device was a monolithic silicone microcatheter approximately 0.5-0.8 mm in diameter, with an internal lumen of approximately 0.2-0.3 mm and an inflatable distal tip. The distal surface of the balloon had calibrated microholes, the diameter and number of which were selected so that the balloon would begin to leak when inflated to a certain volume or pressure. The balloon was inserted into the patient using a propulsion chamber and guided by blood flow.

In 1974, Kerber used calibrated leaky balloons to perform the first intranidal endovascular embolization of a cerebral AVM using cyanoacrylate glue [52].

In 1982, Debrun published a seminal series. 46 patients with cerebral AVMs underwent cyanoacrylate embolization with calibrated leaky balloons. Total occlusion of the AVM was achieved in 8 patients (17%) and subtotal occlusion in 4 patients (9%). Partial occlusion was achieved in 27 cases (59%), and in 7 patients the malformation catheterization failed. The incidence of neurological complications of embolization (mostly transient) was about 20% [53].

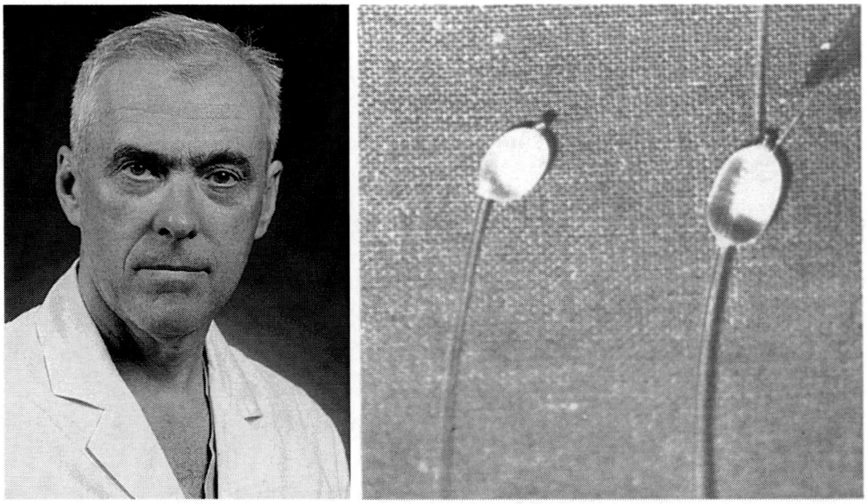

a) b)

Figure 16. a) Charles Kerber b) Kerber's calibrated leak balloon (from the original publication by Debrun, 1978 [34]).

Cyanoacrylate became the primary material for embolization of cerebral AVMs and dAVFs until the introduction of non-adhesive liquid embolic materials in the 2000s. Concurrent with the introduction of cyanoacrylate into neurosurgical practice, the search for other embolic materials continued.

In 1970, Djindjian proposed a crushed polyvinyl alcohol hemostatic sponge ("Ivalon," "Gelfoam") as an embolic agent (Figure 17a). He used it to occlude hemangiomas and other tumors in the external carotid basin and arteriovenous fistulas of the spinal cord. He also had the idea of using lyophilized dura mater for these purposes [48, 54, 55].

In 1975, Murthy Tadavarthy extended Djindjian's concept by finding a way to grind polyvinyl alcohol sponges into a homogeneous fine dust. When mixed with a water-soluble contrast agent, it became liquid and could be injected through a microcatheter directly into the pathological vasculature. Djindjian and Tadavarthy's ground hemostatic sponge embolization became the forerunner of non-adhesive liquid embolic materials developed much later [56].

During this period, significant advances were also made in the diagnosis and treatment of arteriovenous shunts and vascular tumors of the spinal cord. Rene Djindjian was the founder of endovascular spinal cord interventions; from the mid-1960s to the mid-1970s, he systematically studied spinal vascular anatomy and developed applied methods for selective catheterization and embolization of spinal cord vessels [48, 54, 55].

Another outstanding pioneer in spinal embolization is one of Serbinenko's favorite students, the Soviet neurosurgeon Theodor Thiessen (Figure 17b). He has the most extensive experience in endovascular treatment of vascular pathology of the spinal cord in the world. From 1982 to 2018, he performed embolization of more than 400 AVMs and more than 800 dAVFs of the spinal cord using various embolic materials. With embolization, Thiessen improved neurological symptoms in 90% of patients with symptomatic spinal arteriovenous shunts. The results of his work were described in two landmark publications in 2008 and 2019. He is also the author of numerous papers on the vascular anatomy and hemodynamics of the spinal cord, the neurological manifestations and the clinical course of spinal vascular disease [57-59].

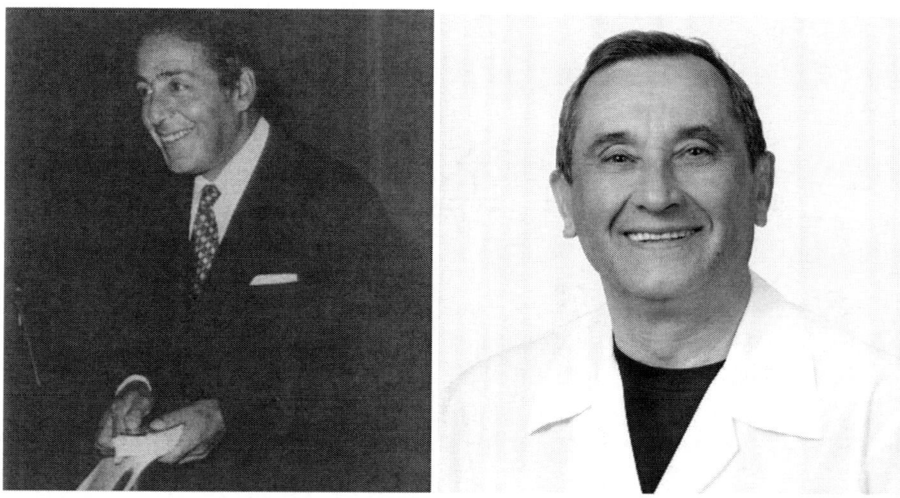

a) b)

Figure 17. a) Rene Djindjian (1918-1974). b) Theodor Thiessen.

Contemporary Endovascular Neurosurgery

Over-the-Wire Microcatheters

As mentioned earlier, instruments and techniques for intravascular interventions using transfemoral and transradial approaches were developed in the 1970s. They were quickly adopted by endovascular neurosurgery for diagnostic cerebral angiography. However, until the 1990s, neurosurgeons continued to prefer direct transcarotid and vertebral approaches for embolization.

One of the main reasons was the modest "traction characteristics" of flow-directed balloons. Long microcatheters created significant drag as they moved through the vascular bed, significantly reducing balloon maneuverability in the cerebral arteries. Direct puncture of the carotid and vertebral arteries could be accomplished with microcatheters approximately 30 cm long, whereas transfemoral interventions required microcatheters 100-110 cm or longer. A complete transition to peripheral vascular approaches in endovascular neurosurgery became possible with the advent of a fundamentally new method of cerebral intravascular navigation - microcatheters of variable stiffness guided by microguidewires.

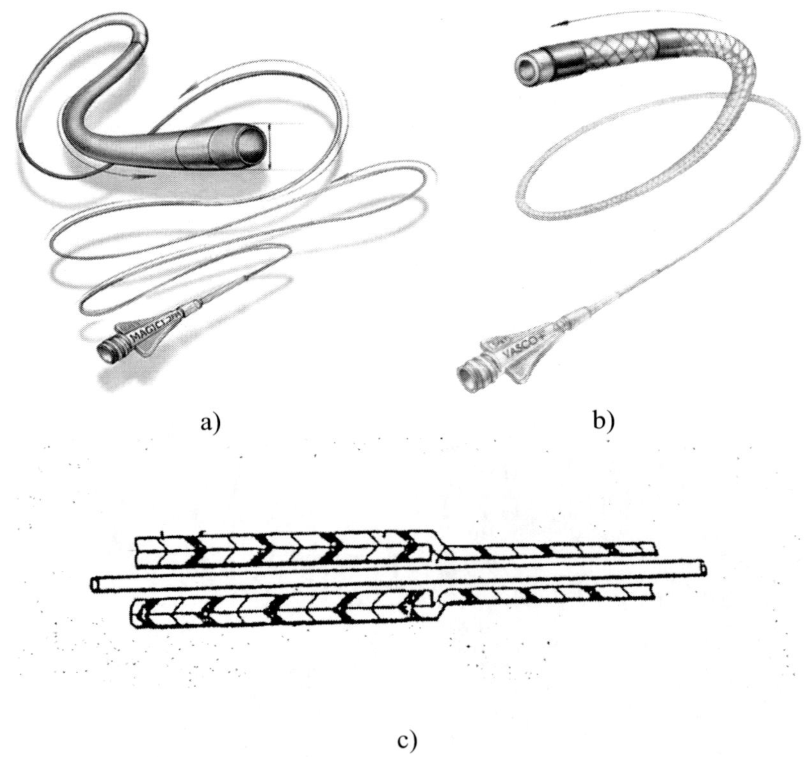

a) b)

c)

Figure 18. Modern variable stiffness over-the-wire microcatheters. a) Magic (Balt extrusion). b) Vasco (Balt extrusion). Note the metal braid under the polymeric coating of the microcatheter. c) A drawing from the original patent of the Tracker microcatheter (Target therapeutics) by Engelson, 1988 [60], showing a telescopic connection of separate polymeric tubes and a wire within the microcatheter lumen.

The first such device - the Tracker microcatheter - was developed in 1986 by Eric Engelson, an engineer at Target therapeutics (now Stryker, USA). The second such microcatheter - Magic (Balt extrusion, France) was introduced into clinical practice in 1987 by Leopold Plowiecki and Luc Picard (Figure 18) [40, 60].

Variable stiffness microcatheters consisted of multiple polymer tubes of different thicknesses and materials telescoped together with a common polymer coating. The proximal segment of such a microcatheter was rigid to provide mechanical support and transmit push force. The distal segment was flexible and atraumatic for safe passage through the bends of the cerebral vessels. The tip of the microcatheter was equipped with multiple radiopaque markers in the form of rings.

An equally important component of the system was the shape-memory micro-guidewire: a thin, hollow tube of nickel-titanium alloy with a rigid steel core at the proximal end and a flexible polymer core and a braid of radiopaque platinum thread at the distal end. The proximal segment of the guidewire assisted in the transmission of shear and torque forces, while the distal segment was atraumatic and retained its former shape, allowing the guidewire to be rotated in the vessel lumen and precisely inserted into the desired arterial branches.

By the early 1990s, such microcatheters had largely replaced flow-directed balloons as a tool for superselective catheterization of cerebral vessels and delivery of embolic materials.

The next step was reinforced microcatheters. The first was the Vasco microcatheter (Balt extrusion) introduced in 2001. These devices have a braid of thin metal filaments between the outer polymer tube and the outer hydrophilic coating of the microcatheter. The thickness of the threads and the density of the weave can vary in different segments of the microcatheter, resulting in different mechanical properties. Reinforced microcatheters are more resistant to longitudinal deformation, twisting and fracture, and provide better mechanical support and transmission of push force [40].

The vast majority of microcatheters used in endovascular neurosurgery today are reinforced variable stiffness microcatheters guided by a shape memory micro-guidewire.

Detachable Coils

We have already mentioned that the technical limitations of detachable balloons were most evident in the embolization of cerebral saccular aneurysms with preservation of the lumen of the affected artery. For safer and more controlled aneurysm occlusion, it was necessary for the embolization material to conform to the shape of the aneurysm sac and have minimal mechanical impact on the aneurysm wall, while being reliably retained within the aneurysm cavity. Thin metal filaments twisted in a spiral shape were best suited for these purposes.

As mentioned earlier, the first procedure in history that can be considered the prototype of spiral embolization was the electrothrombosis of a giant aneurysm of the ophthalmic artery performed by Werner in 1938. During this operation, he introduced almost 10 meters of silver wire with a diameter of 0.16 mm (34 gauge) into the aneurysm cavity (Figure 19) [12].

In 1975, the Italian-American radiologist Cesare Gianturco proposed occluding arteriovenous fistulas in peripheral vessels with spirally twisted metal filaments. Initially, he used the cut ends of endovascular guidewires and later turned to specially designed spirals of platinum braided steel wire. To increase thrombogenicity, Dacron fibers were added between the spiral turns [61].

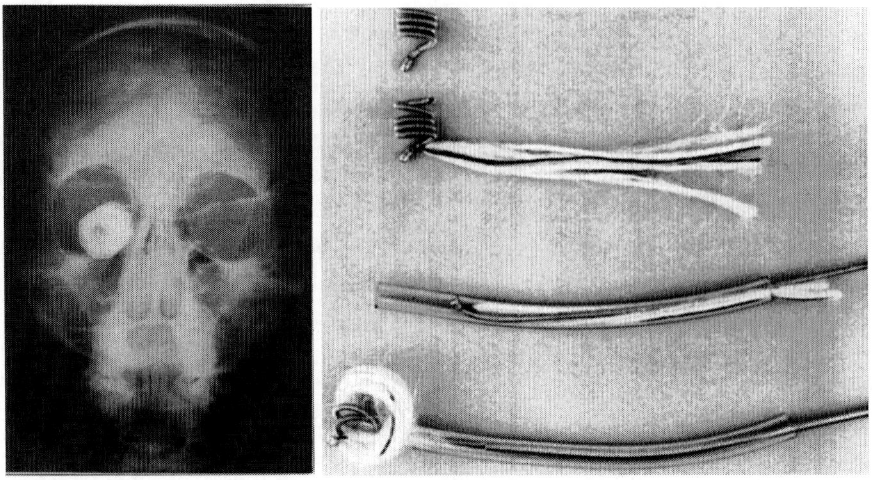

a) b)

Figure 19. a) An image from Werner et al. 1941 [12] showing a thread-like silver electrode inside the patient's skull - a very first known image of "endosaccular aneurysm coiling." b) Early Gianturco coil, 1970s.

Ira Braun first used Gianturco coils for cerebral aneurysm occlusion in 1985. He used it to deconstruct the ICA in a patient with a giant cavernous aneurysm. Large, very rigid Gianturco coils were delivered with peripheral guide catheters, which made them poorly suited for cerebral arteries [62].

In 1988, Peter Yang suggested trying free platinum coils made from the cut ends of tracker micro-guidewires to occlude the anastomosis. These coils were delivered with the same Tracker microcatheter. Yang performed 8 such embolizations, complete occlusion of the fistula was achieved in 6 cases, transient neurological complications were noted in 2 patients [63].

The main disadvantage of free coils was the poorly controlled embolization. In case of unsatisfactory coil position, protrusion or migration of coil turns, repositioning was practically impossible.

The first arbitrarily detachable (and therefore repositionable) coils specifically designed for cerebral aneurysm embolization were invented by the Italian-American neuroradiologist Guido Guglielmi in 1990.

In the second half of the 1980s, he worked on endovascular electrothrombosis based on the earlier experiments of Mullan (1974), Piton (1978), Werner (1941), Thompson (1977) and Salazar (1961). Guglielmi found that platinum filament was the optimal material for intravascular electrodes because it combined high thrombogenicity, biocompatibility, excellent radiopacity, and was sufficiently flexible and atraumatic. In addition, he found that a steel thread placed in the bloodstream is subject to electrolysis and can dissolve under the influence of electric current. In 1989, during one of his experiments on electrothrombosis, Guglielmi's electrode spontaneously detached, which gave him the idea of using this phenomenon for therapeutic purposes.

One year later, Guglielmi, together with Target Therapeutics engineer Ivan Sepetka, presented the first custom-designed detachable microcoil - the Guglielmi Detachable Coil (GDC-10) (Figure 20). The device consisted of a 175 cm long steel wire with a cross-section of 0.25 mm, to the distal end of which a 0.010-inch thick platinum coil with a coil diameter of

2 to 8 mm and a length of 5 to 40 cm was microwelded. The steel wire had Teflon electrical insulation along its entire length, except for the proximal end and the distal 2-3 mm of thread near the coil attachment site where it was to be severed.

Coil embolization was performed via a transfemoral approach using standard endovascular catheters. A Tracker-18 microcatheter was advanced into the aneurysm cavity and the coil was carefully placed loop by loop. The coil could be repositioned and repositioned prior to delivery. Once the entire coil was delivered, if its position was satisfactory, the positive electrode was applied to the bare proximal end of the delivery wire and the negative electrode was applied to the patient's body. The distal portion of the delivery wire, which had no electrical insulation, was electrolyzed and the coil was detached. Electrothrombosis and coil detachment took 10 to 40 minutes in early device models. Coils were placed sequentially until satisfactory thrombosis of the aneurysm was achieved [64].

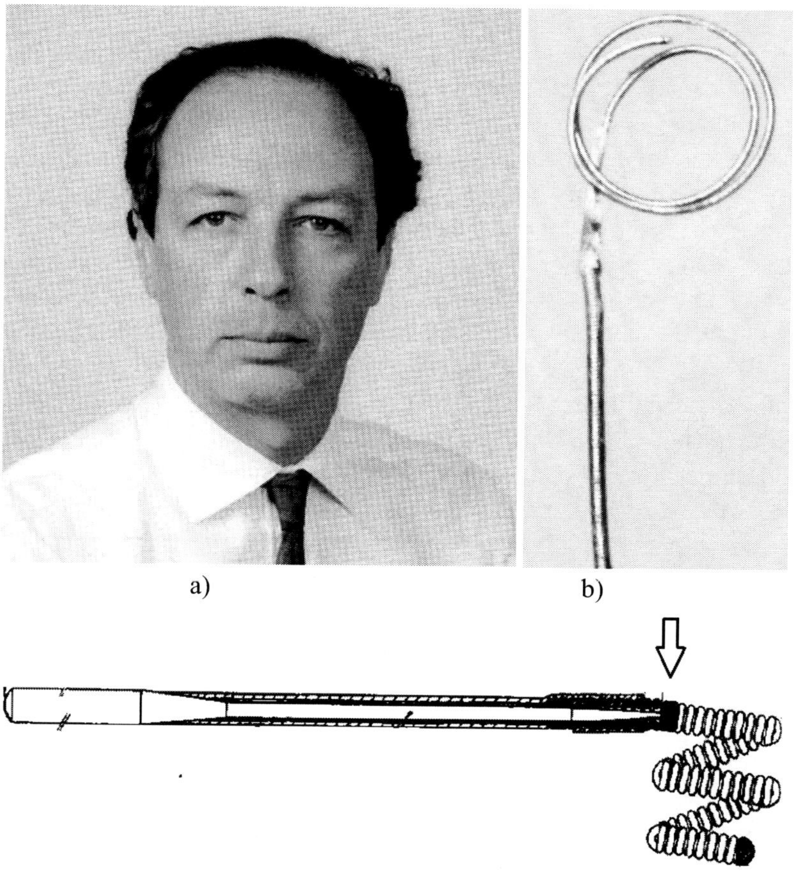

c)

Figure 20. a) Guido Guglielmi. b) Guglielmi's earliest coil (from his original publication, 2009 [32]) c) A schematic drawing of Guglielmi's early coil, black arrow indicates an uninsulated segment of silent wire where electrolysis and detachment are intended to occur (from Guglielmi's original publication, 1991 [64]).

In 1991, Guglielmi published a series of 13 patients with cerebral saccular aneurysms who underwent embolization with detachable coils. Complete aneurysm occlusion was achieved in half of the cases, and incomplete but satisfactory occlusion (more than 70% of the aneurysm volume) was observed in all other cases. Transient neurological complications occurred in 1 patient and there was no surgical morbidity or mortality [65].

It soon became clear that the mechanism of action of detachable coils was based on hemodynamic changes in the aneurysm cavity (reduction of volumetric blood flow velocity, turbulence and blood stagnation) and thrombogenic material of the coils themselves, while electrothrombosis did not play a significant role in stable aneurysm occlusion. Guglielmi rejected electrothrombosis and improved the coil delivery system to reduce coil release time to a few minutes. GDC coils quickly gained popularity and by the mid-1990s had virtually replaced detachable balloons in the embolization of saccular intracranial aneurysms.

In 1997, Vinuela, Duckwiler, and Mawad published the results of coil embolization in 403 patients with aneurysms of various locations and sizes in the acute phase of subarachnoid hemorrhage. The rate of complete occlusion of small aneurysms was 71% compared to approximately 40% for large and giant aneurysms. Morbidity and mortality from surgical complications were 9% and less than 2%, respectively [66].

In 2002, the first results of the large randomized ISAT trial (1493 patients operated on between 1994 and 2002) were published, comparing the results of coil embolization and microsurgical clipping of cerebral aneurysms in the acute phase of subarachnoid hemorrhage. Despite the lower radicality of embolization compared to clipping, the frequency of adverse neurological outcomes was significantly lower in the endovascular group (20% versus 30%), while the frequency of recurrent hemorrhage was negligible in both groups. Due to the good angiographic and clinical results of coil embolization, the proportion of endovascular surgery for cerebral aneurysms increased to 30-50% in the 2000s [67].

Throughout the 1990s and 2000s, coil embolization technologies continued to improve. By the end of the 1990s, thicker 14-gauge (0.014-0.016 inch) and 18-gauge (0.018-0.020 inch) coils were available in addition to the original 10-gauge (0.010 inch) coils. Coils of different calibers had different stiffnesses, which could be selected according to the task at hand, making the embolization process more controllable. At the same time, the so-called “3 F concept” (framing, filling, finishing) was established. The first step was to place the stiffest coil into the aneurysm to create a “frame” in the aneurysm cavity (framing). Next, the main volume of the aneurysm was filled with coils of intermediate stiffness. Finally, the remaining voids between the coils and the aneurysm neck were filled with the thinnest and most pliable coils (finishing).

Early coils in the free state had a ring shape, which is not the best for uniform filling of the aneurysm cavity. In 2000, coils were introduced that had a nickel-titanium alloy core with shape memory in addition to the main platinum filament, allowing for a more favorable spatial configuration. The most popular coils are spherical (3D coils) and cylindrical (helical coils). The first such devices were GDC 3D (Boston Scientific, formerly Target Therapeutics, USA) and Helipaq (Codman, USA) (Figure 21).

Early models of coils often unwound and stretched under excessive mechanical stress (especially under traction). An unwound coil is almost impossible to properly place, reposition or remove, which is a major technical complication. In 2000, the first unwind resistant coils were developed - GDC-10 SR (“stretch resistant”). A thin polymer filament was placed inside such a coil, physically securing the proximal and distal ends of the coil together, significantly reducing the likelihood of unwinding or breakage. This design is currently standard and is used in all modern detachable coils.

Attempts have been made to increase the thrombogenicity of the coil and the radicality of coil embolization with various bioactive coatings. In 2000, GDC VortX coils (Boston

Scientific, later Stryker, USA) with a polyester fiber coating were introduced. Later, other manufacturers tested coils with nylon and polyglycolic acid fibers. In 2002, Microvention (USA) introduced HydroCoil coils with a hydrogel coating based on polyglycolide co-lactide (PGLA). Upon contact with blood, the hydrogel absorbed water and expanded 1.5-2 times, occupying a significantly larger volume in the aneurysm lumen. Later, several randomized trials (MAPS, 2011, HELPS, 2014, and GREAT, 2018) did not show any significant advantages of coated coils over uncoated ones, so coated coils are not widely used at present.

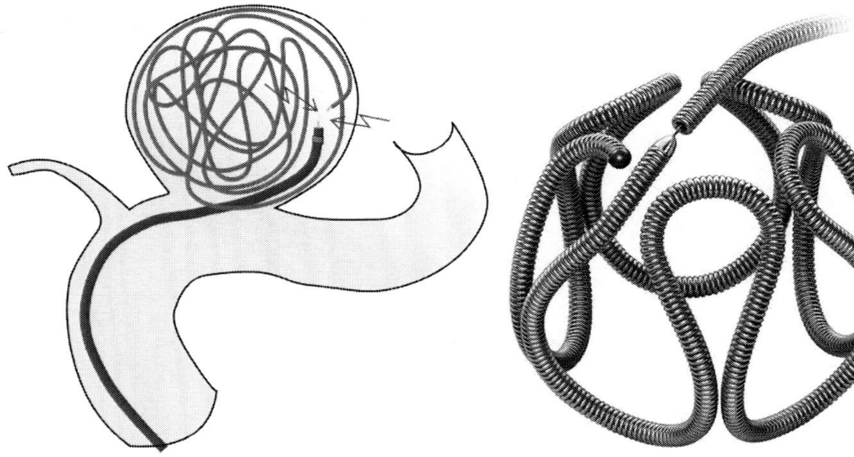

a) b)

Figure 21. a) "Classical" unassisted endosaccular coiling technique. b) Modern detachable spherical coil.

As the coil design evolved, so did the systems for delivering and removing the coils. Electrolytic detachment of the original GDC devices was time-consuming and not always reliable.

In 1993, French neuroradiologist Jacques Moret and Balt Extrusion introduced the first mechanical coil detachment system - the Moret/Mechanical Detachment System (MDS). The proximal end of the coil had a metal ball shaft, while the delivery system thread ended in a small metal "claw." When the ball-claw pair was inside the microcatheter, the coil was securely fixed. When the pair exited the microcatheter, the ball fell out of the claw and the coil separated.

The design was not very successful and did not gain widespread acceptance, but it became the prototype for Axium - a later (2008) and more advanced mechanical separation system (ev3, later Medtronic, USA). This system consisted of a hollow metal tube with a thin polymer thread running through it, attached to a spiral. When the polymer thread was pulled, it tore and the device detached.

In 2002, the first hydraulic separation system was developed - Hydrolink (Microvention, USA). It was also a hollow tube, but at its distal end was a polymer plug to which a coil was attached. When liquid was introduced into the delivery system tube, the plug was pushed out and the spiral separated.

In 2005, the first modern thermomechanical (V-Trak, Microvention, USA) and thermoelectric (Micrus, later Codman, USA) coil separation systems appeared. These systems are similar in design. The coil is fixed to the delivery thread with a fusible bridge made of special glue or polymer. An electrical heating element is located at the distal end of the delivery wire. When an electric current is applied, the heating element melts the bridge, releasing the coil.

Modern detachable coils utilize mechanical and thermomechanical systems that ensure reliable and instantaneous detachment of the device. In particular, the German neuroradiologist Hans Henkes played a key role in the development of modern coil release systems [32, 40, 42, 68-71].

Classical coil embolization of saccular aneurysms with a wide or poorly formed neck is technically difficult. An unfavorable neck configuration prevents reliable coil retention in the aneurysm cavity, creating a risk of protrusion or migration of coil turns from the aneurysm and occlusion of the affected artery.

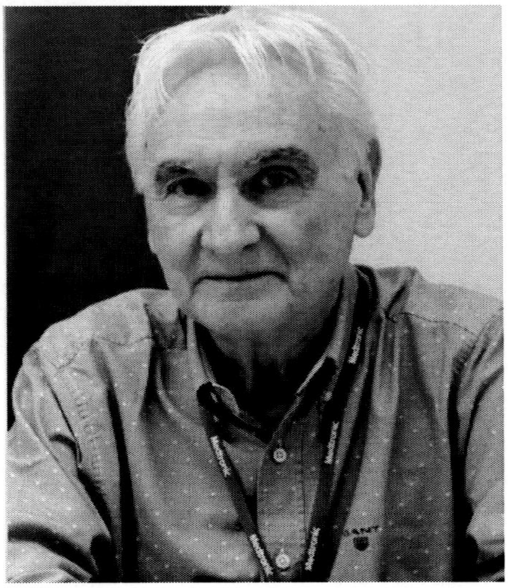

a)

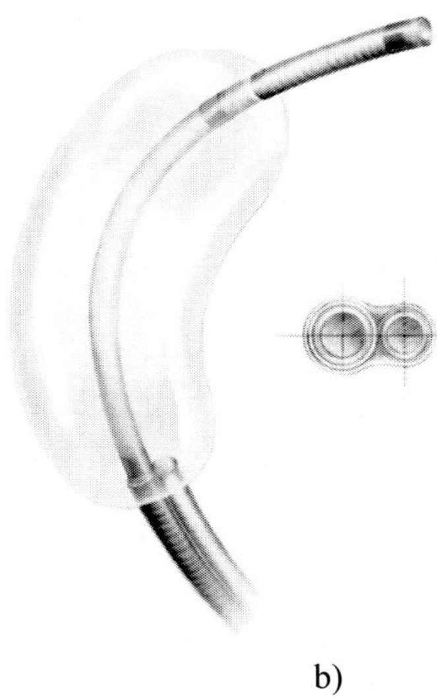

b)

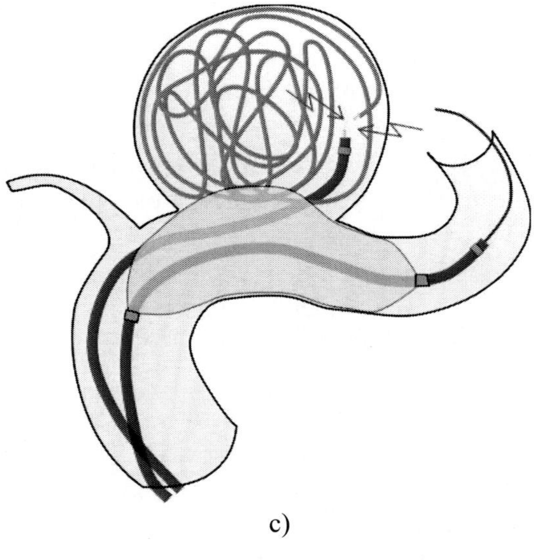

c)

Figure 22. a) Jacques Moret. b) Modern non-detachable double lumen balloon. c) Balloon-assisted coiling technique.

Since 1992, Jacques Moret has been performing coil embolization under temporary balloon occlusion of the aneurysm neck (Figure 22). In his early experiments, he used the "Moret catheters," developed in collaboration with Balt Extrusion. These were a dual lumen modification of the Magic microcatheter with a non-detachable latex balloon attached to the end. These devices were flow-directed and structurally similar to the balloons used in endovascular neurosurgery in the 1980s. Later, Moret began using Cirrus (Medtronic, USA) over-the-wire coronary balloons [40, 72, 73].

In 1997, he published a series of 57 cases of balloon-assisted coiling. Complete aneurysm occlusion was achieved in 40 cases (77%) and satisfactory occlusion in 49 cases (94%), with surgical morbidity in 1 patient (1.5%) and no deaths. These results significantly exceeded the results of "classical" coil embolization, and the balloon-assisted coiling technique quickly gained popularity [72].

In 2002, Boston Scientific developed Grapewine, the first modern balloon support device: a single-lumen, non-detachable over-the-wire balloon. Made from a new, super-pliable polymer, polyether block amide (Pebax), it was far less traumatic than any balloon previously used in endovascular neurosurgery. A year later, Balt Extrusion offered a similar balloon - the Magellan [40, 73].

In 2009 and 2013, the US companies Micrus and Microvention introduced Ascent and Scepter, respectively: dual lumen neurovascular balloons. In these devices, one lumen was dedicated to the inflation and deflation of the balloon, while the second lumen could be used not only for the introduction of the microdevice, but also for the delivery of other intravascular devices (primarily coils and stents) and, in the case of Scepter, also for the introduction of liquid embolic materials [42].

In coil embolization, balloon assist provides critical advantages and is currently considered part of the standard technique for endovascular treatment of cerebral aneurysms. It allows successful embolization of wide-necked aneurysms by preventing coils from falling out of the aneurysm; it provides tighter coil packing in the aneurysm cavity, increasing the radicality of the occlusion; and finally, in the event of intraoperative aneurysm rupture, the balloon minimizes the volume and severity of bleeding [74].

Stent support is another technique that has significantly expanded the technical capabilities of the detachable coils. According to the most popular version, the word "stent" comes from the name of the British dentist Charles Stent. In 1856, he invented a new material called "Stent plastic," which was originally intended for dental impressions, but later found many other applications in surgery [75].

The first intravascular stent for peripheral arteries was developed in 1969 by the aforementioned Charles Dotter [26]. In 1987, radiologists Julio Palmaz and Richard Schatz designed balloon-expandable coronary stents, which later became the first stents used in endovascular neurosurgery.

In 1997, American neuroradiologist Randall Higashida published the first case of stent-assisted coil embolization of a wide-necked cerebral aneurysm. In this procedure, he placed a Palmaz-Schatz coronary stent in the projection of the vertebral artery aneurysm and then catheterized the aneurysm through the stent cell [76].

In 2001, Pedro Lylyk published a series of 8 cases of coil embolization of aneurysms supported by coronary stents. Complete aneurysm occlusion was observed in 7 patients (87%) and no complications were noted. However, he used this technique only for proximal aneurysms of the internal carotid and vertebral arteries (Figure 23) [77].

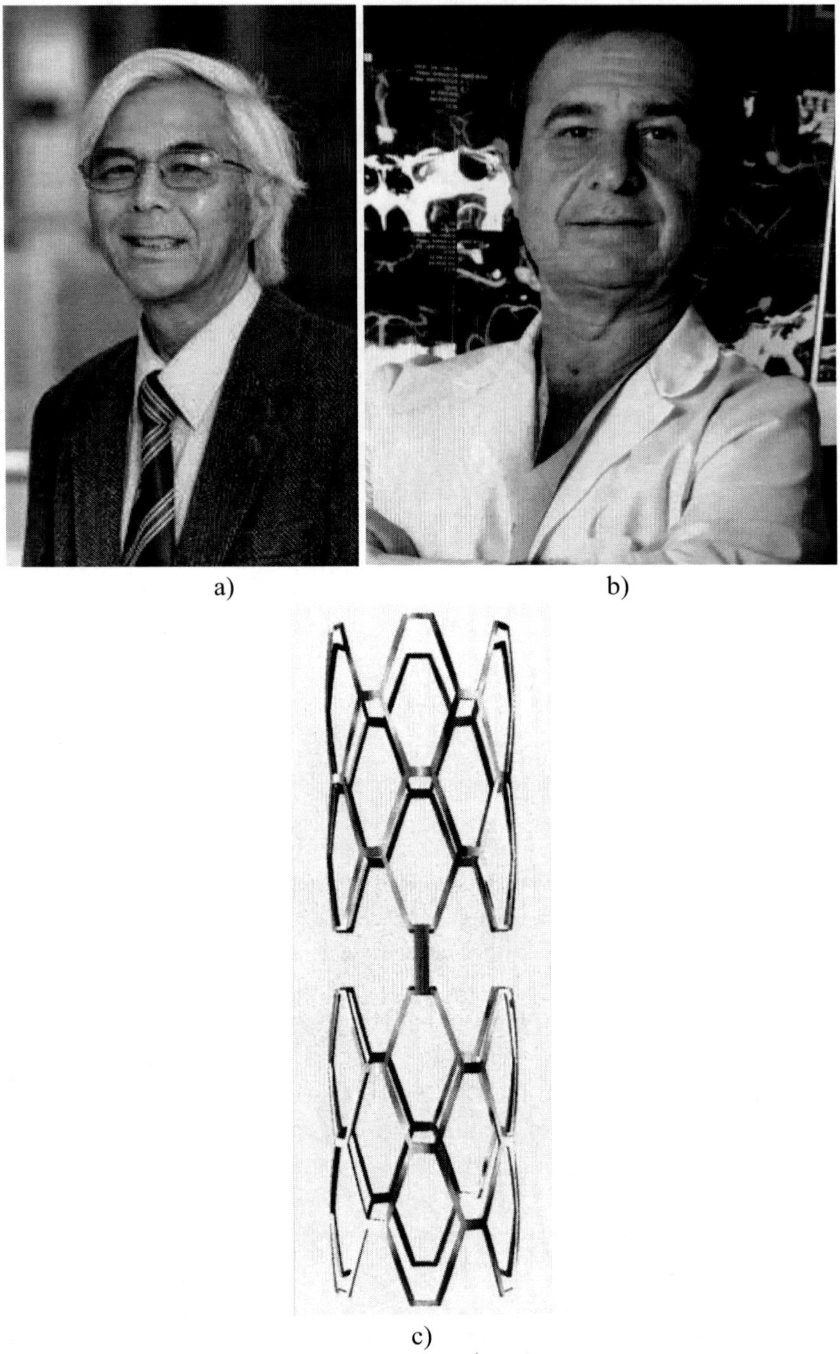

Figure 23. a) Randall Higashida. b) Pedro Lylyk. c) Palmaz-Shatz balloon-mounted stent used in early stent-assisted coiling procedures.

Coronary stents were rigid, traumatic, and had difficulty negotiating the curves of intracranial arteries. Their use in the cerebral vascular bed was associated with a high risk of technical failure and complications.

In 2002, Boston Scientific developed Neuroform, the first stent designed specifically for cerebral arteries (Figure 24). It was a self-expanding, open-cell stent made of a laser-cut nickel-titanium alloy. The device was preinstalled externally on a 2 French microcatheter, which was placed inside another 3 French microcatheter. Delivery was by exchange via a 300-cm micro-guidewire.

Despite a less than successful design, Neuroform has shown good results in coil embolization of cerebral aneurysms. In 2002, Hans Henkes presented the results of using this device in 16 patients with aneurysms of various locations, including ACA, MCA, and BA. Total or subtotal occlusion of the aneurysm was achieved in all cases, with complications in only one patient. Fiorella achieved similar results in one of his early clinical series (2004) [78, 79].

In 2003, Balt Extrusion introduced Leo, the first braided intracranial stent, and in 2005, Codman introduced Enterprise, a laser-cut, closed-cell neuroendovascular stent. Both devices were delivered through standard 2.1 French reinforced microcatheters, a major advantage over Neuroform.

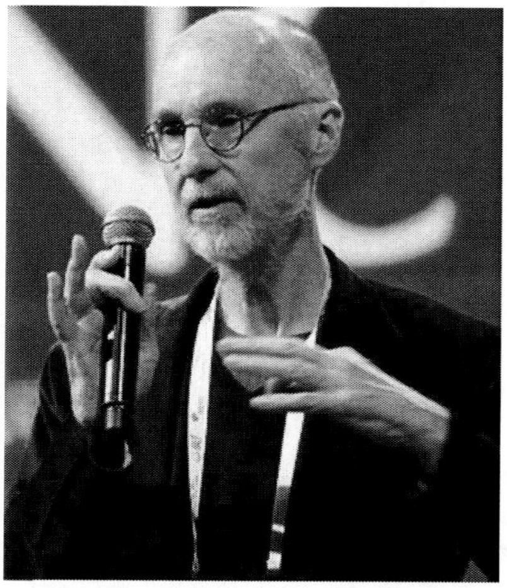

a)

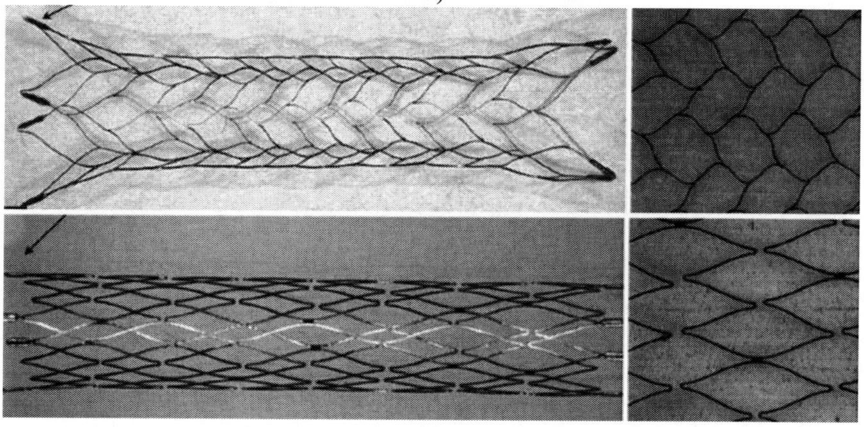

b)

Figure 24. a) Peter Kim Nelson, co-inventor of the Neuroform stent. b) Advanced laser-cut neurovascular stents: Enterprise (top) and Neuroform (bottom), note the difference between open and closed cell design.

In 2006, Juszkat presented initial results of using Leo in coil embolization of 24 aneurysms. The rate of complete aneurysm occlusion was 17 cases (71%) and satisfactory occlusion - 21 cases (81%), complications occurred in 3 patients (12%), one of whom died (4%) [80, 81].

Standard intracranial stents have diameters of 4 to 6 mm and are delivered through rather rigid microcatheters, which limits the use of such stents in aneurysms of small distal cerebral arteries. In 2012, Balt extrusion offered the first low-profile braided intracranial stent - Leo baby, and two years later a similar device - LVIS junior - was introduced by Microvention (Figure 25). In 2019, Neuroform Atlas (Stryker, formerly Boston Scientific, USA) became the first cut-out low-profile intracranial stent [82].

Low-profile stents have a deployed diameter of 2 to 4 mm and are more flexible than standard models. They are delivered through thinner 1.7 French diameter microcatheters - the same ones used to deliver detachable coils. Low-profile devices have significantly expanded the technical capabilities of stent support in small-diameter arteries.

According to the meta-analysis of 4 studies published by Park in 2017 (a total of 217 observations), coil embolization assisted by low-profile intracranial stents achieved satisfactory occlusion of target aneurysms in 80% of cases, with a neurological complication rate of 12.5% and surgical morbidity observed in 2% of cases [83].

The question of which stent - braided or cut - is better remains open. Braided stents can adapt to different diameters and shapes of the arterial lumen and also have a better hemodynamic effect. Cut stents are less thrombogenic and less prone to deformation, twisting, and incomplete opening, especially in highly tortuous vessels.

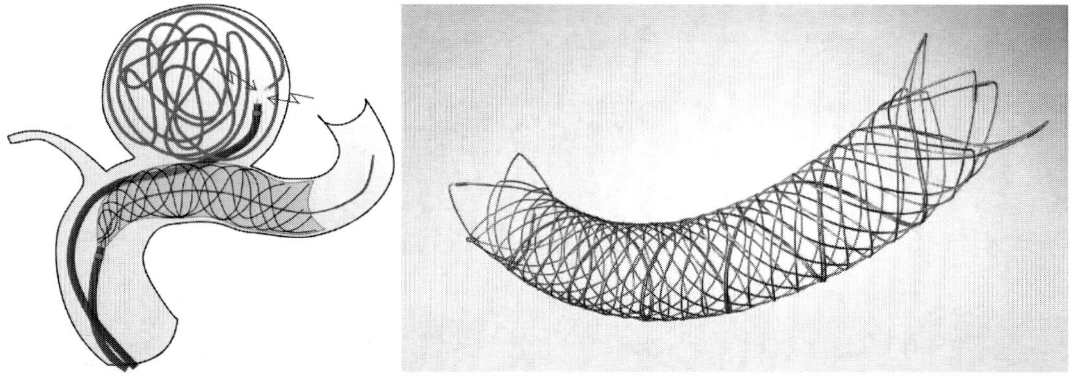

a) b)

Figure 25. a) Stent-assisted coiling technique. b) Modern braided neurovascular stent (LVIS).

In 2020, Mokin reported a multicenter series of 670 observations comparing the results of LVIS braided stents with Enterprise and Neuroform cut stents. The braided stents were characterized by a higher rate of complete target aneurysm occlusion (84% versus 78% and 67%, respectively), while the rate of surgical complications was not significantly different between groups [84].

Stent support significantly increases the radicality of coil embolization. According to meta-analyses by Phan (2016, approximately 33,000 observations) and Nabizadeh (2024, approximately 12,000 observations), the combined rate of complete target aneurysm occlusion without stenting typically did not exceed 60%, compared to 80% with stenting. Stents provide a higher coil packing density within the aneurysm, creating favorable local hemodynamics for stable aneurysm thrombosis and promoting endothelialization of the arterial wall defect. At the same time, the use of stents is associated with a higher rate of surgical complications (10-12% versus 5-6%), which can be a critical drawback in asymptomatic patients with incidental aneurysms. Another disadvantage of stent-assisted coiling is the mandatory prolonged dual antiplatelet therapy (DAPT), which may also have a negative safety effect [85, 86].

A special case for endosaccular coiling are bifurcation aneurysms located at the MCA, BA, and less commonly, ICA. Such aneurysms often have an unfavorable neck configuration; sometimes the neck is absent and the branches of the arterial bifurcation emerge directly from the aneurysm sac. Successful occlusion of these aneurysms requires complex stenting techniques such as the Y stent (first described by Michael Chow, 2004) or the half-T stent (introduced by Young Cho in 2012) [87, 88]. In some cases, the small size of the daughter arteries and the unfavorable bifurcation angle make even these interventions inapplicable.

In the early 2010s, Phenox (Germany) developed the first dedicated device for occluding complex bifurcation aneurysms - the pCONus. The stent was cut from a nickel-titanium alloy, with the distal crown of the stent expanded in a "flower" shape. The stent was placed in the inflow segment of the affected artery with the distal crown inside the aneurysm. The crown held the coil loops in the aneurysm cavity and prevented occlusion of the daughter branches of the arterial bifurcation.

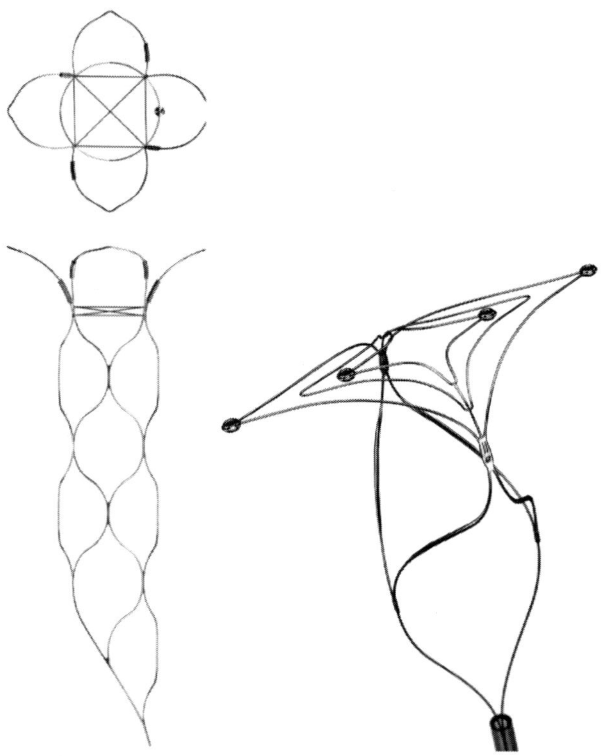

a) b)

Figure 26. Stent-like devices for bifurcation reconstruction. a) pCONus. b) Pulse Rider.

The first clinical experience with the pCONus was reported in 2014 and 2015 by Marta Aguilar-Perez, Francis Turjman and Hans Henkes. They presented the results of embolization of 40 complex bifurcation aneurysms with satisfactory occlusion in 79% of patients, neurological complications in 2 cases (5%) and morbidity in 1 patient (2.5%) [89, 90].

In 2013, Pulsar vascular (later Cerenovus, USA) introduced a second similar device - the Pulse Rider (Figure 26). The first results of bifurcation aneurysm embolization with Pulse Rider were published by Alejandro Spiotta in 2016. Satisfactory aneurysm occlusion was observed in 31 of 34 cases (91%), 1 patient had neurological complications (3%) [91].

Stent-like devices for reconstruction of arterial bifurcations occupy a small but significant niche in the endovascular treatment of cerebral aneurysms and are an important adjunct to stenting.

Flow-Diverters

As early as the mid-1990s, carotid and coronary stents were found to significantly alter hemodynamics in the affected arterial segment and, in some cases, to be capable of inducing aneurysm thrombosis on their own, without the use of detachable coils. The hemodynamic phenomena caused by the presence of a stent in the arterial lumen have been studied in sufficient detail in the experimental work of Ajay Wakhloo, Barukh (Barry) Lieber and M. Aenis and have been collectively termed the "flow-diverting effect" (Figure 27) [92-94].

In the early 2000s, the idea of using this effect to occlude cerebral aneurysms was supported by clinical experience. In a series of observations by Fiorella and Zenteno (2006 and 2008, a total of 30 patients), stenting without detachable coils resulted in partial occlusion of cerebral aneurysms in 70% of cases. The authors used both coronary and neuroendovascular stents and implanted multiple devices (from 2 to 4) in a telescopic fashion to increase the flow-diverting effect [95, 96].

In 2007, Ajay Wakhloo, Barry Lieber and Babu Welch in collaboration with Chestnut medical (later Medtronic, USA) introduced the first device in history designed to occlude cerebral aneurysms based on the flow-diverting effect - the Pipeline Embolization Device (PED). One year later, the second similar device - Silk Flow Diverter (SFD) was offered by Balt Extrusion [97, 98].

Both devices are self-expanding braided stents in the form of a flexible elastic tube consisting of 48 filaments with a cross section of approximately 20 μm, forming a fine mesh (approximately 20-30 cells per 1 mm^2). The mechanism of action of the flow diverter is based on the hydrodynamic properties of such a mesh. The devices are mainly made of shape-memory metals, most commonly cobalt-chromium and nickel-titanium alloys.

The ability to induce aneurysm thrombosis while maintaining patency of the affected artery and its side branches is a fundamental property of flow diversion. The mesh structure of such devices provides minimal resistance to the laminar blood flow present in normal cerebral arteries. The decrease in volumetric blood flow rate in such branches blocked by a flow diverter does not exceed 10-20% and does not lead to their occlusion (Figure 28).

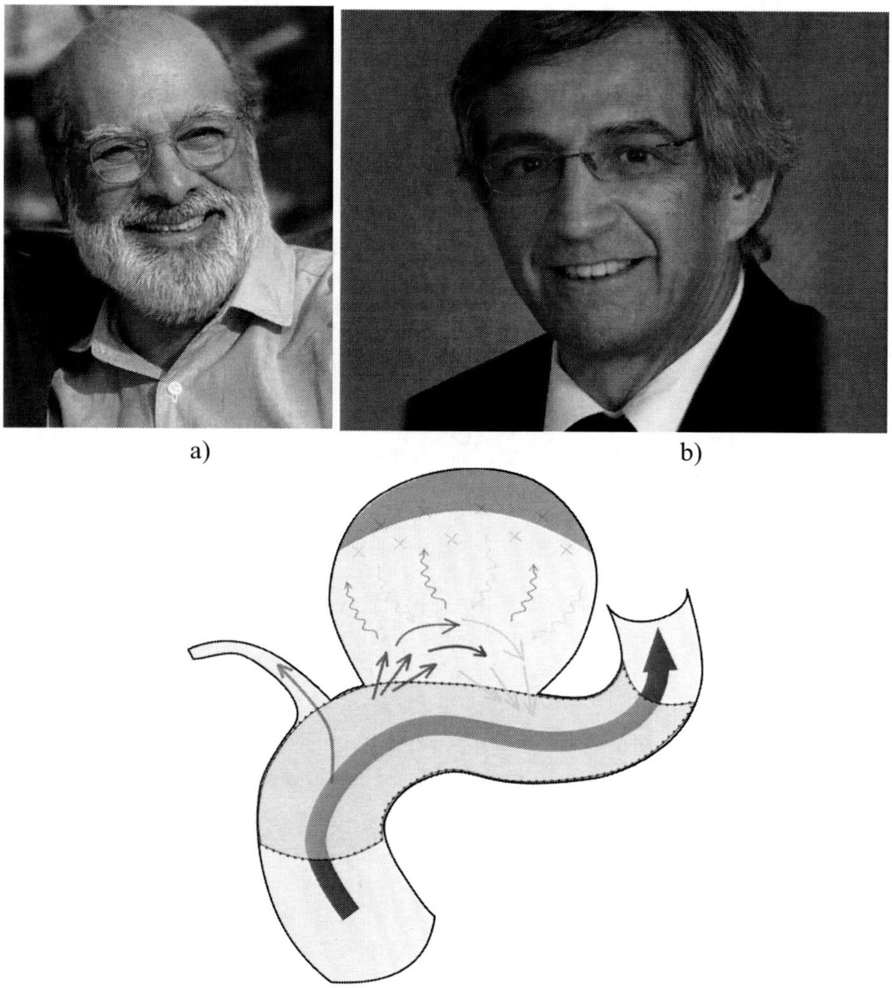

a) b)

c)

Figure 27. a) Ajay Wakhloo. b) Barry Lieber. c) A flow diverter concept.

At the same time, the blood flow in the aneurysm cavity is turbulent and oscillating (constantly changing its intensity and direction), and the blood pressure gradient at the border of the aneurysm and the arterial lumen tends to zero. The flow diverter creates a very high resistance to such a blood flow pattern and reduces the volumetric blood flow velocity in the aneurysm by 50-60%. In this case, the kinetic energy of the flow decreases by 80-90% and the blood dwell time in the aneurysm increases by 2-3 times. These changes represent a special case of "thrombogenic Virchow's triad" and lead to progressive thrombosis of the aneurysm cavity. In addition, flow diverters provide a mechanical scaffold for endothelization and healing of the arterial wall defect, contributing to permanent exclusion of the aneurysm from the circulation [99, 100].

Because flow diverters are implanted within the arterial lumen, there is no need for direct catheterization of the aneurysm cavity and manipulation within it, which reduces technical risks and represents a more physiologic approach to reconstructing the affected artery. A relative disadvantage of the method is the delayed occlusion of the aneurysm (from several days to several months), which can be critical in the case of ruptured aneurysms.

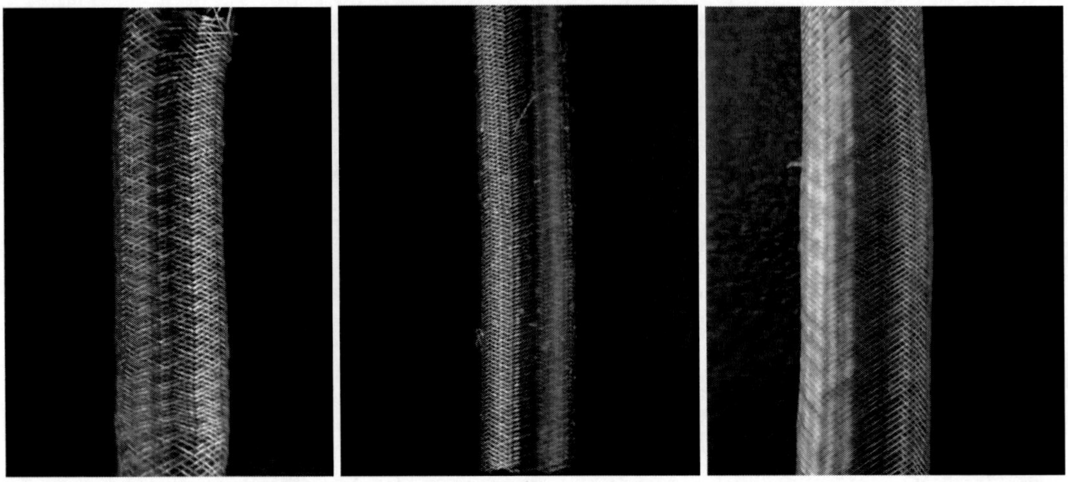

a) b) c)

Figure 28. Modern Flow Diverter Devices.

These devices have evolved in several directions. The flow diversion effect was found to be directly proportional to the area of the vessel wall covered by the stent threads (metal coverage area ratio, MCR) and the number of cells per unit area of the device. To improve these parameters, later models of flow-direction devices incorporated a greater number of threads. For example, the p64 flow diverter from Phenox (Germany), first introduced in 2012, consisted of 64 threads. Stryker's Surpass, developed in 2013, had 72 or 96 threads depending on the diameter [101, 102].

A known limitation of flow diverters is their high thrombogenicity, due to their hemodynamic effects and the large amount of metal in the arterial lumen. The use of these devices necessarily requires prolonged DAPT. To overcome this problem, flow-directed stents with biologically active coatings have been developed.

The first such device was the Pipeline Shield (Medtronic, USA), which entered clinical practice in 2015. It had a coating of phosphatidylcholine covalently bonded to the surface of the device's threads. Later, other coated devices appeared, such as p64-HPC (polyglycan coating, 2020, Phenox) and Fred-X (polymethoxyethyl acrylate coating, 2022, Microvention). Currently, most flow diverters have some type of biologically active coating, although the clinical efficacy of these coatings has not been convincingly demonstrated and DAPT has not been withdrawn [103, 104].

Cobalt-chromium and nickel-titanium alloys have low radiopacity, so early flow-directed stents were characterized by poor visualization. To improve radiopacity, single platinum filaments and small platinum, tungsten, or tantalum markers were used.

Around 2016, Acandis (Germany) introduced Derivo2, the first flow diverter made of bimetallic threads using DFT (drawn-filled tubing) technology. Each thread has a platinum core in a nickel-titanium alloy sheath, giving it high radiopacity while maintaining shape memory properties. Since the early 2020s, most flow diverters have been made from bimetallic DFT threads [105].

Classic models of flow diverter stents have a working diameter of 4 to 5.5 mm and are delivered through thick and rather rigid 2.7 French diameter microcatheters, which limits the possibilities of these devices in the treatment of distal cerebral aneurysms.

In 2012, the first low-profile flow diverter, FRED junior, was introduced. This device was delivered via reinforced 2.1 French caliber microcatheters and was available in diameters starting at 3.5 mm. Later, almost all manufacturers began to offer their own versions of low-profile flow diverters. The smallest low-profile flow diverter to date is the Silk Vista Baby (Balt extrusion), which was introduced into clinical practice in 2022. It is available in sizes from 2.5 mm and is implanted via 1.7 French microcatheters, which are also used to deliver detachable coils [106, 107].

Initially, flow-directed stents were used in large and giant aneurysms, as well as aneurysms that were difficult to treat with other methods (e.g., fusiform and bubble aneurysms). According to the early prospective studies PITA, PUFS and ASPIRe (approximately 350 observations in total), flow-directed stents showed results in the treatment of such "complex" aneurysms that were significantly superior to other treatment methods. Complete aneurysm occlusion was achieved in 70-80% of cases, with rates of neurological complications, morbidity and mortality of 10%, 3-7% and 2-3%, respectively [98, 108, 109].

Naturally, such results have fueled the desire to expand the indications for flow diverters to simpler and more common types of cerebral aneurysms. According to several comparative studies (Chalouhi, 2014 and 2017, DiMaria, 2015, Durst, 2016, Salem 2020), the radicality of aneurysm occlusion with flow diverters is approximately equal to the radicality of stent-assisted coil embolization (70-80% complete occlusion rate) and significantly exceeds the radicality of coil embolization without stent-assistance (50-60% complete occlusion rate) [110-115].

According to the most recent meta-analyses by Fiorella (2020, approximately 2300 observations) and Shehata (2022, approximately 1100 observations), the rate of complete occlusion of cerebral aneurysms using flow-directed stents exceeds 90% at 5 years after surgery, while neurological complications occur in approximately 10% of cases, and the rates of surgical morbidity and mortality do not exceed 5% and 1%, respectively [116, 117].

One of the technical limitations of flow-directed stents is their relatively low efficacy in aneurysms with bifurcation hemodynamics: the frequency of complete occlusion of such aneurysms typically does not exceed 50%. In 2011, a group of engineers from the American company Sequent Medical (later Microvention, USA) developed the WEB ("Woven EndoBridge") specifically for the embolization of complex bifurcation aneurysms, which implemented the principles of the flow-diverting technique more successfully for this category of patients (Figure 29).

WEB consisted of two layers of fine metallic mesh woven from nickel-titanium filaments with a structure similar to the mesh of flow-directed stents. The device had a spherical or cylindrical shape ranging in size from 4 to 12 mm and was intended for direct implantation into the aneurysm cavity. Proprietary Via microcatheters were used for delivery, with calibers ranging from 2.1 to 3.3 French (most commonly 2.4 or 2.7 French), depending on the size of the device. The WEB was self-expanding. Due to its compliance, the device assumed the shape of the aneurysm sac as it was pushed out of the microcatheter. Its mechanism of action was the same as that of flow-directed stents, but because it was implanted in the aneurysm lumen rather than the aneurysm sac, prolonged DAPT was not required.

In 2014, Danial Behme reported the first clinical experience with WEB. In a series of 55 patients, complete aneurysm occlusion was observed in 37 cases (67%) 3 months after surgery, neurological complications occurred in 7 patients (12%), and there was no morbidity or mortality [118].

In 2016, Muskens published a meta-analysis of WEB results in complex bifurcation aneurysms (total of 718 observations). The frequency of complete aneurysm occlusion reached 85%, and neurological complications were observed in 10% of cases [119].

In the following years, other similar devices were introduced, such as pCANvas (Phenox, Germany) and Artisse (Medtronic, USA). This specific category of endovascular devices is referred to in the literature as intra-aneurysmal flow disrupters (IFDs). Together with stent-like devices for the reconstruction of arterial bifurcations, IFDs are finding very successful, albeit niche, applications [120].

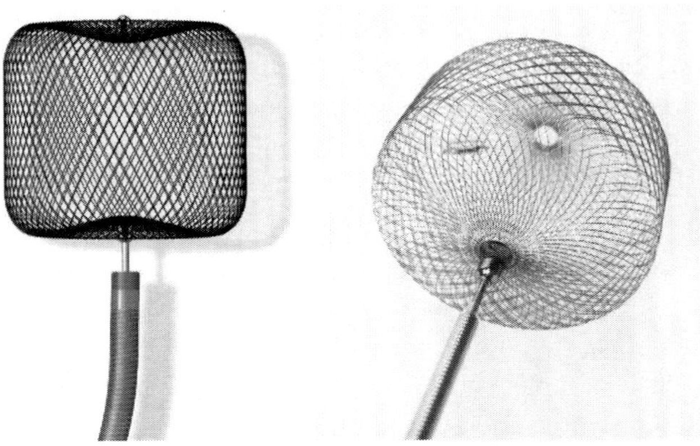

a) b)

Figure 29. Modern intrasaccular flow disruptors - a) WEB, b) Artisse.

Embolization with detachable coils, especially balloon and stent support, flow diverters, as well as intra-aneurysmal flow disrupters and stent-like devices for reconstruction of arterial bifurcations, offer the widest range of minimally invasive treatment options for cerebral aneurysms. Currently, the rate of endovascular treatment of cerebral aneurysms reaches 80-90% in developed countries. At the same time, the current stage of endovascular neurosurgery is characterized by significant progress in the treatment of other, rarer cerebrovascular diseases [121, 122].

As mentioned above, since the second half of the 1970s, the main method of endovascular treatment of cerebral AVMs and dAVFs has been embolization with cyanoacrylate glue using calibrated leaky balloons. In the second half of the 1980s, balloons were replaced by over-the-wire microcatheters as a means of delivering liquid embolic materials.

As early as 1989, Masaki Komiyama described several cases of cerebral AVM embolization using cyanoacrylate (Histoacryl) through Tracker-18 microcatheters. In this publication, he also mentioned multi-stage AVM embolization with an interval of 3-6 months, which is still the standard approach today [123].

Intranidal catheterization of AVMs and dAVFs was not always possible with both the old balloons and the new microcatheters due to the anatomical characteristics of the feeding arteries. In these cases, free emboli made of solid materials, such as plastic beads known since the 1960s, could be useful. Unfortunately, such emboli did not fit into the microcatheter.

Also in 1989, Aldo Benati proposed the use of 3-0 surgical polypropylene sutures as free emboli, which passed freely through the microcatheters available at that time. He reported the results of embolization in 11 patients using this method. In 9 of them, occlusion of more than 50% of the malformation node was achieved [124].

In 1996, Alejandro Berenstein improved on Benati's concept by using platinum coils of his own design as free emboli. Unlike the Guglielmi coils, the Berenstein coils were much softer and smaller, had no delivery system, were delivered through a microcatheter with a stream of liquid, and could move freely with the blood flow. Later, Boston Scientific began manufacturing these devices under the brand name "Berenstein Liquid Coils" and they are still in limited use today [125].

Non-Adhesive Liquid Embolics

The growing popularity of liquid embolic agents with non-adhesive properties has had the most significant impact on the embolization technique for cerebral AVMs and dAVFs.

The pattern of distribution of non-adhesive materials in the lumen of blood vessels differs significantly from that of adhesive substances ("glues"). Unlike glues, which are present in solution as monomers and polymerize upon contact with blood, nonadhesive compounds are polymerized in solution and precipitate (deposit) upon entry into the vasculature. Compared to polymerization, precipitation is a slower and more gradual process, which makes embolization more controllable and allows these substances to spread a long distance from the injection site, especially against the flow of blood. In addition, these substances do not adhere to the vessel wall, which facilitates their penetration into small, branched vessels, but may cause migration and non-target embolization, especially in high-flow arteriovenous shunts.

In 1990, Waro Taki first used Eval, a drug he developed, to embolize cerebral AVMs. It was a 5% solution of ethylene-vinyl alcohol copolymer (EVOH) in dimethylsulfoxide (DMSO) with the addition of metrizamide (a water-soluble contrast agent). Eval was the first modern non-adhesive liquid embolic material and had limited use until the 2000s [126].

By 2004, ev3 (now Medtronic) had developed a new non-adhesive embolic material, Onyx. It is a solution of polyvinyl alcohol copolymer (PVOH) in DMSO to which tantalum powder is added for radiopaque properties. This embolic material is available in different concentrations (Onyx-12-4% PVOH, Onyx-18-6% PVOH, Onyx-34-8% PVOH), which have different precipitation rates in the vascular bed. Due to its favorable properties, it has rapidly gained popularity in the embolization of AVMs, dAVFs, and vascular tumors [127].

In 2023, V. Letchuman published a meta-analysis of the use of Onyx in 1133 patients with cerebral AVMs. According to his data, Onyx embolization resulted in complete AVM occlusion in 47% of patients without other treatment. Various neurological complications were observed in 23% of patients, and the operative mortality was 1.5% [128].

According to CONDOR, a large multi-center prospective study published in 2021, complete occlusion of the anastomosis was achieved in 83% of 911 patients with cerebral dAVFs who underwent embolization with Onyx, and the operative mortality rate was 2% [129].

In 2014, Microvention introduced another liquid embolic material with non-adhesive properties - PHIL (Precipitating Hydrophobic Injectable Liquid). It is a solution of polyglycolide-co-lactide (PGLA) and polyhydroxyethyl methacrylate (PHEMA) copolymer in DMSO and is also available in different concentrations with different precipitation rates (PHIL-15, PHIL-25, PHIL-35). Instead of tantalum powder, iodine compounds covalently bonded to the drug molecules are used for radiopacity. Compared to Onyx, Phil has a significantly lower radiopacity and does not interfere with the visualization of the remaining part of the arteriovenous shunt during multistage embolization [130]. The distribution pattern of this substance in the vascular bed is also different and is preferred by multiple users (Figure 30).

The first relatively extensive clinical experience with PHIL was presented by Stanimir Sirakov in 2018. He performed embolization of cerebral AVMs in 27 patients, with complete occlusion achieved in 14 cases (52%), the incidence of neurological complications was 6 observations (22%), and there were no fatal outcomes [131].

In 2017, Salem Lamin published the results of the occlusion of 26 dAVFs with PHIL. The frequency of complete occlusion of the anastomoses was 23 cases (88%), with one patient experiencing disability (4%) [132].

Technically, Onyx and PHIL are complementary. They are both DMSO soluble and can be combined in the same procedure, even in the same injection [133].

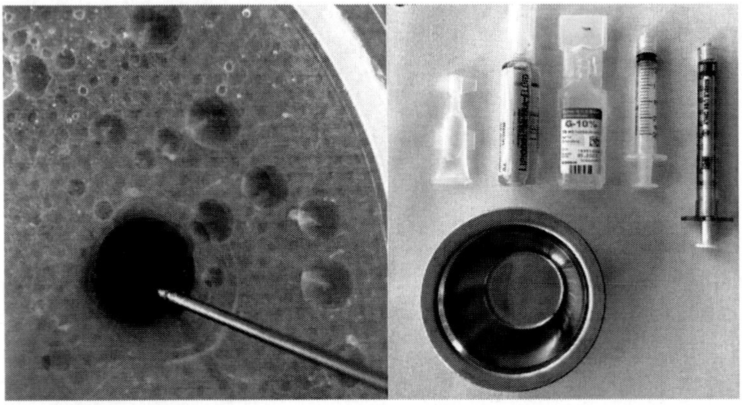

a)

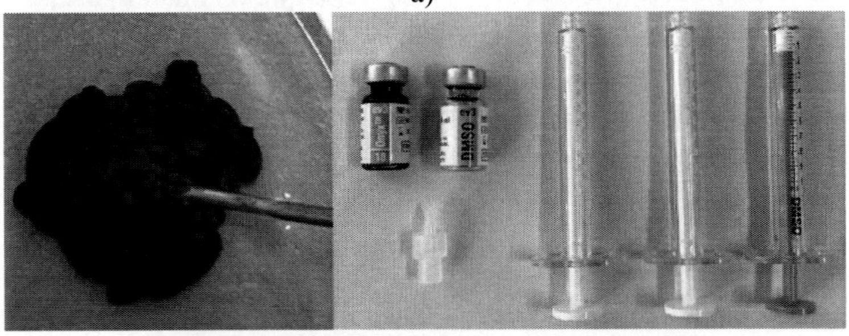

b)

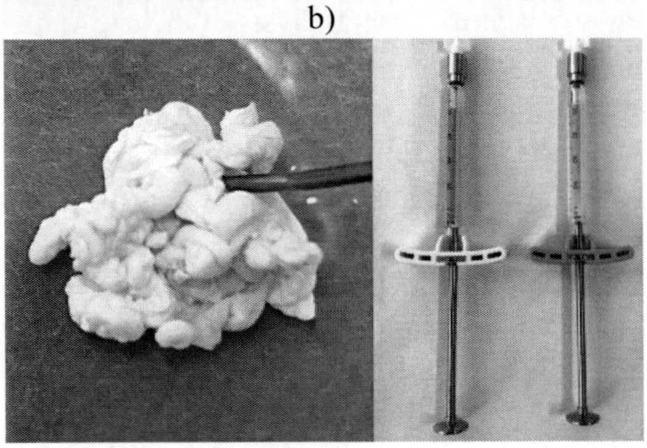

c)

Figure 30. Modern liquid embolic agents and their behavior in water. a) n-BCA b) Onyx c) PHIL.

From the late 1980s to the late 2000s, the main instruments used to deliver liquid embolic agents were the same microcatheters used for coil embolization (Tracker, Magic, etc.) A major drawback of these devices was that they often became lodged in the cerebral arteries during embolization and could not be safely removed, which was a serious technical complication.

In 2006, Balt Extrusion introduced Sonic - the first microcatheter with a detachable tip specifically designed for the delivery of non-adhesive embolic materials. The microcatheter tip was connected to the proximal part of the device by a piece of a special polymer that, when exposed to DMSO, lost its strength and was easily torn off [134].

In 2013, ev3 (Medtronic) introduced a similar microcatheter - Apollo. This device had a tip glued to the proximal part of the microcatheter inside a small polymer sleeve. The release mechanism of the Apollo microcatheter did not require DMSO exposure, making it more suitable for use with adhesive embolization agents (glues) [135].

Detachable-tip microcatheters allow the injection of liquid embolic materials without the risk of microcatheter adhesion for an indefinite period of time, as long as the reflux of embolic material into the afferent does not exceed the length of the detachable tip of the device.

Other methods of delivering liquid embolic materials for cerebral AVMs and dAVFs have also been described. For example, in 2014, Alejandro Spiotta cited a series of 24 patients in whom the aforementioned Scepter dual-lumen balloon (Microvention) was used to deliver Onyx. In this method of embolization, a non-adherent material is delivered through the instrument lumen of the balloon while the afferent is occluded by the same balloon [136]. This technique allows the substance to be injected under high pressure without significant reflux. The method is highly radical, but quite aggressive and should be used with caution.

Non-adhesive liquid embolic agents in combination with modern detachable-tip microcatheters have changed the approach to the treatment of cerebral AVMs and dAVFs. Previously, embolization was considered mainly as an adjunct to microsurgery or as a palliative measure in unresectable cases; now it is the first-line treatment in a multimodal approach to these diseases. Moreover, in almost half of the cases, embolization achieves radical results without other treatment modalities.

References

[1] Tan TC, Black PMcL. Sir Victor Horsley (1857–1916): pioneer of neurological surgery. *Neurosurgery*. 2002;50 (3):607–612.

[2] Dawbarn J. The starvation plan for malignancy in the external carotid area: its failures and success. *JAMA*. 1904;42:792–794.

[3] Hamby WB. Treatment of pulsating exophthalmus with report of two cases. *Arch Surg*. 1933;27:676–685.

[4] Vitek JJ, Smith MJ. The myth of the Brooks method of embolization: a brief history of the endovascular treatment of carotid–cavernous sinus fistula. *J Neurointerv Surg*. 2009;1 (2):108–111.

[5] Arutiunov AI, et al. Surgical treatment of carotid-cavernous fistulas. *Prog Brain Res*. 1969;30:441–444.

[6] Moniz E. L'encéphalographie artérielle, son importance dans la localisation des tumeurs cérébrales. R*ev Neurol* (Paris). 1927;2:72–90.

[7] Moniz E. Cerebral angiography and its application in clinical practice and physiology. *Lancet*. 1933;222 (5751):1144–1147.

[8] Forssmann-Falck R. Werner Forssmann: a pioneer of cardiology. A*m J Cardiol*. 1997;79 (5):651–660.

[9] Seldinger SI. Catheter replacement of the needle in percutaneous arteriography. *Acta Radiol.* 2008;49 (Suppl 434):47–52.

[10] Dotter CT. Catheter access and visualization of the cardiovascular system. In: Viamonte M, ed. *Progress in Angiography*. Springfield: Charles C Thomas; 1964.

[11] Cowley MJ. Tribute to a legend in invasive/interventional cardiology Melvin P Judkins (1922–85). *Catheter Cardiovasc Interv*. 2005;64 (2):259–261.

[12] Werner SB, et al. Aneurysm of the internal carotid artery within the skull: wiring and electrothermic coagulation. *JAMA*. 1941;578–582.

[13] Mullan S, et al. Electrically induced thrombosis in intracranial aneurysms. *J Neurosurg*. 1964;21:539–547.

[14] Gallagher JP. Pilojection for intracranial aneurysms. *J Neurosurg*. 1963;29:129–134.

[15] Samotokin BA, Khilko VA. *Anevrizmy i arteriovenoznyye soustya golovnogo mozga*. Leningrad: Meditsina; 1973:170–185.

[16] Alksne J. Stereotactic thrombosis of intracranial aneurysms. *N Engl J Med*. 1971;284 (4):171–174.

[17] Luessenhop AJ, Velasquez AC. Observations on the tolerance of the intracranial arteries to catheterization. *J Neurosurg*. 1964;21 (2):85–91.

[18] Maiti TK, et al. Alfred J Luessenhop and the dawn of a new superspecialty: endovascular neurosurgery. *J Neurointerv Surg*. 2016;8 (2):216–220.

[19] Luessenhop AJ, Presper JH. Surgical embolization of cerebral arteriovenous malformations through internal carotid and vertebral arteries. *J Neurosurg*. 1975;42 (4):443–451.

[20] Khilko VA, Zubkov YN. *Vnutrisosudistaya neirokhirurgiya*. Moscow: Meditsina; 1982:35–58.

[21] Frei EH, et al. The POD and its applications. *Med Res Eng*. 1966;5 (4):11–18.

[22] Penn RD, et al. Intravascular intracranial EEG recording. *J Neurosurg*. 1973;38 (2):239–243.

[23] Cares HL, et al. Laboratory experience with a magnetically guided intravascular catheter system. *J Neurosurg*. 1973;38 (2):145–154.

[24] Hilai SK, et al. Magnetically guided devices for vascular exploration and treatment. *Radiology*. 1974;113 (3):529–540.

[25] Singh D, Madavan P, Aryala S. The invention of Fogarty embolectomy balloon catheter: a paradigm shift toward minimally invasive vascular surgery. *Indian J Vasc Endovasc Surg*. 2024;11 (1):57–59.

[26] Payne MM. Charles Theodore Dotter: the father of intervention. *Tex Heart Inst J*. 2001;28 (1):28–38.

[27] Rothenberg SF, et al. Angiotactic surgery. J Neurosurg. 1962;19 (10):877–883.

[28] Teitelbaum GP, et al. A tribute to Dr Fedor A Serbinenko, founder of endovascular neurosurgery. *Neurosurgery*. 2000;46 (2):462–469.

[29] Serbinenko FA. Balloon catheterization and occlusion of major cerebral vessels. *J Neurosurg*. 1974;41 (2):125–145.

[30] Madapoosi A, et al. Part 1: pushing the boundaries of neurointerventional surgery—a historical review of the work of Dr Gerard Debrun. *Interv Neuroradiol*. 2024;30 (6):854–861.

[31] Romodanov AP, et al. *Atlas operatsiy na golovnom mozge*. Moscow: Meditsina; 1986:303–315.

[32] Guglielmi G. History of endovascular endosaccular occlusion of brain aneurysms: 1965–1990. *Interv Neuroradiol*. 2007;13 (3):217–224.

[33] Madapoosi A, et al. Part 2: the development and advancement of the detachable balloon catheter. *Interv Neuroradiol*. 2024;30 (6):862–869.

[34] Debrun G, et al. Detachable balloon and calibrated-leak balloon techniques in cerebral vascular lesions. *J Neurosurg*. 1978;49 (5):635–649.

[35] Zubkov YN. Method for treating cerebral arterial aneurysm: *Patent* 812264 USSR. 1976.

[36] Zubkov YN, Nikiforov BM, Shustin VA. Balloon catheter technique for dilatation of constricted cerebral arteries after aneurysmal SAH. *Acta Neurochir* (Wien). 1984;70 (1-2):65–79.

[37] Pevsner PH. Micro-balloon catheter for superselective angiography and therapeutic occlusion. AJR *Am J Roentgenol*. 1977;128 (2):225–230.

[38] DiTullio MV, Rand RW, Frisch E. Detachable balloon catheter. *J Neurosurg*. 1978;48 (5):717–723.

[39] Berenstein A, Song JK, Niimi Y. Personal accounts of the evolution of endovascular neurosurgery. *Neurosurgery*. 2006;59 (Suppl 5):S3-15–S3-21.

[40] Plowiecki L. *Art et savoir-faire en neuroradiologie interventionnelle—mémoire d'un industriel.* Warsaw: Bellona; 2009.

[41] Taki W, et al. The releasable balloon technique with activated high-frequency electrical current. *Surg Neurol.* 1980;13 (6):405–408.

[42] Lauzier DC, et al. A review of technological innovations leading to modern endovascular brain aneurysm treatment. *Front Neurol.* 2023;14:1156887.

[43] Moonsein LH. Detachable balloons. *Endovask Neuroradiol.* 2013;4 (6):1–5.

[44] Debrun GM, et al. Indications for treatment and classification of 132 carotid-cavernous fistulas. *Neurosurgery.* 1988;22 (2):285–289.

[45] Fox AJ, et al. Use of detachable balloons for proximal artery occlusion in unclippable cerebral aneurysms. *J Neurosurg.* 1987;66 (1):40–46.

[46] Higashida RT, et al. Treatment of intracranial aneurysms with preservation of the parent vessel. *AJNR Am J Neuroradiol.* 1990;11 (4):633–640.

[47] Shcheglov VI. Endosaccular detachable balloon catheter treatment of cerebral saccular aneurysms. In: Holtzman RNN, ed. *Endovascular Interventional Neuroradiology.* New York: Springer-Verlag; 1995:298–300.

[48] Djindjian R. Treatment of spinal angiomas by embolization. In: *Spinal Angiomas.* Berlin: Springer; 1978:189–200.

[49] Zanetti PH, Sherman FE. Experimental evaluation of a tissue adhesive for aneurysms and arteriovenous anomalies. *J Neurosurg.* 1972;36 (1):72–79.

[50] Kerber C, Bank W, Cromwell L. Calibrated-leak balloon microcatheter for arterial exploration. AJR *Am J Roentgenol.* 1979;132 (2):207–212.

[51] Kerber C. Balloon catheter with a calibrated leak. *Radiology.* 1976;120 (3):547–550.

[52] Kerber C. Intracranial cyanoacrylate: new catheter therapy for arteriovenous malformation. *Invest Radiol.* 1975;10 (5):536–538.

[53] Debrun G, et al. Embolization of cerebral arteriovenous malformations with bucrylate. J Neurosurg. 1982;56 (5):615–627.

[54] Djindjian R, et al. Superselective arteriographic embolization by the femoral route in neuroradiology. *Neuroradiology.* 1973;6 (3):143–153.

[55] Djindjian R, et al. Superselective arteriographic embolization by the femoral route in neuroradiology. *Neuroradiology.* 1973;6 (3):132–142.

[56] Tadavarthi SM, Moller JH, Amplatz K. Polyvinyl alcohol (Ivalon)—a new embolic material. *AJR Am J Roentgenol.* 1975;125 (3):609–616.

[57] Tissen TP. Clinical signs, diagnostics and endovascular treatment of dural arteriovenous fistulas of spinal cord. *Russ J Neurosurg.* 2016;2:9–15.

[58] Tissen TP, et al. Endovascular surgery of spinal dural arteriovenous fistulas. *Vopr Neirokhir.* 2018;82 (4):15.

[59] Tissen TP. *Endovaskulyarnoye lecheniye arteriovenoznykh malformatsiy spinnogo mozga.* Moscow: Meditsina; 2006.

[60] Engelson ET. Catheter for guide-wire tracking: *US Patent* 4739768. 1988.

[61] Gianturco C, Anderson JH, Wallace S. Mechanical devices for arterial occlusion. *AJR Am J Roentgenol.* 1975;124 (3):428–435.

[62] Braun IF, et al. Use of coils for transcatheter carotid occlusion. *AJNR Am J Neuroradiol.* 1985;6 (6):953–956.

[63] Yang PJ, et al. Platinum wire: a new transvascular embolic agent. *AJNR Am J Neuroradiol.* 1988;9 (3):547–550.

[64] Guglielmi G, et al. Electrothrombosis of saccular aneurysms via endovascular approach. *J Neurosurg.* 1991;75 (1):1–7.

[65] Guglielmi G, et al. Electrothrombosis of saccular aneurysms via endovascular approach. *J Neurosurg.* 1991;75 (1):8–14.

[66] Viñuela F, et al. Guglielmi detachable coil embolization of acute intracranial aneurysms. *J Neurosurg.* 1997;86 (3):475–482.

[67] Molyneux AJ. International Subarachnoid Aneurysm Trial (ISAT). *Lancet*. 2002;360 (9342):1267–1274.
[68] Richling B. History of endovascular surgery: personal accounts. *Neurosurgery*. 2006;59 (Suppl 5):S3-30–S3-38.
[69] Prestigiacomo CJ. Surgical endovascular neuroradiology in the 21st century. *Neurosurgery*. 2006;59 (Suppl 5):S3-48–S3-55.
[70] Prestigiacomo CJ. Historical perspectives. *Neurosurgery*. 2006;59 (Suppl 5):S3-39–S3-47.
[71] Hui FK, et al. A history of detachable coils: 1987–2012. *J Neurointerv Surg*. 2014;6 (2):134–138.
[72] Moret J, et al. The "Remodelling Technique" in wide-neck intracranial aneurysms. *Interv Neuroradiol*. 1997;3 (1):21–35.
[73] Plowiecki L. From the detachable balloon to the endothelial prosthesis. *Interv Neuroradiol*. 2009;15:470–474.
[74] Spelle L, et al. Remodeling technique: indications and limits. *Interv Neuroradiol*. 2008;14 (Suppl 1):52–59.
[75] Hedin M. The origin of the word "stent." *Acta Radiol*. 1997;38 (6):937–939.
[76] Higashida RT, et al. Intravascular stent and endovascular coil placement for ruptured fusiform basilar aneurysm. *J Neurosurg*. 1997;87 (6):944–949.
[77] Lylyk P, et al. Combined stent-coil treatment of dissecting vertebral aneurysms. *J Neurosurg*. 2001;94 (3):427–432.
[78] Fiorella D, et al. Preliminary experience with the Neuroform stent. *Neurosurgery*. 2004;54 (1):6–17.
[79] Henkes H, et al. Endovascular coil occlusion with Neuroform stent assistance. *Interv Neuroradiol*. 2002;8 (2):107–119.
[80] Juszkat R, et al. Leo stent for wide-neck and fusiform aneurysms. *Interv Neuroradiol*. 2007;13 (3):255–269.
[81] Higashida RT, et al. Initial experience with the Cordis Enterprise stent. *AJNR Am J Neuroradiol*. 2005;26 (7):1751–1756.
[82] Negrotto M, et al. Assisted coiling using LEO Baby or LVIS Jr stents. *Interv Neuroradiol*. 2015;21 (5):566–574.
[83] Park SY, et al. Safety and efficacy of low-profile self-expandable stents. *Interv Neurol*. 2017;6 (3-4):170–182.
[84] Mokin M, et al. Stent-assisted coiling: multi-center analysis. *J Neurointerv Surg*. 2020;12 (3):289–297.
[85] Phan K, et al. Meta-analysis of stent-assisted coiling vs coiling-only. *J Clin Neurosci*. 2016;31:15–22.
[86] Nabizadeh F, et al. Stent-assisted vs non-stent-assisted coiling: meta-analysis. World Neurosurg X. 2024;21:100243.
[87] Chow MM, et al. Y-configuration double-stent technique for basilar apex aneurysm. *AJNR Am J Neuroradiol*. 2004;25 (3):509–512.
[88] Cho KC, et al. Prediction of thin-walled areas in unruptured cerebral aneurysms. *Biomed Res Int*. 2018;2018:1–9.
[89] Pérez MA, et al. Use of the pCONus for acutely ruptured aneurysms. *J Neurointerv Surg*. 2017;9 (1):39–44.
[90] Aguilar-Perez M, et al. Coil occlusion assisted by pCONus. *AJNR Am J Neuroradiol*. 2014;35 (5):965–971.
[91] Spiotta AM, et al. Initial experience with the PulseRider for bifurcation aneurysms. *J Neurointerv Surg*. 2016;8 (2):186–189.
[92] Aenis M, et al. Modeling flow changes by stenting in aneurysms. *J Biomech Eng*. 1997;119 (2):206–212.
[93] Lieber BB, et al. Alteration of hemodynamics by stenting. *Ann Biomed Eng*. 1997;25 (3):460–469.
[94] Wakhloo AK, et al. Self-expanding nitinol stents in canine vertebral arteries. *AJNR Am J Neuroradiol*. 1995;16 (5):1043–1051.
[95] Fiorella D, et al. Endovascular reconstruction with Neuroform stent. *Neurosurgery*. 2006;59 (2):291–300.
[96] Zenteno MA, et al. Sole stenting for posterior-circulation aneurysms. *J Neurosurg*. 2008;108 (6):1104–1118.

[97] Byrne JV, et al. Early experience with endovascular flow diversion: multicentre prospective study. *PLoS One*. 2010;5 (9):e12492.

[98] Nelson PK, et al. Pipeline Embolization Device trial. *AJNR Am J Neuroradiol*. 2011;32 (1):34–40.

[99] Dholakia R, et al. Hemodynamics of flow diverters. *J Biomech Eng*. 2017;139 (2):024501.

[100] Ravindran K, et al. Mechanism of action of flow diverters. *Neurosurgery*. 2020;86 (Suppl 1):S13–S19.

[101] Fischer S, et al. Initial experience with p64 flow diverter. *AJNR Am J Neuroradiol*. 2015;36 (11):2082–2089.

[102] Wakhloo AK, et al. Surpass flow diverter multicentre study. *AJNR Am J Neuroradiol*. 2015;36 (1):98–107.

[103] Lenz-Habijan T, et al. Thrombogenicity of bare vs coated flow diverters. *Cardiovasc Intervent Radiol*. 2020;43 (1):140–146.

[104] Girdhar G, et al. Thrombogenicity assessment of Pipeline, Shield, Derivo and P64. *eNeurologicalSci*. 2019;14:77–84.

[105] Ley D, et al. Derivo Embolization Device in elastase-induced aneurysm model. *Clin Neuroradiol*. 2017;27 (3):335–343.

[106] El Naamani K, et al. FRED Jr flow-diverting stent: case series and meta-analysis. *Clin Neurol Neurosurg*. 2022;223:107483.

[107] Gavrilovic V, et al. Silk Vista Baby flow-diverting stent. *Front Neurol*. 2021;12:688702.

[108] Becske T, et al. Pipeline for uncoilable or failed aneurysms: multicentre trial. *Radiology*. 2013;267 (3):858–868.

[109] Kallmes DF, et al. International Pipeline registry study. *AJNR Am J Neuroradiol*. 2015;36 (1):108–115.

[110] Di Maria F, et al. Flow diversion vs standard techniques for unruptured carotid-ophthalmic aneurysms. *AJNR Am J Neuroradiol*. 2015;36 (12):2325–2330.

[111] Chalouhi N, et al. Extending flow diversion to small unruptured anterior-circulation aneurysms. *Stroke*. 2014;45 (1):54–58.

[112] Chalouhi N, et al. Flow diversion vs coiling in large unruptured saccular aneurysms. *Stroke*. 2013;44 (8):2150–2154.

[113] Chalouhi N, et al. Matched comparison of flow diversion and coiling in small noncomplex aneurysms. *Neurosurgery*. 2017;81 (1):92–97.

[114] Durst CR, et al. Ophthalmic artery patency after flow diversion vs coil embolization. *J Neurointerv Surg*. 2016;8 (9):919–922.

[115] Salem MM, et al. Pipeline vs stent-assisted coiling: propensity-matched study. *Neurosurgery*. 2020;87 (3):516–522.

[116] Fiorella D, et al. Meta-analysis of flow diverters for small/medium ICA aneurysms. *J Neurointerv Surg*. 2020;12 (9):869–873.

[117] Shehata MA, et al. Long-term outcomes of flow diversion for unruptured aneurysms: meta-analysis. *J Neurointerv Surg*. 2023;15 (9):898–902.

[118] Behme D, et al. Woven EndoBridge for wide-neck cerebral aneurysms. *AJNR Am J Neuroradiol*. 2015;36 (8):1501–1506.

[119] Muskens IS, et al. Woven EndoBridge systematic review. *World Neurosurg*. 2017;98:809–817.e1.

[120] DeMessie B, et al. Review of endosaccular flow disrupters. *Cardiol Rev*. 2025;in press.

[121] Belavadi R, et al. Surgical clipping vs endovascular coiling for intracranial aneurysms. *Cureus*. 2021;13 (4):e14521.

[122] Hoh BL, et al. Length of stay and charges: clipping vs coiling. *Stroke*. 2010;41 (2):337–342.

[123] Komiyama M, et al. A new microcatheter for endovascular cerebral AVM treatment. *Surg Neurol*. 1989;32 (2):91–97.

[124] Benati A, et al. Endovascular treatment of intracranial AVMs with mobile-wing microcatheter. *J Neuroradiol*. 1987;14 (2):99–113.

[125] Ha-Kawa SK, et al. Berenstein Liquid Coil for transcatheter embolotherapy. *Cardiovasc Intervent Radiol*. 1998;21 (4):297–299.

[126] Nishi S, et al. Embolization of cerebral aneurysms with EVAL mixture. *Acta Neurochir* (Wien). 1996;138 (3):294–300.

[127] Katsaridis V, et al. Curative embolization of cerebral AVMs with Onyx in 101 patients. *Neuroradiology*. 2008;50 (7):589–597.

[128] Letchuman V, et al. Onyx embolization before radiosurgery for cerebral AVMs: systematic review. *World Neurosurg*. 2023;170:90–98.

[129] Li Y, et al. Onyx embolization for dural arteriovenous fistulas: multi-institutional study. *J Neurointerv Surg*. 2022;14 (1):neurintsurg-2020-017109.

[130] Cheung EYH, et al. PHIL and Squid embolization of cerebral AVM: retrospective series. *Neurointervention*. 2022;17 (3):174–182.

[131] Sirakov SS, et al. Initial experience with PHIL in cerebral AVMs. *Interv Neuroradiol*. 2019;25 (1):58–65.

[132] Lamin S, et al. PHIL embolization of intracranial dural AV fistulas: multicenter study. *AJNR Am J Neuroradiol*. 2017;38 (1):127–131.

[133] Tasenko A, et al. E-082 initial experience of combined PHIL and Onyx AVM embolization. *Electronic Poster Abstracts*. BMJ Publishing Group Ltd.; 2018:A89.2–A90.

[134] Öztürk MH, et al. AVM embolization with acrylic glue via detachable-tip microcatheter. *Neuroradiology*. 2008;50 (10):903–904.

[135] Paramasivam S, et al. N-butyl cyanoacrylate embolization with detachable-tip microcatheter. *J Neurointerv Surg*. 2015;7 (6):458–461.

[136] Spiotta AM, et al. Combined balloon-stent technique with Scepter C and LVIS. J Neurointerv Surg. 2013;5 (Suppl 3):iii79–iii82.

Chapter 23

The History of Neurointerventional Surgery in East Asia: China, Japan and Korea

Weiming Kong
and Xianli Lv*, MD
Department of Neurosurgery, Beijing Tsinghua Changgung Hospital, School of Clinical Medicine, Tsinghua University, Beijing, China

Abstract

The development of neurointerventional surgery began in the former Soviet Union (now Russia and Ukraine) and continued in Western Europe. It then spread to some centers in East Asia, such as China, Japan, and Korea. At the start, the only options in East Asia are balloons and liquid embolic agents. The development of new medical tools and surgical techniques has allowed doctors to better treat diseases that affect the blood vessels of the brain and spine. This chapter talks about how neurointerventional surgery has changed in East Asia. It also gives the latest information on improving new techniques and adding new devices used in neurointerventional surgery. In East Asia, China, Japan and Korea have government or non-governmental INR training programs. However, there are some differences between the programs of these three countries, as well as differences in medical education. Specialty (residency) or subspecialty (fellowship) education and training are included in continuing education programs with varied content, format, or period.

Keywords: cerebral angiography, history, neurointervention, cerebral aneurysm, brain AVM, endovascular therapy

Introduction

The earliest documented neurosurgical procedures were skull trephines, which appear to have been performed on both living and deceased subjects. The motivations behind these actions remain ambiguous, as it is uncertain whether they were executed for therapeutic or ritualistic purposes. Numerous trepanned skulls have been unearthed, with dates ranging from the

* Corresponding Author's Email: lvxianli000@163.com

In: World History of Neurointerventional Surgery
Editors: Xianli Lv and Zhongxue Wu
ISBN: 979-8-89530-792-2

Neolithic era to even earlier periods. These findings have been reported from various sites across the globe [1]. The evolution of endovascular neurosurgery in China has been a remarkable one, spanning over six decades. It has progressed from the utilization of cerebral angiography and the employment of handmade balloons to the advent of modern coils, balloon/stent techniques, flow-diverting techniques, and liquid embolization techniques [2]. Since the inaugural utilization of the Guglielmi detachable coil system for cerebral aneurysm embolization in 1998, a plethora of endovascular methodologies have been devised to address a substantial number of aneurysms in China [3]. This chapter provides a comprehensive overview of the historical development and contemporary status of neurointerventional surgery in China, in comparison with Japan and Korea. The following discussion will commence with an introduction to the evolution of diagnostic cerebral angiography, accompanied by a thorough examination of advancements in the treatment of cerebral aneurysms, arteriovenous malformations (AVMs) embolization, and ischemic stroke. During this process, we engaged in discourse on the individuals who played a pivotal role in the development and maturation of this field in East Asia. A pivotal element in the accelerated advancement of this domain is the integration of neurosurgical interventions. The narrative commences with the account of Zhongcheng Wang, a pioneering figure in the field of neurosurgery who, in the year 1955, became the first to perform head and neck angiography in China. Initially, he directly punctured the carotid and vertebral arteries and injected contrast.

Cerebral Angiography

Visualization and acquisition of head and neck blood vessels through diagnostic angiography is a necessary step in the field of neurointervention [4]. The challenges associated with ventriculography in tumor imaging motivated Zhongcheng Wang to explore alternative methods for imaging intracranial lesions. Consequently, he investigated the potential of intracranial angiography (Figure 1). Following the conduction of preliminary research on cadavers, the researcher tested the technique on living patients with the assistance of his colleagues (Figure 2).

The origins of neurointerventional surgery in China can be traced back to the 1950s, a period that coincided with the development of cerebral angiography for the diagnosis of neurological diseases. From 1955 onward, Zhongcheng Wang initiated the clinical application of cerebral angiography and subsequently published his seminal work, entitled Cerebral Angiography, in 1965 [5]. Since that time, significant advancements have been made in the domain of imaging technology, materials, and procedural techniques, thereby expanding its scope and capabilities. His contributions marked the advent of the era of diagnostic and therapeutic angiography. Concurrently, the role of cerebral angiography is expanding in parallel with the growth of neurosurgery as a specialized field in China. A group of researchers, including Yicheng Zhao, Zhongcheng Wang, Yuquan Shi, Qingcheng Xue, Guosheng Duan, and Chengji Liu, are currently engaged in a project to establish neurosurgery as a distinct medical specialty. In this regard, cerebral angiography plays a prominent role. At that time, imaging modalities included plain radiography, ventriculography, pneumoencephalography, and angiography [6]. Angiography is a radiological procedure that generates radiopaque images of the cerebral vascular system. These images can be used to identify vascular occlusion and ultimately identify vascular lesions. The distortion and displacement of vascular anatomical structures can also be used for tumor and hematoma localization.

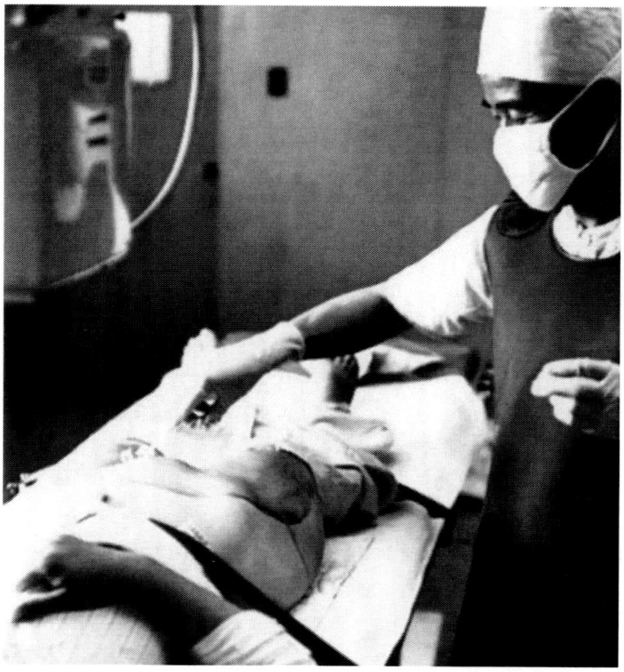

Figure 1. Photograph demonstrating Dr. Zhongcheng Wang was performing cerebral angiography.

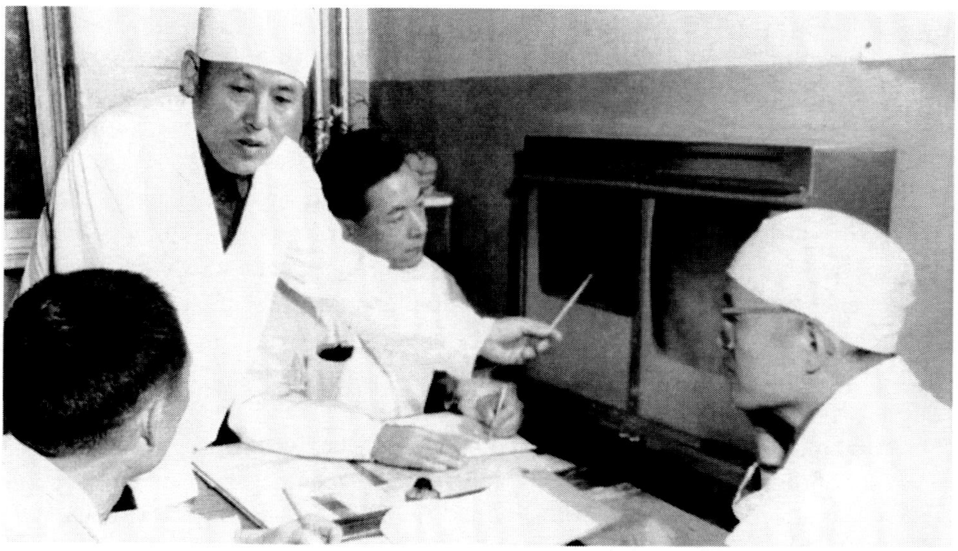

Figure 2. Dr. Zhongcheng Wang was interpreting the cerebral angiogram at the neurosurgery case discussion meeting.

Over the past four decades, the fields of diagnostic imaging and image-based treatment in neurosurgery have undergone continuous development. The advent of computed tomography

(CT) and magnetic resonance imaging (MRI) has led to a symbiotic relationship between neuroimaging and neurosurgery, to the extent that these disciplines have become indistinguishable in many respects. Concurrently, angiography is undergoing constant refinement and innovation. Initially utilized as a diagnostic instrument, it rapidly evolved into a distinct therapeutic modality. For those who undergo diagnostic cerebral angiography, the potential for intervening in neurovascular pathology is evident. However, the tools necessary to achieve distal catheterization—namely, catheters and wires—were not initially available [5].

Pre-Balloon Era

In 1978, Dr. Lianting Ma pioneered the use of a piece of muscle through an open arteriotomy of the carotid artery to embolize a traumatic carotid cavernous fistula (TCCF) under local anesthesia [7]. The specific muscle fiber, measuring between 3 and 10 millimeters in diameter, was meticulously marked with a silver clip and secured using a 4-0 silk thread. Under the guidance of X-ray fluoroscopy, the muscle was carefully maneuvered into the fistula. Subsequent neurosurgeons employed the same method to treat cavernous sinus fistula with embolization [8]. Concurrently, Dr. Qingshun Dai initiated electrocoagulation for the treatment of TCCF and large or giant cavernous aneurysms of the internal carotid artery via craniotomy [9]. The physician inserted 3-6 No. 34 copper wires, measuring 20-30 centimeters in length, into the cavernous sinus or aneurysm. Upon insertion of a copper wire, a direct current of 1mA is established for a duration of five minutes. Following the implementation of electrocoagulation, the copper wire must be severed, with the severed end being left within the cavernous sinus or aneurysm. In 1984, Dr. Guozhen Hui described a procedure for embolizing a TCCF by means of craniotomy, followed by the insertion of a copper wire measuring 0.15 mm in diameter and 60 cm in length into the cavernous sinus [10]. The principle of electric thrombosis is the attraction of negatively charged white blood cells, red blood cells, platelets, and fibrinogen to the positively charged copper wire placed inside the cavernous sinus or aneurysm. Concurrently, Dr. Jiang employed a treatment strategy involving the use of Gelfoam [11] to trap and plug the TCCF. In 1985, Dr. Lianting Ma developed a 7-F catheter for the purpose of catheterization and occlusion of TCCF and major cerebral vessels for pseudoaneurysms through femoral artery puncture using spring coils (COOK MEDICAL LLC, Bloomington, U.S.A.) under local anesthesia [12]. In subsequent years, he advanced this technique to encompass selective spinal angiography and endovascular embolization of maxillofacial and peripheral arteriovenous malformations (AVMs) [13, 14]. In the same year, Dr. Huancong Zuo embolized TCCF using a Fogarty occlusion catheter (Edwards, USA) under X-ray fluoroscopy via arteriotomy of the carotid artery under local anesthesia. This was followed by cutting of the balloon catheter and ligation of the carotid artery [15].

The advent of digital subtraction angiography (DSA) technology in China occurred in the early 1980s. The advent of braided catheters and hydrophilic wires laid the foundation for endovascular catheterization, enabling the catheterizations to be inserted quickly and safely in the 1980s [16]. The subsequent reference to embolic therapy appears in a clinical report from 1982, which details the treatment of a case of middle meningeal arteriovenous fistulas through the injection of povidone iodine (PVP) particles. Upon revisiting the patient 42 years later, he indicated that he was among the initial cases treated. The patient had undergone over 40 years of embolization for dural arteriovenous fistulas, and no recurrences were observed on subsequent control angiograms (Figure 3). The Beijing Neurosurgical Institute and the Wuhan General Hospital of the Guangzhou Military Region were the first medical centers to treat CCF using endovascular methods between 1982 and 1983 [17-37].

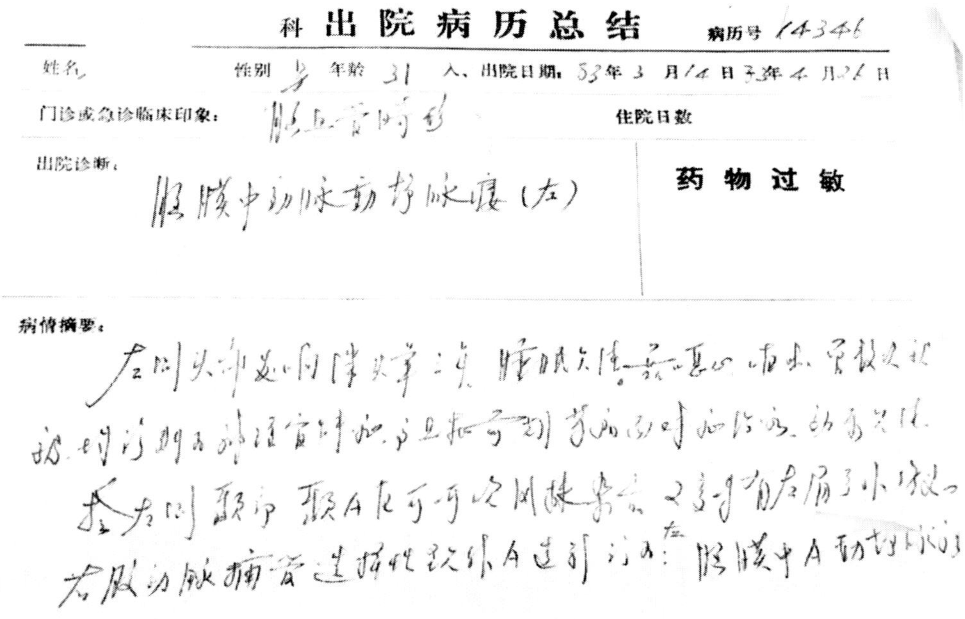
科 出院病历总结 病历号 14346

姓名 性别 年龄 入、出院日期 年 月 日 年 月 日

门诊或急诊临床印象： 住院日数

出院诊断： 药物过敏

病情摘要：

Figure 3. Photograph demonstrating the clinical report of dural arteriovenous malformation embolization in the early of 1983.

The Detachable Balloon

In the 1980s, the most common complaint was that despite better delivery catheters, there was a lack of embolic materials that could be delivered through them. In the early days, doctors were both engineers, inventors, and manufacturers. Dr. Zhongxue Wu has stated the following: In 1985, I was admitted to the doctoral program under the supervision of Academician Zhongcheng Wang. My research focused on the development of interventional treatment methods for cerebrovascular diseases. At that time, no effective methods existed for performing neuroendovascular embolization. The initial phase of my research was conducted at the Beijing Tiantan Hospital and the Beijing Neurosurgical Institute, where I focused on the development of embolic materials, specifically latex balloons (Tables 1 and 2). At that time, tungsten coils in the light bulb were utilized as the embolic material. During the neurointerventional surgery, the use of catheters manufactured by the French company Balt was employed (Figure 4).

As indicated by the reports from the Beijing Neurosurgical Institute, the People's Liberation Army General Hospital, the Guangzhou Military Region General Hospital, and other centers, the use of balloon embolization for the treatment of intracranial aneurysms has been documented since 1985 [18]. From 1986 to 1992, the Beijing Neurosurgical Institute successfully developed and utilized domestic balloon catheters [18], latex balloon (filling liquid silicone) [19], and tungsten coils [23] to treat TCCFs (Figure 5), aneurysms (Figure 6), AVMs (Figure 7), and vein of Galen malformations [38] (Table 3).

Table 1. Specification of latex balloon made by Beijing Neurosurgical Institute in 1988

No.	Balloon Length (mm)	Diameter (mm)	Neck length (mm)	Long diameter after filling (mm)	Diameter after filling (mm)	Volume (ml)
1	2.3	1.3	4	12	8	0.6
2	4.3	1.3	4	16	9	1.2
3	5.3	1.3	4	18	9	1.4
4	5.3	2.5	4	22	14	3.0
5	10.0	1.3	4	25	9	1.8
6	The double balloon: both balloons are 2.3mm in length and 1.3mm in diameter.					

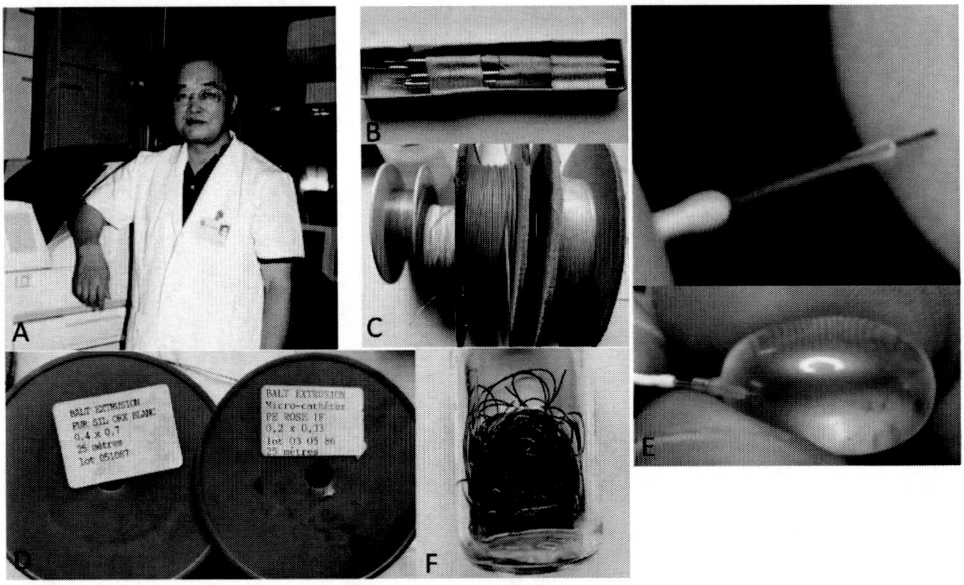

Figure 4. Photographs demonstrating Dr. Zhongxue Wu (A) and the devices were used by him (B-E) in 1980s. B, the molds used for handmade latex balloons. C and D, reels of catheters produced by Balt Extrusion, France. Among them, there are PE ROSE 1F and PURSIL 1.5F. PE means PolyEthylene, it's a kind of polymer. PURSIL 1.5F was 0.5mm outer diameter (0.4mm = inner diameter ; 0.6mm= outer). The PURSIL is the commercial name as it is made of PolyURethane (PUR) and SILicon (SIL), and simply named it “PURSIL.” As for their size, he used the “French gauge (F)” system. "French gauge (F)" comes from the first French manufacturer of rubber urinary catheters. For example, in order to make a 15F catheter (5 mm), a 15 mm wide band had to be cut-out of a sheet of rubber and rolled round a mandrel before its edges were stuck together. The width of the 15 mm band = F = the circumference of the catheter $=\pi\times d = 3.14\times d$. If we consider that 0.14 represents the glue, 3.0 mm remains. Therefore, 15: 3 = a diameter of 5 mm. For example: 3F catheter: 3 = 1 mm in diameter. E, the photo showing the tube is the polyethylene distal tip of the catheter that carried the balloon (0.17mm = inner diameter ; 0.33mm= outer). The balloon was mounted on this tube. F, the tungsten coils soaked in alcohol.

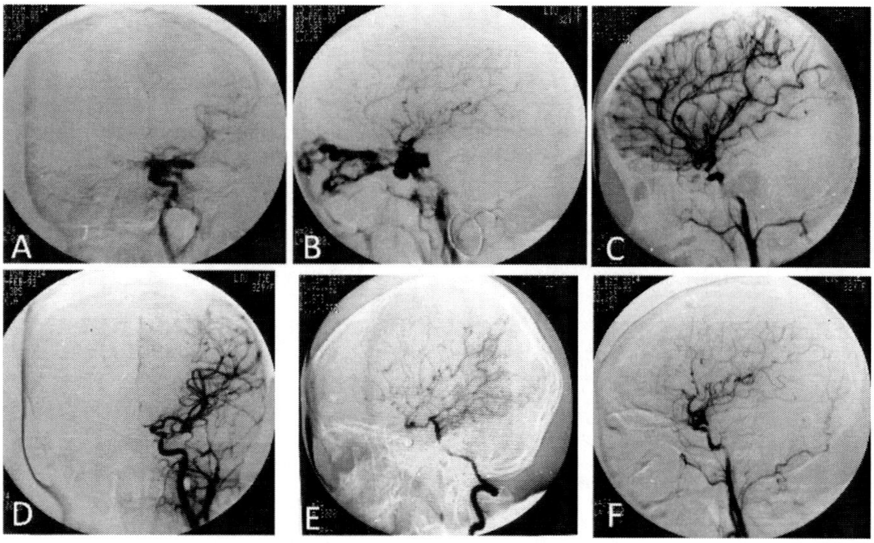

Figure 5. A 32-year-old female patient with left carotid-cavernous fistula (CCF) was treated with handmade latex balloon embolization. A, left carotid artery angiography, anteroposterior view; B, left carotid artery angiography, lateral view. Showing the left CCF, mainly draining forward through the ophthalmic veins. C, left carotid artery angiography, lateral view; D, left carotid artery angiography, anteroposterior view; E, left vertebral artery angiography, lateral view; F. right carotid artery angiography, lateral view. Showing the fistula was completely occluded using one balloon.

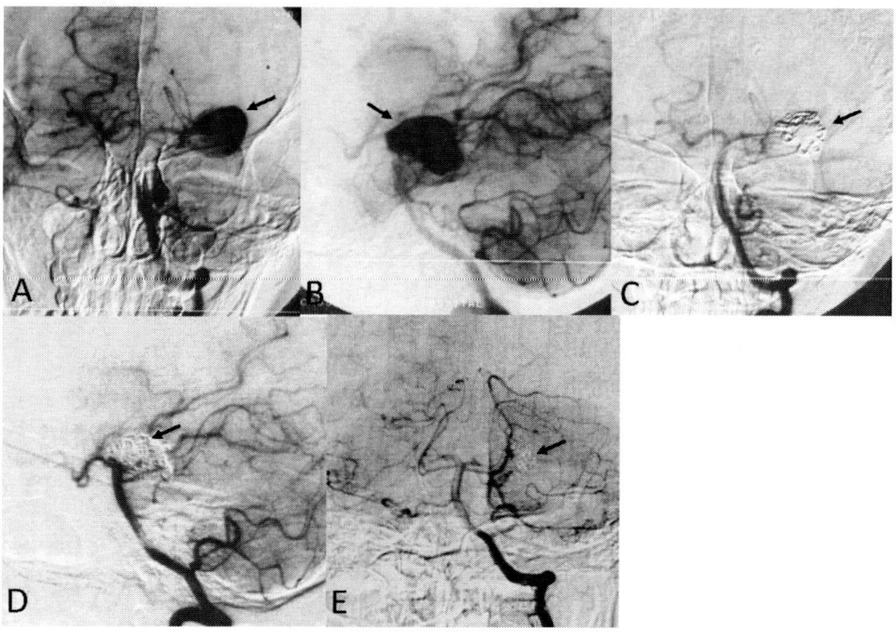

Figure 6. A 6-year-old boy with a giant aneurysm of the left posterior cerebral artery was treated with tungsten coil embolization in 1993. A, left vertebral artery angiography, anteroposterior view. B, left vertebral artery angiography, lateral view. Showing a giant aneurysm in the P2 segment of the left posterior cerebral artery. C, left vertebral artery angiography, anteroposterior view. D, left vertebral artery angiography, lateral view. Showing complete embolization of the aneurysm. E, four years later, a follow-up angiography of the left vertebral artery showing complete occlusion of the aneurysm and absorption of the tungsten coils.

Table 2. Specification of polyethylene balloon catheter made by Beijing Neurosurgical Institute in 1988. Catheter 1: Making detachable balloon catheter can be used to occlude aneurysms and arteriovenous fistulas. Catheter 2: (1) Making a leakage balloon catheter for injection of liquid embolic material for AVMs embolization, such as IBCA. It is characterized by using epoxy resin instead of latex thread to prevent stenosis of catheter lumen; (2) Making an undetachable balloon catheter, which can be used for temporary occlusion of vessels and balloon occlusion test. Catheter 3: Coaxial external cannula for catheter 1. Catheter 4: Coaxial external cannula for the above catheters

No.	Inner diameter (mm)	Outer diameter (mm)
1	0.3	0.5
2	0.4	0.8
3	0.7	1.2
4	2.2	3.0

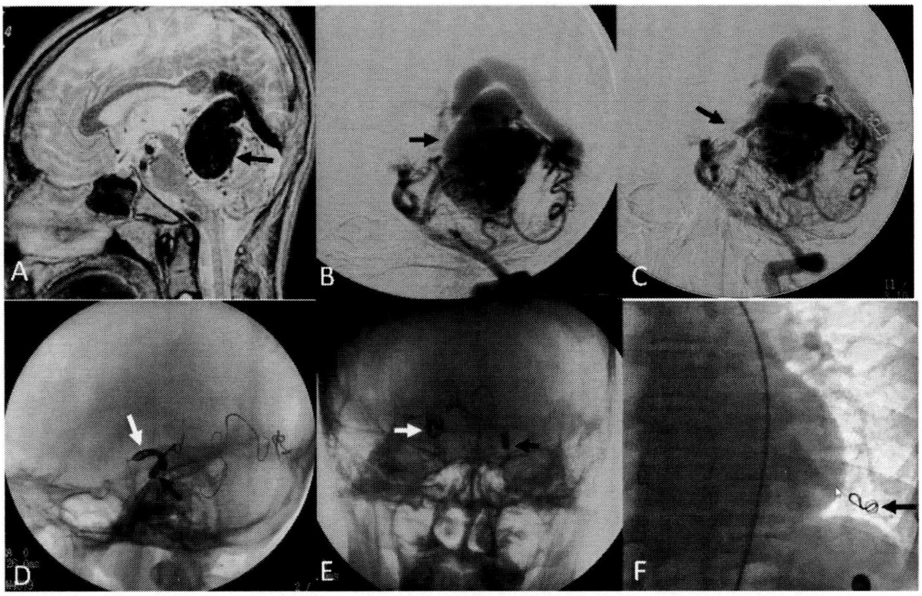

Figure 7. An 18-year-old man had a complex arteriovenous malformation (AVM) with high-flow arteriovenous fistulas (AVFs), which was treated in 1999. A, magnetic resonance imaging (MRI) examination, T2-weighted, sagittal view, showing a giant flow-void signal in the quadrigeminal area, indicating a giant vascular lesion (arrow). B, left vertebral artery angiogram (lateral view) showing a giant AVM fed by bilateral posterior cerebral arteries and drained into a giant venous pouch (arrow). C, left vertebral artery angiogram (lateral view) showing the right posterior cerebral artery was occluded with coils. D, unsubtracted image (lateral view) and E, unsubtracted image (anteroposterior view) showing the right posterior cerebral artery was occluded with coils (white arrow) and the left posterior cerebral artery was occluded with a detachable balloon (black arrow). F, one coil migrated into the left lung because of the high flow fistula (arrow).

The primary constraints associated with the implementation of the balloon occlusion technique are readily apparent. The process of catheterizing an aneurysm is significantly more challenging in the absence of a guide wire. The configuration of the balloon is often inadequate for completely filling irregular aneurysms, resulting in the fundus remaining unprotected or the occurrence of a ball valve effect during aneurysm refilling. Consequently, the paradigm of endovascular treatment has evolved from balloon occlusion to tungsten coil occlusion [18-36]. These tungsten coils function as "free coils" and are advanced through the microcatheter using a specialized metal wire that is equipped with a blunt head, known as a "coil pusher." As illustrated in Figure 8, the coils can be characterized as either straight or exhibiting alternative curves or loops. Once the coil departs from (or even partially departs from) the tip of the catheter, it is not possible to retract it. It is imperative that the coil be fully expelled; failure to do so necessitates the retraction of the microcatheter with the coil partially exposed. At that time, there is a high risk of coil loss during embolization (Figure 7). In the context of arteriovenous fistula or occlusion of major vessels, these non-retrievable coils emerge as a suitable instrument. However, in the context of occluding aneurysms, these devices have proven to be ineffective. In the event that the dimensions or configuration of the coil prove to be suboptimal, it becomes unfeasible to reposition the coil by extracting it. This limitation renders aneurysm treatment a high-risk procedure with minimal probability of achieving complete and stable outcomes. In 2004, a patient with a P2 segment aneurysm of the posterior cerebral artery was treated with embolization using free tungsten coils. The patient subsequently experienced a rupture on day 2, resulting in death one week after the procedure.

In the early 1980s, a significant number of pioneering physicians traveled to Lariboisière Hospital in Paris, France, to observe the novel neuroendovascular treatment techniques that had been developed there. Dr. Feng Ling was a visiting scholar at Lariboisière Hospital from Beijing during the 1982-1983 academic year. In July 1986, she hosted the inaugural National Symposium on Interventional Neuroradiology in Beijing, with distinguished attendees including Dr. Jean-Jacques Merland from Lariboisière Hospital in Paris and Daniel Rufenacht, who was then based in Geneva but had been working at Lariboisière Hospital in Paris. In October 1986, Target Therapeutics, in collaboration with Boston Scientific/Target (Fremont, California), introduced the Tracker microcatheter and associated microwires, a development that significantly enhanced the practicality, effectiveness, and safety of neurointerventional therapy. It is unfortunate that despite the rapid advancement in the development of microcatheters and guide wires, the availability of embolic materials remained deficient.

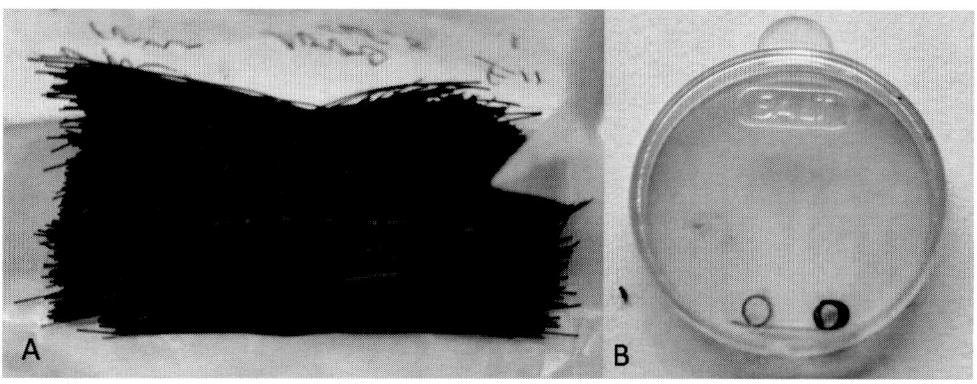

Figure 8. Photograph demonstrating free tungsten coils of straight (A) and curve (B) shapes.

Table 3. 1982-1998 Development of endovascular neurosurgery in China before modern era

Years	Centers	Endovascular Procedures
1982 – 1983	Beijing Neurosurgical Institute, Wuhan General Hospital of Guangzhou Military Region	Begin clinical application of DSA machine and pioneered endovascular embolization of CCF.
1985	Beijing Neurosurgical Institute	Balloon embolized intracranial aneurysms, only 5% of the parent artery was reserved. Local anesthesia; Mata test; carotid or femoral artery puncture Balloon catheter: domestic balloon catheter/Magic-BD/Cook-MF BALT latex balloon
July 1986	Beijing Neurosurgical Institute	Endovascular treatment of CCF Debrun three coaxial system; Magic-BD Balloon catheter was flushed into the internal carotid artery by injecting heparin saline into the delivery catheter through a tee fitting. BALT latex balloon filled with contrast/copper coagulation via craniotomy/ PVA/IBCA
October, 1986	Bethune Medical University, Changchun	Traumatic CCF embolization; Debrun three coaxial system; Magic-BD; BALT balloon filled with contrast agents
1987	Beijing Hospital	Brain AVM Embolization Femoral artery puncture; Leakage balloon catheter/Magic microcatheter IBCA/NBCA
March, 1990	Beijing People's Liberation Army General Hospital	IBCA embolization of brain AVM and DAVF Carotid artery/femoral artery puncture Microcatheter: Magic/red catheter; IBCA/balloon
1991	Beijing Neurosurgical Institute	Traumatic CCF embolization Carotid or femoral artery puncture Microcatheter: Magic-BD/Tracker BALT latex balloon filled with liquid silicone/IBCA/contrast; tungsten coils; silk
1991	Beijing Neurosurgical Institute	Brain AVM embolization IBCA/silk/ coils
August, 1991	Wuhan General Hospital of Guangzhou Military Region	Aneurysm balloon embolization Microcatheter: Magic-BD, Teflon guidewire BALT balloon filled with HEMA
December, 1992	Beijing Neurosurgical Institute	Brain AVM embolization Local anesthesia, the femoral artery puncture Magic/Cook-MF/Tracker catheters; domestic microcoil/domestic IBCA/silk The coil was put into the microcatheter using a small forceps and pushed into the AVM using 1ml syringe filled with saline.
January, 1993	Beijing Neurosurgical Institute	Aneurysm coil embolization Most local anesthesia; Tracker/Cook-MF/TRANSIT/Magic catheters Domestic microcoils/MDS
1993	Tianjin Brain Hospital	Transcatheter embolization of CCF using ophthalmic vein approach Embolic material: balloons/coils/IBCA Local anesthesia; surgical access of the ophthalmic vein
1993	Wuhan General Hospital of Guangzhou Military Region	Detachable balloon filled with domestic filler to embolize intracranial aneurysm
October, 1993	Wuhan General Hospital of Guangzhou Military Region	Domestic micro-tungsten spiral coil embolization of CCF and aneurysm Neuroleptic anesthesia; the femoral artery puncture; 6F guiding catheter Microcatheter: Magic/Tracker/Cook-MF; platinum guidewire. The tungsten coil was mounted on a steel wire with a pushing tube; the pushing tube push the coil into the microcatheter; withdraw the steel wire and pushing tube; and the tungsten spiral coil was pushed into the cavernous or aneurysm using guidewire or syringe.

Years	Centers	Endovascular Procedures
January, 1994	Tianjin Brain Hospital	Domestic 3-D structure of tungsten coil embolization of aneurysm Basic anesthesia; femoral artery or carotid artery puncture; Tracker microcatheter; tungsten coil; pushers push slowly.
March, 1993	Beijing People's Liberation Army General Hospital	Domestic NBCA embolization of brain AVM. Femoral artery puncture; Magic microcatheter; Amytal sodium 50mg function test
February 1995	Beijing Neurosurgical Institute	Domestic coil embolization of spinal cord AVM Tracker/Magic microcatheter; domestic MDS microcoil
February 1998		GDC available in China

In the autumn of 1992, Jacques Moret visited China and documented his observations on the use of tungsten coil embolization for the treatment of intracranial aneurysms. At that time, this type of micro-coils was not available in the Chinese market. Dr. Zhongxue Wu is recognized for his pioneering contributions to the field of endovascular neurosurgery, particularly in the domain of aneurysm treatment. In 1992, he developed a domestic tungsten coil, which was utilized in the treatment of 39 cases of aneurysms within the following years. The Wuhan General Hospital of the Guangzhou Military Region, in conjunction with other medical facilities, also initiated the utilization of tungsten coil embolization as a treatment modality for cerebral aneurysms. From 1993 to 1998, the embolic materials utilized in China were predominantly domestic NBCA, free tungsten coils, spiral coils, detachable balloons, Magic, Cook-MF, and Traker microcatheters [34, 36].

Several key introductions are prominent for endovascular aneurysm embolization, including flexible catheters, steerable wires, detachable balloons, liquid embolic materials, detachable coils, intracranial stents, flow diverters, intrasaccular devices, as well as recent stent retrievers and aspiration catheters [4, 5]. These were all introduced at some point in the past 40 years. Endovascular devices used for cerebral aneurysm embolization in China has gone through the detachable balloon (1985-1992), free tungsten coil (1985-1998), mechanically detachable Spiral coil (MDS) (Balt Extrusion, Montmorency, France) (1993-1998), Guglielmi detachable coil (GDC) system (Boston Scientific/Target, Fremont, California) (since 1998) [4, 5].

In February 1998, GDC system (Guglielmi detachable coil; Boston Scientific/Target Therapeutics, Fremont CA) came into China market and Chinese neurosurgeons accept it quickly. It is widely used because of its good controllability and effective embolization [39]. Professor Zhongxue Wu developed the domestic electrolytic tungsten micro-coils and treated 16 cases of intracranial saccular aneurysms in 1999 [40].

The Detachable Coil

The advent of detachable coils has precipitated a marked increase in the utilization of endovascular treatment for cerebral aneurysms in China since 1998, as evidenced by a substantial rise in documented cases [39]. Coils of varying sizes, three-dimensional configurations, and lengths are all instrumental in the endovascular embolization of aneurysms, as well as arteriovenous malformations (AVMs) (Figure 9 and Table 4). The overall occlusion rate is notably high, though it does not exceed the rate associated with direct surgical clipping, particularly among the selected aneurysm group. For instance, wide-necked and complex cerebral aneurysms remain incurable and demonstrate a high rate of recurrence following endovascular therapies.

Table 4. Imported devices in China

Imported Device	Manufacturer and year of FDA approval	Material	Detachment
Coils			
Target (Guglielmi) detachable coil	Target (Stryker), 1995	Bare platinum	Electrolytic
Micrus microcoil	Micrus, 2001	Bare platinum	Mechanical (using resistive heating)
HydroCoil embolic system	Microvention, 2002	Hydrogel-coated bare platinum coils	V-grip detachment controller with self-contained integral power supply
Orbit detachable coil	Codman, 2003	Bare Platinum	Mechanical/Hydraulic
Matrix bioactive coil	Boston Scientific/Target, 2003	Polyglycolic acid-coated bare platinum coils	Electrolytic
Cerecyte coil	Micrus, 2004	Platinum coils with polyglycolic acid running through lumen of primary platinum wind	Mechanical (using resistive heating)
Orbit Galaxy coil	Cerenovus, 2010	Bare platinum	Mechanical (using resistive heating)
Codman Trufill coil	Johnson and Johnson, 2013	Bare platinum	Mechanical (hydraulic)
Axium	Medtronic, 2014	Bare platinum	Mechanical
Axium prime	Medtronic, 2017	Bare platinum	Mechanical
Stents			
Device	Manufacturer and Year of FDA Approval	Material	Delivery System (size)
Neuroform stent	Boston Scientific/Target, 2002	Nitinol, open-cell design	0.027-inch microcatheter
Enterprise stent	Cordis Neurovascular, 2007	Nitinol, closed-cell design coated with insulating polymer (Parylene C)	0.021-inch microcatheter
LVIS, LVIS Jr	Microvention, 2018	Nitinol, closed-cell braided design	0.021-inch, 0.0165-inch microcatheter, respectively
LVIS EVO	Microvention,	Nitinol, closed-cell braided design	0.0165-inch microcatheter
Neuroform Atlas	Stryker Neurovascular, 2019	Nitinol, laser-cut open-cell design	0.0165-inch microcatheter
Flow diverters			
Device	Manufacturer and year of FDA approval	Material	Delivery catheter size
Pipeline Embolization Device	Medtronic Neurovascular, 2011	36 cobalt-chromium strands, 12 platinum-tungsten strands woven in 3:1 ratio	0.027-inch microcatheter
Pipeline Flex Embolization Device	Medtronic Neurovascular, 2018	36 cobalt-chromium strands, 12 platinum-tungsten strands woven in 3:1 ratio	0.027-inch microcatheter
Pipeline Flex with Shield	Medtronic Neurovascular, 2021	36 cobalt-chromium strands, 12 platinum-tungsten strands woven in 3:1 ratio, phosphorylcholine polymer surface coating	0.027-inch microcatheter

Imported Device	Manufacturer and year of FDA approval	Material	Detachment
Pipeline Vantage	Medtronic Neurovascular	36 or 48 cobalt-chromium strands, 12 or 16 platinum-tungsten strands woven in 3:1 ratio, phosphorylcholine polymer surface coating	0.021-inch or 0.027-inch microcatheter
FRED	Microvention, 2019	Self-expanding braided 66 nitinol wires	0.027-inch microcatheter
FRED Jr	Microvention, 2019	Self-expanding braided 54 nitinol wires	0.021-inch microcatheter
FRED X	Microvention	Self-expanding braided 54 or 66 nitinol wires, protective nano-polymer hydration layer	0.021-inch or 0.027-inch microcatheter
Surpass Streamline	Stryker Neurovascular, 2018	72 or 96 cobalt-chromium wires	0.053-inch intermediate catheter, passed over 0.014-inch microwire
Surpass Evolve	Stryker Neurovascular, 2020	64 cobalt-chromium wires	0.027-inch microcatheter
Other			
Device	Manufacturer and year of FDA approval	Material	Delivery catheter size
WEB	Microvention, 2018	Nitinol wires with platinum coil, now single layer of mesh	0.017, 0.021, 0.027, or 0.033-inch microcatheter
Balloons			
Device	Manufacturer and Year of FDA Approval	Lumen type	DMSO compatible?
HyperGlide	Medtronic Neurovascular, 2010	Single lumen	Yes
HyperForm	Medtronic Neurovascular, 2010	Single lumen	Yes
Scepter	Microvention, 2012	Dual lumen	Yes
Liquid embolic materials			
Names	Manufacturer and year of FDA approval	Component	Radiopaque
Glubran 2	GEMSRL, Viareggio, Italy	nBCA + MS	Lipiodol
Trufill	Cordis Neurovascular, 2023	nBCA	Lipiodol
Onyx	Medtronic, 2005	EVOH and DMSO based	Tantalum
Squid	Emboflu, Fribourg, Switzerland	EVOH and DMSO based	Tantalum
PHIL	MicroVention, Tustin, CA, USA	PLGA, PHEMA and DMSO based	Triiodophenol

nBCA n-butyl cyanoacrylate, MS metacryloxysulpholane, EVOH ethylene vinyl alcohol, DMSO dimethyl-sulfoxide, PHIL precipitating hydrophobic injectable liquid, PLGA Polylactide-co-glycolide, PHEMA polyhydroxyethyl-methacrylate.

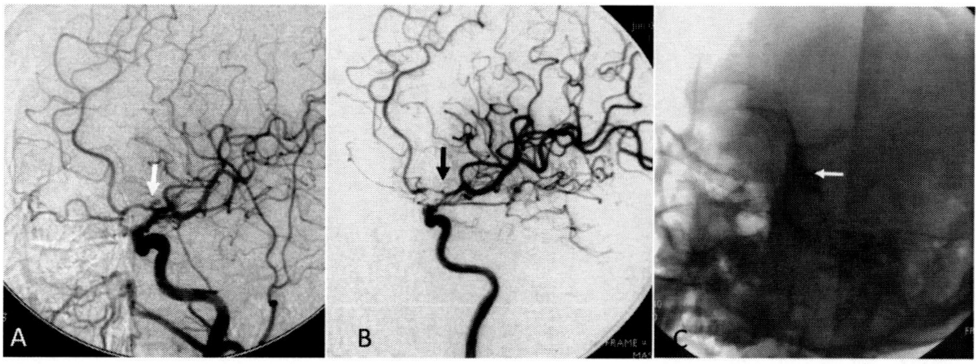

Figure 9. A 45-year-old woman with a ruptured aneurysm of the left anterior cerebral artery was coiled with Microplex coils (Microvention, USA). A, oblique view of the left internal carotid artery injection showing the aneurysm of the A1 segment of the left anterior cerebral artery (arrow). B, oblique view of the left internal carotid artery injection after aneurysm coil embolization showing the aneurysm was completely occluded (arrow). C, unsubtracted image showing the coil mass (arrow).

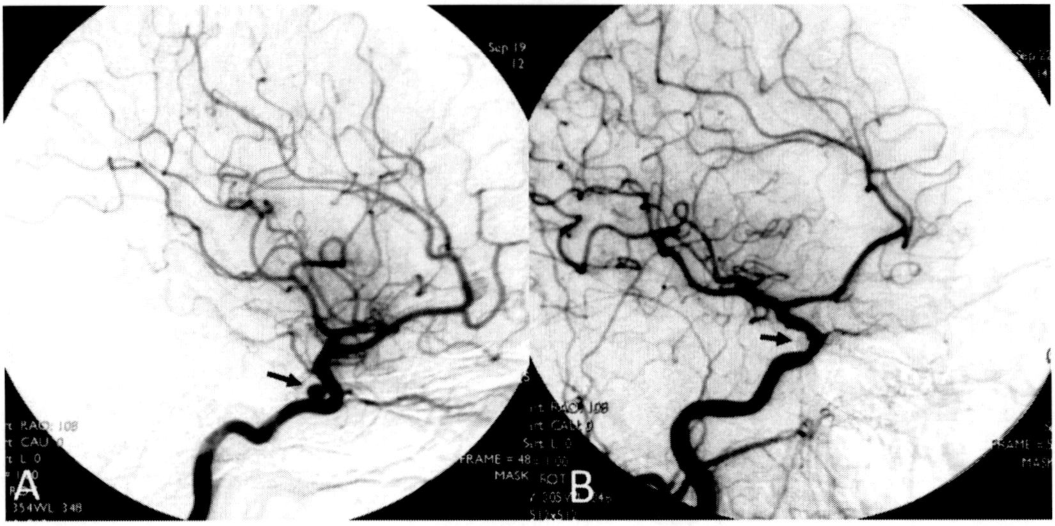

Figure 10. A 38-year-old woman presented with an unruptured ophthalmic segment aneurysm of the internal carotid artery. A, oblique view of the right internal carotid artery injection showing a 4mm×4mm aneurysm of the ophthalmic artery segment (arrow). The aneurysm was coiled (Orbit 4mm×10cm; Microplex 2mm×4cm, 2mm×2cm, 2mm×1cm, 2mm×1cm coils) with assistance of a 4mm×20mm Hyperglide balloon catheter (Medtronic ev3, USA). B. oblique view of the right internal carotid artery injection showing the aneurysm was completely occluded (arrow).

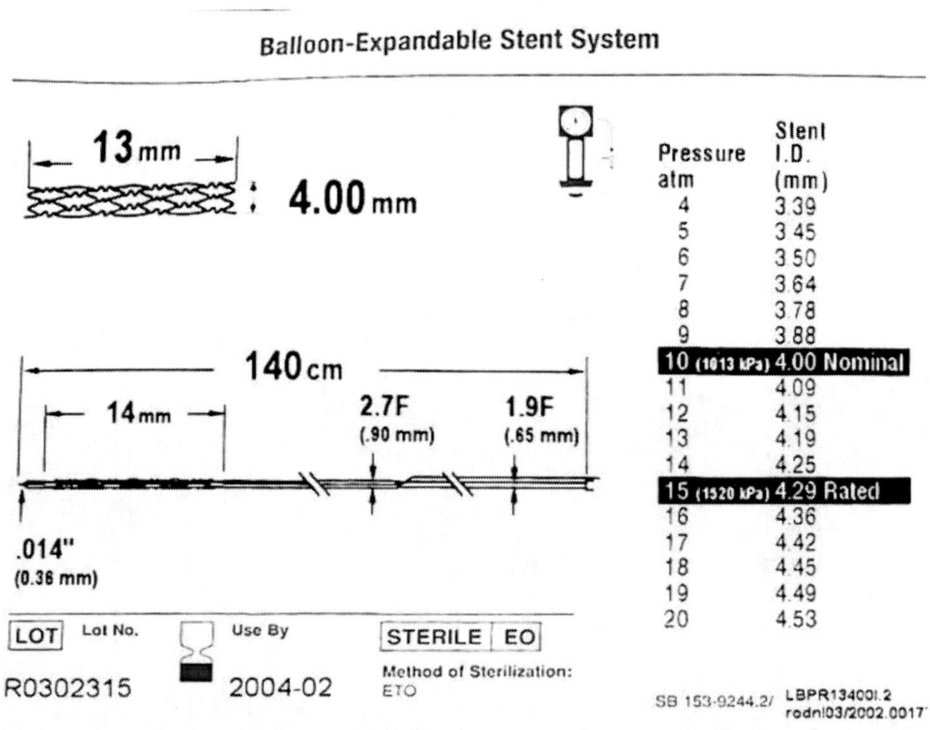

Figure 11. Photographs demonstrating the label of BX coronary artery stent (Medtronic, USA), as used around 1990s.

Notwithstanding the advantages of the GDC system, the treatment of wide-necked and large aneurysms remains challenging [41]. New techniques were developed to keep the detached coils inside the aneurysm sac. In the early 2000s, Chinese doctors initiated the utilization of inflated balloons within the parent vessel to maintain the coils within the aneurysm sac during the delivery process. This approach was employed as a treatment modality for wide-necked aneurysms, constituting a remodeling technique, as illustrated in Figure 10. However, the efficacy of this technique is constrained to saccular aneurysms, the attainment of which necessitates a considerable degree of technical expertise that is acquired over an extended period of time. Furthermore, the increase in the incidence of complications was initially emphasized and noted in clinical practice.

Concurrently, Dr. Zhongxue Wu firstly used stents or covered stents from the interventional cardiology suite to treat complex aneurysms and carotid-cavernous fistulas, with or without additional coils in 1999 (Figure 11) [42, 43]. These devices are specifically designed for cardiac use and are stiffer and more difficult to navigate in tortuous neurovascular anatomical structures. However, if positioned correctly, they can be used with or without detachable coils to obliterate complex aneurysms and carotid-cavernous fistulas. As an increasing number of cerebrospinal vascular diseases become suitable for endovascular treatment, a continuous stream of new devices and concepts has emerged. Subsequently, neuroendovascular surgery underwent rapid development in China, ultimately becoming a subspecialty of neurosurgery in the country.

The Neurostents for Cerebral Aneurysms

The advent of neurostents, such as the Neuroform and Wingspan stents manufactured by Boston Scientific Target, which are expressly intended for intracranial application (see Figure 12), rendered the utilization of cardiac stents largely superfluous [44, 45]. The utilization of stents necessitates that patients adhere to dual antiplatelet therapy (DAPT) for an extended duration. This combination therapy involves the administration of aspirin and clopidogrel, with the aim of mitigating the risk of thromboembolic complications associated with the deployment of neurovascular stents. The utilization of DAPT has become customary over the past two decades [44, 45]. However, the use of intravenous glycoprotein IIb/IIIa inhibitors has been shown to result in a significant reduction of these complications, concurrent with an increase in the overall occlusion rate [46]. Prior to the advent of stents, coil packing was managed through dense packing techniques, irrespective of whether balloon remodeling was performed. In the 2007-2008 period, a series of bioactive coils were developed with the objective of promoting thrombosis and endothelialization. However, these experiments were promptly discontinued due to the limited efficacy of the coils, and no significant advantage was observed when using them in isolation compared to using pure platinum coils [46]. The utilization of polymers in the treatment of cerebral aneurysms has been investigated by others during the 2009-2010 period [46]. However, the elevated risk and morbidity associated with this approach have led to its temporary rejection and impeded its widespread acceptance. The advent of detachable coils and intracranial stents (including Willis covered stents) (Figure 13) has led to a notable increase in the number of aneurysm patients in China who are treated endovascularly following the publication of the International Subarachnoid Aneurysm Trial (ISAT) [47]. This evidence led to the rapid adoption of detachable coils as the primary treatment modality for both ruptured and unruptured aneurysms in China, surpassing open surgery. The number of publications related to aneurysm coiling is increasing exponentially, indicating that this technique has become a standard treatment modality.

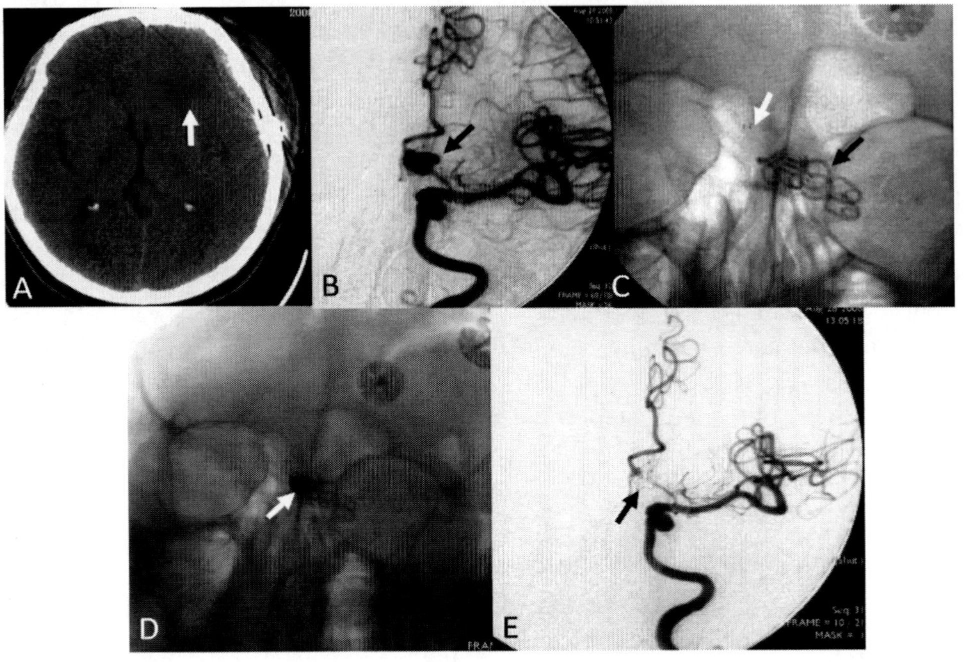

Figure 12. A 43-year-old man presented with a recurrent aneurysm after surgical clipping. A, CT scanning showing an infarction in the left frontal lobe after aneurysm clipping (arrow). B, frontal view of the left internal carotid artery injection showing a 10mm×12mm aneurysm of the left anterior communicating artery (arrow). C, frontal view of the unsubtracted image showing the aneurysm was stented with a 3.0mm×20mm Neuroform stent (white arrow) and clips (black arrow). D, frontal view of the unsubtracted image showing the aneurysm was coiled (black arrow). E, frontal view of the left internal carotid artery injection after treatment showing complete occlusion the aneurysm (arrow).

However, in Japan, a considerable number of patients continue to receive open surgery treatment. However, recent data indicates that endovascular therapy is approaching a 60%-70% success rate [48]. The advent of advanced non-invasive imaging techniques has led to an increase in the detection of unruptured aneurysms, which are defined as small aneurysms that have not yet ruptured. This is further compounded by the reduction in morbidity associated with treatment, which consequently leads to an increase in the number of patients who are deemed eligible for treatment. In response, the industry has allocated substantial resources to the research and development of new endovascular technologies. The concept of flow diversion was initially explored since 2016 [49]. The concept of flow diversion introduces the notion of physiological treatment for aneurysms, emphasizing the treatment of the parent vessel without the necessity of entering the aneurysm dome. The data indicates that, following a one-year observation period, the complete occlusion rate approaches 90%. Additionally, a significant shift has occurred in the proposed treatment recommendations for select intracranial aneurysms (Figure 14) [49]. Consequently, cerebral aneurysms, whether ruptured or unruptured, can be treated with various endovascular tools, including detachable coils, intracranial stents, flow diverters, and intrasaccular devices.

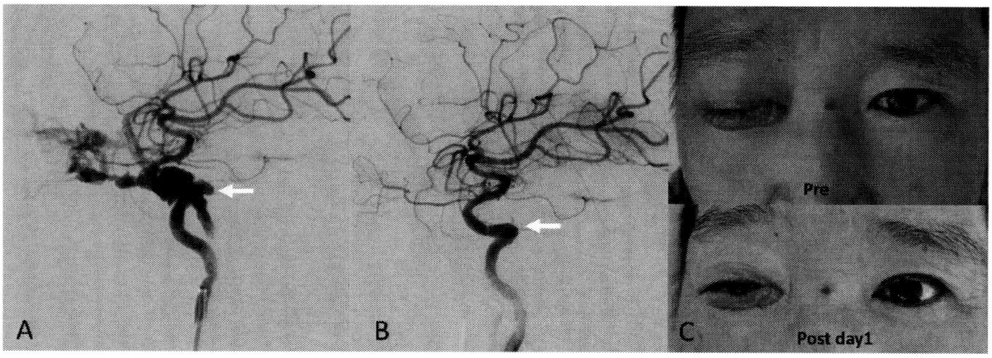

Figure 13. A 52-year-old male patient presented with conjunctival congestion and edema after head trauma. A, lateral view of the right internal carotid artery angiography showing a carotid cavernous fistula (arrow), which is mainly drained forward from the ophthalmic veins. B, the lateral view of the right internal carotid artery angiography showing complete occlusion of the carotid cavernous fistula (arrow) after a Willis covered stent implantation. C, the pre- and post-treatment photos showing a significant improvement in the patient's symptoms.

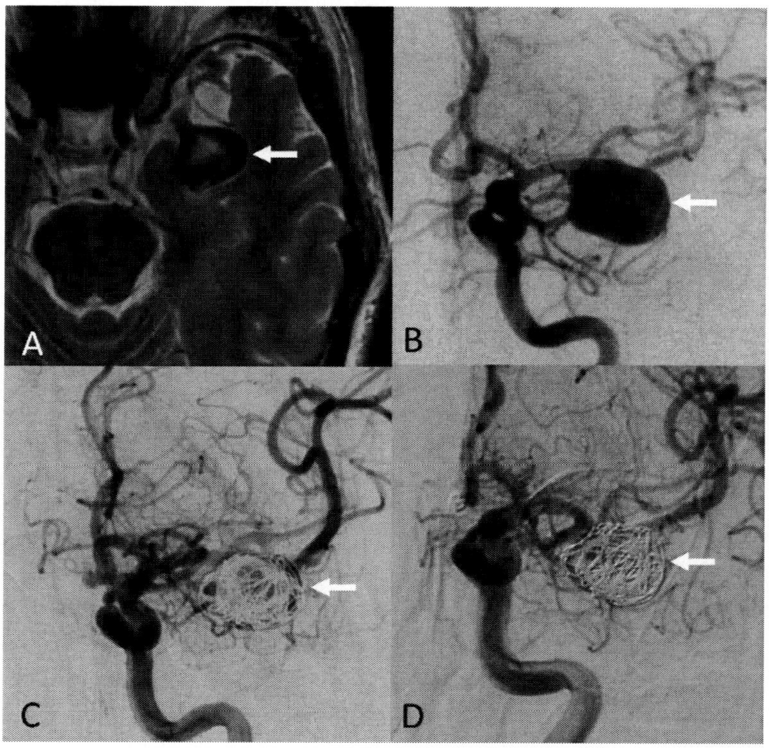

Figure 14. A 56-year-old male patient presented with an incidental aneurysm in the left middle cerebral artery. A, cranial MRI, T2-weighted, axial view, showing a circular mixed signal in the left lateral fissure (arrow). B, the left internal carotid artery angiography, anteroposterior view, showing a large aneurysm in the M1 segment of the left middle cerebral artery. C, immediately after Pipeline flex flow diversion stent and coil embolization, the left internal carotid artery angiography, anteroposterior view, showing partial occlusion of the aneurysm. D, 6-month follow-up angiography of the left internal carotid artery, anteroposterior view, showing complete occlusion of the aneurysm with patency of the left middle cerebral artery and no intimal hyperplasia or stenosis.

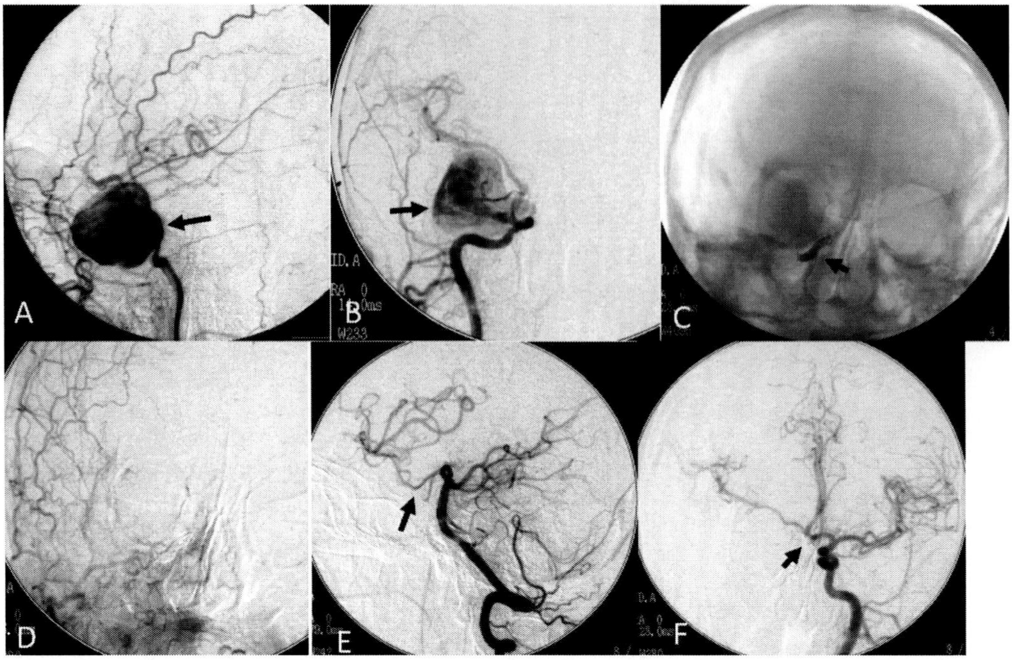

Figure 15. A 54-year-old woman presented with headache, blurred vision of the right eye and diplopia. A, lateral view of the right carotid artery injection. B, frontal view of the right carotid artery injection. Showing a giant aneurysm of the cavernous segment of the internal carotid artery (arrows). C, unsubtracted image, frontal projection, showing the right internal carotid artery was occluded at the proximal of the aneurysm using coils (Microplex 6mm×20cm, 6mm×20cm, 6mm×20cm, 5mm×20cm, 5mm×20cm, Microvention, USA) through an Excelsior SL-10 microcatheter (Stryker, USA) (arrow). D, frontal view of the right carotid artery injection showing the disappearance of the giant aneurysm. E, lateral view of the right vertebral artery injection showing the right middle cerebral artery was filled through the posterior communicating artery (arrow). F, frontal view of the left internal carotid artery injection showing the right anterior cerebral artery and the right middle cerebral artery were filled through the anterior communicating artery (arrow). The patient did not experience any neurological dysfunction after treatment.

The proportion of aneurysms that remain unresolved following endovascular intervention has been observed to decline. A multitude of clinical studies have demonstrated the safety of utilizing stents and flow diverters in the treatment of acute and subacute subarachnoid hemorrhages. Giant aneurysms that were previously treated with balloon test occlusion and parent vessel sacrifice or complex bypass therapy can now be treated with flow diverters (Figure 15). The treatment of giant aneurysms has evolved to a point where the utilization of flow diverters has become a standard procedure. This development has led to a significant reduction in the efficacy and morbidity associated with these procedures, when compared to historical outcomes. Furthermore, the indications for flow diverters have expanded to encompass smaller aneurysms, which are conventionally treated with coiling, stent-coiling, or clipping [50]. Research in the domain of surface modification, delivery mechanisms, and device miniaturization is ongoing, and treatment of even the most distal aneurysms is a possibility. Consequently, the training of endovascular neurosurgeons facilitates the delivery of sophisticated endovascular services in community hospitals, which were previously within the purview of academic and specialty practices. This results in a reduction of the rate at which patients are transferred to more experienced medical centers, leading to an increase in the number of patients receiving endovascular treatment within the community and a decrease in the number of patients receiving open surgical treatment. A high risk of delayed bleeding complications has been identified in flow diversion treatment for intra-dural giant aneurysms. The staged flow diversion treatment has been demonstrated to provide a safe and long-term obliteration of the aneurysms [51]. In the initial phase of treatment, the aneurysm is partially embolized with the use of coils. Subsequent to this procedure, a flow-diversion stent is implanted in a second stage, which occurs one month later. This strategy has been demonstrated to avert the complications associated with delayed rupture, which are precipitated by acute thrombosis within the aneurysm.

Recent advancements in hemostatic technologies, such as collagen plugs, percutaneous devices, and external compression devices, have emerged as promising solutions for achieving hemostasis. It is important to note that while certain techniques may result in a reduction in compression time, they may not necessarily lead to a decrease in the incidence of groin hematomas. Furthermore, these techniques have the potential to induce significant complications. The implementation of these preventive strategies exhibits variation among institutions. The potential benefits of standardizing one or more of these practices, either individually or in combination, in reducing hematoma rates require further investigation.

New Devices for Endovascular Aneurysm Therapy

Intra-aneurismal obliteration devices, such as WEB (Microvention, USA), were approved for use in China at the end of 2020 [52]. The potential consequences of this condition include the rapid formation of blood clots within the aneurysmal sac. The current utilization of this treatment is primarily focused on addressing wide-necked aneurysms that occur at the point where cerebral arteries bifurcate. Its primary indication may be for ruptured aneurysms, as antiplatelet drugs are not required prior to treatment. Preliminary results demonstrated the technique's high success rate; however, complications such as compression deformation and aneurysm recurrence during follow-up were observed [52]. Further validation is required from clinical research to substantiate its safety and efficacy. The development and introduction of such devices has been so persistent and rapid that these new devices have already been available in China (Table 4).

Since 2008, China has witnessed the gradual establishment of a neurointerventional industry capable of producing an array of neurointerventional devices, including but not limited to catheters, guide wires, coils, neck-bridging devices, and liquid embolic agents (Table 5). It is imperative that new products undergo rigorous testing prior to their release, as inadequate testing can potentially result in deleterious long-term effects [53]. The existing products are also quite costly and frequently inaccessible to developing countries. The development of increasingly sophisticated devices that are only accessible to a select group of experts does not represent a viable solution to the underlying problem. These techniques are designed to be straightforward and accessible to a wide range of individuals within the field.

Table 5. Domestic materials in China

Imported Device	Manufacturer and year of FDA approval	Material	Detachment
Coils			
Jasper coil	Jasper, Shanghai, 2008	Bare platinum	Electrolytic
Visee coil	Visee medical, 2014	Hydrogel-coated bare platinum coils	Mechanical
Perdenser coil	TJWY Medical, Beijing, 2015	Bare platinum	Electrolytic
Numen coil	MicroPort NeuroTech, Shanghai, 2020	Bare platinum-tungsten	Electrolytic
Avenir coil	Wallaby Medical, Shanghai, 2021	Bare Platinum	Mechanical
Gekko coil	Ton-bridge, 2021	Bare Platinum	Mechanical
Stents			
Device	Manufacturer and Year of FDA Approval	Material	Delivery System (size)
Apollo stent	MicroPort NeuroTech, Shanghai, 2005	Stainless steel, balloon-expanding	0.014-inch guidwire
Willis coverd stent	MicroPort NeuroTech, Shanghai, 2010	Stainless steel, Tefflon cover	0.014-inch guidwire
Flow diverters			
Device	Manufacturer and year of FDA approval	Material	Delivery catheter size
Tubridge Flow diverter	MicroPort NeuroTech, Shanghai, 2016	Self-expanding braided 66 nitinol wires	0.027-inch microcatheter
Nuva	TJWY, 2021	Self-expanding braided 48/64 nitinol wires	0.027-inch microcatheter
Lattice	Accumedical, 2023	36 cobalt-chromium strands, 12 platinum-tungsten strands woven in 3:1 ratio	0.027-inch microcatheter
Qilin	Ton-bridge, 2024	48, 72 or 96 nitinol wires strands	0.021-inch or 0.027-inch microcatheter
Other			
Device	Manufacturer and year of FDA approval	Material	Delivery catheter size
Tulip	TJWY Medical, Beijing, 2024	Nitinol wires with platinum coil, now single layer of mesh	0.017, 0.021, 0.027, or 0.033-inch microcatheter
Liquid embolic materials			
Names	Manufacturer and year of CFDA approval	Component	Radiopaque
Fuaile	Fuaile, Beijing, China	nBCA and 2-octyl cyanoacrylate (OCA)	Lipiodol
EVAL liquid embolic material system	Success, Jinan, 2008	EVOH/DMSO/ethanol	Tantalum

nBCA n-butyl cyanoacrylate, EVOH ethylene vinyl alcohol, DMSO dimethyl-sulfoxide.

Liquid Embolic Materials

Since 1983, with the advent of digital subtraction angiography in China, Chinese medical professionals have attained a more profound comprehension of brain and spinal arteriovenous malformations (AVMs), vein of Galen malformations, and digital avulsions of the retina (DAVFs) [54-57]. In 1984, Dr. Yuquan Shi developed a modified classification system for brain arteriovenous malformations (AVMs) and discussed its implications for microsurgical strategies. In 1993, Dr. Feng Ling proposed a classification system for spinal AVMs [56]. Intramedullary arteriovenous malformations (AVMs); perimedullary arteriovenous fistulas (AVFs); dural arteriovenous fistulas (AVFs); and Cobb's syndrome. The four categories classification proposed by Ling et al. is a valuable asset. Microsurgery and endovascular strategies remain important treatment options for patients with spinal AVMs, and preliminary data suggests that spinal radiation surgery may play a role in the treatment of certain specific lesions in the future. While some neurosurgeons may possess extensive expertise in microsurgical resection of these lesions, there is an observed trend of referring patients with these lesions to endovascular surgeons.

In 1986, the Beijing Neurosurgical Institute, the Beijing Hospital, and the People's Liberation Army General Hospital initiated the utilization of domestic IBCA, silk sutures, and coils for the embolization of brain and spinal arteriovenous malformations (AVMs), dural arteriovenous fistulas (DAVF), and vein of Galen malformations and tumors [17, 21, 38, 56, 57]. Subsequently, a number of medical centers in China initiated the embolization of brain arteriovenous malformations (AVMs), thereby acquiring substantial practical knowledge in this domain [58, 59].

The Chinese seminar on neuroendovascular surgery, which was held in December of 1993, resulted in the publication of numerous papers pertaining to the embolization of arteriovenous malformations (AVMs) [60]. In China, materials utilized for AVM and tumor embolization have been documented to include silk, detachable balloons, coils, PVA, IBCA, N-butyl-cyanoacrylate (NBCA), and ethylene vinyl alcohol polymer (EVOH) [2, 4, 5]. It has been established that the utilization of silk suture frequently results in the occurrence of severe inflammation of brain tissue. The polymerization of IBCA in AVM vessels has been observed to result in the formation of hard agglomerations. Surgical resection is often challenging due to the local rigidity of IBCA, which is difficult to excise with micro-scissors and is challenging to coagulate with bipolar electrocoagulation. NBCA has been shown to possess a spongy and flexible nature, which renders it amenable to surgical resection following its polymerization in AVM vessels. Consequently, it is being progressively replaced by IBCA.

Following a period of several years, EVOH was introduced to the market as the Onyx embolization system (Medtronic, USA) in 2003. In 2003, the liquid copolymer Onyx (Microtherapeutics, Inc., Irvine, CA) was introduced to the Chinese market [61]. The Onyx liquid embolization system is characterized by its non-adhesive property, a feature that enables its application in the embolization of various vascular malformations and tumors. This system has been demonstrated to offer enhanced control over embolization procedures when compared to cyanoacrylate glue [2]. Examples of the Onyx liquid embolization system's applications include the embolization of arteriovenous malformations (AVMs) (Figure 16), dural arteriovenous fistulas (DAVFs) (Figure 17), and brain aneurysms (see Figure 18). The utilization of liquid embolizing agents for aneurysms necessitates the temporariness of the occlusion of the parent vessel, which is achieved through the injection of the liquid via a specialized microcatheter that is inserted into the aneurysm lumen.

The EVOH is a novel instrument due to its low viscosity and excellent controllability. It can be utilized in conjunction with NBCA in AVM embolization procedures. Another non-adhesive mixture, the EVAL mixture (EVAL, SUCCESS, Shandong, China), was approved for AVM embolization by the State Food and Drug Administration of China in 2012 [62]. EVAL is a combination of EVAL/DMSO/ethanol that functions as an embolic agent for the treatment of arteriovenous malformations (AVMs) (Figure 19).

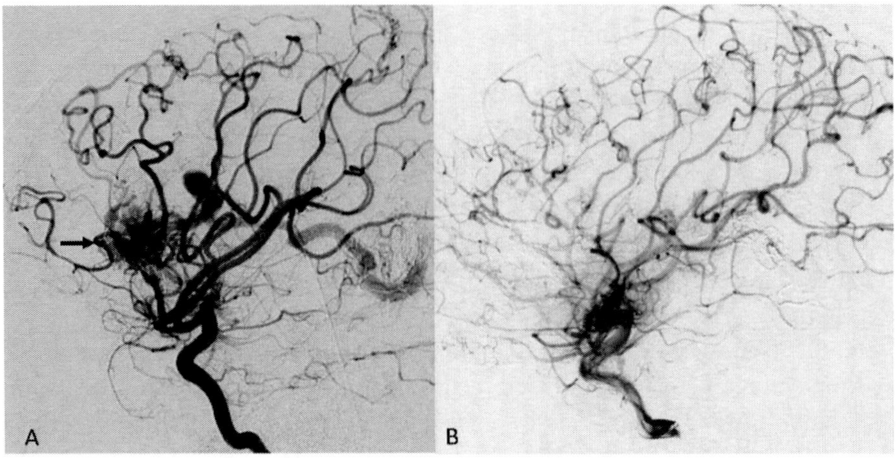

Figure 16. An 18-year-old female patient presented with intraventricular hemorrhage. A, the left internal carotid artery angiography, lateral view, showing an arteriovenous malformation in the frontal lobe (arrow). There is an aneurysm dilation on the drainage vein, which is the site of bleeding. B, the left internal carotid artery angiography after Onyx embolization, lateral view, showing complete occlusion of the arteriovenous malformation. The patient did not experience any complications related to embolization.

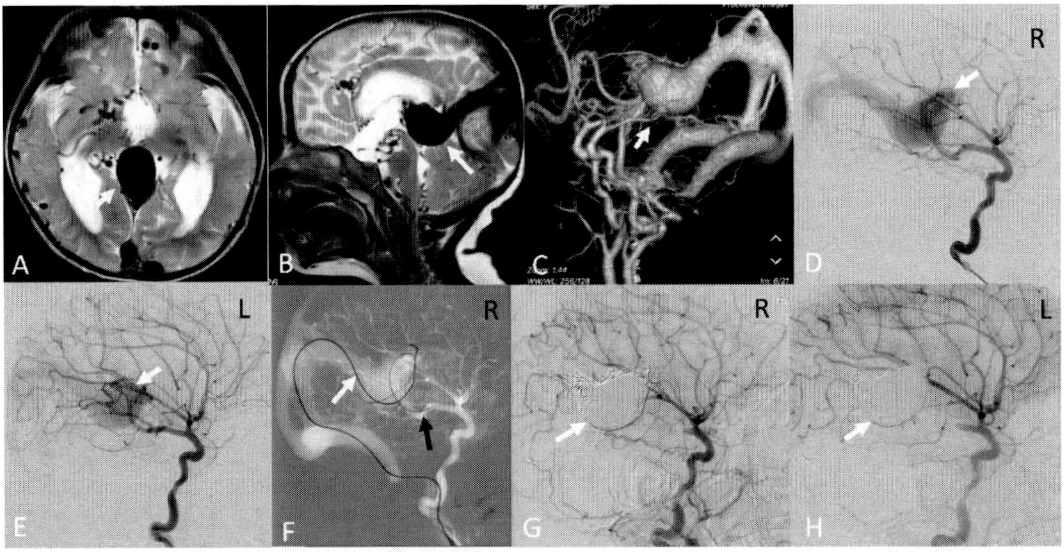

Figure 17. The head circumference of a 9-month-old infant girl was increased. A, cranial MRI examination, T2-weighted, axial view. B, cranial MRI examination, T2-weighted, sagittal view. Showing a giant vascular flow void signal in the quadrigeminal area, indicating a vascular lesion. C, cranial CTA examination suggesting a vein of Galen malformation. D, the right internal carotid artery angiography, lateral view. E, the left internal carotid artery angiography, lateral view. Showing a vein of Galen malformation with bilateral medial posterior choroidal arteries supplying the fistula with significant dilation. F, endovascular embolization is performed through a combination of intraarterial and intravenous pathways, the coils were delivered through the intraarterial microcatheter (black arrow) and Onyx was injected through the intravenous microcatheter (white arrow). G, the right internal carotid artery angiography, lateral view. H, the left internal carotid artery angiography, lateral view. Showing complete obliteration of the vein of Galen malformation. There was no any neurological dysfunction caused by endovascular embolization.

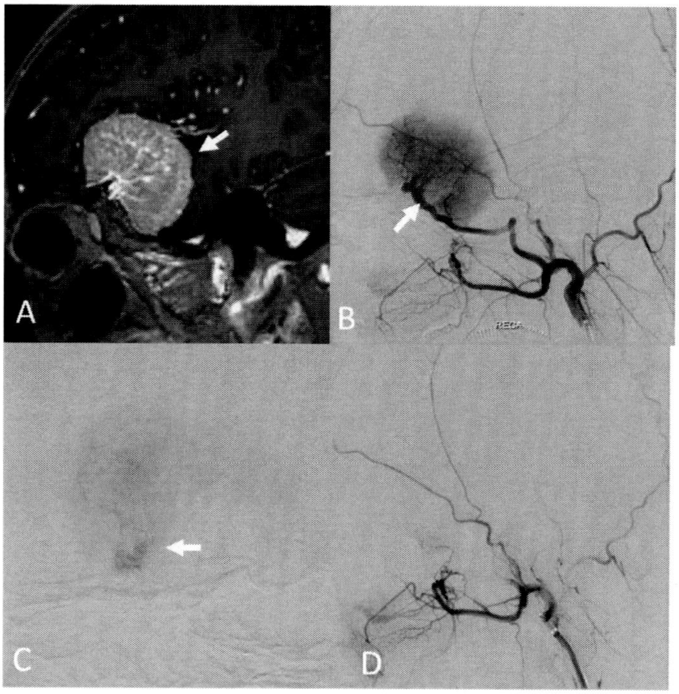

Figure 18. A 27-year-old woman presented with dizziness. A, enhanced cranial MRI, sagittal view, showing the large sphenoid wing meningioma. B, the left external carotid artery angiography (lateral view) showing the dense opacification of the tumor. C, the selective injection showing the dense opacification of the tumor indicating the microcatheter tip in the tumor. D, the left external carotid artery angiography (lateral view) showing the tumor was nearly complete occluded with Onyx injection. The tumor has been completely removed under the microscope, and the intraoperative bleeding is less than 300 ml. the whole process does not use the brain retractor, realizing no brain traction, and the time is greatly shortened to 4 hours.

New tip detachable microcatheters (Sonic, Balt, France; and Apollo, Medtronic, USA) have been shown to reduce the occurrence of microcatheter entrapment. The double lumen balloon catheter (Scepter C, Microvention, USA) has been demonstrated to temporarily obstruct arterial blood flow, thereby averting premature embolic agent flow into the venous system. This augmentation of controllability in high-flow fistula embolization is a notable advancement in the field [63].

The advent of EVOH and detachable tip catheters has led to an increased utilization of transvenous embolization for the treatment of arteriovenous malformations (AVMs). However, the current literature on the subject is limited to a few successful clinical reports from China [64]. Transvenous AVM embolization is an emerging technology [65]. French and German institutions have been particularly innovative in this area [66]. The clinical indications for transvenous embolization of arteriovenous malformations (AVMs) remain confined to small AVMs (maximum diameter <2 cm), the inability to perform arterial embolization, unsuitable resection or radiotherapy, and simple drainage vein structure (single drainage, no stenosis) [65]. Complication and adverse event rates exceed 14%, and more than 4% of patients have poor clinical outcomes in the transvenous approach for the treatment of arteriovenous malformations (AVMs) [64-66]. This proportion significantly exceeds the natural history of AVM. The most common complication is cerebral hemorrhage, which limits the clinical application of intravenous techniques [67].

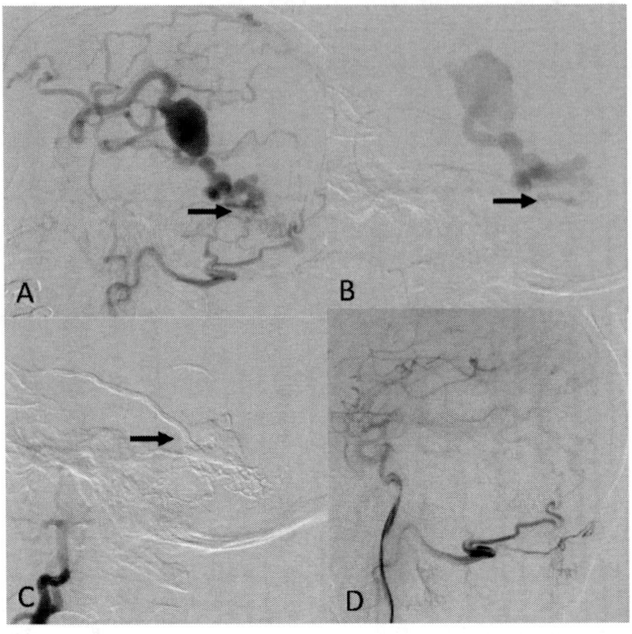

Figure 19. A 62-year-old male patient presented with intracranial hemorrhage. A, the left external carotid artery angiography, lateral view, showing a dural arteriovenous fistula in the left lateral sinus (arrow), with an aneurysm dilation on the drainage vein indicating the location of bleeding. B, the microcatheter angiography showing that the tip of the microcatheter reaches the fistula outlet and can be used for embolization (arrow). C, the subtracted image showing the cast of EVAL (arrow). D, post-embolization angiography of the left carotid artery, lateral view, showing complete occlusion of the lesion. The patient did not experience any complications related to embolization.

A variety of transarterial strategies, including the pressure-cooker technique and the multiple catheters technique, have been proposed to enhance the clinical efficacy of transarterial embolization of arteriovenous malformations (AVMs) [67]. Due to the relative ease with which the veins can be filled with EVOH from the arterial side, Dr. Lv et al. have reported on two methods of treatment: "multiple pedicle embolization for curative AVM embolization" and "no-plug technique." These methods have been shown to result in a high complete obliteration rate and a low complication rate [68]. The following are indications of an arteriovenous malformation (AVM) embolization: ruptured AVM, AVM of small size, or deep location; AVM with coexisting aneurysm and high-flow fistula (Figure 20) [69].

The transarterial embolization of arteriovenous malformations (AVMs) remains the prevailing standard of care. The efficacy of transarterial AVM embolization has been significantly enhanced by the advancement of theoretical and technical knowledge [70]. In cases of small (≤3cm) arteriovenous malformations (AVMs) undergoing embolization, the efficacy of the treatment can reach up to 80%, and the risk of complications is already lower than the risk of natural bleeding. For middle AVMs (defined as those with a diameter between 3 and 6 centimeters), staged embolization (typically two-stage) has been shown to achieve a cure rate of up to 50% [71]. For patients with large arteriovenous malformations (AVMs) measuring at least 6 centimeters, the treatment modality of choice is embolization of hemorrhagic risk structures. These structures include coexisting aneurysms, high-flow arteriovenous fistulas, and lesions with restricted venous drainage [72].

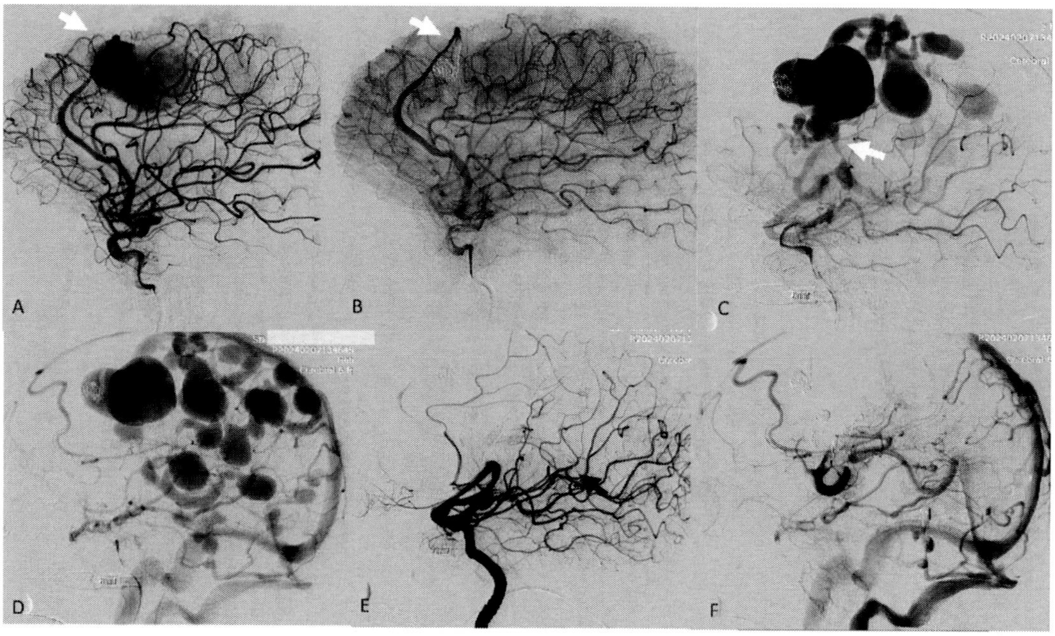

Figure 20. A 49-year-old female presented Hunt-Hess 1 grade SAH. A, the right internal carotid artery angiography, lateral view, showing anterior cerebral artery arteriovenous fistula (arrow) with significant venous dilation. B, the right internal carotid artery angiography, lateral view, showing complete embolization of the anterior cerebral artery arteriovenous fistula with a coil and Onxy (arrow). C, the left internal carotid artery angiography, lateral view, showing arteriovenous fistula of the middle cerebral artery (arrow), with multiple venous aneurysms formed by venous dilation. D, late phase of the left internal carotid artery angiography, lateral view, showing multiple dilated venous aneurysms with grape-like changes. E, arterial phase of the left internal carotid artery angiography, lateral view. F. venous phase of the left internal carotid artery angiography, lateral view, showing complete occlusion of the cerebral arteriovenous fistula.

Cerebrovascular Stenosis

At the beginning of the 21st century, Chinese neurosurgeons initiated the use of endovascular techniques in the treatment of ischemic cerebrovascular disease. In 2000, Zhongrong Miao et al. made an attempt to treat symptomatic intracranial artery stenosis with a soft coronary stent [73]. Self-expanding stents for the treatment of carotid artery stenosis were introduced in 2002 [74]. In 2003, the development of a protective device aimed at reducing the incidence of intracranial embolus thrombosis led to the enhancement of safety measures in the context of carotid artery stenosis stenting treatments [74]. The Apollo stent, the world's first stent designed for intracranial artery stenosis, was developed by Dr. Weijian Jiang from China and was launched in 2005, one month ahead of the launch of the self-expandable Wingspan stent for intracranial artery stenosis in the United States [75]. This stent has been recognized as a global leader in the domain of intracranial vascular stenting in China [75]. In consequence of his contributions, he was elevated to the distinction of distinguished professor at the Cleveland Clinic in the United States (Figure 21).

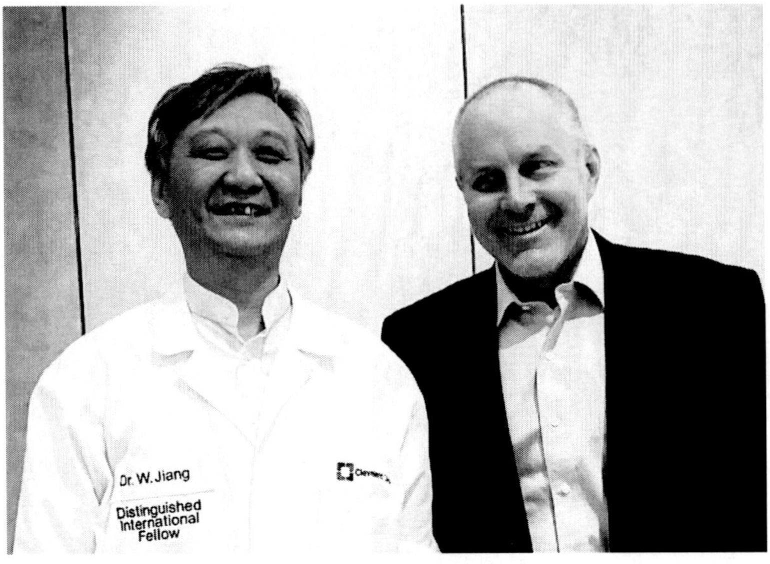

Figure 21. A photo of Dr. Jiang Weijian (left) and Dr. Peter Rasmussen from Cleveland Clinic (right) in Beijing in 2019.

The Wingspan stent, which was the first self-expanding nitinol-composite stent to be approved by the US Food and Drug Administration (FDA), was approved in 2005 for patients with 50% or higher ICAS who were symptomatic despite medical therapy [5]. It has been postulated that endovascular therapy could be a viable treatment option for these patients, as their plaques may not stabilize with conventional medical therapy alone, potentially resulting in recurrent artery-to-artery embolic strokes. The advent of novel angioplasty balloon catheters and flexible stents has profoundly transformed the management paradigm for symptomatic intracranial stenosis. A mounting body of research has documented a low complication profile and a satisfactory rate of angiographic patency at follow-up [5].

Angioplasty with stenting of carotid stenosis does not require general anesthesia and requires only a few seconds of carotid artery occlusion. The utilization of endoluminal revascularization as a therapeutic modality for carotid stenosis in high-risk patients has been proposed. These patients may include those with contralateral carotid occlusion, postendarterectomy stenosis, and/or severe coronary and other systemic diseases [5].

In China, endovascular therapy has been utilized as the primary treatment for patients with symptomatic intracranial atherosclerosis, with surgical revascularization reserved for those patients who have failed endovascular therapy [5]. Endovascular management of intracranial atherosclerotic diseases has gained popularity as a treatment option for patients with such conditions, who frequently exhibit severe and debilitating comorbidities (Figure 22). The field is rapidly evolving, and it is anticipated that endovascular surgeons will assume a pivotal role in propelling the frontiers of contemporary ischemic stroke management and prevention. In select instances of atherosclerotic carotid stenosis, carotid angioplasty and stenting have been shown to supersede open surgical interventions. This trend is anticipated to persist in the foreseeable future.

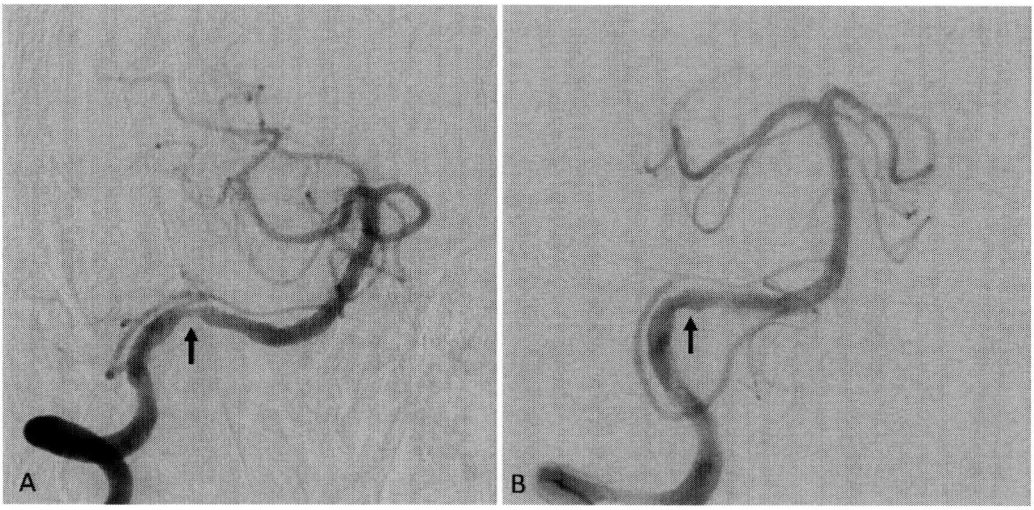

Figure 22. A 73-year-old male patient presented with dizziness. A, the right vertebral artery angiography, oblique view, showing stenosis of the V4 segment of the right vertebral artery (arrow). B, after balloon dilation and stent implantation at the site of stenosis, the right vertebral artery angiography showing an improvement of stenosis and the patient's dizziness symptoms disappeared (arrow).

Thrombolysis and Mechanical Thrombectomy

In China, the administration of intravenous thrombolysis using Alteplase for the treatment of acute ischemic strokes commenced subsequent to the approval of the Food and Drug Administration (FDA) in 1996 [76]. The concept of intra-arterial pharmacologic thrombolysis was initiated in 2000 due to the determination that intravenous alteplase was not an effective treatment for patients with large vessel occlusions [76]. Nevertheless, due to the stringent time window limitations of intravenous thrombolysis (within 4.5 hours), less than 3% of ischemic stroke patients are candidates for treatment. Consequently, Chinese medical practitioners initiated the utilization of the Solitaire AB stent as a clot retrieval device for the treatment of thrombosis in 2013 [76]. This concept has been developed by endovascular neurosurgeons who have employed this device to remove the coils that have become dislodged during the process of embolization of cerebral aneurysms. The endovascular thrombectomy approach was established as the prevailing standard of care for large vessel occlusion following a series of five randomized control trials (RCTs) in 2015 [76]. In 2020, the number of mechanical thrombectomies in China exceeded 40,000 cases, which was more than 10 times higher than the number of cases in 2015. Patients who met the eligibility criteria for mechanical thrombectomy did not demonstrate an increased risk within the extended window of 16 to 24 hours. The second generation of devices, including stent retrievers and aspiration catheters, has demonstrated a significantly improved safety, revascularization, and patient outcome.

Manpower and Training

In China, due to difficulties in distance and transportation, it is impossible for a few technical masters and groups to treat all SAH patients. But in some small countries, such as Japan and Korea, one to two large centers can easily treat all patients with ruptured aneurysms. In Japan and China, most endovascular surgery is carried out by neurosurgeons who carry out cerebral and spinal cord angiography and interpret the images obtained.

Neurointerventional surgery in China has become the largest one in the world in terms of the number of neurointerventional surgeons [77]. In the past 10 years, neurointerventional procedures dramatically have increased in China. Advanced endovascular techniques are confined to big cities such as Beijing, Shanghai, and Guangzhou, where most of the Chinese neurosurgeons have their 6- to 12-month fellowship or 2-year residency of endovascular neurosurgery at major medical centers. In Korea, neurointerventional surgery was originally the domain of neuroradiologists. In China and Japan, endovascular training has already become a component of neurosurgical residencies. Given that most practicing neurointerventional surgeons are within 10 years of training, the current pool of neurointerventional surgeons is relatively young and expanding in China.

The Chinese INR Coordinating Committee of the Chinese Doctor Association was founded at the beginning of 2014 and included 9 members. Every year, 3 major international symposiums are hosted regularly in Beijing and Shanghai, such as China Forum of Cerebrovascular Diseases (CFCVD), Beijing Tiantan Neurointervention Symposium, and Oriental Conference of Interventional Neurovascology (OCIN), for which the number of participants has increased to approximately 1000. Many world-renowned professors, including Fernando Viñuela, Lasjaunias (Figure23), Karel terBrugge, LucPicard, Alex Berenstein, Anton Valavanis, Marco Leonardi, Michel Mawad, and Timo Krings have come to China to deliver lectures. These meetings and symposia offer good platforms for Chinese neurosurgeons to exchange ideas and broaden their views.

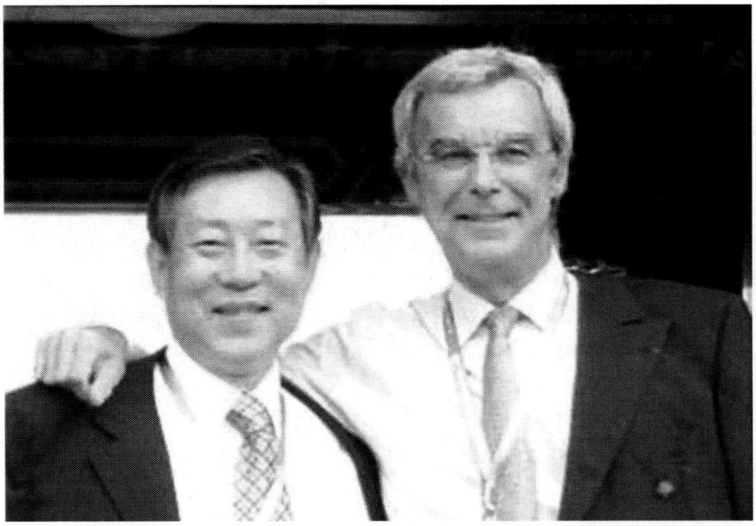

Figure 23. The photo of In Sup Choi (left) and Pierre Lasjaunias (right) in China.

In Japan

Cerebral arteriography by percutaneous carotid injection, first introduced in Japan in 1937 by Kentaro Shimidzu at Tokyo University Hospital, is widely regarded as a significant milestone that contributed to the dissemination of cerebral angiography in general medical practice [78]. The majority of neurointerventional surgeons are affiliated with the neurosurgical department in Japan. Since the establishment of the Japanese Society for Endovascular Neurosurgery in 1982, there has been a historical precedent of endovascular neurosurgeons being trained alongside neurosurgeons, a tradition that persists to the present day [79].

During the 1980s in Japan, a variety of embolic materials were utilized for the treatment of brain lesions, including cyanoacrylates, ethylene-vinyl alcohol copolymer mixtures, Ethibloc, ethanol, estrogen, poly (vinyl acetate), cellulose acetate polymer, poly (vinyl alcohol), gelatin sponges, microfibrillar collagen, surgical silk sutures, detachable balloons, and coils [80]. In 1985, the Osaka Neurological Institute initiated the embolization of spinal arteriovenous malformations (AVMs) by introducing a diagnostic catheter into the origin of the segmental artery and injecting polyvinyl alcohol (PVA) particles (500–1000 μm) in a flow-directed manner (conventional embolization) [81]. In light of the high rate of reperfusion and/or the emergence of new blood supply arteries, the Tracker catheter was introduced for the embolization of arteriovenous malformations (AVMs) in April 1990 [81]. Subsequently, they utilize 180 to 350 μm PVA particles or NBCA to embolize cerebral and spinal AVMs [81, 82].

At the time of the initial introduction of neurovascular therapies to Japan, a lack of widespread acceptance in the field of neurosurgery was observed [83]. Consequently, Japan has not produced a sufficient number of endovascular neurosurgeons to address the increasing demand for timely treatment of lesions that cannot be treated by surgery. The absence of endovascular treatment has been associated with the deterioration of patient outcomes [83]. Prior to 2004, Japan had documented a limited number of cases involving coil embolization treatment for cerebral aneurysms, even subsequent to the implementation of GDC in April 1997 [84]. In the year 2000, researchers at Kyoto University developed isostearyl-2-cyanoacrylate (ISCA), a non-adhesive cyanoacrylate, for the treatment of arteriovenous malformations (AVMs) and aneurysm embolization [85].

In 2004, Japan became the first nation to approve the utilization of stents for the treatment of intracranial aneurysms [86]. Presently, three categories of stents are available in Japan: The Neuroform Atlas, developed by Stryker Neurovascular of Fremont, California, USA, is one such example. Another is the Enterprise 2, created by Cerenovus, and the LVIS, produced by Microvention. A study titled "Dawn of Stent Era" and employing the Japan Neurovascular Therapy Registry (JR-NET3) has revealed a substantial increase in the utilization of stents [86]. The utilization of FD implantation for the treatment of aneurysms has been extensively adopted in Japan, with health insurance coverage becoming a prevalent aspect of this practice. Additionally, the indications for FD implantation have undergone an expansion, encompassing a broader range of medical conditions. Presently, three categories of FD are in operation in Japan: Pipeline, FRED, and Surpass Streamline. The WEB (Microevent, Terumo, Aliso Viejo, CA, USA) and PulseRider (Cerenovus, Johnson & Johnson Medical Devices, New Brunswick, NJ, USA) have been introduced and utilized in select medical centers.

A comparison of the present situation with that of the previous twenty-year period reveals that neurosurgical residents currently have more opportunities to attend neurointerventional treatment. Furthermore, endovascular surgery has achieved an important position in the practice of neurosurgery in Japan [87]. The Japanese Society of Neuroendovascular Therapies has evolved into an organization comprising over 4,000 members and 1,500 specialists, including more than 400 supervisors, as of 2022 [88]. The composition of the society is as follows: 90% neurosurgeons, 5% neuroradiologists, and 5% neurologists and other disciplines. Despite the considerable number of endovascular members, there remains a paucity of faculties that have attained proficiency in complex endovascular techniques (representing a mere 10% of all members), a circumstance that renders the capacity to perform endovascular treatment in all institutions inadequate [89]. A 2022 study revealed that 65.5% of the cerebral aneurysms received surgical treatment. The treatment modality was nonrandomized and determined by the institutes themselves. Despite the increasing prevalence of endovascular treatment, the Japan Neurosurgical Society has persisted in its commitment to the advancement of neurosurgical practice.

A survey conducted in the United States in 2010 to evaluate the status of neurointerventionalists and basic trends of the physicians' backgrounds in this subspecialty found similar trends as in Japan and China [90]. The aggregate number of graduates is increasing, particularly in the fields of neurosurgery and neurology. Despite the fact that the majority of the current faculty are neuroradiologists, there will be a decline in the number of graduates in radiology over the next five years. This decline reflects a trend toward greater subspecialization within the fields of neurosurgery and neurology.

Neurovascular therapy, a minimally invasive surgical procedure, has gained significant traction in China, Japan, and Korea, with a steady increase in demand observed on an annual basis. However, in many Asian and Middle Eastern countries, the number of experts in neuroendovascular therapy is limited, thereby limiting the number of patients who can benefit from this therapy. One of the main reasons for this situation is the lack of sufficient educational systems to train experts in neuroendovascular therapy.

In South Korea

A parallel can be drawn between the status of neurointerventional surgery in South Korea and its counterpart in Europe. The majority of early neurointerventional physicians were neuroradiologists who received training in neurointerventional surgery in North America or Europe in 1994 [53]. The Korean Society of Interventional Neuroradiology (KSIN) was founded in 1994 [53]. As of 2024, the KSIN had a membership of over 300 individuals, with 75% being neuroradiologists, 22% being neurosurgeons, and 4% being neurologists. A comparative analysis of neurointervention practices in South Korea reveals that they emerged at a comparatively later stage and have maintained a comparatively smaller number of practitioners compared to China and Japan. With respect to medical education, there are notable discrepancies in the fundamental medical education curriculum. These include premedical education (Japan and South Korea), long-term service (South Korea), internships (Japan and North Korea), and long-term residencies (China) [91].

The Korean Neuroendovascular Society (KoNES), formerly known as the Korean Society of Intravascular Neurosurgery (KSIN), was founded in December 1995 [92]. In July 2012, it was renamed the Korean Society of Endovascular Neurosurgeons (SKEN), and in December 2019, it was renamed the current Korean Society of Neurovascular Surgeons (KoNES). In recent years, there has been a notable surge in the number of South Korean neurosurgeons and neurologists who have entered this field. As of 2024, the KoNES membership has surpassed 400 individuals from diverse backgrounds, including neurosurgery, neuroradiology, and neurology.

According to data collected from SKEN members over the 5-year period from 2013 to 2017 [93], the number of endovascular treatments conducted in collaboration with SKEN members has continued to increase during this time. This trend has been particularly evident in major metropolitan areas such as Gyeonggi-do, Seoul, and Busan, although it has also been documented on a national scale. In the domain of endovascular treatment, conventional cerebral angiography is the most prevalent procedure, followed by endovascular treatment for cerebral aneurysm embolization and ischemic stroke, and finally, endovascular treatment for arteriovenous malformations (AVMs) and tumor embolism. For the past five years, endovascular neurosurgeons have been the primary providers of endovascular treatment in South Korea.

Despite having received approval from both the European Union and the US Food and Drug Administration, the pre-market access process for new medical devices may be mandated in the Asian market, given the potential for racial disparities among Asian populations. In contrast to the rapid development and implementation of useful new devices in China and Japan, it has become increasingly challenging to obtain insurance coverage for new products in South Korea [94]. For instance, protective devices utilized during carotid stent implantation or glue employed for AVM embolization are not encompassed within the insurance coverage.

China, Japan, and South Korea are regarded as pivotal East Asian countries that have demonstrated remarkable contributions to the domain of neurointerventional surgery. Despite the existence of a substantial domestic market for medical devices in these countries, a significant reliance on imported medical devices is in place. The East Asian Conference of Neurointervention (EACoN) is an annual event that fosters international collaboration and the exchange of knowledge among Asian countries in the field of neurology. The members present their research topics at academic conferences, both domestically and internationally, and have published numerous papers in leading academic journals around the world.

Conclusion

This chapter provides a historical overview of the rapid development of neurointerventional surgery in East Asia. A discussion was held regarding the process of innovative developments that have made endovascular treatment of cerebrospinal vascular diseases possible. It is evident that there are discernible discrepancies in this process among China, Japan, and South Korea. The initial pivotal step in the evolution of endovascular techniques in China was the implementation of detachable balloons, a development that is not evident in Japan and South Korea. For particular neurovascular diseases, including arteriovenous fistulas, particularly chronic cavernous fistulas (CCFs), detachable balloon therapy has been shown to be both efficient and safe when compared with surgical intervention. In East Asia, the advent of GDC has precipitated a substantial escalation in the realm of neurointervention, particularly in China. In East Asia, neurointerventional surgery has emerged as a prominent modality for the treatment of cerebral and spinal vascular diseases.

References

[1] Lv X, Li Z, Li Y. Prehistoric skull trepanation in China. *World Neurosurg*. 2013;80 (6):897-899.

[2] Lv X, ed. *Arteriovenous Malformations of the Brain*. Nova Science; 2020.

[3] Ji Y, Wang ZG, Ding X, Qu CC, Zhang QL. Recurrence of intracranial aneurysms after endovascular embolization: study of 70 cases. *Zhonghua Yi Xue Za Zhi*. 2008;88 (19):1303-1305.

[4] Lv X, Zhao W, Jiang W. A brief history of neurointerventional development. In: Zhao J, ed. *Hybrid Operation of Neurosurgery*. Beijing: People's Health Publishing House; 2022:8-16.

[5] Lv X. The history and development of endovascular neurosurgery. In: *Frontiers in Clinical Neurosurgery*. IntechOpen; 2021.

[6] Zhao J. A brief history of neurosurgery. In: Zhao J, ed. *Hybrid Operation of Neurosurgery*. Beijing: People's Health Publishing House; 2022:1-7.

[7] Ma LT. Treatment of internal carotid-cavernous sinus fistula with a "flying kite." *Zhonghua Wai Ke Za Zhi*. 1983;21 (10):618-620.

[8] Lang GL. Carotid-cavernous fistulas treated surgically by the so-called flying kite method—report of 4 cases. *Zhonghua Shen Jing Jing Shen Ke Za Zhi*. 1984;17 (3):155-157.

[9] Dai QS, Yue W, Liu XZ. Treatment of aneurysm of the cavernous carotid artery by electrothrombosis: report of 4 cases. *Zhonghua Wai Ke Za Zhi*. 1985;23 (10):589-591.

[10] Hui GZ. Post-traumatic bilateral carotid-cavernous fistulas—a case report. *Zhonghua Wai Ke Za Zhi*. 1984;22 (8):501-502.

[11] Jiang ZQ. Treatment of carotid-cavernous fistula by trapping and plugging with gelatin sponge—report of 3 cases. *Zhonghua Shen Jing Jing Shen Ke Za Zhi*. 1984;17 (3):158-160.

[12] Ma LT, Li YG, Yu Z. Treatment of aneurysm or arteriovenous fistula with an occluding spring coil via catheter. *Zhonghua Wai Ke Za Zhi*. 1985;23 (1):27-29.

[13] Ma LT. Clinical uses of vascular embolism by means of the spring coil. *Zhonghua Yi Xue Za Zhi*. 1987;67 (6):330-333.

[14] Ma LT, Yu Z, Zhang JZ. Percutaneous transfemoral catheterization in selective spinal angiography: report of 12 cases. *Zhonghua Wai Ke Za Zhi*. 1986;24 (1):13-15.

[15] Ma LT. Clinical treatment of traumatic false aneurysm and arteriovenous fistula. *Zhonghua Wai Ke* Za *Zhi*. 1989;27 (6):361-363.

[16] Zuo HZ, Zuo F, Jiao SX. Treatment of carotid-cavernous sinus fistula using the Fogarty balloon catheter. *Zhonghua Wai Ke Za Zhi*. 1987;25 (9):544-547.

[17] Ling F, Liu S, Duan G. Intravascular IBCA embolization therapy for cerebral arteriovenous malformation. *Chinese J Neurosurg*. 1988;4 (3):144.

[18] Wu Z, Wang Z. Domestic balloon catheter embolization for carotid-cavernous fistula. *Chinese J Neurosurg*. 1989; (4):7-9.

[19] Wu Z, Wang Z, Zhu Y, et al. Development of latex-producing balloon, performance experiment and balloon catheter preparation. *Chinese J Neurosurg*. 1989; (4):65-66.

[20] Wu Z, Sun Y, Wang Z, et al. Preliminary clinical application of domestic electrolysis detachable micro-coil. *Chinese J Neurosurg*. 2000; (01).

[21] Wang D, Lu J. A brief overview of new progress in neurological intervention. *Chinese J Surg*. 2016;54 (5):328-331.

[22] Lv X, He H, Wu Z. China's medical education and interventional neuroradiology training. *World Neurosurg*. 2015;84 (5):1462-1465.

[23] Yu Z, Ma L, Qin S, et al. Domestic tungsten micro-helical embolization for traumatic carotid-cavernous sinus fistula. *Chinese J Neurosurg*. 1995;11 (4):187-188.

[24] Ling F, Duan G. Endovascular treatment of internal carotid-cavernous fistula (report of 27 cases). *Chinese J Neurosurg*. 1989;5:224.

[25] Yin L, Huang W, Sun R, et al. Transcatheter embolization for carotid-cavernous sinus fistula. *Chinese J Neurosurg*. 1995;11 (4):191-194.

[26] Shang J, Wu Z, Dai J. Traumatic carotid-cavernous fistula balloon embolization. *Chinese J Neurosurg*. 1995;11 (4):198-199.

[27] Ma L. The detachable balloon filled with domestic filler for intracranial saccular aneurysms. *Chinese J Neurosurg*. 1993;31:36.

[28] Wang Z, Wu Z, Zhang Y. Treatment of 132 cases of intracranial aneurysms with detachable balloon occlusion. *Chinese J Neurosurg*. 1997;13 (6):319-322.

[29] Wu Z, Wang Z, Zhang Y. Treatment of 205 cases of intracranial saccular aneurysms by intravascular embolization with microcoils. *Chinese J Neurosurg*. 1997;13 (6):323-326.

[30] Wu Z, Wang Z, Dai J. Experimental study of intravascular embolization of self-made tungsten wire coil. *Chinese J Neurosurg*. 1994;10:5.

[31] Wu Z, Wang Z, Dai J. Domestic micro-coil embolization for intracranial aneurysms (three preliminary reports). *Chinese J Neurosurg*. 1993;9 (3):161-162.

[32] Huang S, Ling F, Dai L, et al. Mechanical detachable coil embolization for intracranial aneurysms (report of 18 cases). *Chinese J Radiol*. 1996; (9):591-594.

[33] Wu Z, Wang Z, Dai J. Micro-coil embolization for cerebral arteriovenous malformations. *Chinese J Neurosurg*. 1994;10 (3):127-129.

[34] Ma L, Wang Q, Zhang L, et al. Treatment of basilar artery bifurcation aneurysms. *Chinese J Neurosurg*. 1994;10 (3):132-134.

[35] Huang Z, Suo J, Liu F, et al. Treatment of traumatic carotid-cavernous fistula with detachable balloon embolization. *Chinese J Neurosurg*. 1994;10 (3):151.

[36] Ma L, Li S, Yu Z, et al. Treatment of 6 cases of intracranial aneurysms with domestic tungsten filament micro-helical embolization. *Chinese J Neurosurg*. 1994;10 (3):155-156.

[37] Wu Z, Wang Z, Dai J. Endovascular embolization for complex traumatic carotid-cavernous fistula. *Chinese J Neurosurg*. 1994;10 (3):157-158.

[38] Shen C, Ling F, Meng X. Angiographic classification and endovascular therapy of vein of Galen aneurysmal malformation. *Zhonghua Wai Ke Za Zhi*. 1996;34 (8):488-491.

[39] Wang D, Ling F, Zhang H, et al. Endovascular treatment of intracranial aneurysms with GDC: report of 8 cases. *Zhonghua Wai Ke Za Zhi*. 1998;36 (7):389-391.

[40] Wu Z, Wang Z, Sun Y, et al. Electrolysis of detachable micro-coil embolization for intracranial aneurysms. *Chinese J Neurosurg*. 1999;42 (2):90-93.

[41] Fan Y, Yan S, Wang S, et al. Treatment of wide-necked cerebral aneurysms using stent and balloon-assisted technique. *Zhonghua Wai Ke Za Zhi*. 2007;45 (4):220-222.

[42] Lv X, Jiang C, Li Y, et al. Intracranial pseudoaneurysms, dissections and carotid-cavernous fistulas: repair with covered stents. *Interv Neuroradiol*. 2008;14:435-440.

[43] Ding H, He M, You C, Deng L. Application of endovascular covered stent for vertebral dissecting aneurysm and carotid-cavernous fistula. *Zhongguo Xiu Fu Chong Jian Wai Ke Za Zhi*. 2009;23 (2):215-218.

[44] Wu Z, Lv X, Yang X, He H. Ruptured vertebro-inferoposterior cerebellar artery dissecting aneurysm treated with Neuroform stent and vertebral artery occlusion. *Eur J Radiol Extra*. 2009;70:e100-e103.

[45] Zhang J, Lv M, Lv X, et al. Endovascular treatment using stents for cerebral aneurysms. *Neuroradiol J*. 2010;23:730-736.

[46] Lv X. *Understanding and Managing Cerebral Aneurysms*. Nova Science; 2024.

[47] Zhang J, Wu Z, Liu A, et al. Endovascular stent implantation for wide-necked intracranial aneurysms. *Zhonghua Yi Xue Za Zhi*. 2006;86 (3):148-151.

[48] Irie K, Murayama Y, Urashima M, et al. Japanese Subarachnoid Aneurysm Trial: clipping vs coiling in 1863 ruptured aneurysms. *Neurol Med Chir* (Tokyo). 2022;62 (5):231-237.

[49] Lv X, Yang H, Liu P, Li Y. Flow-diverter devices for intracranial aneurysms: meta-analysis and systematic review. *Neuroradiol J*. 2016;29 (1):66-71.

[50] Zhang H, Ren J, Wang J, Lv X. Off-label pipeline use for complex cerebral aneurysms: mid-term follow-up. *Interv Neuroradiol*. 2022;15910199221148800.

[51] Liang S, Yuan R, Lv X. Giant ruptured MCA aneurysm treated by acute coiling plus scheduled Pipeline Flex. *Neuroradiol J*. 2020;33 (6):517-519.

[52] Lv X. Editorial: advances in flow-diversion devices for cerebral aneurysms. *Front Neurol*. 2023;14:1195367.

[53] Jia Z, Shi H, Miyachi S, et al. Development of new endovascular devices for aneurysm treatment. *J Stroke*. 2018;20 (1):46-56.

[54] Shi YQ. A proposed scheme for grading intracranial arteriovenous malformations. *Zhonghua Shen Jing Jing Shen Ke Za Zhi*. 1984;17 (2):65-68.

[55] Shi YQ, Chen XC. A proposed scheme for grading intracranial arteriovenous malformations. *J Neurosurg*. 1986;65 (4):484-489.

[56] Ling F. Classification and embolization of spinal cord arteriovenous malformation. *Zhonghua Wai Ke Za Zhi*. 1993;31 (1):13-16.

[57] Ling F, Wu J, Zhang H. Classification of intracranial dural arteriovenous fistula. *Zhonghua Yi Xue Za Zhi*. 2001;81 (23):1439-1442.

[58] Lin G, Gao F, Hu S. Endovascular treatment of brain arteriovenous malformation. *Zhonghua Wai Ke Za Zhi*. 1997;35 (2):117-118.

[59] Li X, Qi T, Guo S, et al. Therapeutic effect of embolization of brain AVM with non-adhesive liquid embolic agent. *Nan Fang Yi Ke Da Xue Xue Bao*. 2008;28 (12):2192-2195.

[60] Wang Z. Progress and prospects of endovascular treatment in neurosurgery in China. *Zhonghua Shenjing Wai Ke Za Zhi*. 1994;10 (3):125-126.

[61] Xu F, Ni W, Liao Y, et al. Onyx embolization for brain AVMs. *Acta Neurochir* (Wien). 2011;153 (4):869-878.

[62] Zhang H, Su Y, Lv X. Transarterial embolization of sinus dural AVF using non-adhesive liquid embolic material. *Neuroradiol J*. 2023;19714009231224439.

[63] Zhang H, Liang S, Lv X. Proof-of-principle for AVM embolization complications by proximal occlusion using Onyx. *Neurol India*. 2022;70 (4):1443-1447.

[64] He Y, Bai W, Xu B, et al. Perioperative complications of transvenous embolization of ruptured intracranial AVMs. *Front Neurol*. 2022;13:873186.

[65] Lv X, Song C, He H, et al. Transvenous retrograde AVM embolization: indications, techniques, complications and outcomes. *Interv Neuroradiol*. 2017;23 (5):504-509.

[66] Saal-Zapata G, Visconti-Lopez FJ. Worldwide trends on transvenous embolization of brain AVMs: bibliometric study. *World Neurosurg*. 2023;178:20-27.

[67] Lv X, Zhang Y, Wang J. Systematic review of transcatheter arterial embolization of AVM. *Neurol India*. 2020;68 (6):1285-1292.

[68] Lv X. Comparison of NBCA and Onyx for AVM embolization. *Oper Neurosurg*. 2017;13 (6):E37-E38.

[69] Zhang H, Liang S, Lv X. Radio-clinical grading system for transarterial AVM embolization: Tsinghua AVM grading system. *Neurosci Inform*. 2021;1 (3):100021.

[70] Lv X, Wu Z, Li Y. AVM in the brain: theoretical study on liquid embolic behavior. *Neuroradiol J*. 2013;26 (6):661-668.

[71] Lv X, Liang S. Update Onyx embolization for plexiform AVM: ante-grade drifting technique. *Neuroradiol J*. 2020;33 (5):386-392.

[72] Lv X, Wu Z, Jiang C, et al. Angioarchitectural characteristics of brain AVMs with/without hemorrhage. *World Neurosurg*. 2011;76:95-99.

[73] Miao Z, Huo X. The future has come: current situation of endovascular treatment for acute ischemic stroke in China. *Chin J Stroke*. 2021;16 (11):1085-1090.

[74] Jiang W, Dai J, Du B, et al. Symptomatic intracranial artery stenosis stenting. *Chin J Neurosurg*. 2005;21 (2):75-79.

[75] Gao F, Du B. Apollo stents fill the domestic gap. *Chin Med J*. 2005;85 (17):1221.

[76] Huo X, Lv X. Mechanical thrombectomy. In: Lv X, Wang G, Wang J, eds. *Craniospinal Vascular Diseases and Endovascular Neurosurgery*. Nova Science; 2021:455-480.

[77] Lv X, He H, Wu Z. China's medical education and interventional neuroradiology training. *World Neurosurg*. 2015;84 (5):1462-1465.

[78] Cohen ER, Meyers PM, Lavine SD, Higashida RT. Historical account of interventional neuroradiology. In: Lanzer P, ed. *Textbook of Catheter-Based Cardiovascular Interventions*. Springer; 2018.

[79] Miyachi S, Okamoto T, Kobayashi N, et al. Nagoya university training system for neuroendovascular therapists. *Interv Neuroradiol*. 2004;10 (Suppl 1):103-106.

[80] Matsumaru Y, Hyodo A, Nose T, et al. Embolic materials for endovascular cerebral lesions. *J Biomater Sci Polym Ed*. 1997;8 (7):555-569.
[81] Touho H, Karasawa J, Ohnishi H, et al. Superselective embolization of spinal AVMs using Tracker catheter. *Surg Neurol*. 1992;38 (2):85-94.
[82] Miyachi S, Tanaka T, Kobayashi T, et al. Embolization of cerebral AVMs to enhance radiosurgery success. *Interv Neuroradiol*. 1998;4 (Suppl 1):121-126.
[83] Kobayashi S, Teramoto A. The current state of neurosurgery in Japan. *Neurosurgery*. 2002;51 (4):864-870.
[84] Ueno J, Sugiyama K, Naitou H, et al. Endovascular treatment for ruptured cerebral aneurysms in acute stage. *Interv Neuroradiol*. 1999;5 (Suppl 1):195-198.
[85] Oowaki H, Matsuda S, Sakai N, et al. Non-adhesive cyanoacrylate as embolic material. *Biomaterials*. 2000;21 (10):1039-1046.
[86] Haryu S, Sakata H, Matsumoto Y, et al. Endovascular treatment of wide-neck bifurcation aneurysm. *J Neuroendovasc Ther*. 2024;18 (3):75-83.
[87] Ebisudani Y, Sugiu K, Murai S, et al. Questionnaire survey of neurointerventional simulation training. *J Neuroendovasc Ther*. 2023;17 (9):181-187.
[88] Japanese Society for Neuroendovascular Therapy. *Documents & guidelines*. http://jsnet.website/documents.php?id=646.
[89] Hayakawa M. How interventional neurologists function in the clinical setting. *Rinsho Shinkeigaku*. 2013;53 (11):951-955.
[90] Sakai N, Yoshimura S, Taki W, et al. Recent trends in neuroendovascular therapy in Japan: JR-NET 1 and 2. *Neurol Med* Chir (Tokyo). 2014;54 (1):1-8.
[91] Zhao LB, Miyachi S, Shi HB, Suh DC. Comparison of medical education in interventional neuroradiology among China, Japan, and Korea. *Neurointervention*. 2013;8 (1):3-8.
[92] Korean Neuroendovascular Society. Official website. https://www.konesonline.or.kr/english/
[93] Kim TG, Kwon O, Shin YS, et al. Endovascular treatments by Korean neuroendovascular surgeons: nationwide survey. *J Korean Neurosurg Soc*. 2019;62 (5):502-518.
[94] Shin SH, Kwon SC, Suh DC. Recent update of guidelines for neurointerventional procedures. *Neurointervention*. 2013;8 (2):68-72.

Chapter 24

The History of Neurointervention in North America

Pouria Abolfazli[1,*]
Cristina Nkene Apue Nchama[1]
Mahonri Rushton[2]
Behnam Ahmadi[3]
and Brandon Lucke-Wold[4], MD

[1]College of Medicine, Xi'an Jiaotong University, Xi'an, China
[2]Utah Valley University, Orem, UT, USA
[3]Student Research Committee, Ahvaz Jundishapur University of Medical Sciences, Ahvaz, Iran
[4]University of Florida Department of Neurosurgery, Gainesville, FL, USA

Abstract

The history of neurointervention in North America began in the mid-20th century, with early interventions focused on open surgical procedures for conditions such as aneurysms and arteriovenous malformations (AVMs). This article explores the key milestones in the development of neurointervention in the U.S., highlighting advancements from early surgical interventions to the modern era of catheter-based techniques. In 1938, Dr. Walter Dandy performed the first successful surgical clipping of a cerebral aneurysm, particularly targeting internal carotid artery aneurysms, marking a critical milestone in vascular neurosurgery. In the 1970s, digital subtraction angiography (DSA) significantly advanced imaging technologies, improving the diagnosis and treatment of cerebrovascular conditions, particularly aneurysms and AVMs. Key innovations in the 1980s, such as the development of endovascular techniques and microcatheter systems, provided a safer and less invasive alternative to open surgery for conditions like AVMs and carotid-cavernous fistulas (CCFs). In the 1990s, advancements like balloon angioplasty and the Tracker Catheter System further revolutionized the field, enabling more precise treatment and enhancing clinical outcomes. The 2000s witnessed a significant shift in the treatment of aneurysms with the widespread adoption of coiling and the development of embolic agents, reducing the need for surgical clipping. More recently, the advent of thrombectomy devices has revolutionized acute stroke treatment, providing life-saving interventions for patients with large vessel occlusions. Today, neurointervention in North America stands at the intersection of neurosurgery, interventional radiology, and neurology, offering patients

* Corresponding Author's Email: Abolfazli.pouria@gmail.com

In: World History of Neurointerventional Surgery
Editors: Xianli Lv and Zhongxue Wu
ISBN: 979-8-89530-792-2

more effective and less invasive treatment options for complex cerebrovascular conditions. This article traces the history of neurointervention in the U.S., examining its transformative impact on the treatment of cerebrovascular diseases.

Keywords: neurovascular interventions, North America, endovascular neurosurgery, endovascular techniques

Introduction

Endovascular intervention for the diagnosis and treatment of disease of the nervous system has an evolving history in North America. This field is closely linked to the evolution of technology in medical imaging, and catheter-based therapies. Many of these developments unfolded on the global stage, but North America was pivotal to many and helped to define the trajectory of the field.

In 1938 Dr. Walter E. Dandy performed the first successful surgical clipping of a cerebral aneurysm [1]. This marked the birth of modern vascular neurosurgery. Dandy's technique involved isolating the aneurysm from the parent artery using a clip to prevent further blood flow into the weakened vessel [2]. His approach influenced later surgical strategies for aneurysm management. Despite its effectiveness, aneurysm clipping remained a highly invasive procedure, requiring a craniotomy and carrying significant risks such as brain tissue injury, vessel damage, and hemorrhage. Nonetheless, it became the gold standard for the treatment of aneurysms and laid the foundation for future advancements in neurovascular care.

In the mid-20th century, key advancements like angiography, introduced by Arthur Elvidge in the U.S., offered more accurate diagnoses for cerebrovascular diseases [3]. He also expanded on Bailey and Cushing's work on brain tumor, correlating clinical and histological data, and created an updated classification for neuroepithelial tumors, including a modern definition of glioblastoma multiforme [3]. By the 1950s, iodinated contrast agents improved patient safety, and in the 1970s, Digital Subtraction Angiography (DSA) revolutionized vascular imaging with real-time, high-contrast visualization [4, 5]. The rise of non-invasive imaging technologies such as CT and MRI in the late 1970s and 1980s further reshaped the field, offering clearer, non-invasive alternatives to older techniques [6-10].

The 1990s witnessed a breakthrough in endovascular treatment with Guido Guglielmi's development of the Guglielmi Detachable Coil (GDC), a safer, less invasive alternative to aneurysm clipping [11]. This innovation significantly improved patient outcomes and paved the way for the use of catheter-based interventions in treating a range of cerebrovascular disorders, including AVMs, ischemic stroke, and carotid-cavernous fistulas [12, 13]. By the 2010s, the advent of thrombectomy devices revolutionized stroke treatment, offering life-saving options for patients with acute ischemic stroke [14]. Balloon angioplasty and stenting also became essential tools in managing conditions like intracranial stenosis, further cementing the role of neurointervention in modern neurological care [15].

Today, neurointerventional surgery stands as a multidisciplinary field at the intersection of neurosurgery, interventional radiology, and neurology. The collaboration among these specialties ensures that patients benefit from broader treatment options, from surgical clipping to utilizing advanced endovascular techniques. As technology continues to evolve, neurointervention promises even greater precision, safety, and efficacy in managing complex cerebrovascular disorders. With innovations in imaging, catheter technology, and embolic agents, this field further advances, offering hope for even more patients in the future. In this article, we aim to explore the history of neurointervention in North America, tracing the development of the field and its profound impact on the treatment of cerebrovascular diseases.

Discussion

Foundational Developments in the Treatment of AVMs and AVFs

The history of neurointervention in the U.S. has been shaped by early work on AVMs and AVFs. In the early 20th century, Harvey Cushing and Bailey documented brain AVMs, noting their clinical symptoms such as seizures and hemorrhages [16]. Walter Dandy further advanced the field with his research and anatomical insights, recognizing AVMs as a distinct clinical entity requiring surgical intervention [17]. In the 1950s and 1960s, McKissock and Paterson published a series on 110 AVM cases, highlighting the variability of symptoms and the need for early diagnosis [18]. Pilcher in 1946 advocated for radical surgical removal of AVMs with severe symptoms, [19] while Pool in 1961 explored both surgical and conservative treatment options [20]. In addition to AVMs, early research on AVFs, particularly those involving the CCF, was essential in advancing neurointervention. Hanford and Wheeler in 1930 and Hamby and Gardner in 1933 contributed significantly to the treatment of these fistulas, focusing on surgical techniques such as the ligation of affected arteries. Their work provided crucial insights into the management of CCF [21-23].

While surgery played a central role in the treatment of AVMs and AVFs during the early decades of neurointervention, the field has since evolved with the introduction of minimally invasive endovascular techniques, which have reduced morbidity and mortality. In the early development of endovascular intracranial embolization, much of the pioneering work was initially focused on treating aneurysms. However, these techniques were later adapted for use in addressing AVMs and other intracranial vascular conditions. [24] In contrast to today's minimally invasive procedures, early embolization techniques relied on open surgical methods, which required direct puncture of target vessels for catheter and embolic material insertion. As a result, these early procedures were associated with high morbidity and mortality, much like the open neurosurgical techniques of that era. [24, 25] The foundation for endovascular treatment of AVMs was laid in the early 1960s, particularly through the work of Luessenhop and William Spence (1908–1992) in the United States, who proposed the concept of blocking hypertrophied, abnormal feeding vessels. [26] This approach, known as "artificial embolization," involved using embolic material to obstruct the enlarged feeding vessels without affecting the smaller vessels within the AVM nidus.

Emergence of Endovascular Treatments: A Paradigm Shift in Neurosurgery

The evolution of endovascular treatments for intracranial pathologies represents one of the most significant advancements in modern neurosurgery. Beginning in the mid-20th century, these minimally invasive techniques revolutionized the management of conditions such as aneurysms and AVMs [27]. From the early days of surgical clipping to the widespread adoption of coiling and embolization, endovascular treatments offered new options for patients, reducing morbidity and mortality while improving recovery times [27].

In the late 1970s and 1980s, the primary treatment for many non-CCF cranial dural arteriovenous fistulas (DAVFs) involved open surgery to disrupt the fistula connection and, in some cases, to resect the affected dura and venous sinus [28, 29]. These procedures were technically demanding and carried significant risks, including substantial blood loss, venous stroke, and other complications. Similar to AVM surgery, open surgery for DAVFs benefited from advancements in the operative microscope, microinstruments, and microsurgical techniques. While surgical intervention remains a key option for treating DAVFs today, endovascular embolization is now typically the first-line treatment at most institutions [30].

Building upon decades of foundational work, the evolution of neurointerventional techniques in the United States has led to significant advancements in the treatment of like aneurysms. In 1975, researchers at the University of Pittsburgh began developing a method to track the movement of catheters and guidewires. This technique, widely referred to as "road mapping," enabled the simultaneous display of a static subtracted image of the intracranial vessels alongside the real-time fluoroscopic view [31].

Neurointervention, which began as a relatively specialized and limited field, advancement significantly over the past few decades. These innovations, largely driven by research and clinical practice, have transformed patient care and treatment outcomes. an analysis by Lin and colleagues, published in the Journal of NeuroInterventional Surgery (JNIS) in 2012, revealed a significant increase in endovascular treatments between 1998 and 2007, with coiling rates rising from 9% to 21% for ruptured aneurysms and from 43% to 62% for unruptured cases. Importantly, their findings highlighted reduced disparities in treatment across demographics, hospital types, and regions, reflecting improved accessibility and uniform care delivery. Over the last decade, JNIS has played a critical role in driving neurointerventional innovation, ensuring that aneurysm management remains at the forefront of research and clinical practice [32].

From Embolization to Coiling

In 1960, Luessenhop and Spence performed the first successful embolization of a brain AVM using spherical methyl methacrylate emboli. [33] Building on this early work, Sergei Serbinenko in 1974 developed methods for endovascular balloon occlusion to treat AVMs and other cerebrovascular conditions [34]. His innovation included reporting endovascular treatment of over 300 patients using detachable and non-detachable balloons, initiated what became known as the "balloon era" in neuroendovascular therapy and had a profound influence on the global neurosurgical community [34]. His methods paved the way for significant advancements in North America. In Canada, Debrun, Viñuela, and Fox in London, Ontario, applied Serbinenko's techniques to perform proximal artery occlusion using detachable balloons for treating unclippable cerebral aneurysms. Their research demonstrated that this method was both safe and effective, achieving permanent occlusion in most cases and establishing it as a viable alternative to surgical clipping [35].

Kerber, based in Portland, further refined these methods in the 1970s by introducing a calibrated leak balloon microcatheter that allowed precise delivery of liquid embolic agents into AVM feeding arteries [36]. The 1980s and 1990s saw exponential progress in microcatheter design and embolic agents, enabling more effective and targeted treatments [37].

Later, in 1995, Neil Miller and his team in the Maryland reported the successful combined microsurgical-endovascular approach for treating CCFs, using the superior ophthalmic vein as an access route into the cavernous sinus [38].

The introduction of the Guglielmi Detachable Coil a breakthrough originated outside the United Statesin in 1991 marked a turning point in the treatment of intracranial aneurysms [11]. This device allowed for the safe and effective endovascular occlusion of aneurysms through coiling [11]. Coiling quickly gained traction as the preferred method for managing unruptured aneurysms and became a critical tool in the management of ruptured aneurysms as well. By the early 2000s, coiling had surpassed clipping as the leading treatment modality for intracranial aneurysms in the United States, with over 34,000 aneurysms treated with coiling between 2001 and 2008 compared to 29,866 managed with clipping [39, 40].

Expanding Endovascular Applications: AVMs and Other Pathologies

Endovascular techniques have not been limited to aneurysms. The management of AVMs has also benefited significantly from early advancements [41, 42]. In addition to embolization with liquid agents and coils, newer techniques involving Onyx, a liquid embolic agent, provided greater precision and control during AVM occlusion [43]. The refinement of these methods has allowed for pre-surgical embolization, reducing AVM size and minimizing bleeding risks during resection [44].

Beyond aneurysms and AVMs, endovascular treatments have expanded to address other cerebrovascular pathologies. For example, in the case of CCFs, endovascular occlusion using coils or liquid embolic agents has become the standard treatment for these abnormal connections between the carotid artery and the cavernous sinus [45]. Additionally. Stroke management has changed based upon the development of thrombectomy devices and stent retrievers in the 2010s. Endovascular thrombectomy, guided by advanced imaging and catheter techniques, allowed for the rapid removal of clots from large vessel occlusions, significantly improving outcomes for stroke patients [14]. In cases of intracranial stenosis the use of balloon angioplasty and stenting has provided effective treatment for patients with symptomatic intracranial atherosclerotic disease, reducing the risk of recurrent strokes [15].

The Introduction of Microcatheters and Embolic Agents

Higashida and colleagues explored the use of percutaneous balloon embolization to treat intracranial aneurysms while preserving the parent artery. The study included 84 patients and demonstrated that balloon embolization could successfully occlude aneurysms without damaging the parent vessel, thus offering a less invasive alternative to traditional surgical methods. This innovation expanded the potential for treating aneurysms in locations that were previously difficult to access or considered high-risk for surgery [46]. Additionally, their innovative efforts extended to posterior circulation aneurysms, where direct balloon embolization or parent vessel occlusion was performed, demonstrating the potential of these methods as alternatives for surgically complex cases [47].

Meanwhile, in a related study conducted San Francisco by Hieshima, Higashida, and Halbach, who focused on endovascular embolization of intracranial aneurysms, particularly in surgically challenging locations such as the cavernous segment of the internal carotid artery. Between 1981 and 1989, their team utilized endovascular detachable balloon techniques to treat 87 patients with intracavernous aneurysms of the internal carotid artery [48].

The Tracker Catheter System, developed and mass-produced by Target Therapeutics in Fremont, California, in 1986, revolutionized endovascular treatment by providing the first alternative to balloon-directed catheters. It enabled more precise navigation with advanced guidewires, enhancing the consistency and effectiveness of endovascular procedures [49].

A major advancement behind this system was the work of engineer Engelson, who addressed the challenges of neurovascular navigation. He developed a variable-stiffness microcatheter with a radiopaque marker at its tip, which was steam-shapeable for greater adaptability. In addition, he introduced a steerable micro-guidewire featuring a deformable, shapeable tip that could maneuver through complex vascular bends and bifurcations. These innovations led to the creation of the "over-the-wire Tracker" microcatheter, which became the ideal delivery system for detachable coils and transformed the catheterization of cerebral arteries, marking a key milestone in endovascular treatment [50].

In 1976, the "Gianturco coils," small stainless steel coils with the inner core removed, were first introduced as embolic materials [51]. Originally, they were used for the treatment of renal arteriovenous fistulas and various tumors. Over time, their application in expanded, particularly in transvenous procedures like the treatment of dural fistulas and carotid-CCF [52]. Furthermore, one of the earliest tissue adhesives used as an embolic material was IBCA (isobutyl-2-cyanoacrylate), [53] first described in 1972 by Zanetti and Sherman in the University of Pittsburgh School of Medicine for embolizing renal arteries and surgically created aneurysms in dogs [54]. IBCA is injected through a microcatheter and quickly polymerizes upon contact with blood, which can sometimes lead to catheter adhesion within the feeding artery. Despite this rapid polymerization, retained catheters have generally been well tolerated, with only a few reports of thrombotic or neurological issues arising from this complication [55].

In 1990 Onyx (Micro Therapeutics, Inc., Irvine, CA) was first described by Taki et al. [56] and Terada et al. [57] from Japan. Onyx is a liquid embolic agent made from a combination of ethylene-vinyl alcohol copolymer and dimethyl sulfoxide (DMSO). It is used in endovascular procedures to block blood flow in specific vessels, such as in treating aneurysms or AVMs. The copolymer solidifies upon contact with blood, while DMSO keeps it in liquid form for precise delivery [58].

Conclusion

The history of neurointervention in North America has advanced by continuous discoveries in imaging technologies and minimally invasive techniques, transforming the management of cerebrovascular diseases. From the early introduction of cerebral angiography to the developments such as DSA, microcatheters, and embolic agents, the field has steadily moved toward safer, more precise treatments. The introduction of endovascular coiling, embolization techniques, and thrombectomy devices has significantly reduced the need for invasive surgeries, offering improved outcomes and faster recovery times for patients with conditions such as aneurysms, AVMs, and acute ischemic stroke. Furthermore, the expansion of neurointerventional treatments to address other pathologies like CCFs and intracranial stenosis has further solidified the role of endovascular approaches in modern neurological care. As the field continues to evolve with innovations in imaging, catheter technology, and therapeutic agents, the future of neurointervention promises even greater precision, safety, and efficacy, ensuring that patients with complex cerebrovascular diseases continue to benefit from advanced, less invasive treatment options.

References

[1] Kretzer RM, Coon AL, Tamargo RJ. Walter E. Dandy's contributions to vascular neurosurgery. *J Neurosurg*. 2010;112 (6):1182-1191.

[2] Dandy WE. Intracranial aneurysm of the internal carotid artery: cured by operation. *Ann Surg*. 1938;107 (5):654-659.

[3] Preul MC, et al. Arthur Roland Elvidge (1899–1985): contributions to diagnosis of brain tumors and cerebrovascular disease. *J Neurosurg*. 1998;88 (1):162-171.

[4] Tondreau RL. The retrospectoscope: Egas Moniz 1874–1955. *Radiographics*. 1985;5 (6):994-997.

[5] Crummy AB, Strother CM, Mistretta CA. The history of digital subtraction angiography. *J Vasc Interv Radiol*. 2018;29 (8):1138-1141.

[6] Webb S. Historical experiments predating commercially available computed tomography. *Br J Radiol*. 1992;65 (777):835-837.

[7] Castillo M. History and evolution of brain tumor imaging: insights through radiology. *Radiology*. 2014;273 (2S):S111-S125.

[8] Abbara S, Shaw LJ. Past, present, and future of CTA. *Circulation*. 2024;150 (2):87-90.

[9] Clow H, Young I. Britain's brains produce first NMR scans. *New Scientist*. 1978;80 (588):26.

[10] Hartung MP, Grist TJ, François CJ. Magnetic resonance angiography: current status and future directions. *J Cardiovasc Magn Reson*. 2011;13 (1):19.

[11] Dovey Z, et al. Guglielmi detachable coiling for intracranial aneurysms: the story so far. *Arch Neurol*. 2001;58 (4):559-564.

[12] Richling B. History of endovascular surgery: personal accounts of the evolution. *Neurosurgery*. 2006;59 (5):S3-30-S3-38.

[13] Loh Y, Duckwiler GR. A prospective trial of Onyx vs NBCA for cerebral AVM embolization. *J Neurosurg*. 2010;113 (4):733-741.

[14] Goyal M, et al. Endovascular thrombectomy after large-vessel ischaemic stroke: meta-analysis. *Lancet*. 2016;387 (10029):1723-1731.

[15] Luo J, Wang T, Gao P, Krings T, Jiao L. Endovascular treatment of intracranial atherosclerotic stenosis: current debates and future prospects. *Front Neurol*. 2018;9:666.

[16] Harvey SC. Tumors arising from the blood-vessels of the brain: angiomatous malformations and hemangioblastomas. *Yale J Biol Med*. 1930;2:403-405.

[17] Dandy WE. Arteriovenous aneurysm of the brain. *Arch Surg*. 1928;17:190-243.

[18] McKissock W, Paterson JH. A clinical survey of intracranial angiomas. *Brain*. 1956;79 (2):233-266.

[19] Pilcher C. Angiomatous malformations of the brain: successful extirpation in three cases. *Ann Surg*. 1946;123:766-784.

[20] Pool JL. Treatment of arteriovenous malformations of the cerebral hemispheres. J Neurosurg. 1962;19:136-141.

[21] Hamby WB. Carotid-cavernous fistula: report of 32 surgically treated cases. *J Neurosurg*. 1964;21:859-866.

[22] Hamby WB, Gardner WJ. Treatment of pulsating exophthalmus: report of two cases. *Arch Surg*. 1933;27 (4):676-685.

[23] Hanford JM, Wheeler JM. Pulsating exophthalmus. *Ann Surg*. 1930;92 (1):8-22.

[24] Bristol RE, Albuquerque FC, McDougall CG. Evolution of endovascular treatment for intracranial AVMs. *Neurosurg Focus*. 2006;20 (6):1-5.

[25] Kanaan Y, Kaneshiro D, Fraser K, Wang D, Lanzino G. Evolution of endovascular therapy for aneurysm treatment—historical overview. *Neurosurg Focus*. 2005;18 (2):E2.
[26] Luessenhop AJ, Spence WT. Artificial embolization of cerebral arteries. *JAMA*. 1960;172 (11):1153-1155.
[27] Agner C, Dujovny M. Historical evolution of neuroendovascular surgery of intracranial aneurysms. *Neurol Res*. 2009;31 (6):632-637.
[28] Sundt TM, Piepgras DG. Surgical approach to AVMs of the lateral and sigmoid dural sinuses. *J Neurosurg*. 1983;59 (1):32-39.
[29] Hugosson R, Bergström K. Surgical treatment of dural AVMs of the sigmoid sinus. *J Neurol Neurosurg Psychiatry*. 1974;37 (1):97-101.
[30] Giannopoulos S, et al. Treatment of ethmoidal dural AVFs: meta-analysis. *World Neurosurg*. 2019;128:593-599.e1.
[31] Horowitz M, et al. An endovascular primate model for MCA infarction. *Interv Neuroradiol*. 2001;7 (3):223-228.
[32] Lin N, et al. Treatment of ruptured and unruptured cerebral aneurysms in the USA: paradigm shift. *J Neurointerv Surg*. 2012;4 (3):182-189.
[33] Luessenhop AJ, Spence WT. Artificial embolization of cerebral arteries. *JAMA*. 1960;172:1153-1155.
[34] Serbinenko FA. Balloon catheterization and occlusion of major cerebral vessels. J Neurosurg. 1974;41 (2):125-145.
[35] Fox AJ, et al. Use of detachable balloons for proximal artery occlusion in unclippable cerebral aneurysms. *J Neurosurg*. 1987;66 (1):40-46.
[36] Kerber C. Balloon catheter with a calibrated leak. *Radiology*. 1976;120 (3):547-550.
[37] Triano MJ, et al. Embolic agents and microcatheters for cerebral AVMs. *World Neurosurg*. 2020;141:383-388.
[38] Miller NR, et al. Treatment of carotid-cavernous fistulas via superior ophthalmic vein. J Neurosurg. 1995;83 (5):838-842.
[39] Nasra M, et al. Clipping vs coiling: critical re-examination. *Interv Neuroradiol*. 2024;30 (1):86-93.
[40] Brinjikji W, et al. Effect of age on outcomes of unruptured cerebral aneurysms. *Stroke*. 2011;42 (5):1320-1324.
[41] El-Abtah ME, et al. Endovascular management of AVM-associated intracranial aneurysms. *World Neurosurg*. 2022;164:257-269.
[42] Ognard J, et al. Endovascular management of brain arteriovenous malformations. *Semin Neurol*. 2023;43 (3):323-336.
[43] Ayad M, Eskioglu E, Mericle RA. Onyx: a unique neuroembolic agent. *Expert Rev Med Devices*. 2006;3 (6):705-715.
[44] Ozden M, et al. Surgery in intracerebral AVMs: role of preoperative embolization. *Turk Neurosu*rg. 2023;33 (6).
[45] Gemmete JJ, Ansari SA, Gandhi DM. Endovascular techniques for carotid-cavernous fistula. *J Neuroophthalmol*. 2009;29 (1):62-71.
[46] Higashida RT, et al. Percutaneous balloon embolization of intracranial aneurysms with parent-vessel preservation. *AJNR Am J Neuroradiol*. 1990;11 (4):633-640.
[47] Higashida RT, et al. Detachable balloon therapy of posterior-circulation aneurysms. *J Neurosurg*. 1989;71 (4):512-519.
[48] Higashida RT, et al. Endovascular detachable balloon therapy of cavernous carotid aneurysms. *J Neurosurg*. 1990;72 (6):857-863.
[49] Kerber CW, et al. Rapid intracranial clot removal with the Alligator Retriever. *AJNR Am J Neuroradiol*. 2007;28 (5):860-863.
[50] Engelson ET. Catheter for guide-wire tracking. *US Patent* 4,739,768; 1988.
[51] Wallace S, et al. Therapeutic vascular occlusion utilizing steel coil technique. *AJR Am J Roentgenol*. 1976;127 (3):381-387.
[52] Halbach VV, et al. Transvenous embolization of dural fistulas involving cavernous sinus. *AJNR Am J Neuroradiol*. 1989;10 (2):377-383.

[53] Bank WO, et al. Treatment of cerebral AVMs with isobutyl 2-cyanoacrylate. *Radiology*. 1981;139 (3):609-616.

[54] Zanetti PH, Sherman FE. Experimental evaluation of tissue adhesive for aneurysms. *J Neurosurg*. 1972;36 (1):72-79.

[55] Debrun GM, et al. Glued catheters during embolisation of brain AVMs with acrylic glue. *Interv Neuroradiol*. 1997;3 (1):13-19.

[56] Yamashita K, et al. Characteristics of ethylene vinyl alcohol copolymer (EVAL) mixtures. *AJNR Am J Neuroradiol*. 1994;15 (6):1103-1105.

[57] Terada T, et al. Embolization of AVMs with peripheral aneurysms using EVOH. *J Neurosurg*. 1991;75 (4):655-660.

[58] Szajner M, et al. Onyx in endovascular treatment of cerebral AVMs. *Pol J Radiol*. 2013;78 (3):35-41.

Chapter 25

The Evolution of Endovascular Neurosurgery in India: A Historical Overview

Arunkumar Sekar[1,*]
and Nandita Kujur[2]
[1]Department of Neurosurgery, All India Institute of Medical Sciences, Bhubaneswar, India
[2]Endovascular Neurosurgery, Department of Neurosurgery, All India Institute of Medical Sciences, Bhubaneswar, India

Abstract

The history of endovascular neurosurgery in India reflects the significant advancements driven by pioneering neurosurgeons and neuroradiologists. The foundation of neuroradiology in India was laid in the early 1950s, with the first percutaneous carotid angiography performed in 1952 by Professor Dr. B. Ramamurthy and Dr. Mahadevan Pillai. This early work established the stage for the development of endovascular techniques. In the 1970s and the 1980s, transfemoral angiography and interventional procedures emerged. Pandya et al. contributed to the growth of this field. The establishment of interventional neuroradiology departments at institutions such as the NIMHANS, SCTIMST, and AIIMS further advanced diagnostic and therapeutic capabilities.

A pivotal figure in the growth of endovascular neurosurgery in India is Professor Dr. Karapurkar, who, after training in France and Canada, introduced modern vascular neurosurgical techniques in India. Over the decades, improved hardware, including high-resolution biplane imaging, and innovations, such as stent-assisted coiling, have expanded the scope of treatable conditions.

Currently, endovascular neurosurgery in India is used to treat a wide range of conditions, including stroke, aneurysm, AVMs, and tumors. The establishment of accredited training programs, such as the National Board of Education's 2-year fellowship in interventional neuroradiology, promises to further enhance the field. Despite challenges, such as cost and access, India's journey in endovascular neurosurgery continues to be marked by progress and global leadership.

Keywords: history, evolution, endovascular neurosurgery, India

---

* Corresponding Author's Email: neurosurg_arun@aiimsbhubaneswar.edu.in

In: World History of Neurointerventional Surgery
Editors: Xianli Lv and Zhongxue Wu
ISBN: 979-8-89530-792-2

Introduction

The history of endovascular neurosurgery in India is a story of remarkable evolution, driven by innovation, perseverance, and collaboration among pioneers in the fields of neurosurgery and neuroradiology. From its humble beginnings in the mid-20th century to its current state as a cutting-edge subspecialty, endovascular neurosurgery has significantly transformed the treatment of complex neurological conditions, including aneurysms, arteriovenous malformations (AVMs), and ischemic strokes, among others.

Early Beginnings in Neuroradiology (1950s - 1960s) [1, 2]

The roots of endovascular neurosurgery in India were traced back to the 1950s, when neuroradiology was established as a distinct discipline. In 1952, the first percutaneous direct carotid angiography was performed in India, which marked a pivotal moment in the country's neurosurgical landscape. This achievement came from the collaborative efforts of Professor Ramamurthy, a pioneering neurosurgeon, and Dr. Mahadevan Pillai, a radiologist trained in England. Dr. Pillai's work on diagnostic imaging, especially in cerebral angiography, laid the foundation for the eventual development of therapeutic endovascular procedures.

In 1958, Dr. Pillai and Dr. Ramamurthy published a review of the first 1,000 diagnostic angiograms, which became a cornerstone in the field's growth. Dr. Pillai later moved to the National Institute of Mental Health and Neurosciences (NIMHANS) in Bangalore, where he established the Department of Neuroradiology in 1958, further advancing diagnostic capabilities and contributing to the development of therapeutic neurointerventions.

Rise of Endovascular Neurosurgery (1970s - 1980s)

While early efforts were primarily focused on diagnostic angiography, the true emergence of endovascular neurosurgery occurred in the 1970s and the 1980s, when interventional procedures began to take root. Dr. S. K. Pandya, a key figure in the field, introduced transfemoral angiography at King Edward Memorial Hospital (KEM) in Mumbai in 1976, under the guidance of Dr. Mutjaba Tayabali, a radiologist who had been trained in the UK. This innovation opened the door to performing interventional procedures, a practice that would gradually grow in India in the following decades.

In the late 1970s, Dr R. K Goulatia and Dr N. K. Mishra of All India Institute of Medical Sciences (AIIMS) in Delhi and DR V. R. K Rao at Sree Chitra Tirunal Institute for Medical Sciences and Technology (SCTIMST) in Thiruvananthapuram started offering advanced diagnostic and therapeutic angiography, including the early stages of interventional neurovascular procedures.

Pioneering Endovascular Neurosurgeons [2]

Professor Dr. Anil Karapurkar was one of the most significant contributors to the development of endovascular neurosurgery in India. After completing his neurosurgical training in 1975, Professor Karapurkar developed a strong interest in vascular neurosurgery. In 1980, he trained under Professor Bernard Pertuiset at La Pitié-Salpêtrière Hospital in Paris, an institution with expertise in vascular neurosurgery. He also trained under Professor Luc Picard in neuroradiology at Nancy, France and spent time with Professor Charles Drake in Canada, who was instrumental in advancing the field of vascular neurosurgery.

Professor Karapurkar's work in India revolutionized the practice of endovascular neurosurgery, especially with his emphasis on minimally invasive procedures. He adopted and actively propagated the use of new techniques and tools such as the telescoping guide catheter and liquid embolic materials such as isobutyl-2-cyanoacrylate, which replaced earlier methods such as sialic spheres. His department at KEM Hospital became a center of excellence, and he was instrumental in advancing the use of embolization techniques for treating conditions, such as intracranial aneurysms, arteriovenous malformations (AVMs), and tumors.

The Expansion of Interventional Procedures (1990s - Early 2000s)

As the availability of medical technology improved during the 1990s, the range of treatable conditions expanded significantly. Guglielmi detachable coils (GDC) have become available for the treatment of aneurysms, which is a significant advancement in the field. Other innovations include balloon remodeling for aneurysms (introduced in 1999), stent-assisted coiling, and the advent of carotid stents in 2002.

The introduction of Onyx, an advanced embolic agent for the embolization of AVMs and fistulas, in 2005, further revolutionized the treatment landscape in India. Indian neurosurgeons, including Professor Karapurkar and others, have received training in Ankara, Turkey, to master the use of this novel embolic material.

By the late 2000s, the imaging equipment used for endovascular procedures had also significantly improved. Less efficient biplane machines with low-resolution images were replaced by high-quality flat-panel biplane angiography machines, offering clearer images and real-time subtraction techniques.

Broadening the Scope of Endovascular Neurosurgery (2000s - Present) [3]

With the advent of more refined tools and techniques, the scope of conditions treated with endovascular neurosurgery in India has expanded dramatically. Acute ischemic strokes, intracranial aneurysms, brain and spinal AVMs, angioplasty, stenting, tumor embolization, thrombolysis, and venous stenting for idiopathic intracranial hypertension are now regularly treated using endovascular procedures.

By 2020, the National Board of Education accredited a 2-year program in interventional neuroradiology aimed at training both neurosurgeons and neurologists. This program, along with other post-doctoral fellowships in prominent institutions, including our current workplace, has been pivotal in the development of specialized expertise in India.

Challenges and Future Directions

Despite considerable progress, endovascular neurosurgery in India still faces several challenges. The high costs of medical equipment and treatment coupled with regional disparities in healthcare infrastructure mean that access to advanced care remains limited, particularly in rural areas. Furthermore, the field's growth is hindered by the lack of standardized training programs, although the recent establishment of dedicated fellowships and training programs is a positive step toward improving the situation.

As the field continues to evolve, India's contributions to endovascular neurosurgery will likely remain at the forefront of innovation with growing access to state-of-the-art technology and increased collaboration between international and Indian institutions.

Conclusion

India's journey in this field reflects a blend of innovation, dedication, and collaboration from its first diagnostic angiogram in 1952 to the present-day practice of complex endovascular neurosurgery. The contributions of pioneering neurosurgeons, neuroradiologists, and institutions have paved the way for India to become a global leader in vascular neurosurgery. As technologies continue to evolve and training programs become more standardized, India will undoubtedly remain at the cutting edge of endovascular neurosurgical practices.

References

[1] Karapurkar AP. Our experiences with neurovascular intervention at King Edward VII Memorial Hospital, Mumbai 1976-1996. *Neurol India*. 2021 Jan-Feb;69 (1):4-11.

[2] Anonymous. Cerebral angiography: a review of 1000 cases. *Neurol India*. 1958;6:38-41.

[3] Chaganty SS, Ozair A, Rahman F. State of accredited endovascular neurosurgery training in India in 2021: challenges to capacity building in subspecialty neurosurgical care. *Front Surg*. 2021 Aug 31;8:705246.

Chapter 26

The History of Interventional Neuroradiology and the Latino-American Contribution

Angel Ferrario[1]
Pablo Villanueva[2,*]
Villa Platas[3]
and Alery Liebet[3]
[1]Department of Interventional Neuroradiology, FLENI institute, Buenos Aires, Argentina
[2]Hospital Regional Ramon Carrillo, Neuquen, Argentina
[3]Universidad Nacional Autónoma de México, Distrito Federal, Mexico

Abstract

Interventional neuroradiology is a relatively new term in the field of neuroscience, but it has a rich history that is closely linked to significant developments in radiology, neurology, neurosurgery, and neuroethics. Understanding this history is essential for readers to appreciate how the practice has evolved over time, the importance of technological advancements, and the ongoing effort to balance the advantages and disadvantages of these procedures. This balancing act is crucial as it can lead to drastically different decisions based on varying social and economic contexts.

The purpose of this chapter is to outline the evolution of interventional neuroradiology from its inception, highlighting key milestones, its impacts, and future prospects for this minimally invasive method. Numerous countries have played pivotal roles in developing techniques and advancing technology in this field, driving it towards greater independence and the emergence of specialized operators. Regions such as France, China, Russia, the USA, Argentina, and Mexico have contributed unique conceptual and technical innovations that have shaped the history of interventional neuroradiology in diverse ways, while still aiming for the same goals. This paper will provide a brief overview of some of these regional developments.

Keywords: interventional neuroradiology, history, neuroethics, Latin-America contribution

---

* Corresponding Author's Email: pvillanuevach@gmail.com

In: World History of Neurointerventional Surgery
Editors: Xianli Lv and Zhongxue Wu
ISBN: 979-8-89530-792-2

Introduction: The Concept

Interventional neuroradiology (INR), also known as neurointerventional surgery (NIS), endovascular therapy (EVT), endovascular neurosurgery, and interventional neurology, is a medical subspecialty that combines elements of neurosurgery, neuroradiology, interventional radiology, and neurology. This field specializes in the use of minimally invasive, image-guided techniques and procedures for the diagnosis and treatment of diseases affecting the head, neck, and spine [1].

The term "neurointerventionism" is a compound word: "neuro" refers to the specific tissues and organs that are the focus of diagnosis and treatment in this field. While it might seem obvious, part of the history involves a distinct separation from general radiologic interventionism, which existed earlier and previously included interventions within the neurological system. "Interventionism," on the other hand, represents a set of minimally invasive procedures primarily utilized through direct percutaneous puncture and catheterization, with fluoroscopy serving as the main imaging method during these procedures.

Following this opening paragraph, we can highlight several key aspects related to the history of this field:

- A shared root with radiology
- The evolving technology that serves as a major facilitator for the development of new procedures
- The necessity for sub-specialization to address specific needs, analyses, and protocols

A timeline can be created, detailing significant events from these areas. This timeline will serve as a guide to understanding the fascinating and rapidly evolving history of Interventional Neuroradiology.

The Roots

As it is precisely written at The British Institute of Radiology's article:

> 'Medical radiology has now existed for over a century. It all started in 1895 when Wilhelm Rönt, (Wilhelm Conrad Röntgen) discovered x-rays (figure 1). On 28 December 1895 his manuscript "On a New Kind of Ray" was submitted to the Würzburg Physical Medical Institute.
> The essential features of x-rays were described and the new discovery aroused tremendous interest. Because the apparatus was readily available in most physics departments his results could easily be repeated. The apparatus gradually improved and hospitals started to acquire the equipment' [2].

Even since that early stages, the concept of "apparatus" has been closely linked to radiology, along with its development and progress.

In the previously named article [2], several noteworthy individuals in the field of radiology are highlighted. They were making strides in the neurological field by utilizing various techniques, such as A. Schüller's work on sub-arachnoid cisterns and their demonstration using a positive contrast agent, and E. Lysholm's (Figure 2) research on sub-tentorial tumors. Additionally, H. Kemp has explored the risks associated with ionic contrast agents and thrombosis, while E. Barclay has contributed to improvements in cine-radiology, among others.

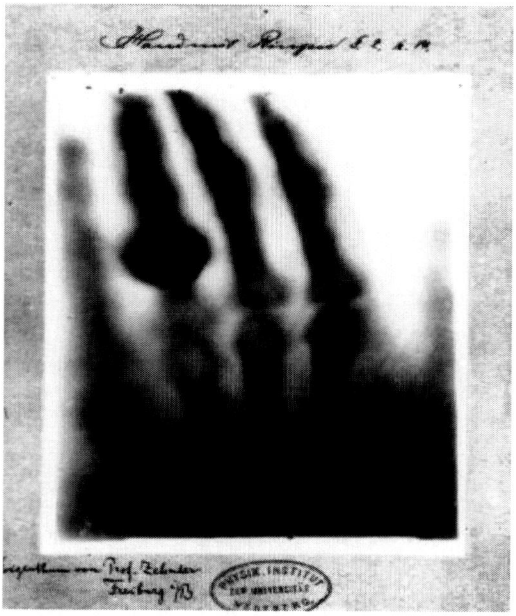

Anna Bertha Ludwing's hand. The first X ray, showing Wilhelm Röntgen's wife as model. Freigburg University. January 1896.

Figure 1. Beginning of X-Ray era.

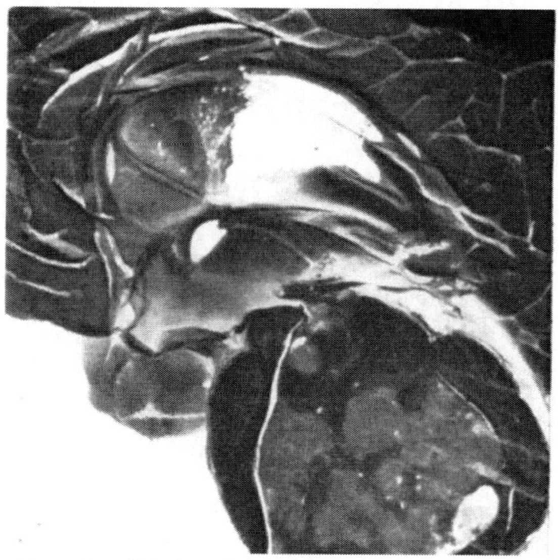

Erik Lysholm, Stockholm, Sweeden. Mackenzie Davidson Memorial Lecture, 1946 about sub-tentorial tumors using contrast agents.

Figure 2. One of the first images showing brain tumors using contrast agents.

The early years of the 20th century saw significant progress in the era of X-rays; however, this topic is beyond the scope of this chapter. Instead, we will focus on Interventional Neuroradiology, which will be discussed in the following sections.

The Interventional Neuroradiology on Its Own Pathway

Cerebral angiography was developed by the Portuguese neurologist Egas Moniz at the University of Lisbon to identify diseases of the central nervous system, such as tumors and arteriovenous malformations. In 1927, he performed the first brain angiography (Figure 3) in Lisbon by injecting an iodinated contrast medium into the internal carotid artery and using X-rays to visualize the cerebral vessels [3]. Before the advent of CT and MRI imaging, this technique was the only method available for observing structures within the skull and was also employed to diagnose extravascular pathologies.

Moniz's work not only led to significant advancements in the technique itself but also had a profound impact on clinical practice, including its indications, risks, and benefits. Furthermore, it contributed to the teaching of anatomy and revealed anatomical details that were previously unknown, which Moniz referred to as "encéphalographie artérielle."

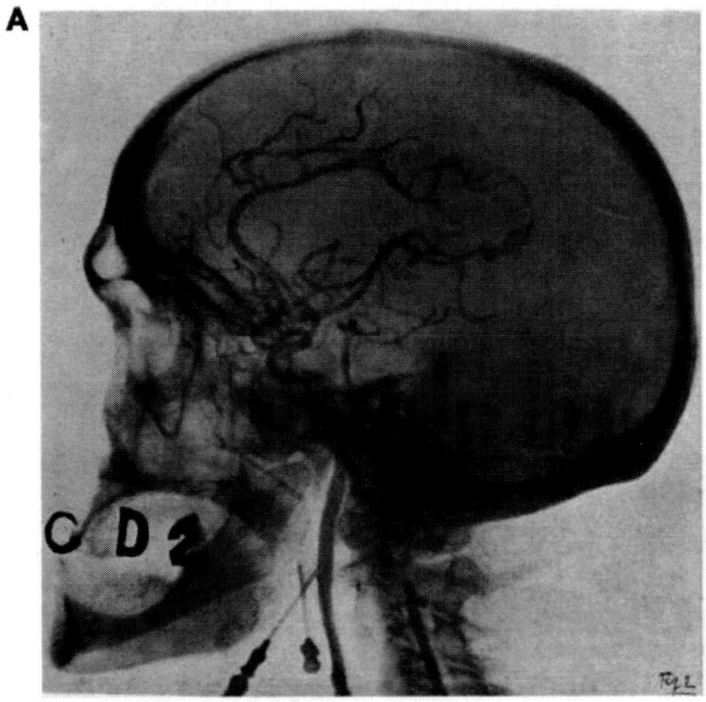

"L'encéphalographie artérielle, son importance dans la localization des tumeurs cérébrales," Egas Moniz (de Lisbon), Nuerology society, July 1927.

Figure 3. First angiography by Carotid access.

European radiologists advanced angiographic techniques by replacing the traumatic direct puncture method with catheterization. In 1953, Swedish physician Sven Ivar Seldinger introduced the arterial and venous catheterization technique, now known as the Seldinger Technique [4].

The many advantages of the Seldinger technique are best encapsulated by the author's own words, which he used to begin his publication, reflecting on the origins of this method.

> '... 1) The contrast medium may be injected into a vessel at any level desired. 2) Risk of extravascular injection of the contrast medium is minimized. 3) The patient may be placed in any position required. 4) The catheter may be left in situ without risk while the films are being developed, thus facilitating re-examination if necessary.
> Until recently, however, the use of the catheter method was restricted because of the lack of a suitable flexible thin-walled catheter which could be used percutaneously. FARINAS, in 1941, described a method in which a urethral catheter was passed up into the aorta through a trocar inserted in the exposed femoral artery. In 1947, RADNER catheterized the exposed and ligated radial artery and performed vertebral angiography and later thoracic aortography. Since then, many authors have catheterized arteries for various purposes, by surgical exposure followed by ligature or suturing of the artery. In 1949, JONSSON performed thoracic aortography after puncture of the common carotid artery by means of a blunt cannula provided with an inner sharp needle.' [4].

It is remarkable how a current issue was addressed by Seldinger in 1953. The lack of proper technology and the varying levels of availability between medical centers have not disappeared. It seems that history was conveying a message not only about technique but also about logistics, equity, and accessibility. The challenges of neuroethics that existed during that time are still present today.

In 1964, the Norwegian radiologist Per Amudsen became the first to perform a complete brain angiography using a transfemoral approach, which is still the standard today. He later moved to San Francisco to teach this technique to American neuroradiologists [5]. These advancements laid the groundwork for modern invasive vascular diagnostics and the subsequent therapeutic developments.

Charles Dotter, known as the father of angioplasty and considered by many to be the pioneer of all interventional radiology, was the first to carry out a true endovascular procedure. On January 16, 1964, he performed a therapeutic angioplasty on a superficial femoral artery [6].

However, Dotter's contributions extended beyond catheter manipulation. His work represents one of the most significant milestones in the history of interventional radiology, as he explored limits and sought ways to transcend them. In 1950, Dotter developed an automatic X-ray roll-film magazine capable of producing images at a rate of two per second [6], highlighting his innovative spirit.

> 'My favorite conceptual trademark is a sketch that I did years ago of a crossed pipe and wrench (Figure 4). It's a gross over simplification, of course, but what it means to me is that if a plumber can do it to pipes, we can do it to blood vessels.' (Charles Dotter)

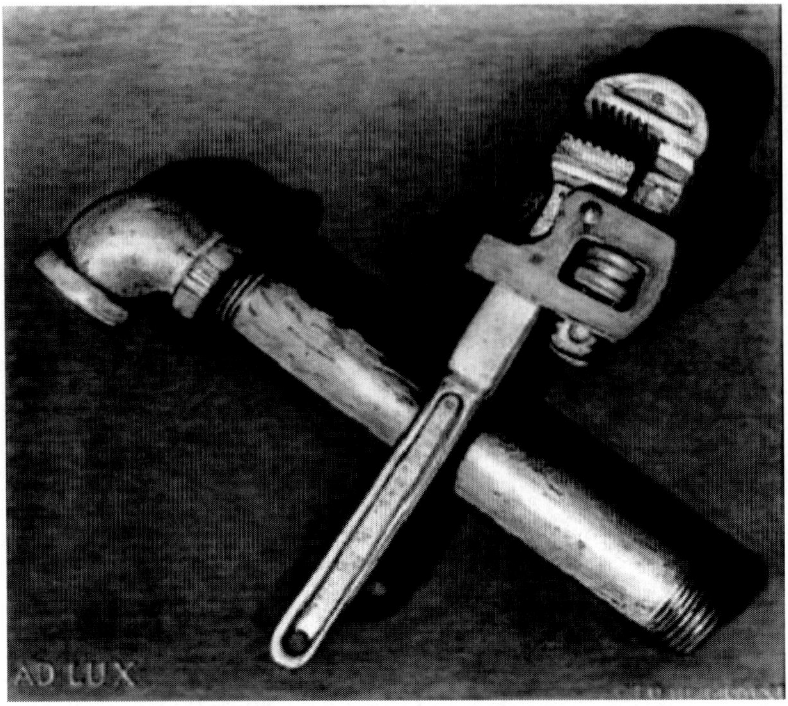

Charles Dotter minimalistic concept of what can be done with blood vessels in 1950s.

Figure 4. Charles Dotter trademark concept.

In the 1970s, Fedor Serbinenko, a Russian neurosurgeon, developed a technique for closing intracranial aneurysms using balloons that were introduced into the internal carotid artery by occluding the lumen [7]. The first procedure took place in 1970 in Moscow when he occluded an internal carotid artery to treat a carotid-cavernous fistula. Therefore, he can be regarded as the first interventional neuroradiologist.

The idea of using balloons to treat cerebrovascular lesions was inspired by a May Day celebration in Red Square, Moscow, in 1959. While observing children using tether lines to manipulate helium balloons, Dr. Serbinenko envisioned small balloons navigating through tortuous arteries. His research on this subject was published in Russian literature in 1971 and 1974 in the Journal of Neurosurgery.

This technique was later refined by neuroradiologists around the world, particularly in France, where interventional neuroradiology (INR) developed significantly. A special mention should be made of Rene Djindjian, former Professor and Chief of the Department of Neuroradiology at Hôpital Lariboisière in Paris, for his contributions to understanding neurovascular diseases of the spinal cord during this pivotal period in the history of INR.

Dr. Djindjian implemented the relatively new technique of selective angiography to study the spinal cord and its diseases [8]. His contributions are well-documented through numerous peer-reviewed papers and his classic text, "L'Angiographie De La Moelle Epinière" (Angiography of the Spinal Cord), which he co-authored with Hurth and Houdart. The preface of this work was written by Guy Lazorthes, former Chief of Neurosurgery and Dean of the University of Medicine and Pharmacy of Toulouse. It was translated into English by Irvin I. Kricheff (New York) and published in 1970.

Pierre Lasjaunias, a neuroanatomist, published his first book on Interventional Neuroradiology titled "Surgical Neuroangiography" in 1986. While this book conveyed a singular message, it showcased Lasjaunias's significant influence in the field of Interventional Neuroradiology, earning him recognition and affection worldwide. He was named Visiting Professor in London, Berlin, New York, and Toronto. In 1998, he received honorary membership from the American Society of Neuroradiology. Additionally, one of his later articles, titled "Cerebral Proliferative Angiopathy," was published in Stroke magazine. This original work stemmed from careful analysis and extensive discussions with colleagues, leading to the identification of a new entity distinct from other brain arteriovenous malformations.

It's important to acknowledge the significant contributions of several French authors to the field and their historical impact. The Cognard classification of dural arteriovenous fistulas (dAVFs) is based on the direction of dural sinus drainage, the presence or absence of cortical venous drainage, and the architecture of venous outflow, which can include non-ectatic cortical veins, ectatic cortical veins, or spinal perimedullary veins [9].

Jacques Moret developed the balloon-assisted technique for treating wide-neck intracranial aneurysms. Charbel Mounayer has published numerous works on the treatment of arteriovenous malformations (AVMs) via the venous route. René Chapot described the pressure cooker technique for the treatment of cerebral AVMs.

Looking back, as technological advancements progressed alongside the development of catheters, imaging technology also saw dramatic improvements. In 1979, Charles Mistretta invented digital subtraction angiography (DSA), a technique that is widely used today. This method involves taking skull radiography under standard conditions, which are then "subtracted" after contrast media is injected. As a result, an image is produced that displays only the brain's blood vessels, significantly enhancing diagnostic capabilities.

Mistretta's findings and the recognition gained by the subtraction method (figure 5) led to patients frequently requesting to have their angiograms performed by him. On one occasion, despite Dr. Strother explaining that Chuck (Charles Mistretta) was not a physician, a patient remarked, "When I go to Rome, I want to see the Pope [10]."

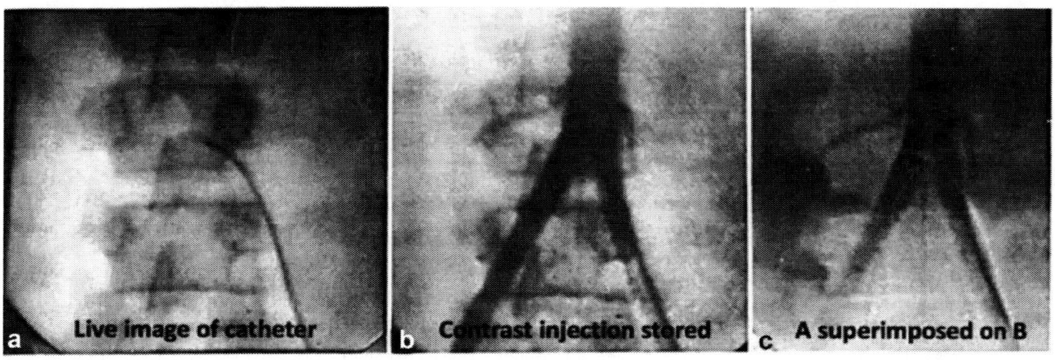

From "An Inexpensive Storage System for Selective Catheterization Procedures." Radiology llO: 3G9-372, February HJ74. Doi: 10.1148/110.2.369.

Figure 5. The first published example of x-ray subtraction after contrast injection.

Between the late 1980s and early 1990s, INR underwent a revolution thanks to the contributions of two Italian physicians: Cesare Gianturco and Guido Guglielmi.

> The use of coils delivered by the endovascular route to occlude vessels started with the introduction of Gianturco's coil in 1975. In 1989, Hilal reported the first case of an intracranial aneurysm treated with embolization with coils. Although some successes were reported, it was difficult to control these coils properly and they were associated with a significantly increased risk of occlusion of the parent vessel and distal embolization.
> At this point it became essential to have a controllable delivery system, with the possibility of recovering, repositioning, and redistributing the coil, arranging it with satisfactory configuration before its detachment, to improve the safety of the procedure. As Guglielmi was to say the idea of catheterizing an aneurysm and applying an electric current to thrombose it was conceived in the early 1980s in the experimental laboratory of the Institute of Neurosurgery, University of Rome. Despite the scarce results obtained with intra-aneurysmal thrombosis, one detail was noted that was to make a difference:
> a 'rat tail' erosion of the intra-aneurysmal stainless-steel electrode was noted, due to the passage of the electric current. This phenomenon, of inducing electrolysis of an endovascular intra-aneurysmal stainless-steel guidewire, was applied almost 10 years later for the detachment mechanism of detachable coils. It was precisely the discovery of this mechanism of release, exploited by other researchers, that entered clinical practice in 1990 with what was to be called the Guglielmi detachable coil. [11]

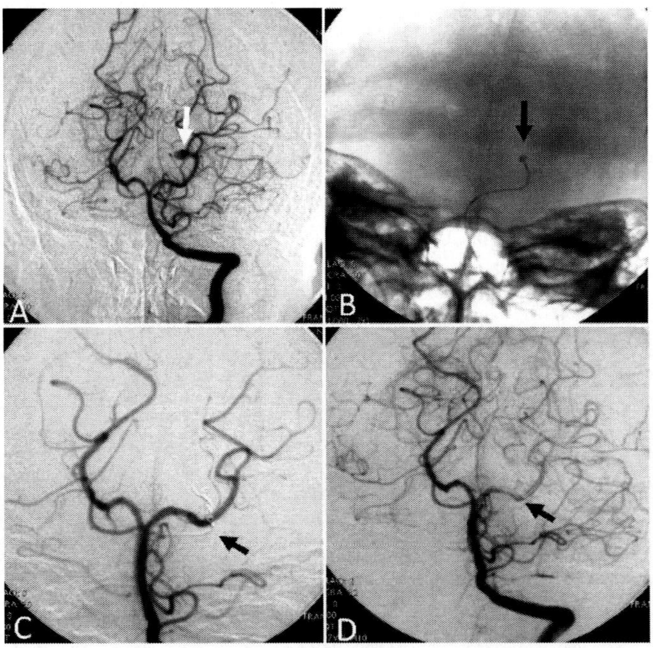

Figure 6. A 20-year-old female presented with headaches and diplopia caused by a superior cerebellar artery aneurysm, which was coiled with Microplex coils (Microvention, USA). A, frontal view of the left vertebral artery injection showing the aneurysm of the distal left superior cerebellar artery (arrow). B, unsubtracted image showing the aneurysm was coiled through a Prowler10 microcatheter (Cordis, USA) (arrow). C, frontal view of the left vertebral artery injection after the last 2mm×1cm Microplex coil was delivered (arrow). D, frontal view of the left vertebral artery injection showing the aneurysm was completely occluded (arrow).

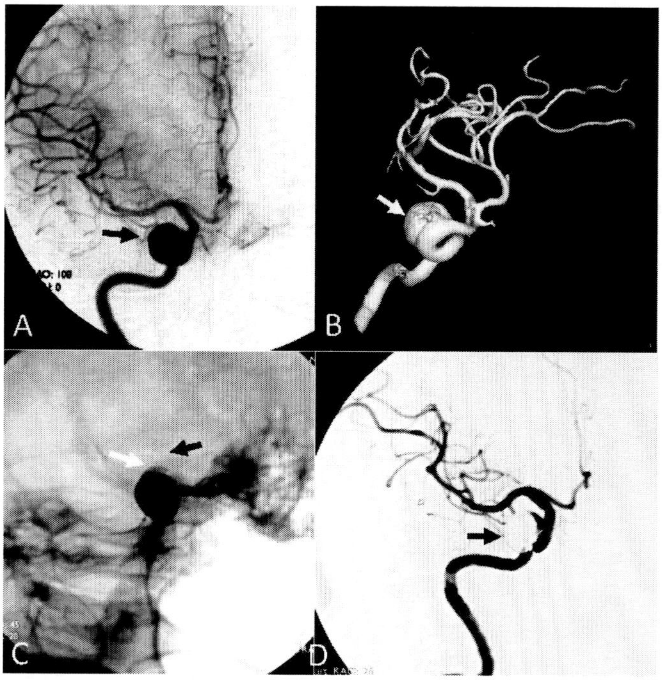

Figure 7. A 71-year-old woman presented with a large cavernous aneurysm of the internal carotid artery. A, frontal view of the right internal carotid artery injection showing a large cavernous aneurysm of the right internal carotid artery (arrow). B, 3-D reconstruction of the right internal carotid artery injection showing the large aneurysm (arrow), which was treated with 4mm×30mm Neuroform stent and coils. C, the unsubtracted image showing the Neuroform stent (black arrow) and intra-stent balloon-assisted coiling (white arrow). D, frontal view of the right internal carotid artery injection after treatment showing the aneurysm was occluded completely (arrow).

Coil embolization was revolutionized by Guido Guglielmi at UCLA, who discovered that electricity could serve as a controlled release mechanism for coils. In 1991, he published two significant papers on the use of detachable platinum coils, known as Guglielmi's coils, for embolizing brain aneurysms. This advancement made the treatment of aneurysms more accessible and safer.

The invention of the Guglielmi detachable coil system in the 1990s sparked the growth of modern neurointervention and endovascular neurosurgery. Initially, the results of coil embolization were challenged by unacceptably high occlusion rates. However, the neuroendovascular field responded by making substantial advancements in coil design, resulting in coils with various lengths, shapes, pliability, coatings, and detachment mechanisms, as well as devices to assist in coil embolization (Figure 6 and 7).

Endovascular coiling has become a viable and effective treatment option for both ruptured and unruptured aneurysms. It is often preferred over surgical clipping, which is associated with higher rates of morbidity and mortality. New devices designed to enhance coil embolization include balloon-assisted techniques and intracranial stents. These innovations aim to increase coil packing efficiency and maintain parent artery patency, while also reducing the risk of coil herniation. Significant improvements in coil properties have also been implemented to increase aneurysm occlusion rates.

State-of-the-Art Today

In the past decade, endovascular treatment has emerged as an evidence-based core approach for addressing neurovascular pathologies. Advances in imaging technology and the development of highly sophisticated catheters have pushed this field to new limits, expanding the range of treatable conditions and improving patient outcomes.

However, finding the right balance between experience and technology can be challenging, given the rapid advancements in the latter and the long learning curve associated with the former. Nevertheless, the results remain safe and encouraging.

Several trials are currently underway to evaluate the effectiveness of new devices, while others have already been established for safe and widespread use. For example:

Stenting and Flow Diversion Stents

In the early 1990s, Guido Guglielmi introduced detachable coils for the treatment of cerebral aneurysms. After receiving approval in 1995, endovascular coil embolization gained global popularity. The emergence of micro-coil embolization was considered groundbreaking in this field, and it began to be assessed through long-term case series. However, the results were not as promising as anticipated.

New devices and innovative techniques led to the development of balloon and intracranial stent-assisted methods, which broadened the indications for endovascular treatment of cerebral aneurysms. Despite these advances, wide-neck cerebral aneurysms continued to pose significant technical challenges, and rates of obliteration and recurrence remained less than optimal.

As noted by Dong-Seong Shin et al. in the Journal of Korean Neurosurgical Society [12]:

> "Early series sought to push the boundaries of stent-assisted coil embolization techniques to achieve more satisfactory clinical and radiographic outcomes. Traditional intracranial stents were designed to facilitate coil embolization. These stents have low metal surface-area coverage and high porosity to maintain both parent vessel and branch vessel patency. Additionally, these stents serve as a buttress supporting the coil mass and were designed with high radial force. While these characteristics support a coil mass, traditional stents remain vulnerable to coil prolapse and technically challenging to deploy across significant curves or tortuous segments. Unfortunately, unacceptably high recurrence rates persisted. Intracranial flow-diverting stents (FDS) were developed to address these challenges by targeting aneurysm hemodynamics to promote aneurysm occlusion—a significant departure from traditional intracranial stent design. This design innovation meant FDS were developed as a single-stent treatment solution for intracranial aneurysms not amenable to traditional coiling and assisted-coiling techniques. To achieve this goal, FDS eschewed high radial force designs to buttress coils in favor of low radial force to promote conformability and navigability in tortuous vessels. Additionally, FDS were woven with increased metal surface- area coverage to promote flow along the parent vessel and decrease flow into the aneurysm while maintaining sufficient porosity to maintain branch vessel and perforators patency."

The technical changes in the use of intracranial stents evolved into the early 2000s. Initially, these stents were used to prevent coils within the aneurysmal sac from protruding into the parent artery. This eventually progressed to the development of flow-diverting devices, which aim to reconstruct the vessel's normal anatomy without directly closing the neck of the aneurysm. As a result, side branches of the artery were better preserved, reducing the risk of ischemia.

The concept of the flow diverter was initially explored by Ajay Wakhloo, but it was Kim Nelson and his colleagues who developed the first commercially available device. The introduction of flow diverters made it possible to treat previously unmanageable aneurysms, such as giant wide-necked, blister, or fusiform aneurysms. This area of medical technology is still actively evolving, thanks to ongoing advancements in technology and imaging (Figure 8).

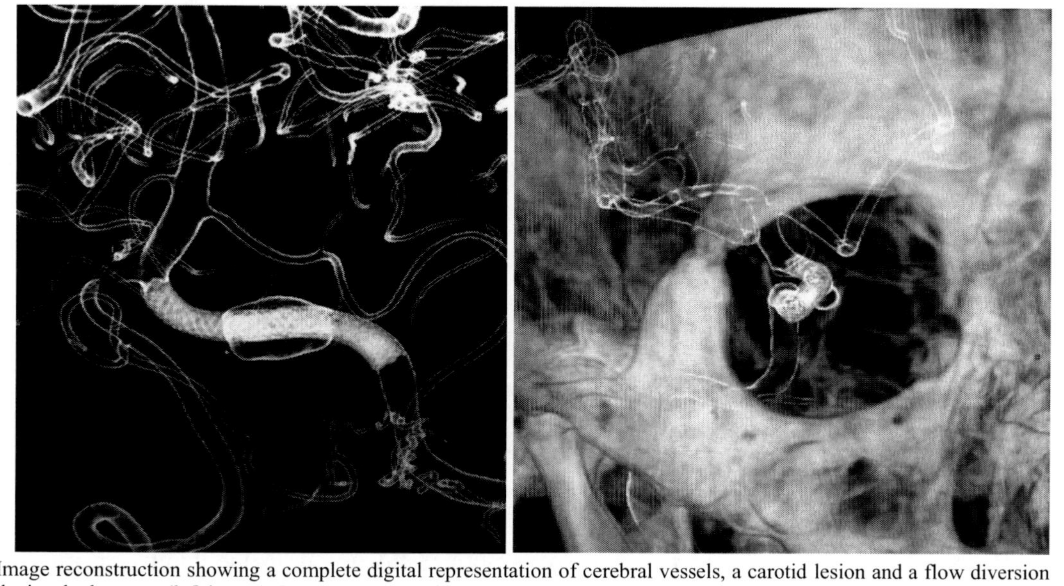

Image reconstruction showing a complete digital representation of cerebral vessels, a carotid lesion and a flow diversion device deployment (left image). Image reconstruction showing the anatomical definitive placement view (right image).

Figure 8. Imaging advances nowadays.

Not Just Hemorrhages: The Treatment of Ischemic Stroke

Recanalization refers to the process of opening an artery that has been blocked by a thrombus. Pharmacological thrombolysis began to face competition from mechanical methods after Dr. Y. Pierre Gobin at the University of California, Los Angeles, patented a corkscrew-like device designed for retrieving foreign bodies, such as misplaced coils. Although this device did not see widespread use, it marked the inception of mechanical thrombectomy.

Subsequently, the Mechanical Embolus Removal in Cerebral Ischemia (MERCI) retriever was tested. Concentric utilized the FDA 510-K regulatory pathway to obtain clearance for the device. The approval process for the MERCI device was based on substantial equivalence, as it was deemed capable of removing foreign bodies and clots (considered as foreign bodies). The device demonstrated a superior ability to open occluded vessels compared to the natural progression of similar cases and was shown to be safe for use in stroke patients.

From January to June 2015, five major randomized trials were published in the New England Journal of Medicine (NEJM) with contributions from interventional neuroradiologists and stroke neurologists from the Netherlands [13], Canada [14], Australia [15], the United States [16], and Spain [17].

Using the PROACT-II control recanalization rate of 18% as a benchmark, the single-arm MERCI trial achieved the primary outcome of the study with significant recanalization rates. In August 2004, the FDA cleared the MERCI retriever as the first device approved for clot removal in acute ischemic stroke [18].

All of the studies aimed to assess the role of mechanical thrombectomy in treating ischemic stroke. They demonstrated that when performed at centers with proven expertise, intra-arterial mechanical thrombectomy is more effective than traditional treatment methods, such as intravenous thrombolytic injection.

The promising results of these mechanical thrombectomy trials were highlighted in an editorial by the New England Journal of Medicine (NEJM), which concluded with the statement: "Endovascular equipoise no longer exists. It's about time." [19].

As a result, thrombectomy is currently recommended by the guidelines established by leading American (AHA/ASA) and European (ESO-ESNR-ESMINT) societies of stroke neurologists and interventional neuroradiologists.

The Latino-American Contribution to This History

I In the late 1980s, several South American radiologists and neurosurgeons who had trained in interventional neuroradiology abroad, mainly in French centers, returned to their home countries. In the late 1990s, Ronie Leo Piske from Brazil and Luis Lemme Plaghos from Argentina, while attending a course in interventional radiology in Brazil, initiated a friendly dialogue to organize an informal meeting focused on morbidity and mortality in interventional neuroradiology. Their initial idea was to hold a regional meeting after the annual meeting in Val d'Isère, featuring an "international guest" to lead the various presentations and keep participants informed about the latest techniques and standards through short lectures.

Following this proposal, 19 interventional neuroradiologists from South America met for the first time in May 1991 at the Department of Radiology of the Hospital Portuguesa in São Paulo, Brazil [24]. The first "international guest" was Professor Pierre Lasjaunias from Paris, who proved to be an excellent moderator during the discussions of difficult cases. Although the first meeting was very informal, it was deemed a success, leading to the decision to organize annual meetings in the future to foster continental integration.

It became clear among the South American interventional neuroradiologists that they shared similar technical and academic developments, as well as common regional challenges in daily practice. In line with these goals, a second meeting was held in Buenos Aires, Argentina, in December 1992, coordinated by local interventionalists Luis Lemme Plaghos and Claudio Schonholz. On this occasion, 14 neuroradiologists from Argentina, Brazil, and Uruguay participated in oral presentations of cases, with Professor Jacques Moret serving for the first time as an esteemed guest presenter. By this time, the group had already identified itself as the "South American Group for the Diagnosis and Treatment of Neuroangiomas."

All participants in this group will apply for membership in the WFITN. It was also voted and approved to take the name "South American Group for Interventional Neuroradiology Work (GSANIT)."

Argentina

Pedro Lylyk, a neurosurgeon from the University of Buenos Aires and an honorific member of the American Society of Neuroradiology, performed the first endovascular treatment of a cerebral aneurysm in Buenos Aires using the Guglielmi Detachable Coil [20, 21], which was developed at UCLA, in 1990.

In 1996, he placed the first intracranial stent—a coronary stent—for a dissecting vertebral aneurysm in a young female patient. In 2002, he began using the Neuroform stent for the endovascular treatment of cerebral aneurysms with wide necks [22, 23].

The next significant advance was the introduction of flow diverter stents in Argentina. While the concept of flow diversion was initially explored by Ajay Wakhloo, it was Kim Nelson and his colleagues who developed the first commercially available flow diverter device. The introduction of flow diverters made it possible to treat previously untreatable aneurysms, including giant wide-necked, blister, and fusiform aneurysms. The first case in Buenos Aires was performed at the ENERI institution by Pedro Lylyk and his collaborators in March 2006 [24].

Mexico

Mexico and Peru may have been the first places in the New World with evidence of neurosurgical practices, particularly through the practice of cranial trepanation. The Zapotec civilization, during the Classic period (200–300 AD) [25], was notably prolific in performing this procedure.

Recent reports indicate that over 1,500 prehistoric neurosurgical specimens have been found and examined. The oldest examples of trepanation, dating back to around 10,000 BC, were discovered in North Africa. Excavations in the Jericho area of the Near East and in parts of Asia have uncovered specimens from approximately 8000 to 6000 BC. The earliest examples in Europe are over 10,000 years old, likely from the late Paleolithic period and certainly from the Neolithic age. Early Danubians conducted cranial surgery around 3000 BC, and ancient peoples in the Seine-Oise-Marne area of France were active in this practice around 2000 BC. Based on the number of skulls found in France, it is likely that a "surgery center" existed there between 1900 BC and 1500 BC. Trepanation specimens have also been found in various other regions of Neolithic Europe, including the Balkans and Russia [26].

In 1964, the National Institute of Neurology and Neurosurgery (NINN) was founded in Mexico, marking a significant milestone in the field. Two prominent figures in Mexican neurosurgery emerged during this time: Dr. Clemente Robles-Castillo and Dr. Manuel Velasco-Suárez. Under the exceptional leadership and expertise of Robles-Castillo and Velasco-Suárez, neurosurgery in Mexico made significant advancements.

INR (Interventional Neuroradiology) began to develop in Mexico during the late 1980s and early 1990s, coinciding with global advancements in imaging and catheter technology.

These advancements included the endovascular embolization of cerebral aneurysms and arteriovenous malformations (AVMs), utilizing techniques that had been refined in North America and Europe. The success of these initial procedures demonstrated the potential of INR to provide less invasive treatment options compared to traditional open surgery.

In Mexico and throughout Latin America, a significant challenge for neurointerventional practices is the unequal access to healthcare. While major urban centers are equipped with advanced facilities and skilled practitioners, rural and less developed areas often lack access to these specialized services. This gap is widening and is closely linked to improvements in technology and techniques.

Practitioners in Mexico have taken the field of neurointerventional radiology seriously, considering all its implications. Ethical, legal, and social issues arise from our understanding of the brain and the application of neurotechnology. Neuroethics provides a framework for navigating this complex landscape and ensures that the development and application of neurointerventional techniques are guided by ethical principles that prioritize patient well-being, autonomy, and dignity [27].

Mexico has significantly contributed to neuroradiology, especially in the area of neuroethics, through various technological applications in this field:

- The use of MRI as a powerful neuroimaging tool used by neuroradiology to map brain activity and match timing and outcomes to indicate certain procedures [28].
- Preoperative planning with functional MRI, identifying critical brain regions, thereby minimizing the risk of damage during the intervention [29, 30].
- Management of incidental findings while performing diagnostic or treatment procedures, protocoling how to handle this situation with a corresponding need to properly inform patients and the emotional situation that this information may cause [31].
- Financial and legal issues should be approached, aiming to assure accessibility, proper management, prompt diagnosis, and best-option treatment [32].

Brazil – Chile

Caldas et al. from the University of São Paulo in São Paulo, Brazil, have been using a microcatheter and GDC coils for endovascular embolization of cerebral aneurysms since 1998. This technique aims to completely exclude the aneurysm from circulation while preserving the internal carotid artery [33].

In the ongoing quest for the "gold standard" in aneurysm treatment, liquid embolic materials remain in the testing phase. The new Onyx polymer, which has been utilized for aneurysm treatment, was described by Piske et al. at the Beneficência Portuguesa Hospital in São Paulo between 2002 and 2006. This study represents one of the largest single-center experiences in embolization of intracranial aneurysms using Onyx.

Following this, the Clinical Hospital of the Pontifical Catholic University of Chile applied this technique, but due to unfavorable factors, it was not widely adopted [34].

As of 2017, a Brazilian multicenter study evaluated the efficacy of the Pipeline Embolization Device (PED) with Shield technology for treating aneurysms. This study, conducted by seven centers from November 2017 to December 2018, enrolled 151 patients with a total of 182 aneurysms. The study concluded that PED shielding is safe and effective for treating intracranial aneurysms, with results regarding complete occlusion and ischemic complications comparable to previous versions of the PED [35].

In 2000, Campos et al. at the Beneficência Portuguesa Hospital in São Paulo embolized cerebral arteriovenous malformations using n-butyl-2-cyanoacrylate (NBCA) [36]. Additionally, Abud et al. from the Faculdade de Medicina de Ribeirão Preto, University of São Paulo, employed simultaneous double arterial catheter insertion starting in 2008 as a method for complete lesion exclusion [37].

Piske has been working at the Hospital Beneficência Portuguesa in São Paulo, Brazil, since 1995, focusing on venous access to treat dural sinus lesions, excluding cavernous sinus lesions [38]. In 1996, he performed the first case of removable coil sealing of the dural sinus septum, which successfully healed the lesion while preserving the sinus cavity.

Additionally, Piske published the first article on AVOS in the cavernous sinus in 1986, three years prior to its actual publication [39]. In 2011, Castro-Afonso and colleagues at the University of São Paulo began evaluating the safety and efficacy of the Solitaire AB stent for the treatment of acute ischemic stroke [40].

Conclusion

History could be confusing if certain concepts are not clearly established from the outset. Paradoxically, history often generated new concepts as well. In this article, we discussed the field of Interventional Radiology (IR), a medical specialty that gained widespread recognition and encompassed many key events previously mentioned.

It was essential to connect information from various parts of the world, as there were additional links that could have strengthened and clarified this narrative. This brief overview did not intend to overlook or dismiss other significant facts.

As we aimed to illustrate in this review, Interventional Radiology was a broad and dynamic field characterized by numerous innovative ideas, outstanding individuals, and impressive technological advancements up to that time. Ultimately, this history led to a focus on the primary goal: providing the highest quality care for individuals who required specialized medical attention.

This chapter aimed to clarify the concept, evolution, and imminent progression of this art and science. The contributions from Latin America played a significant role in this field, which we highlighted. The relationships between radiology, neurology, neurosurgery, and neuroethics represented just a few pieces of this complex puzzle.

References

[1] Chen M, Nguyen T. Emerging subspecialties in neurology: endovascular surgical neuroradiology. *Neurology*. 2008;70 (6):e21-e24.

[2] The British Institute of Radiology. The origins of radiology. *British Institute of Radiology*. 2024.

[3] Artico M. Egas Moniz: 90 years (1927-2017) from cerebral angiography. *Front Neuroanat*. 2017;11:81.

[4] Seldinger SI. Catheter replacement of the needle in percutaneous arteriography: a new technique. Acta *Radiol.* 1953;39 (5):368-376.

[5] Rosenbaum AE, et al. In re: Amundsen P. cerebral angiography via the femoral artery. *AJNR Am J Neuroradiol.* 2001;22 (3):584-589.

[6] Payne MM. Charles Theodore Dotter: the father of intervention. *Tex Heart Inst J.* 2001;28 (1):28-38.

[7] Alaraj A. Balloons in endovascular neurosurgery: history and current applications. *Neurosurgery.* 2014;74 (Suppl 1):S163-S190.

[8] Russell EJ. Spinal cord angiography and René Djindjian. *J Neurointerv Surg.* 2012;4 (3):234.

[9] Cognard C, et al. Cerebral dural arteriovenous fistulas: clinical and angiographic correlation. *Radiology.* 1995;194 (3):671-680.

[10] Crummy AB, Strother CM, Mistretta CA. The history of digital subtraction angiography. *J Vasc Interv Radiol.* 2018;29 (8):1138-1141.

[11] Peschillo S, Delfini R. Endovascular neurosurgery in Europe and in Italy: what is in the future? *World Neurosurg.* 2012;77 (2):248-251.

[12] Shin DS, et al. The evolution of flow-diverting stents for cerebral aneurysms. *J Korean Neurosurg Soc.* 2020;63 (2):137-152.

[13] Berkhemer OA, et al. A randomized trial of intraarterial treatment for acute ischemic stroke. *N Engl J Med.* 2015;372 (1):11-20.

[14] Goyal M, et al. Randomized assessment of rapid endovascular treatment of ischemic stroke. *N Engl J Med.* 2015;372 (11):1019-1030.

[15] Campbell BCV, et al. Endovascular therapy for ischemic stroke with perfusion-imaging selection. *N Engl J Med.* 2015;372 (11):1009-1018.

[16] Saver JL, et al. Stent-retriever thrombectomy after intravenous t-PA vs. t-PA alone in stroke. *N Engl J Med.* 2015;372 (24):2285-2295.

[17] Jovin TG, et al. Thrombectomy within 8 hours after symptom onset in ischemic stroke. *N Engl J Med.* 2015;372 (24):2296-2306.

[18] Smith WS, Furlan AJ. Brief history of endovascular acute ischemic stroke treatment. *Stroke.* 2016;47 (2).

[19] Furlan AJ. Endovascular therapy for stroke—it's about time. *N Engl J Med.* 2015;372 (24):2347-2349.

[20] Guglielmi G, et al. Endovascular treatment of posterior-circulation aneurysms by electrothrombosis. *J Neurosurg.* 1992;77 (4):515-524.

[21] Lylyk P, et al. Treatment of a vertebral dissecting aneurysm with stents and coils. *Neurosurgery.* 1998;43 (2):385-388.

[22] Lylyk P, et al. Buenos Aires experience with the Neuroform stent. *J Neurosurg.* 2005;102 (2):235-241.

[23] Lylyk I, et al. Pipeline embolization devices for 1000 aneurysms. *Neurosurgery.* 2021;89 (3):443-449.

[24] Piske RL, Lemme-Plaghos L. To the editor. *Interv Neuroradiol.* 1999;5 (1):83-85.

[25] Beltrán JQ, Carrillo-Ruiz JD. Neurological functional surgery in Mexico. *World Neurosurg.* 2019;122:549-558.

[26] Lv X, Li Z, Li Y. Prehistoric skull trepanation in China. *World Neurosurg.* 2013;80 (6):897-899.

[27] Chatterjee A, Farah MJ, eds. *Neuroethics in Practice: Medicine, Mind, and Society.* Oxford University Press; 2013.

[28] Logothetis NK. What we can do and cannot do with fMRI. *Nature.* 2008;453 (7197):869-878.

[29] Petrella JR, et al. Preoperative functional MR imaging localization. *Radiology.* 2006;240 (3):793-802.

[30] Raichle ME. Behind the scenes of functional brain imaging. *Proc Natl Acad Sci USA.* 1998;95 (3):765-772.

[31] Illes J, et al. Ethical considerations in managing incidental findings in fMRI. *Brain Cogn.* 2002;50 (3):358-365.

[32] Midtlien JP, et al. Conflicts of interest and neurointerventional surgery. *J Neurointerv Surg.* 2024;16 (6):537-540.

[33] Caldas JG, et al. Endovascular treatment of intracavernous carotid aneurysm with hyperprolactinaemia. *Interv Neuroradiol.* 1998;4 (3):253-256.

[34] Tevah J, et al. Endovascular treatment of complex cerebral aneurysms with Onyx HD-500. *J Neuroradiol.* 2011;38 (5):283-290.

[35] Manzato LB, et al. Safety and effectiveness of Pipeline Flex with Shield Technology. *Neurosurgery*. 2020;87 (1):104-111.

[36] Campos C, et al. Single-hole high-flow arteriovenous fistula. *Interv Neuroradiol*. 2002;8 (1):55-60.

[37] Abud DG, et al. Treatment of brain AVMs by double arterial catheterization with simultaneous Onyx injection. *AJNR Am J Neuroradiol*. 2011;32 (1):152-158.

[38] Piske RL, et al. Dural sinus compartment in dural AV shunts. *AJNR Am J Neuroradiol*. 2005;26 (7):1715-1722.

[39] Uflacker R, Lima SS, Ribas GC, Piske RL. Carotid-cavernous fistulas: embolization via superior ophthalmic vein. *Radiology*. 1986;159:175-179.

[40] Castro-Afonso LH, et al. Mechanical thrombectomy with Solitaire stent retrieval for acute ischemic stroke in Brazil. *Clinics* (Sao Paulo). 2012;67 (12):1379-1386.

Chapter 27

The History of Interventional Neuroradiology in Thailand: A Part of Southeast Asia

Sirintara (Pongpech) Singhara Na Ayudhaya*, MD
Department of Radiology (INR), Mahidol University, Thailand

Abstract

The history of interventional neuroradiology in Thailand dates back to cerebral angiography in 1964. Of course, at the same time, it has also undergone the development process of neuroimaging through aeroencephalography and ventriculography. In 1985, detachable balloons were used to embolize carotid-cavernous fistula (CCF), but the results were not ideal at that time. After 1995, there was a significant improvement in the treatment of CCF. The technique of liquid embolization for cerebral arteriovenous malformations was developed in 1993. The Department of Angiography and Interventional Radiology was established in 1999. With the establishment of the National Interventional Neuroradiology (INR) Certification Committee by the first batch of well-trained physicians, the Thai Medical Council began recruiting certified neuroscientists (neuroradiologists, neurosurgeons, and neurologists) for training in neurointerventional techniques in 2006. Endovascular thrombectomy started in 2008. Onyx embolization of AVMs began in 2009. Since 2010, flow diversion devices have been used to treat intracranial aneurysms. With the development of new equipment, materials, technologies, and radiation devices, as well as comprehensive standardization of training, education, and research support, coupled with strong regional and global cooperation, Thailand's neurointerventional surgery is rapidly developing and establishing itself.

Keywords: history, interventional neuroradiology, Thailand, training

Introduction

In Thailand, the very first diagnostic cerebral angiography was performed by Professor Emeritus Udom Posakrissana (Neurosurgeon) in 1953. Professor Emeritus Romsai Suwannik, our very first diagnostic radiologist, was interested in neuroradiology. Professor Udom

* Corresponding Author's Email: sirintarapongpetch2@gmail.com

In: World History of Neurointerventional Surgery
Editors: Xianli Lv and Zhongxue Wu
ISBN: 979-8-89530-792-2

Posakrissana reported in the Siriraj Journal in February 1980 that at that time the diagnostic procedures for neuroradiology were mainly pneumoencephalography and ventriculography. Arteriography was performed through an open incision to the carotid artery for contrast injection [1-3].

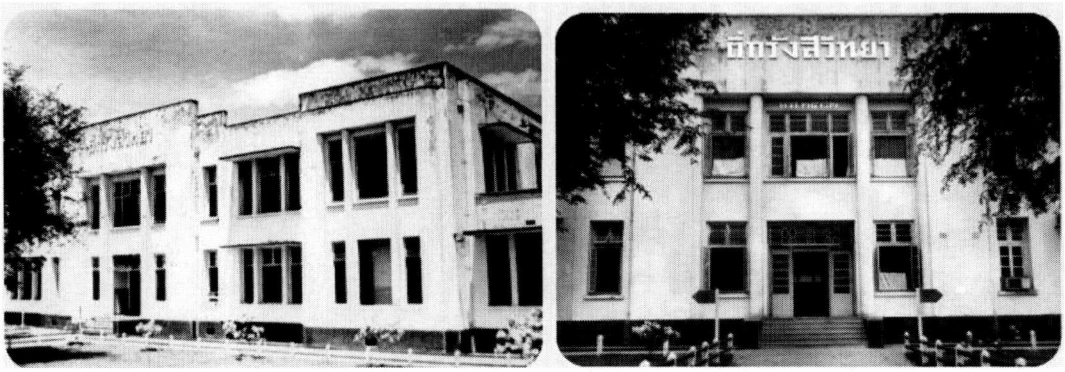

Figure 1. The Siriraj Hospital and the Chulalongkorn Hospital.

In January 1943, a group of U.S. doctors visited Thailand to evaluate Thai neurosurgical capabilities. Dr. Wilson, a thoracic surgeon, encouraged Professor Udom to further develop his skills, which led to his training at the Lahey Clinic in Boston in 1953. Upon his return to Thailand, the development of cerebral angiography was improved using a percutaneous technique with the Poppen-Prahad needle. By this time, the quality of X-ray equipment had also improved. The procedures were performed in collaboration between Siriraj Hospital and Chulalongkorn Hospital (Figure1).

Regarding X-ray machines in Thailand, Professor Pinpart Pittayapet was the first doctor to bring the first X-ray machine to Siriraj (the 8th machine in Thailand) after graduating in radiology from Harvard University. In 1928, William Alfred Kunatelake donated funds for the machine. At that time, the best quality brand was Kellekoette, for which he assembled parts himself. The first x-ray was taken on January 28, 1928 [4-11]. The Department of Radiology was then opened, and in 1933 a medical curriculum for medical students was started [4-11]. Professor Preeya Karnjanuttithi became the head of neuroradiology.

Professor Udom and Professor Vichai Bumrungpol (both neurosurgeons) together performed direct cervical carotid punctures and strong manual injections of contrast media, while the radiology technician had to quickly change the film cassettes to obtain images of the arterial, capillary and venous phases [12-19]. However, the quality of the images was not good. Professor Romsai developed a contrast injection system by creating an ejector beam on the syringe to apply force for bolus injections, which greatly improved image quality.

In 1964, Professor Preeya Karnjanut became the first neuroradiologist to work with neurosurgeons to perform cerebral angiograms using single-plane radiography with two manual injections, one for antero-posterior views and another for lateral views. In 1967, they began using the Sanchez rapid cassette changer for greater efficiency.

In 1970, the first biplane angiography (Philips) with an automatic pressure injector was introduced, allowing the first right brachial injection for both carotid and vertebrobasilar system angiograms [6]. At that time, both neuroradiologists and neurosurgeons were still performing direct puncture procedures [7]. Later, the radiology staff began performing transcatheter cerebral angiography.

In 1976, the polytome machine was introduced for pneumoencephalography, and water-soluble contrast (radiculography) replaced oil myelography (omnipaque was the first contrast) for myelography [19-21].

Also in 1976, interventional neuroradiology procedures were initiated by Professor Wiyada Bhupat and Professor Sutthisak Sutthipongchai, starting with trans (femoral) arterial embolization of the external carotid artery in patients with nasopharyngeal angiofibroma, targeting the internal maxillary artery or the ascending pharyngeal artery using Gelfoam or Ivalon (Figure2). These procedures were designed to reduce intraoperative bleeding and were very successful [22-23].

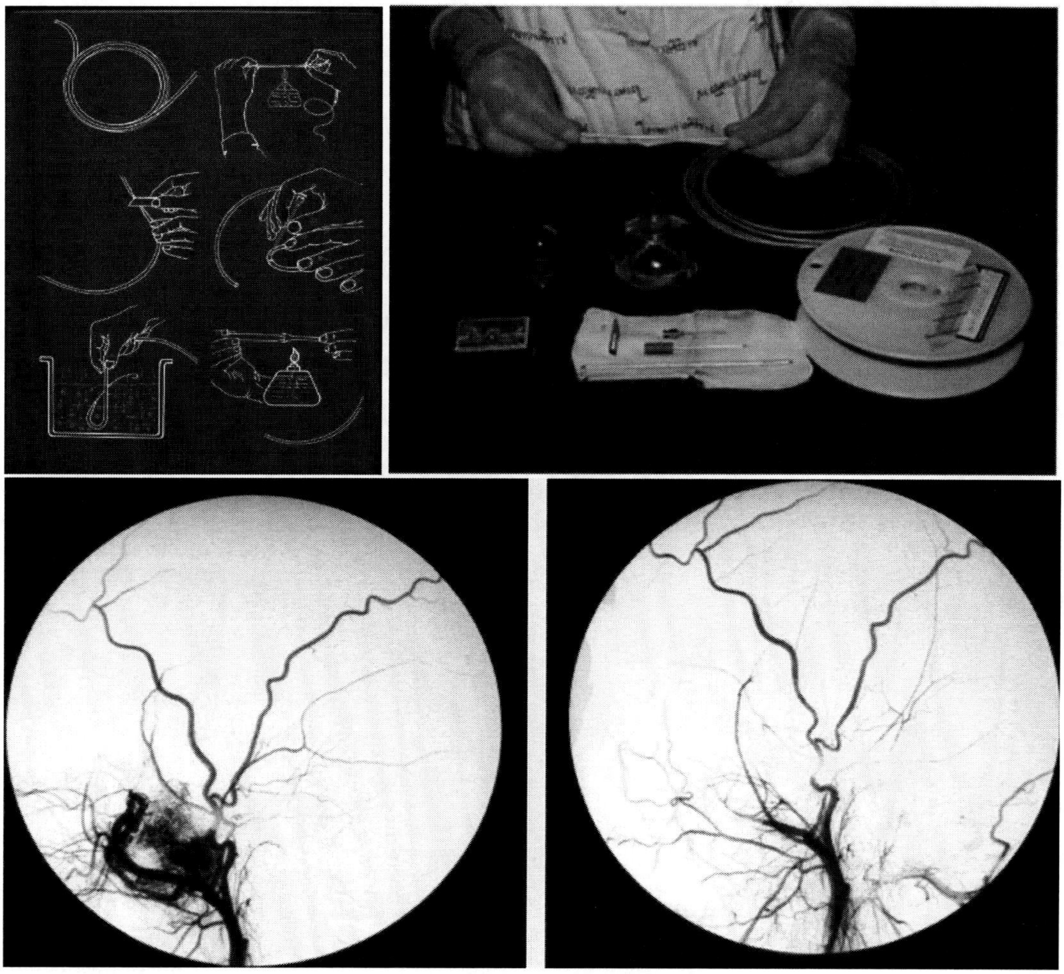

Figure 2. Lt picture: ECA angiogram showing arterial supplies to the Juvenile Nasopharyngeal Angiofibroma. Rt picture: DSA after Gelfoam embolization into ECA showing occlusion of the Internal Maxillary artery.

In 1984, after graduating from U. C. San Francisco and Massachusetts General Hospital, Professor Sutthisak performed animal experiments in collaboration with Professor Voravut

Junyavanich in the dog lab. He performed interventional neuroradiology for the embolization of artificial A-V fistulas in dogs using a ligation balloon until he gained full experience with animal models (Figure 3). In 1985, Professor Sutthisak and his team began using ligation balloons to treat direct carotid-cavernous fistulas (Figure 4) [23]. However, the results were not very satisfactory due to the unpredictability of the detached balloons, which often did not remain at the fistula site [23-26].

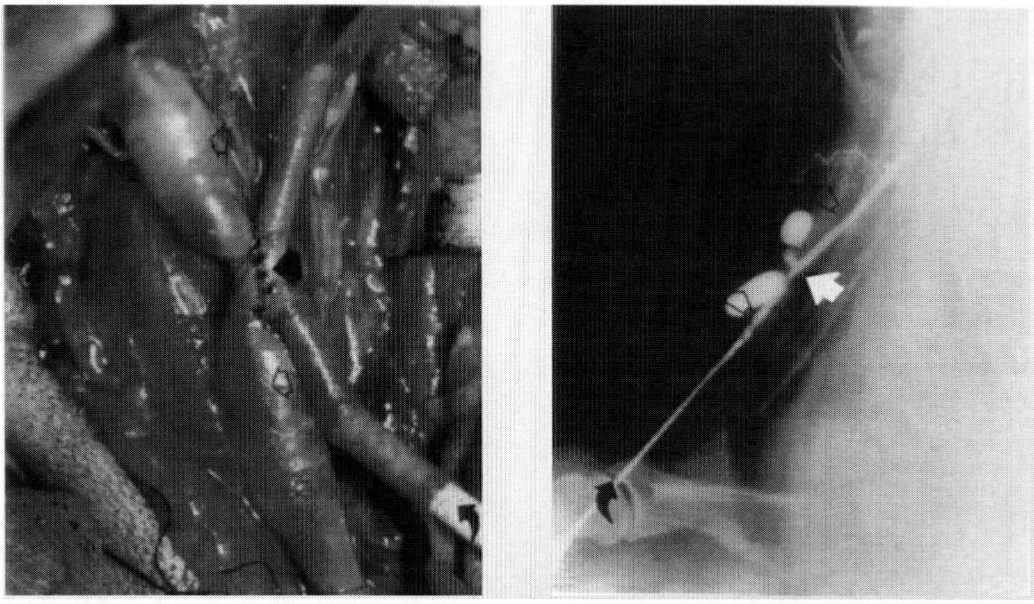

Figure 3. Lt picture: Internal Carotid artery of a Dog that was created arterio-venous fitula to the Jugular Vein (by Prof. Vorawut Junyavanich). Rt Picture: after 2 balloons were detached showing obliteration of the Arterio-venous fistula. Some residual venous pouch was noted.

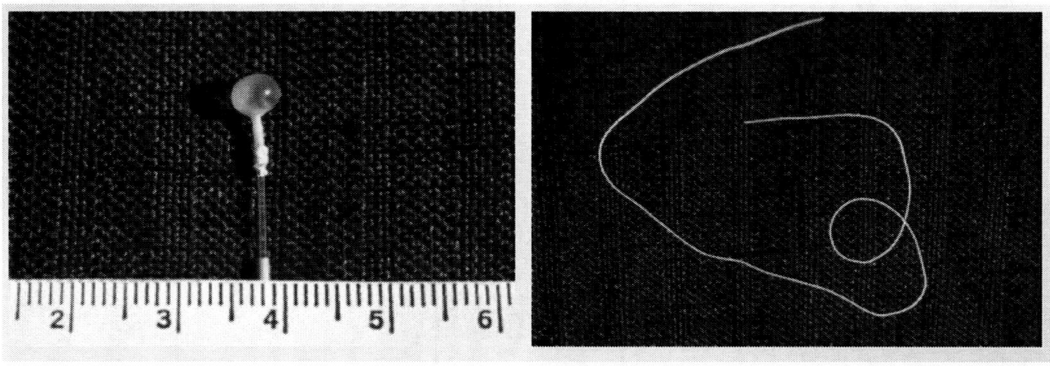

Figure 4. Lt picture: A mini-balloon was tired to microcatheter tip. Rt picture: The elastic thread that was used to tire the balloon to microcatheter tip.

During this period, Professor Sutthipongchai and Associate Professor Wiyada Bhupat were trained by Professor Lasjaunias at the Bicetre Hospital, University of Paris Sud (Figure5). They returned to Thailand and began treating cerebral arteriovenous malformations using transarterial superselective microcatheterization (size 1.5-1.8 Fr.) for permanent liquid embolization in 1993 [27-33].

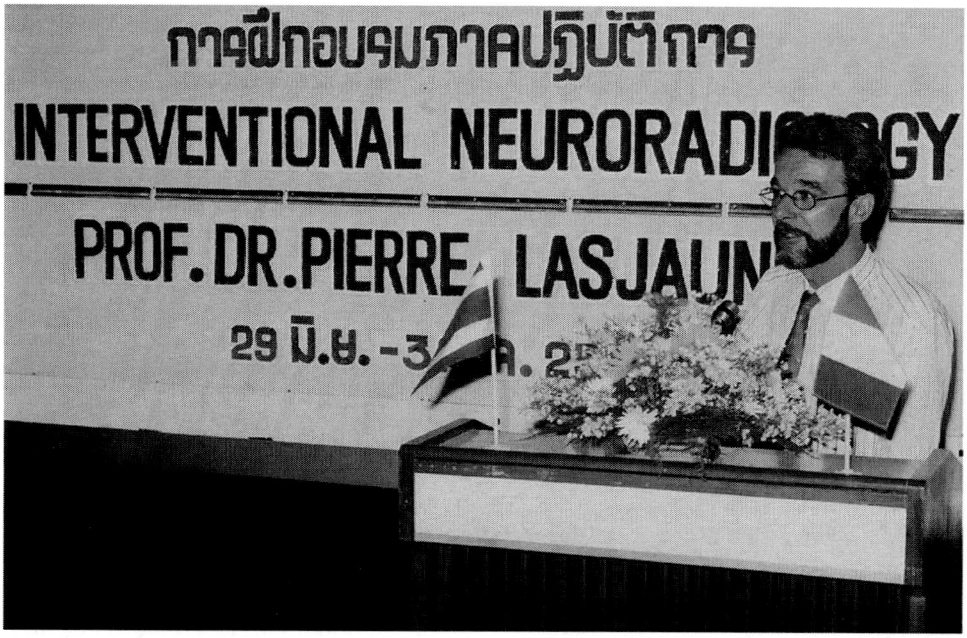

Figure 5. Then, in 1990, Professor Pierre Lasjuanias, a prominent interventional neuroradiologist from the University of Paris Sud, representing the French Society of Neuroradiology and AMFA, came to provide the first short course of lectures in interventional neuroradiology from September 25 to 27, 1990.

Information from the Department of Radiology, Faculty of Medicine, Chulalongkorn University, King Chulalongkorn Memorial Hospital

Interventional procedures for cerebrovascular disease have been performed at the Department of Radiology since 1993 under the supervision of the then Chairman of the Department, Professor Nitaya Suwanwela, following the installation of a hybrid film-digital subtraction angiography unit with endovascular treatment of a case of carotid cavernous fistula (CCF) using customized embolic material. A training workshop on neuroendovascular techniques was held at King Chulalongkorn Memorial Hospital with prominent invited interventional neuroradiologists such as Professor Pier Lasjaunias from Bicetre Hospital, Paris-Sud University, France and Professor in Sup Choi from Harvard Medical School, USA. The first detachable balloon embolization for CCF was performed by Associate Professor Somjai Wangsupachart in 1995 [34, 35]. Since then, many cases of CCF and various neurovascular arteriovenous fistulas have been treated.

In 1994, a new detachable balloon, the gold valve balloon, known as the Nycomed Ingenor gold valve balloon, was introduced [3, 19]. This balloon did not require tying with elastic thread or rubber. There was a valve at the bottom of the balloon that allowed us to inject fluid into the balloon to inflate it or to withdraw fluid to deflate it. Professor P. Lasjaunias came to Siriraj

Hospital, Mahidol University, every six months from 1992 to 1994 to help discuss and treat difficult cases (Figure6).

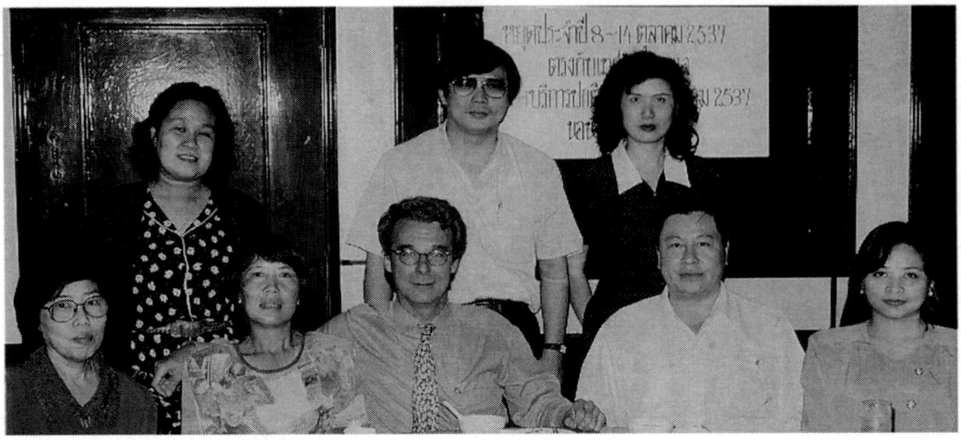

Figure 6. In 1994, during a trip to Bangkok, Professor Pierre Lasjaunias was sitting among Thai doctors: Professor Wiyada Bhupat (second from the left), Professor Sutthisak Sutthipongchai (second from the right), and Professor Sirintara Pongpech Singhara Na Ayudhaya (standing first from the right).

The second phase of the collaboration between Paris Sud University and Mahidol University began in 1994 with the participation of Ramathibodi Hospital. This initiative received the full support of Professor Emeritus Atthasit Vejajiva, then President of Mahidol University and former Dean of the Faculty of Medicine at Ramathibodi Hospital. He envisioned a long-term plan to establish Interventional Neuroradiology at Ramathibodi. Associate Professor Sirintara (Pongpech) Singhara Na Ayudhaya, a neuroradiologist, was the pioneer of this project with the 6 months training at Bicetre Hospital, followed by another 3 years follow-up twice a year, 1 week each trip - during which Professor Lasjaunias would come to assess the work at Ramathibodi and discuss interesting cases from other hospitals (Figure7).

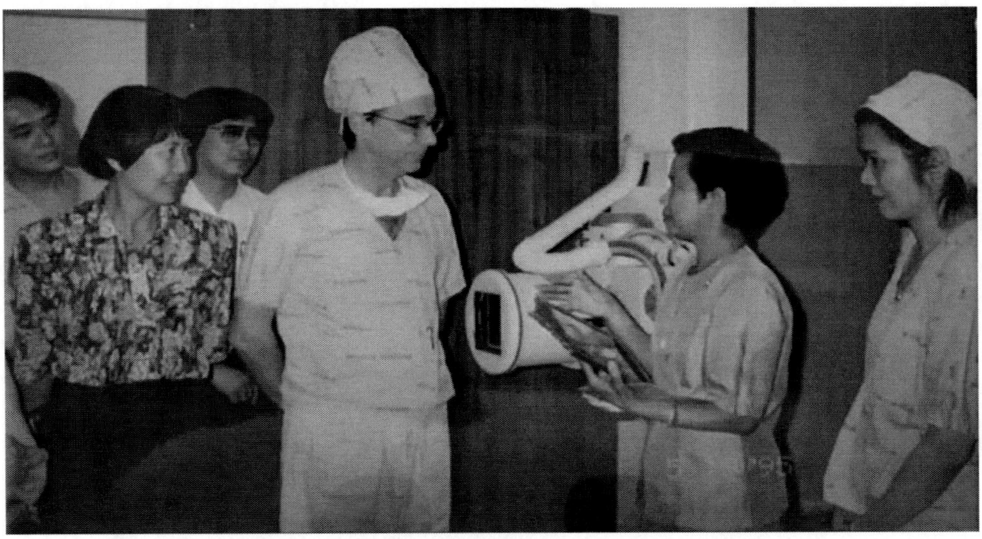

Figure 7. Professor Lasjaunias discussed interesting cases.

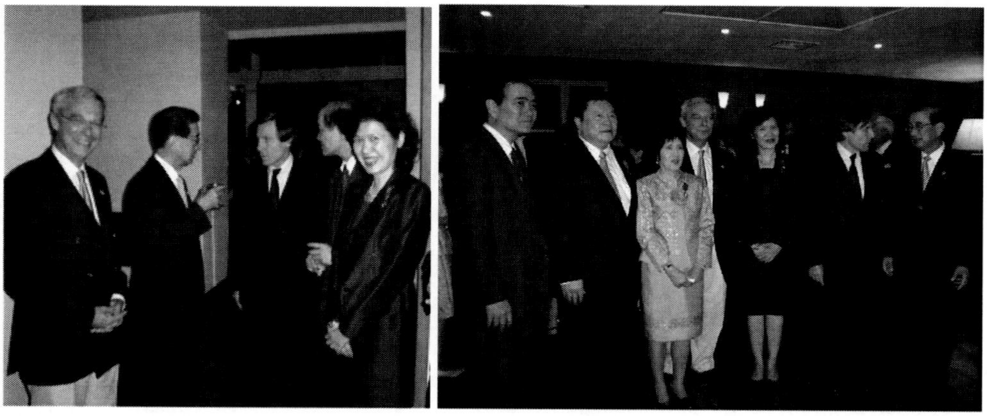

Figure 8. Under the collaboration between the French Embassy in Thailand and Mahidol University, the French Ambassador to Thailand at the time, along with three former-deans of the Faculty of Medicine Ramathibodi Hospital (two of whom were Presidents of Mahidol University), attended the ceremony for the French Decorations (Chevalier dans l'Ordre des Palmes Académiques) awarded to Professor Sutthipongchai and Professor Pongpech Singhara Na Ayudhaya. RT Picture: Professor Pierre Lasjaunias (first standing from the right), Professor Atthasit Vejajiva (second from the right), His Excellency the French Ambassador to Thailand (third from the right), Professor Rajata Rajatanavin (fourth from the right), Professor Sirintara Pongpech Singhara Na Ayudhaya (second from the left), and Professor Prakit Vateesathokit (first standing on the left).

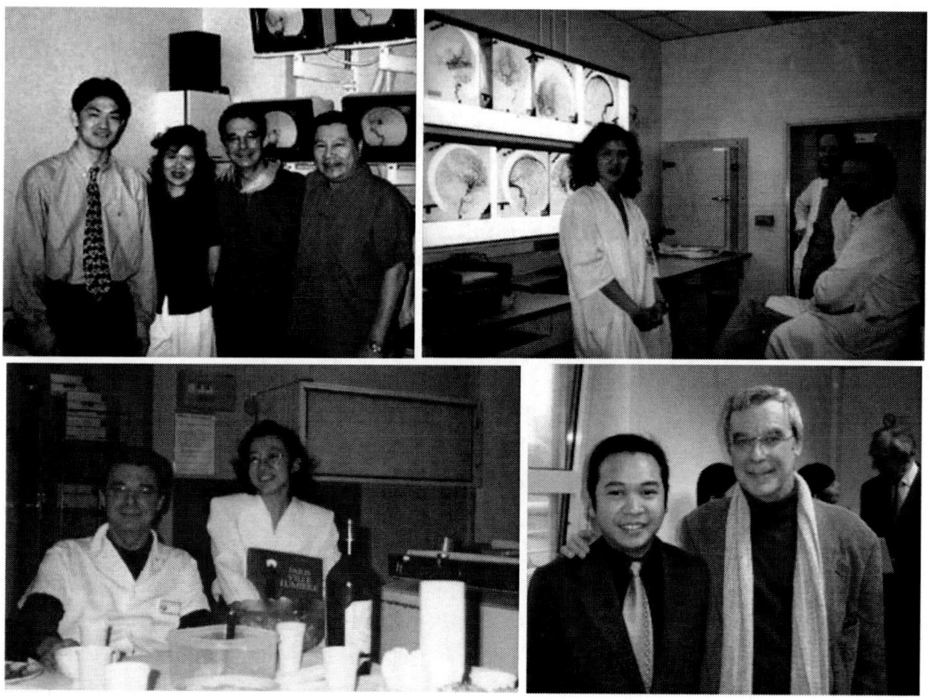

Figure 9. Above 2 pictures: 1994-1995; training time in Bicetre Hospital, Paris Sud, France under Professor P. Lasjaunias. Rt picture: Professor Pongpech S. (Thai fellow) was standing with Dr. Wendy Taylor (UK fellow) and Professor Rodesch G. was sitting. Lt picture: Professor Sutthipongchai S. and Dr. Siriwimolmas S. were visiting the angiosuite in Bicetre. Lower 2 pictures: example of 2 Thai Radiographers (technicians) who received grants to work and train in INR unit in Bicetre hospital France too.

During this period, more Thai neuroscientists were sent for training to Bicetre Hospital in France, and some to the United States and Canada (Figure8). This training started with staff from major medical university hospitals, including the Prasart Neuro Institute under the Ministry of Health (Dr. Somkiet Siriwimolmas), and others from Siriraj Hospital (Associate Professor Pipat Chiewit and Professor Anchalee Churojana), Chulalongkorn University (Assistant Professor Jaturon Tuntiwatana), and Prince Songkhla University (Assistant Professor Kittipong Riabroi from the southern region). Subsequently, many more participants from Chiang Mai University (the main university in the north) and Khon Kaen University (the main university in the northeast) were trained mainly by the first group of Thai teachers. Not only Thai physicians were trained at the University of Paris Sud, but also nurses and radiology technicians from various universities in Thailand (Figure 9).

Information from Department of Radiology, Faculty of Medicine, Chulalongkorn University, King Chulalongkorn Memorial Hospital

The Department of Angiography and Interventional Radiology was formally established in 1999 by Associate Professor Permyot Kosolbhand, an interventional radiologist. The unit included neurovascular, peripheral vascular, visceral vascular, non-vascular and interventional oncology practices. A modern biplane digital subtraction unit was installed in 2000, enabling the rapid growth of comprehensive practices for advanced and complex neurointerventional procedures at King Chulalongkorn Memorial Hospital. Assistant Professor Jarturon Tantivatana, an interventional radiologist and interventional neuroradiologist trained by Professor In Sup Choi, performed the first case of detachable coil embolization for the treatment of a ruptured cerebral aneurysm that year. In addition, the first case of NBCA glue embolization for the treatment of cerebral arteriovenous malformation and the first case of NBCA glue embolization for spinal arteriovenous malformation were performed in the same year.

As the first group of fully trained physicians, the National Certified Board in Interventional Neuroradiology (INR) Training was established, the full 2-year curriculum recruited board-certified neuroscientists (neuroradiologists, neurosurgeons, and neurologists) under the Thai Medical Council starting in 2006, and it is now certified by WFME criteria.

The final outcome of this project is to establish Thailand as an international center for INR teaching courses under Professor Lasjaunias and his team, which includes Professor Karel Terbrugge from Toronto Western University, Canada; Professor In Sup Choi from Tufts University, USA; Professor J. Dion from USA; Professor Georges Rodesch from France; and Professor Philippe Mercier from France. The International Master Course in Neurovascular Diseases was established in Thailand in collaboration with Paris Sud University and Mahidol University with Professor Sutthisak Sutthipongchai and Professor Sirintara (Pongpech) Singhara Na Ayudhaya as co-directors and staff from Chiang Mai University as co-host team. This initiative ran from 2000 until 2008 when Professor Lasjaunias passed away. The course was adapted to become the "PLANET (Pierre Lasjaunias Neurovascular Educational Team) Course" from 2008 to the present, with more educational committee members, including Professor Timo Krings from Canada and Associate Professor Allan Taylor from South Africa (Figure 10). It is still running successfully with more than 800 registered students from all over the world coming to Thailand to study.

Through this regular course, Thailand has also become a training center for many doctors from around the world. Initially, these included Vietnamese doctors (Dr. Luan, Dr. Tran-Chi-Cuong, Dr. Tuan) and radiologists from South Vietnam, as well as Dr. Jeya Mahadevan from Malaysia, along with elective rotations for doctors from South Africa, Japan, USA, etc.

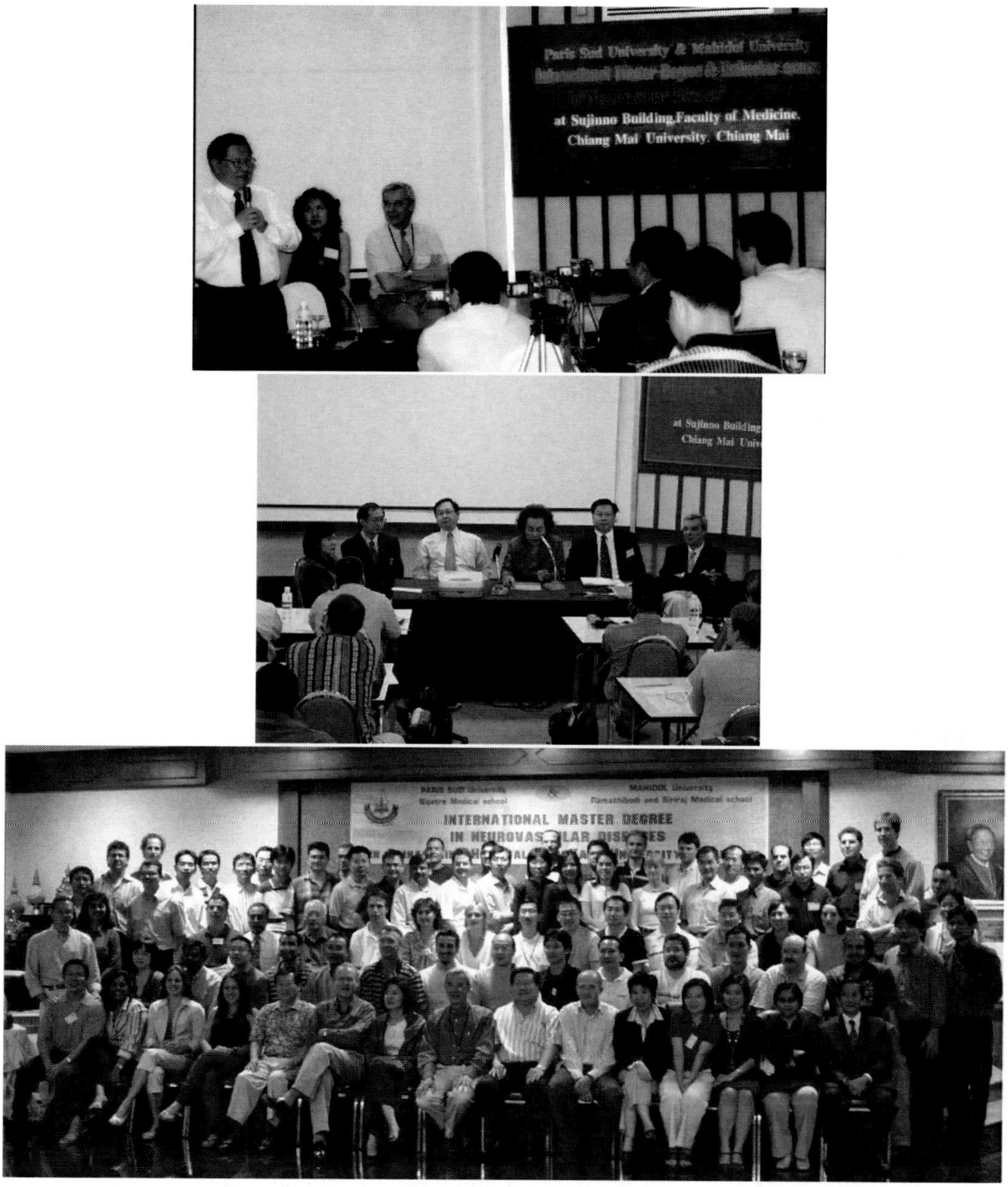

Figure 10. Pictures taken from many sessions during International Master degree Neurovascular courses in Chiangmai, Thailand: collaborated between Paris Sud and Mahidol University (2000-2008) and later on with Toronto Western University Canada and Tuft University USA. (PLANET course since 2008). Lower picture, sitting row from left to right: 5th Professor In Sup Choi, 6th Professor Karel Terbrugge, 7th Professor Sirintara Pongpech Singhara Na Ayudhaya, 8th Professor Pierre Lasjaunias, and 9th Professor Sutthisak Sutthipongchai.

Information from Department of Radiology, Faculty of Medicine, Chulalongkorn University, King Chulalongkorn Memorial Hospital

In 2008, a stent retrieval device was introduced for the treatment of acute ischemic stroke, with the first successful middle cerebral artery thrombectomy performed at the hospital. Ethylene vinyl alcohol (EVOH) in DMSO solution (Onyx) became available in 2009 and has been used for embolization of cerebral arteriovenous malformations, achieving good obliteration with low complications.

Endovascular treatment of cerebral aneurysms with flow-directed stents began in 2010 when the device became available. Precise planning of device placement was made possible by the upgraded 3D angiographic workstation, allowing expanded treatment of wide-neck, bleb and dissecting aneurysms.

In 2013, aspiration thrombectomy was performed using a suction technique through a large soft distal access catheter, successfully removing large thrombi in the distal internal carotid, middle cerebral, vertebral and basilar arteries. The stroke treatment program has been enhanced through good collaboration with the Chulalongkorn Stroke Center of Excellence under the direction of Professor Nijasri Charnnarong Suwanwela.

The Department of Angiography and Interventional Radiology started a two-year fellowship training program in interventional neuroradiology in 2015, under the course supervision of the Royal College of Radiologists of Thailand (RCRT). The service team consisted of two radiologists, a neurosurgeon, and a neurologist, all certified by the Board of Interventional Neuroradiology of the Royal College of Radiologists of Thailand.

Academic Society (National and International Ones)

In 1994, Professor Ling Feng from the Republic of China (ROC) and representatives from many countries in the Asia-Pacific region came together to form a non-profit society called the "Asian-Australasian Federation in Interventional and Therapeutic Neuroradiology" or AAFITN. The founding members and their team consisted of:

- Professor Ling Feng and Professor Hong Qi Zhang from China
- Professor Akira Takahashi and Professor WaroTaki from Japan
- Professor Dong Ik Kim and Professor Dae Suh from South Korea
- Professor Michael Teng and Dr. Luo ChaoBao from Taiwan
- Prof. Sutthisak Sutthipongchai and Professor Sirintara (Pongpech)Singahara Na Ayudhaya from Thailand
- Professor Anil Karapurka and, Dr. Uday Limaye from India
- Professor Winston Chong from Australia
- Professor John Kwok and Dr. George Wong from Hong Kong
- Dr. Prijo Sidipratomo and Dr. Cindy Sadikin from Indonesia
- Dr. Francis Hui, Dr. Winston Lim from Singapore
- Dr. Umair Rashid from Pakistan

(Later on, Dr. Jeya Mahadevan and Dr. Josephin Subramaniam from Malaysia, and Clinical Professor Anchalee Churojana from Thailand jointed the team).

Several more country representatives have joined the Executive Committee during the biennial scientific meetings to date. Thailand has hosted the AAFITN Congress twice: the first time in 2004, and the second time will be in Bangkok in 2025 (Figure11).

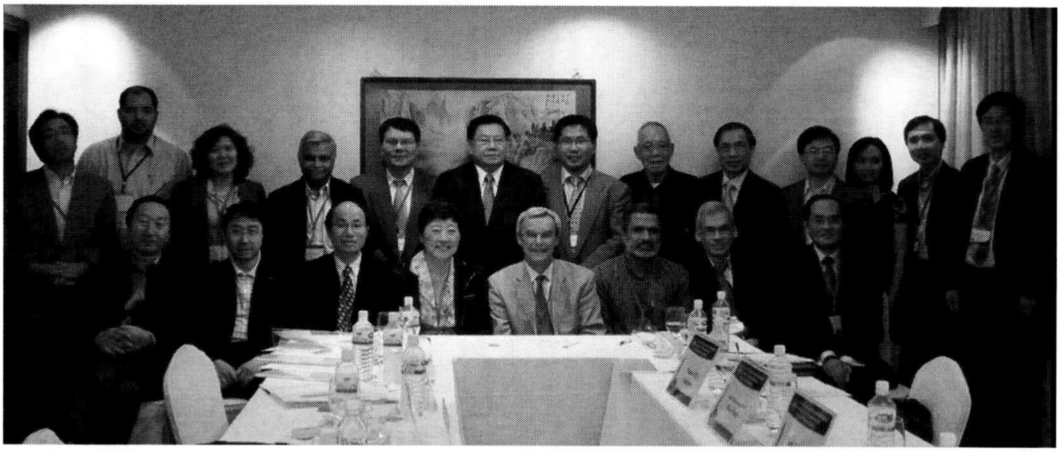

Figure 11. Group photo taking during one of the early AAFITN meeting: Standing from left to right: 1st Professor Takahashi A., 3rd Professor Pongpech Singhara Na Ayudhaya S., 4th Professor Karapurka A., 5th Professor ChaoBao L., 6th Professor Sutthipongchai S., 7th Professor Zhang HQ, 9th Professor Francis Hui, 11th Dr. Sadikin C., 13th Professor Suh D. Sitting from left to right: 1st Professor Kim DI, 2nd Professor Taki W., 3rd Professor Han MH, 4th Professor FENG L., 5th Professor Lasjaunias P., 6th Professor Rashid U., 7th Professor Chong W., 8th Professor Kwok J.

In 2012, we established the official "Association of Thai Interventional Neuroradiology" (ATIN), a national non-profit academic society, starting with 12 full members (2 women and 10 men). The society has grown larger every year with regular scientific activities up to the present.

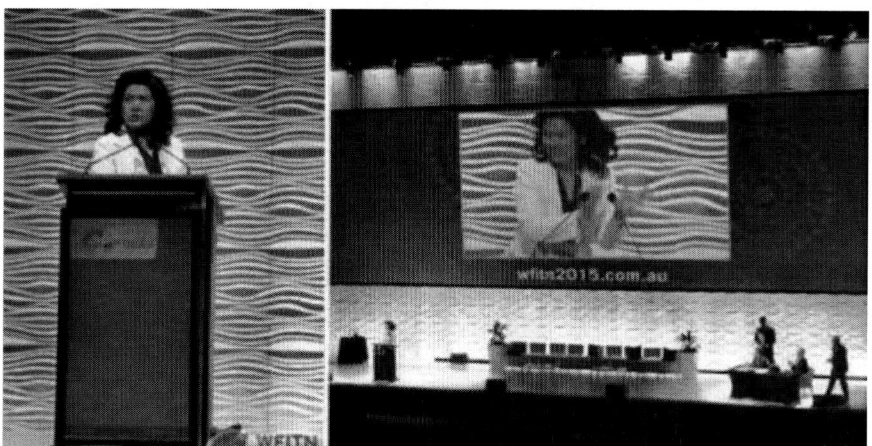

Figure 12. (Continued).

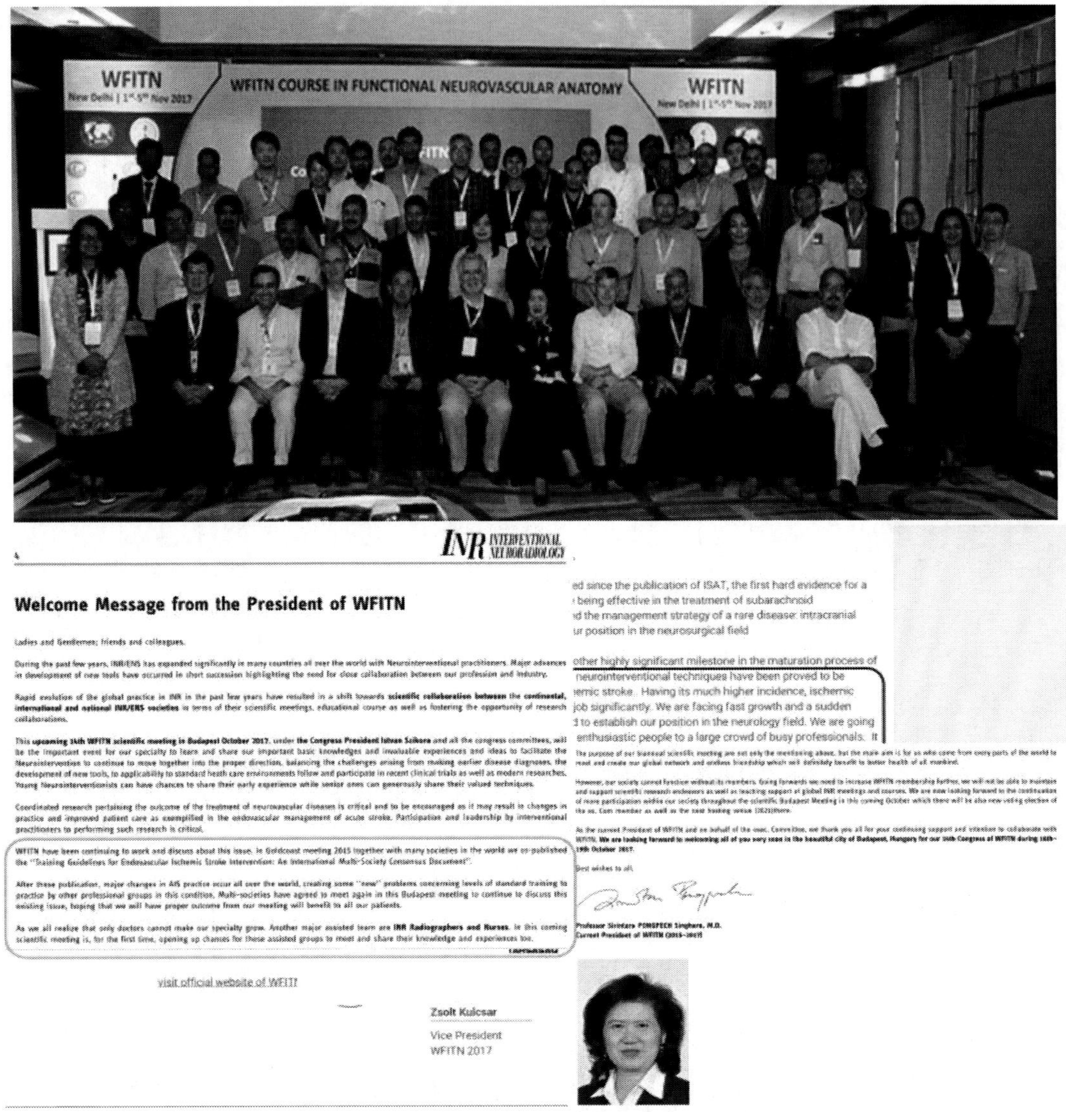

Figure 12. Professor S. Pongpech Singhara Na Ayudhaya was elected as President of WFITN (2015-2017) and was the first woman to hold this position. An example of academic activities organized by WFITN (WFITN Neurovascular Anatomy Course).

In 2005, Professor Sirintara (Pongpech) Singhara Na Ayudhaya began to serve on the Executive Committee of the World Federation of Interventional and Therapeutic Neuroradiology (WFITN), starting with the Ad Hoc Committee. Ten years later, after holding various positions in this society, she became the first woman to be elected president of WFITN (2015-2017) (Figure12). During her tenure, she accomplished numerous tasks and initiatives, and produced many guidelines and standards for training and practice in interventional neuroradiology, including the multi-society consensus on endovascular treatment of AIS, published in various journals worldwide in 2015. After serving as Past President, she continued to be involved in many academic activities and worked to bridge the collaboration between AAFITN and WFITN.

Current Status of Thai INR (2024)

ATIN now has many more members (70 full members and over 150 others). It conducts regular monthly scientific activities and hosts a large annual scientific congress, including some international meetings.

Since 2006, a strong training program for the National Certified Board in Interventional Neuroradiology has been established under the Thai Medical Council, offering a full two-year program. In 2016, another shorter one-year program was implemented (under RCNS) following a five-year neurosurgical residency program.

Collaborations have been established for special training courses for INR nurses (under the Thai Nurse Council) and for practical rotation training for radiographers (technicians).

We are in the process of accepting regular submissions on INR topics to the existing journal of the Royal College of Radiology (Figure 13).

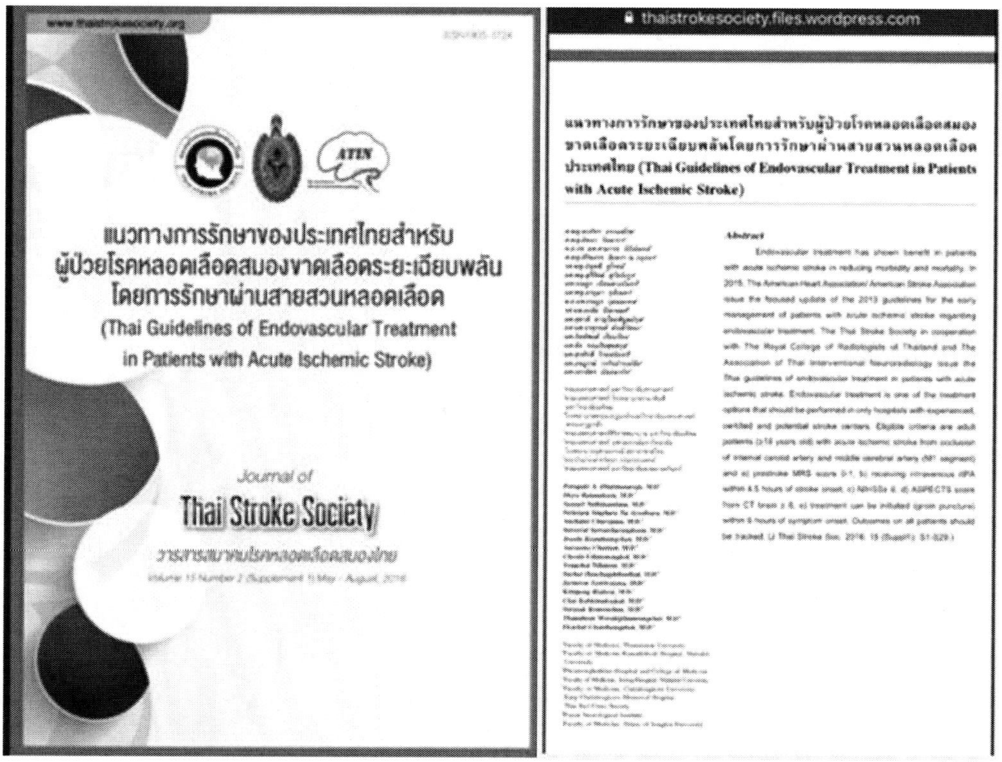

Figure 13. Publication on INR topics in the existing journal of the Royal College of Radiology.

Collaboration with TSVIR (Thai Society of Vascular and Interventional Radiology) and RCRS for regular academic activities includes hosting international meetings such as AAFITN, LINNC Asia, etc. Scholarships have been established for young members to attend academic meetings abroad. With the development of new devices, materials, technologies, and radiological equipment, along with full standards in training, education, and research support, combined with strong regional and global collaboration, the specialty of neurointervention is rapidly growing and becoming well established in Thailand (Figure 14).

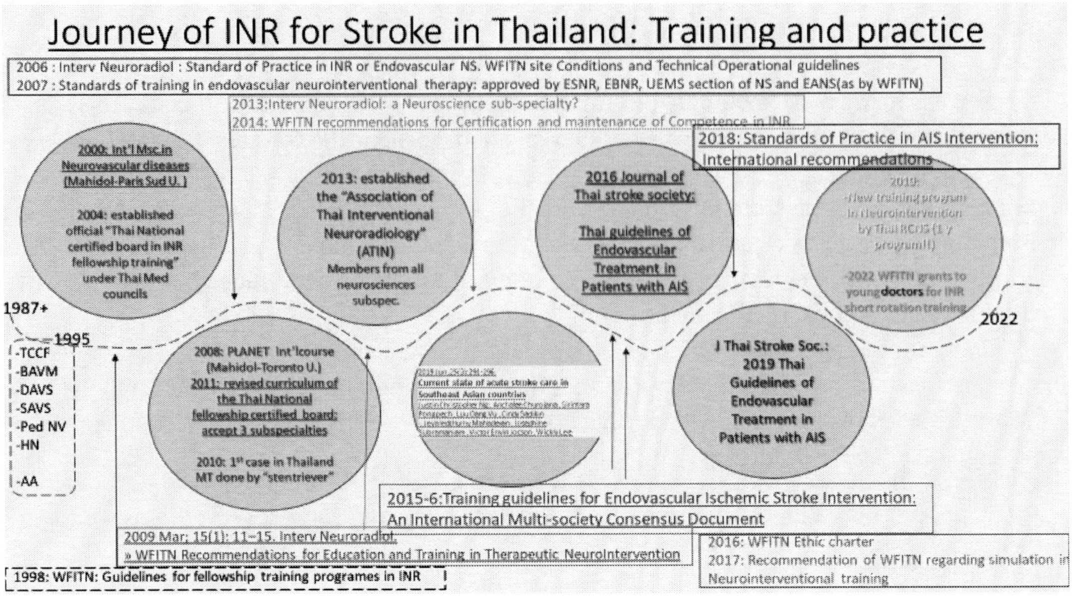

Figure 14. The journey of INR for stroke in Thailand.

Conclusion

The history of interventional neuroradiology in Thailand dates back to cerebral angiography in 1964. After 1995, there was a significant improvement in the treatment of CCF. The technique of liquid embolization for cerebral arteriovenous malformations was introduced in 1993. Endovascular thrombectomy was introduced in 2008. Onyx embolization of AVMs began in 2009. Since 2010, flow diversion devices have been used to treat intracranial aneurysms. With the development of new equipment, materials, technologies, and radiation devices, as well as comprehensive standardization of training, education, and research support, coupled with strong regional and global cooperation, Thailand's neurointerventional surgery is rapidly developing and establishing itself.

Acknowledgments

Courtesy of Professor Sutthisak Sutthipongchai, Prof.Nitaya Suwanwela, Clin. Professor Anchalee Churojana, Asst. Professor Jarturon Tuntivatana, and Asst. Professor Pakorn Jiarakongmun.

References

[1] Serbinenko FA. Balloon catheterization and occlusion of major cerebral vessels. *J Neurosurg* 1974;41:125-145.

[2] Guglielmi G, Vinuela F, Dion J, et al. Electrothrombosis of saccular aneurysms via endovascular approach. Part 2: Preliminary clinical experience. *J Neurosurg* 1991;75:8-14.

[3] Bull JWD. History of neuroradiology. *Br J Radiol* 1961;34:69-84.
[4] Taveras JM. Neuroradiology: Past, Present, Future. *Radiology* 1990;175:593-602.
[5] Loman J, Myerson A. Visualization of cerebral vessels by direct intracarotid injection of thorium dioxide (Thorotrast). *AJR* 1936;35:188-193.
[6] Takahashi M. Pioneers and history of Japanese neuroradiology. *AJNR* 1995;16:741-744.
[7] Shimidzu K. Beiträge zur Arteriographie des Gehirns—einfache percutane Methode. *Arch Klin Chir* 1937;188:295-316.
[8] Shimidzu K, Sano K. Pulseless disease. *J Neuropathol Clin Neurol* 1951;1:37-47.
[9] Seldinger S. Catheter replacement of the needle in percutaneous arteriography: a new technique. *Acta Radiol* 1953;39:368-376.
[10] Roentgen WC. *General Electric Medctclopedia. Textbook of Radiology* 1996-2000.
[11] Roentgen WC. Ueber eine neue Art von Strahlen: Vorläufige Mittheilung. *Sitzungsberichte der Physikalisch-Medizinischen Gesellschaft in Würzburg* 1895;137:132-141.
[12] Orrin HC. *The X-ray Atlas of the Systemic Arteries of the Body*. London: Bailliere; 1920.
[13] Schindler E. Arthur Schüller: Pioneer of Neuroradiology. *AJNR* 1997;18:1297-1302.
[14] Schüller A. *Roentgen Diagnosis of Diseases of the Head.* St Louis, MO: Mosby; 1918.
[15] Picard L, Cabanis EA, Iba-Zizen MT. *A History of Neuroradiology, 1895-2002.* 17th Symposium Neuroradiologicum, Europa Edition: Toulouse.
[16] Dandy WE. Ventriculography following the injection of air into the cerebral ventricles. *Ann Surg* 1918;68:4-11.
[17] Dandy WE. Roentgenography of the brain after the injection of air into the spinal canal. *Ann Surg* 1919;70:397-403.
[18] Lysholm E, Ebernius B, Sahlstedt H. Das Ventrikulogramm. I. Röntgentechnik. *Acta Radiol* 1935;24 (Suppl)
[19] Newton TH, Adam JE. Angiographic demonstration and nonsurgical embolization of spinal cord angioma. *Radiology* 1968;91:873-876.
[20] Doppman JL, Di Chiro G, Omaya A. Obliteration of spinal cord arteriovenous malformation by percutaneous embolization. *Lancet* 1968:477.
[21] Hilal SK, Michelsen J, Michelsen J, Driller J, Lee A. Magnetically guided devices for the vascular exploration: potentials and limitations. Presented at the IX Symposium Neuroradiologicum, Gothenburg, Sweden, 1970.
[22] Djindjian R, et al. Embolization by super selective arteriography from the femoral route in neuroradiology. Review of 60 cases. *Neuroradiology* 1973;6:20-26.
[23] Suthipongchai S, et al. Interventional Neuroradiology in Thailand: 1989-1997. *Interventional Neuroradiology* 1997;3:185-198.
[24] Debrun G, Lacour P, et al. Experimental approach to the treatment of carotid cavernous fistulae with an inflatable and detachable balloon. *Neuroradiology* 1975;9:9-12.
[25] Debrun G, Lacour P, et al. Detachable balloon and calibrated-leak balloon techniques in the treatment of cerebral vascular lesion. *J Neurosurg* 1978;49:635-649.
[26] Debrun G, Lacour P, et al. Treatment of 54 traumatic carotid-cavernous fistulas. *J Neurosurg* 1981;55:578-692.
[27] Debrun G, Varos V, et al. Obliteration of experimental aneurysms in dogs with isobutylcyanoacrylate. *J Neurosurg* 1984;61:37-47.
[28] Lasjaunias P. A revised concept of the congenital nature of cerebral arteriovenous malformations. *Intervent Neuroradiol* 1997;3:275-281.
[29] Lasjaunias P. Arterial aneurysms. In: Lasjaunias P (ed). *Vascular Diseases in Neonates, Infants, and Children.* Berlin, Heidelberg: Springer; 1997. pp 373-393.
[30] Lasjaunias P. *Vascular Diseases in Neonates, Infants and Children.* Berlin, Heidelberg: Springer; 1997.
[31] Lasjaunias P. From aneurysms to aneurismal vasculopathies. *Interventional Neuroradiology* 1997;5:105-108.
[32] Kalumpaheti T. *Cerebral Angiograms.* Bangkok: Siam-Aksorn; 1984.
[33] Posakrisna U. History of Thai Neurosurgery. *Siriraj Hosp Gaz* 1980;32 (2):86-92.

[34] Suthipongchai S, et al. Preoperative transcatheter embolization of juvenile nasopharyngeal angiofibroma. *Royal Thai Airforce Medical Gazette* 1986;32:85-89.

[35] Lussenhop AJ, Spence WT. Artificial embolization of cerebral arteries. Report of use in a case of arteriovenous malformation. *JAMA* 1960;172:1153-1155.

About the Editors

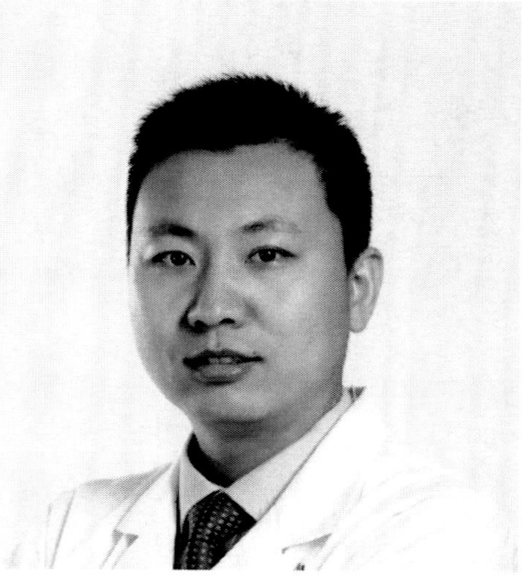

Dr. Xianli Lv, MD, is an associate professor of endovascular neurosurgery, at the Department of Neurosurgery, Beijing Tsinghua Changgung Hospital, School of Clinical Medicine, Tsinghua Medicine, Tsinghua University, China. From 2021 to 2024, he is selected for the "Yearly and Career-Long Top 2% Global Scientists List" released by Stanford University in the United States. His research focuses on neuroendovascular therapy of intracranial aneurysm, cerebral arteriovenous malformation, intracranial dural arteriovenous fistula, spinal vascular malformation, and pediatric cerebrospinal vascular malformation. He has one national invention patent and one utility model patent to his credit and has authored 195 peer-reviewed scientific articles and edited 16 books. His h-index is 31 in 2025 (Scopus). He is an editorial member of *Interventional Neuroradiology*, *Stroke and Vascular Neurology*, *Journal of Neuroradiology*, *The Neuroradiology Journal*, and *World Journal of Radiology*. He is also a deputy editor of *Neuroscience Informatics* and *Frontiers in Neurology*. Dr. Lv is a member of the World Stroke Organization (WSO) and the World Federation of Interventional Therapeutic Neuroradiology (WFITN). He was featured on the cover of *World Journal of Radiology* in April 2022 and June 2024, and journal of *China Science and Technology Achievements* in August 2023.

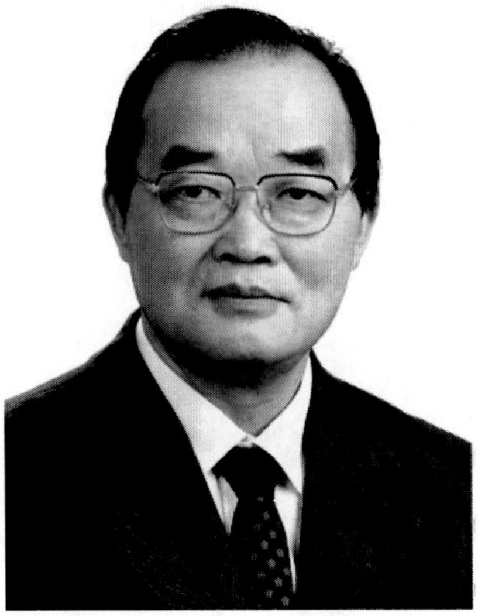

Dr. Zhongxue Wu is vice director of Beijing Neurosurgical Institute (BNI), a founding member of Chinese Societies of Neurosurgery, recipient of "Medal of May Day." He is an expert with outstanding contributions from the Ministry of Health and enjoys special government allowances. He also won the "National Outstanding Medical Workers" and "Young and Middle-aged Experts with Outstanding Contributions by the Ministry of Health." He has presided over the research of major national "Seventh Five-Year Plan," "Eighth Five-Year Plan" and "Ninth Five-Year Plan" major medical science and technology research support projects, the National Natural Science Foundation of China, and the Ministry of Health's special scientific research projects in the health industry. He has published nearly 200 academic papers in core journals at home and abroad. He engaged in neurointervention work for more than 30 years, trained 3 master students, 18 doctoral students, participated in the editing of "Neurosurgery" edited by Academician Wang Zhongcheng.

Index

A

B

C

D

E

F

G

H

I

L

M

N

P

R

S

T

V

W